Child and Adolescent Mental Health

This textbook provides an overview of child and adolescent mental health. The text covers all core aspects on the subject, from the importance of knowing why mental health in children is important, to how to assess, formulate and treat a variety of presentations seen in children and young people.

Beginning with an overview of conditions and the background to emotional and behavioural problems, the book examines the different models and tools used to assess and treat children and young people and provides an outline of the practitioners working to help this population. Chapters consider the many diverse identities and groups within the population, addressing specific problems encountered in children, young people and their families from different cultural backgrounds. This revised edition addresses issues of current public debate such as gender identity and the role of social media in children's and young people's development and behaviour.

Featuring authors from a variety of clinical and research backgrounds, this fully revised third edition is an important resource for all professionals working with children, young people and their families, including student and practitioner psychiatrists, clinical psychologists, mental health nurses and social care specialists.

Cathy Laver-Bradbury, SRN, RSCN, HV cert, MSc Nursing Non-Medical Prescriber, has worked in CAMHS in the UK for the last 27 years specialising in neurodevelopmental disorders.

Margaret J.J. Thompson, MBChB, MD, FRCP, DCh, DRCOG, is a retired clinical academic. She has worked in CAMHS in the UK since 1973. Her particular research and clinical interests are in mental health in pre-schoolers, attention deficit hyperactivity disorders, parenting and in-service delivery. She has published extensively in these areas.

Christopher Gale, RNMH, PhD, MSc, BA (Hons), has worked in child and adolescent mental health services since 1999, developing student nurses to registration since 2008.

Christine M. Hooper, CQSW, MSc, worked as a CAMHS social worker prior to gaining an MSc in Family and Marital Therapy. She left CAMHS to work in the private sector.

Child and Adolescent Mental Health

Theory and Practice

Third Edition

Edited by Cathy Laver-Bradbury, Margaret J.J. Thompson, Christopher Gale and Christine M. Hooper

Routledge
Taylor & Francis Group
NEW YORK AND LONDON

Third edition published 2021
by Routledge
605 Third Avenue, New York, NY 10158

and by Routledge
2 Park Square, Milton Park, Abingdon, Oxon, OX14 4RN

Routledge is an imprint of the Taylor & Francis Group, an informa business

First edition published by Hodder Arnold 2005

Second edition published by CRC Press 2012

Library of Congress Cataloging-in-Publication Data
Names: Laver-Bradbury, Cathy, editor.
Title: Child and adolescent mental health: theory and practice/edited by
Cathy Laver-Bradbury [and three others].
Description: Third edition. | New York, NY: Routledge, 2021. | Includes
bibliographical references and index.
Identifiers: LCCN 2020048554 (print) | LCCN 2020048555 (ebook) |
ISBN 9780367537395 (hardback) | ISBN 9780367537388 (paperback) |
ISBN 9781003083139 (ebook)
Subjects: LCSH: Child mental health. | Teenagers–Mental health.
Classification: LCC RJ499 .C48224 2021 (print) | LCC RJ499 (ebook) |
DDC 618.92/89–dc23
LC record available at https://lccn.loc.gov/2020048554
LC ebook record available at https://lccn.loc.gov/2020048555

ISBN: 978-0-367-53739-5 (hbk)
ISBN: 978-0-367-53738-8 (pbk)
ISBN: 978-1-003-08313-9 (ebk)

Typeset in Galliard
by Deanta Global Publishing Services, Chennai, India

Contents

Contributors

Kirsteen Anderssen
Family Nurse Partnership
Southampton, UK

Jo Barker
Consultant Child and Adolescent Psychiatrists
Solent NHS Trust

Jonathan Bigg
Consultant Forensic Child and Adolescent Psychiatrist
Hampshire and Isle of Wight
Forensic CAMHS

Melissa Bracewell
Retired Community Paediatrician
Southampton, UK

Valerie Brandt
Lecturer
Academic Unit of Psychology
CIMH
University of Southampton
Southampton, UK

Anne Brewster
Family Therapist
Dorchester CAMHS

Vicki Bright
Senior CAMHS Nurse
Solent NHS

Sheila Burton
Educational Psychologist
Consultant to ELSA

Pam Campbell
Consultant Nurse
Homeless Healthcare Team Southampton

Helen Carlow
Educational Psychologist
Hampshire & IoW Educational Psychology (HIEP)

Wai Chen
Child and Adolescent Psychiatrist
Professor of Child Psychiatry
The University of Western Australia
Perth, Australia

Pathiba Chitsabesan
Consultant Child and Adolescent Psychiatrist
Pennine Care NHS Foundation Trust
and
Honorary Professor
Manchester Metropolitan University
Manchester, UK

Alex Christie
Clinical Nurse Specialist
Basingstoke CAMHS

Georgia Chronaki
Senior Lecturer
Developmental Neuroscience
University of Central Lancashire
Preston, UK

Samuele Cortese
Professor of Child and Adolescent Psychiatry
CAMHS
Solent NHS Trust
University of Southampton
Southampton, UK

Anthony Crabb
Consultant Child and Adolescent Psychiatrist
Devonshire Partnership Trust

Karen Davies
Locality Manager
Solent NHS Trust

Suyog Dhakras
Consultant Child and Adolescent Psychiatrist
Solent NHS Trust

Joanne Doherty
Clinical Lecturer
Wales Clinical Academic Track (WCAT) Fellow in Child and Adolescent Psychiatry
Division of Psychological Medicine and Clinical Neurosciences
Cardiff, UK

Bernidka Dubicka
Consultant Child and Adolescent Psychiatrist
Honorary Reader University of Manchester
Consultant in Adolescent Inpatient Unit Lancashire

Anan El Masry
Consultant Child and Adolescent Psychiatrist
Winchester CAMHS

Sue Evans
Independent Occupational Therapist

Graeme Fairchild
Lecturer in Clinical Psychology
University of Southampton
Southampton, UK

Val Forster
Child and Adolescent Psychotherapist
Sussex Partnership

Loz Foskett
Independent Play Therapist

Christopher Gale
Lecturer in MH
University of Winchester

Sarah Gale
Intensive Support Worker
Street Homelessness Prevention Team
Southampton City Council
Southampton, UK

Stuart Gemmell
Senior Practitioner
Solent NHS Trust
Southampton, UK

Anna Gibson
Child and Adolescent Psychiatrist
Solent NHS Trust

Di Glackin
Community Practitioner CAMHS
CAMHS Solent NHS

Dennis Golm
Lecturer
Academic Unit of Psychology
University of Southampton
Southampton, UK

Sally Gray
Cognitive Analytic Psychotherapist
Solent NHS Trust

Jack Groom
Doctor BM BCh
Southampton University NHS Trust

Julie Hadwin
Associate Professor
Developmental Research Group
School of Education
Liverpool Hope University
Liverpool, UK

Chris Hardie
Community Paediatrician
Solent NHS Trust

Diane Henty
Family Nurse Partnership
Solent NHS Trust

Catherine Hill
Honorary Consultant in Paediatric Sleep Medicine and Associate Professor of Child Health
University Hospital Southampton
Southampton, UK

Sarah Holden
Play Therapist
Solent NHS Trust

Chantal Holman
Service and Quality Manager
Solent NHS Trust

Christine M. Hooper
Retired Family and Marital Therapist

Emma House
Art Therapist
Solent NHS Trust

Carlos Hoyos
Consultant Child and Adolescent Psychiatrist and Senior Lecturer in Medical Education
Solent NHS Trust
Southampton University of Winchester
Winchester, UK

Helena Hoyos
Independent Educational Psychologist
Solent NHS Trust

Tony James
Consultant Adolescent Psychiatrist and Honorary Senior Lecturer
University of Oxford
Oxford, UK

Margaret Josephs
Art Therapist
Hampshire CAMHS

Jacqui Kelly
Counsellor
University of Southampton
Southampton, UK

Ellis Kennedy
Consultant Child and Adolescent Psychiatrist and Director of Research
The Tavistock and Portman NHS Foundation Trust

Hannah Kovshoff
Associate Professor
Academic Unit of Psychology
University of Southampton
Southampton, UK

Jana Kreppner
Associate Professor in Developmental Psychopathology
Centre for Innovation in Mental Health – Developmental Laboratory
School of Psychology
University of Southampton
Southampton, UK

Cathy Laver-Bradbury
Consultant Nurse
Solent NHS Trust
Southampton, UK

Gabrielle Loades
CAMHS Social Worker
Solent NHS Trust

Roxanne Magdalena
Consultant Child and Adolescent Psychiatrist
Basingstoke CAMHS

Lucy Manger
Educational Psychologist

Anna Masding
CAMHS Service Manager and NFPP Lead
Nottingham City Early Help Services
Children and Adults Directorate
Nottingham City Council
Nottingham, UK

Liz McCaughey
Retired Community Paediatrician
Southampton, UK

Martin McColl
Consultant Child and Adolescent Psychiatrist
Solent NHS Trust
Southampton, UK

Hollie McGloughlin
ST 6 Child and Adolescent Psychiatrist

Melissa McKimm
CAMHS Nurse
Specialist CAMHS Andover

Alice Mooney
Service Manager
No Limits
Southampton, UK

Sarah Mottram
Senior CBT Therapist
Solent NHS Trust

Jayne Muldowney
Behavioural Advisor
CAMHS Solent NHS Trust

Lakshmeesh Muttur Somashekhar
Specialty Doctor CAMHS
Highfield Unit
Warneford Hospital
Oxford, UK

Phill Nagle
Senior CAMHS Nurse
North Hampshire Specialist CAMHS

Laura Nisbet
Lead Nurse ADHD
CAMHS Solent NHS

Cathie O'Brien
Gestalt Psychotherapist and Gestalt Practitioner in Organisations

Lynne Oldman
Consultant Child and Adolescent Psychiatrist
Community Child and Adolescent Mental Health Services
Isle of Wight NHS Trust

Andrew O'Toole
Family Therapist
Poole CAMHS

Naomi Pang
Health Visitor
Solent NHS

Miranda Passey
Child and Adolescent Psychotherapist

Julia Pelle
Lecturer in Mental Health

Jonathan Prosser
Consultant Child Psychiatrist
Portsmouth CAMHS
Solent NHS Trust
Southampton, UK

Charlotte Pyatt
Senior Nurse Practitioner
Southern Health

Stephanie Ramsey
Commissioner
Southampton CCG
Southampton, UK

Sue Ricketts
Child and Adolescent Psychotherapist
Southampton, UK

Monica Roman-Morales
Senior Family Therapist
CAMHS Solent NHS Trust

Salvatore Rototendo
Community Paediatrician
Solent NHS Trust
Southampton, UK

Anastasia Sedikides
Principal Clinical Psychologist
Solent NHS Trust
Southampton, UK

Michelle Simmonds
Senior CAMHS Nurse
BRS Solent NHS

Liz Smith
Independent Educational Psychologist

Roy Smith
Family Therapist
CAMHS Ashurst
Southampton, UK

Becky Sparks
Learning Disability Nurse
Southern Health NHS Trust

Ann Spooner
Business Manager
Homeless Healthcare Team Southampton
Southampton, UK

Janet Stephens
Senior Speech and language Therapist
Southampton, UK

Cara Sturgess
Senior Practitioner
South West i2i
Hampshire CAMHS Urgent Assessment and Home Treatment Service

Hannah Stynes
Assistant Research Psychologist
Tavistock Centre

Eric Taylor
Emeritus Professor of Child and Adolescent Psychiatry
Institute of Psychiatry
King's College London
London, UK

Sandra Teale
Retired Teacher of Children with Autism

Anita Thapar
Professor of Child and Adolescent Psychiatry
Division of Psychological Medicine and Clinical Neurosciences
and
MRC Centre for Neuropsychiatric Genetics and Genomics
Cardiff, UK

Catherine Thompson
Visitor Academic Unit of Psychology
University of Southampton
Southampton, UK

Margaret J.J. Thompson
Honorary Professor of Child and Adolescent Psychiatry
University of Southampton
Solent NHS Trust

Andrea Thwaites
Family Nurse Partnership
Solent NHS Trust
Southampton, UK

Jeremy Turk
Consultant Child & Adolescent Psychiatrist
Emeritus Professor of Developmental Psychiatry
CAMHS
Isle of Wight NHS Trust
Kings College London

Julie Waine
Consultant Psychiatrist
Southern Health

Alison Wallis
Consultant Clinical Psychologist
Clinical Director
Children and Young Peoples Service
Sussex Partnership NHS Foundation Trust

Gill Waring
Re:Minds Parent Support Group
Southampton, UK

Siobhan West
Named Nurse for Safeguarding
Solent NHS Trust

Oliver White
Consultant Child and Adolescent Forensic Psychiatrist
Southampton & Bristol Bluebird

Sally Wicks
Child and Adolescent Psychiatrist
Southampton University NHS Trust

Lucy Wilford
Child and Adolescent Psychiatrist
Solent NHS Trust

Charlotte Young
Community Mental Health Nurse
Southampton, UK

Foreword

Child and adolescent mental health services have changed greatly in recent years. Basic knowledge has continued to evolve to give an understanding of the importance of genetic influences and their interaction with environmental stresses. Bio-psycho-social formulations have become the rule in practice. Psychological interventions are based on cognitive and behavioural principles as well as psychodynamic. Pharmacology plays a larger role in modern practice than it used to. Guidelines from NICE have been able to draw on an increased evidence base of trials and accordingly to make practice more codified. International schemes of classification have been revised and re-revised in efforts to take account of the dimensional and multi-dimensional nature of the influences on mental development and their consequences.

These are real advances. They have increased the complexity of practice. Collaboration between disciplines is all the more needed for service provision and is sometimes well achieved. Too often, however, recent austerity has made it difficult for professionals to meet and discuss. That same austerity has ensured lower capacity, and correspondingly a trend for cases at clinics to have more severe and complex conditions. Professionals need to have an understanding of the contributions that other disciplines can make and the conceptual approaches they can bring.

This book is written by experts who have good records in collaboration. They are all highly competent in their own fields and well used to teaching them to others. As examples, the chapter on how mental health professionals can learn developmental assessments is likely to create much-needed rapprochement between paediatricians and psychiatrists. The chapter on emotional processing should unify the worlds of neuroscience and family influences and the changes in different disorders. The chapter on autism spectrum disorders should convey the modern concepts of expanded diagnosis and an emphasis on how much can be achieved in education to enhance independence.

Another example of recent changes needing explanation is that of the problems of inattentive and impulsive behaviour. As recently as 40 years ago, 'hyperkinetic disorder' was a rare disorder and to many an unwelcome term. It was seen as an Americanism and a signal that the person using it had an inappropriately medicalised attitude. Twenty years ago, it had become clear that individuals with inattentiveness, impulsiveness and overactivity are marred in their cognitive performance by being less vigilant, variable and requiring more immediate and stronger reinforcement than typical individuals. Brain research and genetic information led to professional recognition of ADHD as a medical disorder. The situation now is very different to that of the 1980s. Attention deficit hyperactivity disorder (ADHD) is one of the commonest child mental health conditions treated by the NHS. In the first part of Part V, interventions are described for ADHD across a wide range of ages, covering pre-school, school-aged children, adolescents and adults.

For all the disorders of mental health, clinical research has demonstrated their heterogeneity and complexity in both children and adolescents. The frequency of multiple morbidity complicates the tasks of clinicians and educators. The commitment of this book's authors to collaborative and multidisciplinary work has enabled them to give a comprehensive account, in Parts III and V, of the variety of presentations. Readers can use them for a narrative about the multiple processes that can engender psychological problems. These chapters will also serve as references for those who are seeking to understand a complex case. They bring in both the insights of clinical science and the practicalities of expert clinicians. Understanding is not yet complete, and these chapters indicate what still has to be learned, as well as what is established.

Part IV takes the guidance on coping with complexity further, into a useful account of how to assess children, adolescents and adults who are struggling with unwelcome differences in their psychological makeup and social environment. In Part VI, different modalities of treatment are discussed (e.g. cognitive training, art therapy, cognitive analytic therapy), and a fair review is provided without being dismissive. Pharmacological treatments as well as stimulant and non-stimulant medications are covered in an up-to-date review. Differences across age groups are emphasised, and the need to individualise and adapt treatments over time is discussed. Systematic algorithms are described for delivering evidence-based treatment.

In Part VII, a variety of community- and residential-based interventions are discussed.

In all these parts, one emphasis is on the developmental aspects of disorders and their implications for treatment.

If attitudes have changed in England it is in no small part due to the willingness of psychiatrists, nurses, psychologists and other disciplines to work together and in partnership with families.

The future is no clearer than it ever was. Nevertheless, it remains clear that advances come when different fields spark across each other. The interdisciplinary focus of this book should therefore be an excellent resource for the education of many professionals and students. To them I recommend it strongly.

Professor Eric Taylor

Part I

An Introduction to Children and Young People's Mental Health

Cathy Laver-Bradbury

This section provides an overview of the history and the ongoing development of Child and Adolescent Mental Health services, its framework and how it is commissioned. It considers the wider legal context and considers the needs of some of our most vulnerable children whilst setting out our paradigm for understanding of mental health and how we understand the importance of putting theory into practice.

1 A Brief History of Child and Adolescent Mental Health Services (CAMHS) to the Present Day

Christopher Gale and Margaret J.J. Thompson

Just as the field of psychiatry is a relatively new discipline within medicine overall, what was then 'child psychiatry', now child and adolescent mental health, was only recognised as a discipline in 1937. This is not to say that services did not exist prior to this for children and young people with mental health difficulties. The first hospital-based service developed for children opened at the Maudsley Hospital in London in 1923, followed by the first community-based child guidance service in East London in 1927. Initially these services were staffed by social workers, psychologists and psychiatrists.

The growth of such services was limited through the 1930s and during the years of World War II, with any co-ordinated effort to provide services for children and young people in mental distress coming in the late 1940s. Blacker (1946) recommended that community child guidance services should predominantly deal with children experiencing educational difficulties and be run by the local education authority. The new hospital-based clinics were to deal with the issues of 'abnormal' behaviour in children and young people.

The 1950s and 1960s saw a greater emphasis on the involvement of families in the treatment of mental health problems, with Emmanuel Miller at the Tavistock Clinic widely regarded as leading the way. Even in these early years of services for children and young people, emphasis was placed on the 'multidisciplined approach', with the whole team sharing clinical responsibility. The psychiatrist as clinical lead would develop later. Despite this being considered the heyday for child guidance clinics, there was no overarching model of practice or any meaningful policy driving the development of services by central government.

The shift towards a health service provision for children and young people did not come until the 1970s, when local government reorganisation focused resources more on generic social and educational issues. In 1974, the National Health Service became the major provider of child and adolescent mental health services, with specialised teams working with discrete groups of children and often adopting a particular model or approach to care delivery.

The 1980s and 1990s saw a dramatic increase in demand for services, with greater identification of conditions, e.g. ADHD and autistic spectrum disorders. A major epidemiological study, funded by the Office for National Statistics in 1999 (Meltzer, 2000), revealed that approximately 10% of children and young people would experience a diagnosable mental disorder. The birth of the modern-day child and adolescent mental health service (CAMHS) came with the publication of *Together We Stand* (Health Advisory Service, 1995). This document introduced the four-tier model of service.

Tier 1 would provide the first line of service and consisted of non-specialist primary care workers, i.e. school nurses, health visitors, general practitioners, teachers, social workers and educational welfare officers. Problems seen at this level could be the common problems of childhood and adolescence, e.g. sleeping or feeding problems, temper tantrums, parent–child interaction, low-level issues with mood and anxiety, behaviour problems at home and school and bereavement.

Tier 2 consisted of specialist primary mental health workers (PMHWs) who, by working relatively independently from other services, would take referrals and provide support to primary care colleagues and if appropriate, offer assessment and treatment on a short- to medium-term basis, e.g. family work, bereavement support, drop-in groups for parents, parenting groups, behaviour problems, anger management and other low-level psychological interventions. Educational psychologists or clinical psychologists might operate at this level. The PMHW would mediate between the primary care level at **Tier 1** and specialist CAMHS at **Tier 3**.

Tier 3 would consist of multi-disciplinary teams, who would work in specialist child mental health services (CAMHS). Problems seen here would be issues too complex to be addressed at **Tier 2** (assessment of developmental problems, autism, hyperactivity, chronic or severe depression and anxiety, early psychosis and severe eating disorders). Joint working with other agencies, family therapy and individual psychotherapeutic work could be offered.

Tier 4 consisted of specialist day- and inpatient units, where children and young people with more severe mental health difficulties could be assessed and treated (e.g. adolescent acute and forensic units and specialist social services therapeutic homes).

The late 1990s until 2010 witnessed an unprecedented interest in children and young people's mental health, with a co-ordinated national policy (National Service Framework for Children DfES, 2004) and a steep rise in investment for services. This was not entirely into specialist CAMHS, but with an important focus on prevention and early intervention with families (**Tiers 1 and 2**). There was a drive for families to be able to seek help locally and be seen quickly, with initiatives such as the Family Nurse partnership for first-time young mothers and families and the creation of SureStart centres for all families with under fives. Developments during this period signalled an attempt to move away from the rigidity of the four-tier system to create a comprehensive and integrated CAMHS service with joint planning and the potential for pooled funding.

Since 2010, there has been a real terms reduction in the investment into CAMHS, i.e. £79 million between 2010 and 2013 according to The Children's Society (2015), and other statutory support services have experienced pressures on funding, for instance, SureStart centres now operate only in areas of highest deprivation. Arguably, this has impacted on the ambition of an integrated comprehensive CAMH service, as agencies scale back their range of activity to deal with 'core business'.

In the wake of the UK 2015 General Election, additional investment in CAMHS was promised and has resulted in emerging new services, e.g. Improving Access to Psychological Therapies for Children and Young People (CYP-IAPT) to work with children and young people with difficulties related to behaviour, depression and anxiety, and specialist eating disorder community teams to work with families to avoid unnecessary inpatient admissions (NHS England, 2015).

The overall rates of diagnosable mental disorder continue to rise, estimated at 9.7% to 11.2% in 5–15-year olds between 1999 and 2017 (NHS Digital, 2018). The challenge for government, health commissioners, CAMHS professionals and communities is how to respond, so that children, young people and families feel empowered and not de-skilled, but nor do they become dependent on professionals. Access to the right support in a timely manner is crucial to the future wellbeing of our children and young people.

This book has been written as a practical and, we hope, pragmatic manual for professionals working with children, young people and their families across a range of health, social care and educational settings, where the issue of mental health is everyone's business.

Key References

NHS Digital, (2018). *Mental Health of Children and Young People in England: Summary of Key Findings*. London: The Health and Social Care Information Centre.

NHS England, (2015). *Future in Mind: Promoting, Protecting and Improving Our Children and Young People's Mental Health and Wellbeing*. London: Department of Health.

The Children's Society, (2015). *Children's Mental Health: Priorities for Improving Children and Adolescent Mental Health Services in England*.

2 The Conceptual Basis of Mental Health Practice

Carlos Hoyos

Introduction

The title of this book, *Child and Adolescent Mental Health Theory and Practice*, refers specifically to two aspects of the activities of people who work in mental health, **theory,** i.e., what you think and what you know and **practice**, i.e., what you do. Here we are aiming to clarify the meaning of *Mental*, *Health*, *Theory*, and *Practice* in addition to other concepts crucial to 'Knowing what you are doing'.

Let's start with the last word 'Practice'. This usually refers to as 'Doing' and is linked to the word 'practical' meaning expedient or to the point, e.g., 'We need to be practical about this, let's not waste too much time thinking about it' and not be 'bogged down' by too much 'theory'.

This is slightly misleading. The Greeks made a distinction between 'Technos', as in technology, meaning the making of something, following instructions but not really knowing or understanding what you are doing and Praxis, or poiesis, meaning the application of all available knowledge to creating something new, good and worthwhile.

By way of illustration, most McDonalds restaurant workers are trained in the techniques of cooking burgers on a grill. They can leave the patty for two minutes then flip it, following detailed instructions. All other decisions, e.g., which meat, what thickness, what temperature and so on, are made for them. Michelin star chefs, however, understand every detail of the chemical processes involved in cooking meat and the effects it will have on the palate of the consumer and the importance of sourcing the right meat, and the effects of ageing on meat. The Greeks would describe the McDonalds' cook as a 'technician', the Chef as a 'Practitioner' of cooking burgers. The purpose here is to help readers set the foundations of the theory that is necessary to become a Mental Health Practitioner, i.e., someone who 'knows what they do' as opposed to a Mental Health Technician, i.e., someone who follows instructions.

Mental Health

Considering how often these two words are used in common parlance, it is remarkable how little attention is paid to their precise meaning by those who work in this area. Some people would associate the word 'mental' with the word 'madness', as in: 'that person is mental'. Similarly, the term 'health' is often likened to 'wellbeing' as in 'this is detrimental to mental health, meaning it causes unhappiness.

Mental refers to the mind, a broad psychological concept. It refers to what drives behaviour. We can observe behaviour and perhaps understand it by inferring what the mind behind it does. Likewise it is a more complex concept than merely the absence of distress. It is important for Mental Health practitioners to understand these two concepts in some more detail.

Key Concepts

The Mind

The Mind is one of those concepts whose meaning is often assumed, yet rarely defined. Many people refer to the mind and the brain indistinctly. Some people refer to the mind as a metaphysical transcendental entity akin to the soul. We, however, situate our understanding of the mind, away from the realms of biology or metaphysics and within the science of psychology. The mind is the collection of psychological processes that underpin behaviour. The brain is the biological support that makes those processes possible. The mind is to the brain what vision is to the eye.

Behaviour

The starting point to understand those processes is to understand what we mean by behaviour. At its fundamental level, behaviour is movement. All living organisms whose survival depends on movement will have evolved a motor system that enables them to move i.e. muscles, bones, joints and a nervous system that enables them to control that movement, so that it is effective and contributes to their survival i.e. sensors, processors, nerves. Living beings that do not move do not have nervous systems.

However, behaviour is not the same as movement. A planet moves, sometimes in complex ways, following orbits, but we do not refer to the behaviour of planets. Behaviour is movement that responds to a control system. The study of behaviour, psychology, has produced a series of complex concepts like perception, motivation, emotion, causality, memory, orientation and so on that help us understand, explain and predict behaviour. Our understanding of behaviour borrows ideas that precede the development of psychology as an empirical science. For thousands of years philosophers have tried to describe and make sense of what a mind is and what it is like to have one. Ideas like consciousness, logic, experience or phenomena existed before and helped shape our understanding of the mind as the driver of behaviour.

Psychological Processes

Since we have defined the Mind as a collection of psychological processes that underpin behaviour, we should explain what those processes are. Explaining every psychological process would make this chapter into a psychology textbook, which is not what we intend, but at least we should list some of them. Psychological processes have become more sophisticated as the complexity of the underpinning nervous systems has evolved. All nervous systems share some structural characteristics. They have sensory elements, processing elements and motor elements. Most psychological processes involve processing information, but the processes involved in acquiring the information to be processed, are also psychological.

When mental health workers conduct a Mental State Examination, they are systematically evaluating these functions, just as physicians examine the different functional systems of the body when they conduct a physical examination.

Perception is the generic psychological process that describes the creation of sensory information. At a time when our phones are equipped with light, motion, GPS, magnetic, cameras and fingerprint sensors, it is easy to think of our own sensors, i.e. vision, sound, taste, smell, touch and proprioception, as passive, mechanical receptors. But whilst there is a receptor component, perception itself involves the processing of information. When light creates an image on our retina, we see shapes and colours. We perceive colour as an attribute of the external world, but it is really a psychological construct.

'Green' is an idea that we need to understand before we can 'see' it. It is important to understand that our perception of reality responds to our pre-existing understanding of that reality. The psychological mechanisms involved in visual perception are the same as those found in hallucinations. Both vision and hallucinations are mental processes.

Spatial and time orientation follow from perception. We may see images, but we perceive and construct internal four-dimensional representations of the world. Knowing what is up, what is down, what is right, what is left, how far things are and how long ago or into the future events are, is what allows us to have sense of reality that allows us to move and orientate ourselves in the world.

Being able to orientate ourselves in time and space is crucial for movement, but it is not possible without a mechanism that allows us to keep this representation of reality in time. Otherwise we would have to perceive the world anew every second. Memory is another crucial psychological process. It allows a permanent representation of reality, but for learning and then eventually a sense of self.

We are used to thinking of a survival instinct and a sexual drive as key, drivers of behaviour. Both are in fact instincts and drivers; instincts because we are born with them and drivers because they drive behaviour. They move us to do things. All animals are born with these behavioural drivers. They are often linked to subjective mental experiences that we call 'emotions' i.e. e-motion as in movement.

These three basic, emotions, hunger, fear and lust, are essential for survival and reproduction and are clearly built into our biology. How we experience them is a psychological phenomenon as are the mechanisms that enable us to perceive, manage and communicate them.

Emotional management and communication are two more crucial psychological functions that add on to these basic emotions. But these basic emotions give rise to more complex ones that have evolved with time, such as envy, love, guilt or responsibility, that motivate behaviour to a no lesser extent.

Most animals have evolved brains that support the perception, memory and orientation necessary to have an internal representation of the external world and a set of emotions that motivate behaviour towards survival and reproduction. Some animals have evolved ways to communicate and influence each other's behaviour. This has represented a huge evolutionary advantage and so-called social animals, those that have minds that allow for interaction with others, have been very successful. Humans are one of these animals. We have psychological mechanisms that allow for automatic communication, such as empathy, or through symbols, such as language. We have adapted our perception to be able to read social clues and our emotions to negotiate our motivation with those of others. We have developed behavioural control mechanisms, both biological and cultural, in order to fit in societies.

The development of communication via chemicals like pheromones or signals like threats or courting rituals, evolved into the much more versatile communication through symbols, and eventually language. This triggered the development of much more complex psychological processes such as thought, the ability to understand abstract concepts, operate with them in imagination and creativity, giving rise to entire worlds of experience beyond that of the physical world. These psychological processes created a world beyond that of physical experience, the world of other beings like us, the social world.

We share psychological processes necessary to fit in society with many animals. Understanding dominance, threats or warnings are crucial for most social species from wolves to whales. But human minds have developed psychological mechanisms that go beyond those basic understandings of each other's minds.

From birth, and possibly through the process of establishing emotional bonds and attachment relationships in early infancy, humans have developed the ability to understand that every other human has a mind of their own. We have become very good at understanding what is in each other's minds, and we have used our language in order to create concepts that allow us to share our minds further. We are not just able to perceive others, but we understand how others perceive. We do not just have emotions linked to others but have an understanding that other people have emotions. We are not just able to think, but we are able to guess what someone else is thinking. We have a 'theory of mind'. We can guess what is in each other's minds.

The psychological function of understanding the behaviour of others is important and central. It is a fundamental function for our survival in a social world. Knowing who to trust, who to help, who to fight and who to mate with, have been key determinants of survival and thus of evolution for millennia. One could argue that the biological and psychological mechanisms that allow us to find food or stay warm have been less important to our survival than knowing who to trust. Being in contact with individuals whose behaviour we do not understand is deeply unsettling. Our natural response when faced with behaviour we cannot understand is to move away or exclude whoever is showing it. Another response is to mobilise all our own psychological resources to understand them.

Functioning

Now that we understand what a psychological process is, we can introduce another tricky word, function. A performer will tell you that a function is a social event or a play, for instance; a mathematician will say that a function is an expression involving one or more variables, y = (bc + x); a social scientist that it is something dependent on another factor, class shame is a function of social power. All these definitions are relevant, but when we refer to function in psychology, we generally mean an activity that fits the purpose of a thing or a person.

Function is often used instead of process when describing psychological processes. Thought is a psychological process, i.e. a sequence of events, but we often refer to it by the activity that that process generates, the thinking function. In this context, function means doing what it is meant to do well enough.

Function is an important word because we often use it to describe how well psychological processes, or complex behaviours emanating from them, work. For instance, we may describe how a child's emotional regulation problems do not allow him or her to function in school.

Health

Health is one of those concepts that are seldom discussed. We take for granted what it means. Doctors and nurses who work with people's bodies seldom question what healthy means. We all know what a healthy lung is. We can tell by taking a history, examining, ordering an X-ray or a biopsy. It is only when we apply the concept of healthy to a mind that we begin to question what it really means. Is the mind of a criminal healthy or just evil? Are narcissistic psychopaths ill or just difficult? Is autism a disorder or a variation of normality?

The WHO famously defines health as ' a state of complete physical, mental and social well-being and not merely the absence of disease or infirmity'. The fact that wellbeing is then defined as a state of 'health, happiness and comfort', leaves us, once the circularity has been eliminated with 'happiness and comfort', as signifiers of what health means. This is not helpful. By this definition, someone on a morphine drip or in a manic episode. would be the epitome of health. We all know that there is much more to health than comfort and that there is much more to mental health than happiness.

Perhaps it would be more helpful to look at the origin of the word Health and to the Germanic roots of the old English word 'hǣlth' meaning whole. When we refer to a body as healthy, we often mean that there is nothing missing, that is as it should be. This is a very similar idea to that of functioning, i.e., that it does what it should do. Whilst this definition feels more consistent with what most professionals think, it is still problematic. How do we then define what 'should be' or what it 'should do'? The answer is clearly we do, society does. Health is a socially constructed idea, something we agree on so that we can understand the physical, i.e. biological, world, rather than a scientific concept describing the physical world, like gravity, for instance.

Health, like beauty or good, is one of those words that allows us to make judgements. It depends on our common understanding of what they mean, but cannot be scientifically measured. They refer to how societies and individuals ascribe value. Good has more value than evil, beauty has more value than ugliness, health has more value than illness. They are all debatable, consensus fading away when we try to pin things down. They are useful in making judgements of value along a scale.

The Health of the Mind

We have defined the mind as a collection of psychological processes that enable us to behave as we should. It follows that when behaviour does not allow us to function, it is because there is a problem with the mind. Since understanding other people's behaviour is crucial to our survival, an individual whose behaviour we do not understand creates a considerable amount of stress, leading to exclusion and avoidance.

For centuries, individuals whose behaviour was not functional or was not understood were separated from society, either hidden in their families or confined into asylums. The explanations for those behaviours ranged from the influences of the planets on their minds. The description Lunatic Asylum referred to those influenced by the moon, to supernatural influences, like spirit possessions. They included judgements along the good-evil value system. Asylum inmates were often referred as morally defective, or as being the recipients of punishments for the sins of their ancestors.

With the Enlightenment, at the end of the Eighteenth Century, health professionals were recruited to look after and try to understand the minds of those individuals confined in asylums. They brought with them a new value system in which to make judgements, not based on moral value but on health value. Their way of thinking, that the health of the nervous system was the explanation for this otherwise unfathomable behaviour, was a revolutionary breakthrough that helped millions. The morally defective became the mentally ill.

The whole of psychiatry and much of normal and abnormal psychological science emerged from the effort to understand the minds of the individuals previously confined to these institutions. In this process, a new idea emerged. They created, not only a medicine of the brain i.e. neurology, but a medicine of the mind i.e. psychiatry. This discipline studied behaviour and mind processes scientifically i.e. psychology, but focused on describing, or inventing, pathological entities that explained behaviour, using the health-illness value system. The explanation for behaviour was not only a pathology of the nervous system, but a pathology of the mind.

A healthy mind is thus a mind free of pathological processes as defined by psychiatry, but one that allows the behaviour of the individual to be functional, i.e. behave as he should do, in each society. An ill mind is therefore a collection of psychological processes that drive dysfunctional, i.e. not as it should be, behaviour. A mental illness is a defined pathological entity, a pattern of behaviour and psychological processes, that we have defined as an illness and that can be identified through the behaviour or mental experiences of an individual.

To use a real-life example, homosexuality is a set of behaviours and a set of mind functions (desire, love, identity…) underpinning that behaviour, that for centuries were not understood and produced fear in society to the point of persecution and exclusion. Society did not understand or accept this behaviour or the minds that underpinned it. Homosexual behaviour was codified as a crime that meant exclusion. The mind behind the behaviour was explained through the moral value system.

The advent of psychiatry brought a new understanding. Homosexuality was not an evil of morally defective individuals, but a disorder of the brain, from moral value to health values. It was codified as a mental disorder and treated as such. The study of this mental disorder showed that not only were the brains of these individuals no different to heterosexuals, but that their functioning in society was identical in any other domain. This contributed to the re-definition of what behaviour should be. Society has now a better understanding of homosexuality. It is no longer seen, in most societies, as a moral choice or a disorder.

Many people that we may define as on the autism spectrum see their predicament in similar terms. They see themselves as different, but not pathological. They see neuro-diversity as a set of mind processes different from most of the population, but not necessarily as impairment to normal functioning, similar to being left-handed.

Health is not the ideal term or value system to use to make judgements on the minds of people who behave in ways that we do not understand, but is what we have. It is a much healthier concept than the alternatives.

Mental Health Practice

What is the practice of mental health workers? What do they do? Nominally it is to contribute to the mental health of a population. But what does this mean in turn? If we take the WHO definition, it involves increasing people's happiness and comfort. Most people would understand the task as helping individuals function in society, that is, behave as they should, *and* to have the mind that enables them to behave as they should.

Most mental health consultations however, especially those in Child and Adolescent Mental Health settings, address one specific aspect of those mental processes, that is, the understanding of behaviour. Parents presenting their children with oppositional behaviour may say that all they want is for their children to be happy and comfortable. What they really crave, and what mental health professionals see as their job, is to help parents understand their children's, or their own, mind so that they can first understand and then change how they behave. Adolescents with unbearable anxiety or recurrent self-harm, want to feel better or to stop. But the job is to understand the cause of the anxiety or the behaviour so that things can change. People who are uncomfortable or unhappy, but who understand why that is the case, do not seek the help of mental health professionals, unless their explanation for their own distress is that their discomfort is the product of a mental illness.

The success of the mental health model at explaining psychological discomfort, the generalisation of the term mental health to include all kinds of psychological discomfort and the long established fear of behaviour or mental experiences we do not understand, have combined in recent years to create an explosive demand for this service. The making sense of behaviour and mental processes has become a huge industry. This has become particularly relevant as children and adolescents have become increasingly distressed and unhappy.

Framing this distress as a health condition has entitled people to seek understanding through publicly available health services. It has become relevant to the practice of mental health work to frame distress and its understanding in terms other than health. This is relevant for work with individual patients, where we may need to say things like, 'your child is not depressed, he is just very sad and troubled because he does not get enough attention'. It is relevant to those practising at service development or commissioning level, where services for children experiencing social deprivation need to be addressed separately from the mental health domain.

Summary

The task of mental health workers is to offer an understanding of the mental processes involved in behaviour that most people are unable to explain. We do this within the health/illness domain rather than in the moral or spiritual one. This activity builds on a natural drive to understand other people's behaviour and constitutes 'practice', an activity that requires theoretical knowledge and skill beyond that of applying a technique.

Reference

Preamble to the Constitution of WHO as adopted by the International Health Conference, New York, 19 June–22 July 1946; signed on 22 July 1946 by the representatives of 61 States (Official Records of WHO, no. 2, p. 100) and entered into force on 7 April 1948.

3 Medico-Legal Frameworks in Making Treatment Decisions with Children and Young People

Suyog Dhakras

The treatment of children and young people with mental disorders and mental health problems involves balancing the need, on the one hand, to give due weight to the views of children and young people themselves and on the other hand, to ensure that the treatment decisions achieved are safe and in their best interests.

KEY CONCEPTS

- The development of human rights law has contributed to the increasing recognition that greater weight should be given to the views of children and young people.
- This involves considering the developing understanding and ability of children and young people to make decisions for themselves.
- Decision-making with regards to the treatment of children and young people with mental disorders occurs within a legal framework that includes statute law, i.e. laws passed in Parliament, i.e. Children Act, Family Law Reform Act, Human Rights Act, Mental Capacity Act, Mental Health Act, in addition to case law or common law, i.e. precedents created through judgements in specific cases, e.g. Gillick competence.
- In addition to statute and common law, every child and young person, up to the age of 18 years, is subject to the inherent jurisdiction of the court which can supersede parental authority.
- The enactment of statutes, such as the Family Law Reform Act, Human Rights Act, Mental Capacity Act and Mental Health Act, has helped to ensure that health care professionals ensure active participation and collaboration with children and young people in achieving treatment decisions, obtain assistance and input from persons with parental responsibility and ensure that safety and safeguarding issues are appropriately addressed.

UN Convention on the Rights of the Child 1989 (UNCRC)

The UN Convention on the Rights of the Child (UNCRC) sets out a range of civil and political, socio-economic and cultural rights that apply to all persons, up to the age of 18 years. Although this charter is not a part of UK law, the Government of the UK, by ratifying the charter, has agreed to take all the steps it can to implement it. Courts in the UK and the European

Court may take into consideration the UNCRC charter when making decisions about the rights of a child.

The UNCRC guiding principles are:

Article 2: All of the rights in the convention apply equally to all children.
Article 3: The best interests of the child shall be a primary consideration in all actions considering the child.
Article 5: States should respect the responsibilities, rights and duties of parents to make decisions in relation to their children 'in a manner consistent with the evolving capacities of the child'.
Article 6: Every child has a basic and unequivocal right to life and to survival and development.
Article 12: All children have the right to express their views and have their views given due weight in all matters that affect them.

Human Rights Act 1998 (HRA'98)

The Human Rights Act 1998 (HRA'98) incorporates the rights set out in the European Charter of Human Rights (ECHR) into UK domestic law. The HRA'98 places an obligation on public bodies to work in accordance with the key relevant rights set out in the ECHR.

Article 3: Freedom from torture and inhuman or degrading treatment.
Article 5: The right to liberty.
Article 6: The right to a fair hearing.
Article 8: The right to private and family life.
Article 10: Freedom of expression.
Article 14: Freedom from discrimination.

Following the implementation of the Human Rights Act 1998 in the UK, individuals working for statutory and public authorities, whether in the delivery of services or in making policy, must ensure that decisions taken do not contravene the articles of the Human Rights Act.

The developments on human rights law are now recognised in relation to the admission to hospital and treatment of mental disorder in young people, for example, through the amendments to the Mental Health Act 1983.

In spite of the increased recognition of the rights of young people to make decisions regarding their treatment, the role of persons with parental responsibility, usually the parents or the local authority if the child or young person is under a Care Order, is still an important one. The Children Act 1989 is useful in determining who has parental responsibility with regards to a particular child or young person.

Consent

Consent is defined as the act of saying that one is willing to do something or allow what somebody else wishes, i.e. giving permission or agreement. In the medical sense, consent to treatment is defined as acquiescence to treatment.

Consent can be implied in certain circumstances and does not always have to be in the written form. A patient who consults a doctor about a sore throat and then opens his mouth for examination will be considered to have given his consent for the examination. In this case, consent is implied and the patient could not then complain if the doctor puts a spatula in his mouth. In the absence of consent, the intervention may be liable to be considered as an assault on the patient.

In order for a patient's consent to be valid, the following are required:

- Capacity/competence to make the decision.
- Sufficient information to decide.
- The decision should be made of his/her own free will and be free from pressure from others.

Historically, health care providers usually looked to parents/those with the responsibilities of a parent to provide consent for health care on behalf of a child/young person. This was understandable and continues to happen appropriately for younger children. However, with changes in society and the development of the notional rights of children and young people, this gradually changed.

The Children Act 1989

The guiding concepts of the Act are:

- Welfare of the child is paramount in all legal proceedings in court.
- Participation of the child.
- Partnership with parents or people with parental responsibility.
- Race, culture, religion, language issues, i.e. equality and diversity.
- Only positive intervention.

An important aspect of the Children Act and requiring consideration when making decisions about children is the Welfare Checklist. An important feature of this list is that the wishes and feelings of the child need to be taken into consideration in addition to the child's age and understanding.

Parental Responsibility (PR)

Parental responsibility is defined under the Children Act as 'all the rights, duties, powers, responsibilities and authority which by law a parent of the child has in relation to the child and his or her property'.

Those who may hold parental responsibility include:

- The child's mother. She loses PR if the child is adopted and the adoptive parents gain parental responsibility.
- Both parents if they are married to each other at the time of the child's birth.
- Both parents if married to each other at any time since the child's conception.
- Mother only, if the parents are not married to each other. Unmarried fathers can acquire parental responsibility by making a formal agreement with the mother or via a court order. The Adoption and Children Act 2002 provides that an unmarried father acquires parental responsibility when he and the child's mother register the birth of their child together. This only applies after 0/12/2003.
- Anyone holding a residence order.
- Special Guardian via a Special Guardianship Order of a child.
- Adoptive parents.

- The local authority, if the child is subject to a Care Order or Emergency Protection Order. Parental responsibility is then shared with the parents and the exercise of PR by parents may be limited.
- Any person granted an Emergency Protection Order, e.g. the police, medical teams.

More than one person can have parental responsibility for the same child, and in these cases, parental responsibility is shared with the mother, who cannot lose parental responsibility, except in the case of adoption.

In cases where treatment is to be given under parental consent and parental responsibility is shared, the consent of only one person/agency with parental responsibility is required. This will still be the case even when the parties do not agree. It is good practice to try to achieve an agreement between parties. In case of disagreements between persons holding parental responsibility, it may become necessary to seek legal advice and authority from the court.

Family Law Reform Act 1969

Section 8 of the Family Law Reform Act (FLRA) states:

> The consent of a minor, who has attained the age of sixteen years, to any surgical, medical or dental treatment which in the absence of consent would constitute a trespass to the person, shall be as effective as it would be if he were of full age. And where the minor has by virtue of this section given effective consent, it shall not be necessary to obtain any consent for it from his parent or guardian.

Thus, capacity to give consent without the need for consent from persons with parental responsibility was made available to young people aged 16 years and over. However, the FLRA did not address the issue of what might happen if a 'minor' refused to give consent to treatment that was considered necessary for them. This resulted in a number of cases, where the courts, High Court and the Law Lords ruled that young people could consent to treatment, but could not refuse treatment that was consented to by persons having parental responsibility.

Mental Capacity Act 200

Capacity is a legal term denoting a patient's ability to consent to an intervention. Capacity is a statutory concept following the enactment of the Mental Capacity Act (MCA). The MCA applies to all persons aged 16 and over. Within the meaning of the Act, all persons aged 16 and over are presumed to have the capacity to make decisions about their health care, including treatment for mental disorder, unless proven otherwise.

The assessment of capacity is a two-stage test:

1. Does the person have an impairment of or disturbance in the functioning of the mind or brain?
2. Does the impairment/disturbance mean that the person is unable to make a specific decision when they need to? This means they cannot understand and retain the information in their mind or use or weigh that information in the balance as a part of the decision-making process or communicate the decision.

The Mental Capacity Act 2005 applies to all young people 16 years old and over in all aspects apart from the following exceptions; young people under 18 years are not able to:

- Make advance decision in regard to treatment refusal.
- Make a Lasting Power of Attorney (LPA).
- Have a statutory will made by Court of Protection.
- Additionally, Deprivation of Liberty Safeguards (DoLS) do not apply to under-18s.

Treatment including for mental disorder 'under' the MCA (2005) means:

- Person lacks capacity to consent to that treatment at that time despite all assistance.
- Treatment given in their 'best interests'.
- Treatment does not involve 'deprivation of liberty'.

Deprivation of Liberty (DOL)

The concept of deprivation of liberty arose from the European Convention of Human Rights (HCHR) and was subsequently embedded and enacted through the Human Rights Act 1998, in particular Article 3 of EHCR, the Right to Liberty. The Code of Practice of the Mental Capacity Act gives us the framework of what might constitute 'DoL' in the treatment of children and young people:

- Use of restraint, sedation, for a resisting patient.
- Complete or effective control over care and movement, assessments, treatments, contacts or residence.
- Prevented from leaving if a meaningful attempt is made.
- Request by carers to be discharged is refused.
- Inability to maintain social contacts because of restrictions on access to other people.
- Loss of autonomy due to being under continuous supervision and control.

The essential components of DoL are:

- Objective: confinement + restricted place + duration.
- Subjective: lack of valid consent.
- Involvement of the state, e.g. as part of treatment in the NHS.
- It is not relevant whether the individual shows compliance/lack of objection, the relative normality of placement or the purpose behind placement.

Scope of Parental Responsibility (Code of Practice of the Mental Health Act)

In certain situations, persons with parental responsibility may consent on behalf of a child under the age of 16 or young people, 16 or 17 years of age, who may not be able to consent due to lack of capacity. In those circumstances, health professionals can rely on such consent only if it is within 'the scope of parental responsibility (SPR)'. The concept of SPR derives largely from case law from the European Court of Human Rights in Strasbourg. The Code of Practice for the Mental Health Act (2015 ed.) gives some guidelines, but it is difficult to have clear rules. SPR is not within the body of the Mental Health Act. Whenever there is doubt, legal advice should be sought.

There are a number of points to be considered before relying on parental consent:

- Parental responsibility.
- Are the parents acting in the best interests of the child/young person?

- Competence/capacity of the child or young person.
- Type of decision: the more invasive the treatment, the more likely it will fall outside SPR.
- Views of child/young person + age and maturity. The more resistance from the child/young person, the more likely the treatment decision would fall outside SPR.
- Validity of consent of the parents in regard to mental capacity, disagreement.

To assess whether a decision falls within the SPR, two key questions must be answered:

1. **Is this a decision a parent should be reasonably expected to make?_**
   - Type and invasiveness of proposed intervention
   - Age, maturity, understanding of patient
   - Wishes and/or resistance of patient
2. **Issues that might undermine validity of parental consent**
   - Parent(s) lack(s) capacity under MCA
   - Unable to focus on best interests of child or young person, distress
   - One parent agrees, the other disagrees_

The parameters of the SPR will vary from case to case. Mental health professionals might find it helpful to consider the following factors:

- The nature and invasiveness of what is to be done and the extent to which the liberty of the patient is to be curtailed. The more extreme the intervention, the more likely it is to fall outside the zone.
- Whether the patient resists. Treating a child or young person who is consistently resisting treatment needs more justification.
- General social standards in force at the time concerning the sorts of decisions it is acceptable for parents to make. Anything beyond the kind of decisions parents routinely make will need scrutiny.
- The age, maturity and understanding of the child or young person. The greater these are, the more likely it will be that it should be the child or young person who takes the decision.
- The extent to which a parent's interests may conflict with those of the child or young person. This may suggest that the parent may not act in the child or young person's best interests.
- Where the decision cannot be made on the basis of falling within the SPR, consideration should be given to alternative methods of treatment.

It is helpful to consider the issues of consent, capacity and decision-making, including treatment in hospital, with regard to mental disorders for young people aged 16–17 and those children and young people under the age of 16.

Decision-Making with Young People 16–17 Years of Age

This age group is considered separately due to the significant changes to the legal frameworks in health care decision-making for 16–17-year olds.

Mental Health Act 1983: Amended in 2007

The amendments to the MHA in 2007 built upon the rights given to young people regarding consent to treatment through the Family Law Reform Act (FLRA), as well as through the MCA. Section 131 of the MHA, i.e. regarding informal treatment of mental disorder, provides that:

- A 16–17-year old with capacity, according to the MCA, can consent to treatment or refuse treatment.
- Their consent or their refusal cannot be overridden by anyone with parental responsibility.
- In a case of refusal, if treatment is thought to be necessary, the options are:
  - Consider whether the young person would satisfy the conditions of the MHA for treatment under compulsion or
  - If MHA conditions are not satisfied, and treatment is needed, then it may be necessary to seek authorisation from the court.

16–17-Year Old without Capacity

If the young person does not have capacity, treatment may still be given using the following legal frameworks:

- Section 131 of the MHA will not apply.
- Treatment may be given under the MCA, in the best interests of the patient, using the best interests checklist provided in the MCA Code of Practice, as long as there is no deprivation of liberty.
- If there is deprivation of liberty, then consideration needs to be given to whether criteria for the Mental Health Act are met.
- If the MHA is not applicable, it may be necessary to seek authorisation from the court.

Case Study (1): Lily

Lily is a 16-year-old girl with anorexia nervosa and depression, who was referred to the Community Specialist CAMHS clinic. In spite of assertive outreach treatment, her weight and physical state deteriorated along with a worsening of the symptoms of depression. Lily lived with her mother, who was not closely involved in her treatment due to the pressure of her job. Parents were divorced and had emphatic disagreements about the treatment options. Lily was admitted to the paediatric ward in the General Hospital. She needed nasogastric tube-feeding because of the physical problems. Lily resisted tube-feeding and threatened to call her solicitors.

The paediatricians and the mental health professionals assessed Lily's capacity to consent to treatment. Their opinion was that Lily did not have capacity to consent due to the severity of the mental disorder. As treatment would involve deprivation of liberty (insertion of nasogastric tube against Lily's wishes), treatment could not be given under the MCA.

Due to the strained relationship between Lily and her mother, the parents' acrimonious relationship, the invasive nature of the proposed treatment and Lily's consistent strong resistance, the professionals' view was that treatment with nasogastric tube-feeding did not fall within the SPR.

Consideration was given to the MHA. Given the severity of the anorexia nervosa, the presence of a co-morbid depressive illness and the risk to her mental and physical health and well-being, Lily was considered to satisfy criteria for compulsory treatment under the MHA and treated accordingly under Section 3 MHA.

Decision-Making with Children below 16 Years of Age

In the case of children below 16 years, the FLRA and MCA would not apply. The legal concept of capacity is not used. Instead the concept of 'Gillick competence' is used to reflect the child's increasing development to maturity. In the case of Gillick, the court held that children, who have 'sufficient understanding and intelligence to enable them to fully understand what is involved' in a proposed intervention will have the 'competence' to consent to that intervention. This is referred to as the child being 'Gillick competent'. A child may be 'Gillick competent' to consent to admission to hospital, medical treatment, research or any other activity that requires their consent. If a child is 'Gillick competent' and gives consent to a particular treatment, it is not necessary to gain consent from a parent/person with parental responsibility. However, it is good practice to involve parents/carers in the decision-making process, if the child consents to information being shared.

In the past, if a child who is 'Gillick competent' refuses admission or treatment, courts have held that a person with parental responsibility can overrule the refusal. There is no post-Human Rights Act decision on this. The Code of Practice for the MHA states that the trend in recent cases is to reflect greater autonomy for competent children. It would be unwise to rely on the consent of a person with parental responsibility. In such cases, consider whether the child would meet the criteria for compulsory treatment under the MHA. If not suitable to use the MHA, it would be appropriate to seek authority from the court.

If the child is not 'Gillick competent':

- It would be appropriate to gain consent from a person with parental responsibility, if the matter falls within the SPR.
- If the matter falls outside the parameters of the SPR, consider whether criteria are met for the MHA.
- If not, it would be appropriate to seek authority from the court.

Case Study (2): Jordan

Jordan (17), who was in care until age 16, was referred to the CAMHS clinic for repeated self-harm in the form of self-cutting and repeated overdoses. He presented to accident and emergency having taken an overdose of a large number of paracetamol tablets several hours earlier. The paediatricians were concerned regarding the risk of serious, potentially fatal, damage to Jordan's liver. Jordan refused to have any blood tests or any treatment. Professionals in accident and emergency were concerned that, on assessment, Jordan seemed to understand the need for treatment and the risks if he did not receive treatment.

In the past, Jordan had accepted treatment for his self-harm. Due to the time elapsed since the overdose, accident and emergency doctors were extremely worried. They wondered whether they would need to treat Jordan under the MHA, but were concerned that arranging this would take up valuable time. Similarly, obtaining a treatment order from the court would cause further delay in treatment that was needed as soon as possible.

Emergency Treatment

CoP MHA (2015 edition, 19.71, 19.72)

- A life-threatening emergency. Treatment urgently needed.
- Not possible to rely on the consent of the child, young person or person with PR.
- No time to seek authorisation from the court or MHA.
- Failure to treat would be likely to lead to death/severe permanent injury.

in which case

- Treatment may be given without consent.
- Or overriding the competent/capacious refusal/capacity and of those with parental responsibility.

- In such cases, the courts have stated that doubt should be resolved in favour of the preservation of life, acceptable to undertake treatment to preserve life or prevent irreversible serious deterioration.
- Only for under-18s.

Proportionate Treatment

This is an example of the use of 'case law or common law' (significant precedents established through court decisions in similar cases). Health professionals can rely on this particular framework to provide treatment lawfully in such emergency circumstances.

Common Law

Common law is not legislation, but a body of law based on custom and law court decisions. In health care, this defines the rights and duties of patients and health care professionals in areas untouched by legislation.

Guiding Principles

There must be a degree of urgency together with safety/protection issues.

The intervention must end immediately once the emergency situation is resolved.

The rights of the patient must be protected at all times.

Secure Accommodation

Where a child or young person needs to be detained, but the primary purpose is not to provide medical treatment for mental disorder (for example, if the young person is behaviourally disturbed but there is no need for them to be hospitalised), their needs might be more appropriately met within secure accommodation under the Children Act 1989, Section 25, Secure Order. The Secure Order does not authorise medical treatment. This option is used when the primary aim of the intervention is to achieve a measure of safety and protection for the young person rather than to provide medical treatment for mental disorder.

Case Study (3): Asha

Asha, a 15-year-old girl in the care of the local authority, was placed in foster accommodation in a neighbouring city. She was in care because her mother was unable to keep her safe and Asha had been part of a group of young people abused by a gang of adults. She was extremely distressed and angry at being moved away from her home town and not being in contact with her peers. She began repeatedly self-harming by cutting herself, threatening to harm herself more severely if she was not moved back to her home city.

She absconded frequently from the foster placement. Asha was known to associate with older males and she was being exploited. She was admitted to the paediatric ward of the local General Hospital after being found in a park, having been severely beaten up. During assessment, Asha expressed her anger and distress at her current placement and repeatedly stated her intention to self-harm and to abscond if she was sent back to the foster placement, and if not moved back to her home city. The social workers wondered whether Asha needed to be admitted to an adolescent psychiatric unit in view of the self-harm.

Repeated mental health assessments from the Paediatric Liaison team and community CAMHS team highlighted emotional distress and anger, though no evidence of a mental disorder. At the request of the local authority, a Mental Health Act assessment was carried out, and the outcome was that the criteria for detention under the Act were not met. However, the assessment highlighted the significant safeguarding needs and Asha's determination to go back to her home city and peers, despite the high risk of inevitable exploitation.

Following a planning meeting, it was agreed that, in view of the repeated and frequent absconding and the risk of significant harm to Asha when she ran away, and the repeated and frequent self-harm, Asha needed protection and safety.

As the criteria for detention under the Mental Health Act were not met, the local authority agreed to consider Section 25 Secure Order under the Children Act to ensure Asha's safety, as it was accepted that she would definitely abscond from any other accommodation that she was placed in. Section 25 was applied for, and Asha was placed in a welfare bed in the local Secure Unit for six weeks. The self-harm stopped. On discharge, Asha was moved into specialist supported accommodation where she has managed to significantly reduce the self-harm and has not absconded.

Mental Health Act 1983 (2007 Amendments) MHA 2007

The Mental Health Act provides for compulsory admission, detention and treatment of a patient deemed to have a mental disorder. In the past, the mental disorders were specified as mental illnesses, commonly diagnosed using ICD-10 criteria, psychopathic disorder, i.e. treatable personality disorder, mental impairment, learning disability or severe mental impairment in the terms of the 1983 Act.

According to MHA 2007, the definition of mental disorder has been broadened to 'any disorder of the mind'. The above sub-categories have been removed.

It is important to remember that sections of the MHA can be applied to all ages, except a Guardianship Order, which only applies to those 16 years old and over.

The MHA 2007 Code of Practice highlights issues specific to the care and treatment of children and young people:

- The best interests of the child or young person must always be a significant consideration.
- Children and young people must be kept as fully informed as possible, just as an adult would, and should receive clear and detailed information about their care and treatment in a format appropriate to their age and development.
- The views of the child or young person and their wishes and feelings should always be considered.
- The intervention for the treatment of the mental disorder should be the least restrictive, least stigmatising, consistent with effective care and treatment, resulting in the least possible separation from family and friends and with least possible interruption of their education.
- All children and young people should receive the same access to education as their peers.
- Children and young people have as much right to expect their dignity to be respected as anyone else.
- Children and young people have as much right to privacy and confidentiality regarding information pertaining to them as anyone else.

The MHA 2007 has introduced the duty on hospital managers to provide age-appropriate hospital environment for the admission and treatment of children and young people. In all MHA Section assessments, it is important to consult with the patient's nearest relative, i.e. spouse, oldest parent, next of kin or legally appointed nearest relative, although only Section 3 requires permission from the nearest relative.

Section 136: This is an **Emergency Police Power** that they use for:

- 'Removal' of a patient to place of safety from a public place, i.e. a place the public have access to.

Table 3.1 Common Applications of the MHA (1983) in Children

Purpose	*Section*	*Requirements in Addition to Mental Disorder*	*Powers*
Assessment	2	Admission necessary for patient's own health and safety or the protection of others. Two doctors, one with Section 12 Approval, and an approved social worker needed to make the assessment.	Up to 28 days' admission for assessment, or assessment followed by medical treatment. Not renewable. Patient may appeal against the Section within 14 days.
Emergency order for assessment	4	As for Section 2: used when only one doctor is available.	Up to 72 hours admission for assessment. Not renewable.
Emergency detention of a voluntary inpatient	5.4	This is a nurse's holding power and can be used if necessary for the patient's own health and safety or the protection of others if no doctor or social worker is available. Patient must have been a voluntary inpatient who is no longer willing to stay. The nurse must be a Registered Mental Health Nurse (RMN).	Up to 6 hours admission. Not renewable and must be reviewed by a doctor
Emergency detention of a voluntary inpatient	5.2	Necessary for patient's own health and safety or the protection of others. Only one doctor needed. Patient must be a voluntary inpatient for this to be applied – cannot be used on patients in A&E.	Up to 72 hours which includes time of 5.4 if applicable. Not renewable.
Treatment	3	Inpatient treatment is appropriate and admission is necessary for patient's own health and safety or for protection of others. It is important that compulsory admission and treatment are considered to alleviate the mental disorder or prevent further deterioration. The patient's nearest relative must give consent for the Section to be applied.	Up to six months' admission and is renewable. Treatment may be enforced for the first three months, but the patient would need to consent after this. If the patient does not consent, a second opinion is required from a doctor recommended by the MHA commission. Patient has the right to appeal against the Section after three months.

- Police believe person is suffering from mental disorder.
- Needs 'care or control'.
- Necessary in interests of that person.
- Protection of others.
- Patient has to be assessed for either consideration of another appropriate.
- Section or discharge within 24 hours. This was previously 72 hours.

Supervised Community Treatment/Community Treatment Order (SCT/CTO)

The MHA 2007 introduced the supervised community treatment/community treatment order (SCT/CTO), that provides a framework for the management of suitable patients, allowing them to be safely treated in the community. This treatment occurs in the context of the Responsible Clinician having the power of recalling the patient to hospital for treatment if necessary. Only patients who have been treated in hospital under Section 3 MHA can be considered for SCT/CTO.

The SCT/CTO has several conditions that the patient must comply with in the community. The Responsible Clinician holds the power to recall the patient to hospital if he considers that the patient can no longer be treated safely in the community. The SCT/CTO may be successful in providing the least restrictive alternative for suitable patients, promoting recovery and participation in age-appropriate activities.

Lily (Case Study 1) was treated successfully in hospital under Section 3 MHA. After she had made a good recovery, she was given increasing periods of leave. She was then put on SCT/CTO. The conditions were that she would have weekly physical monitoring, take medication and meet members of the community team as required.

Lily complied with the conditions and was able to successfully sit for her GCSE exams and go on to college. After five months, she was discharged off the SCT/CTO.

Appeals against Detention and Compulsory Treatment under the MHA

Under the structure of the MHA 2007 patients can appeal against their detention. The appeals are heard by the independent Mental Health Review Tribunals (MHRT) under the aegis of the Department of Justice. The Act and the Code of Practice give details of the processes and time scales at which tribunal reviews of detention and compulsory treatment of children and young people would be carried out.

Changes to Frameworks in the Future

Mental Capacity Act: This was reviewed and amended by Parliament in May 2019, Mental Capacity (Amendment) Act 2019. The provisions under this Act are expected to be applied into practice in 2020. The Code of Practice is due to be reviewed and published in 2020. The main change expected is that the Liberty Protection Safeguards (LPS) would replace the Deprivation of Liberty Safeguards (DoLS) and would apply to 16- and 17-years olds as well.

Mental Health Act: The government has sought consultation for review of the Mental Health Act, and this review process will continue.

Multiple-Choice Questions

See answers on page 666.

1. For a patient's consent to treatment to be valid they must have:

a. Information presented in written form to make the decision
b. An IQ of 100 or more
c. Agreement of their next of kin
d. The capacity to make the decision

2. Which legislation introduced a statutory concept of 'capacity' for young people and adults over age 16?
   a. The 1989 Children Act
   b. The Human Rights Act
   c. The Mental Capacity Act (2005)
   d. Gillick competence

Key References

Department of Constitutional Affairs, (2007). *Code of Practice Mental Capacity Act 2005.* London: TSO.

Department of Health, (2015). *Code of Practice Mental Health Act 1983.* London: TSO.

Hale, B., (2010). *Mental Health Law* (5th edition). Andover: Sweet & Maxwell.

National Institute for Mental Health England, (2009). *The Legal Aspects of the Care and Treatment of Children and Young People with Mental Disorder: A Guide for Professionals.* NIMHE.

4 Safeguarding within Child and Adolescent Mental Health Services

Siobhan West

> Real children are more than just their brain structure, their physiology, their caregiving history, their attachments or their genetics in isolation.
>
> (Woolgar, 2013)

KEY CONCEPTS

- A Think Family approach: consider the other agencies involved with the child and the family. What information do they hold? How does what is happening for other family members impact on the child and the family functioning?
- The voice of the child is paramount. This includes 16–17-year olds, who are legally still children. What is their behaviour telling you if not words themselves?
- Looked after children. Consider the accumulative impact of transition and loss including changes within their named professional network. Continuity of care is crucial where possible and, if change is unavoidable, should be managed carefully and involve the child/young person at all stages.

The duty to safeguard children and young people from harm, abuse and neglect is one held by all professionals in whatever discipline they work. The safeguarding agenda is largely underpinned by the Children Act (1989, 2004) and Working Together to Safeguarding Children (2018), the statutory framework which sets out the legislation relevant to safeguarding. Statutory guidance is issued by law and must be followed unless there is a good reason not to do so.

Safeguarding and promoting the welfare of children are defined as:

- Protecting children from maltreatment.
- Preventing the impairment of children's health or development.
- Ensuring that children grow up in circumstances consistent with the provision of safe and effective care.
- Acting to enable all children to have the best outcomes.

It is essential that all practitioners understand their roles and responsibilities with regard to safeguarding, including how to spot the signs, interpret behaviours and consider the wider picture, known as 'contextual safeguarding', of what life is like for a child and young person. This includes considering how their family and community circumstances influence their safety.

By virtue of the children and young people who access child and adolescent mental health services (CAMHS), practitioners working in this speciality are regularly in the privileged position of working with our most vulnerable children and young people in society and often over protracted lengths of time. This means that CAMHS have an ideal opportunity to explore and consider many aspects of children and young people's lives and circumstances in a broad and contextual manner. This chapter aims to support and develop CAMHS practitioners' understanding of some of the principles of safeguarding children and young people.

The Current National Picture: Child and Adolescent Mental Health

It is important to stress that, although children who are looked after or those who are involved with child protection procedures will invariably have been exposed to trauma, this does not mean that they are destined to be traumatised. All children respond differently to adverse experiences, and the responses to the same trauma will vary between each child.

The proportion of children aged 5–15 with any mental health issue has increased slightly, from just fewer than 10% in 1999 to just over 11% in 2017. The rising prevalence of emotional disorders has been mostly, but not entirely, offset by falling prevalence of behavioural disorders. There has been a faster increase in the prevalence of mental health issues among girls aged 11–15: from 9% in 1999 to 13% in 2017. This includes an increase of more than 50% in the rate of emotional disorders, e.g. anxiety and depression (Children's Commissioner 2019).

A Think Family Approach

'Think Family' is a national agenda first introduced by the Cabinet Office's Social Exclusion Taskforce in 2007. The 'Think Family' approach aims to increase the understanding by the multi-agency partnership of the effect of the family situation on the child, identifying early risk to children and ensuring that the support provided by all services is co-ordinated and focused on problems affecting the whole family (SCIE 2009). The framework to support the child and family is provided in the 2018 guidance, 'Working Together to Safeguard Children'.

All practitioners should follow the principles of the Children Act (1989 and 2004), both of which state that the welfare of the child is paramount and that they are best looked after within their families. Having said this, focusing on the full range of needs within a family should not detract from the over-riding duty to safeguard and promote the welfare of the children.

It is important is to consider the child as part of a wider family and community network. A child is not an island but part of an intricate and complex system of relationships, all of which will inevitably impact on all areas of the child's physical and emotional development. A 'Think Family' approach enables individual needs to be looked at in the context of the whole family. All agencies should avoid focusing only on the individuals to whom they have a responsibility to offer their services. Support needs to be tailored to meet the identified needs, so that families with the most complex needs receive the most intensive support. Where possible, and if not exposing a child to additional increased risk, services should aim to build on the strengths of families, increasing their resilience.

In a system that 'thinks family', contact with any service offers an 'open front door' into a broader system of joined-up support. This enables practitioners to see moments of engagement as an opportunity to identify wider need and direct support to the individual and their family. Within this approach, frontline practitioners are alert to individual and family risk factors and practitioners consider the causes and wider impact of presenting problems. Practitioners consider the ways in which different family members and their problems interrelate and might offer family services which work with both parents and children (Social Exclusion Task Force 2008).

Close collaboration between services and mental health professionals is vital, and this includes adult services that sometimes forget that their patients are parents (Hall and Williams, 2008).

Case Study (1): Jane And Alex

Jane is a single mother. She was previously a habitual user of class A drugs, but has been 'clean' for some years, following her work with the substance misuse team. Jane has emotionally unstable personality disorder (EUPD) that has at times been debilitating. She was referred by her GP to the Adult Mental Health team. Jane has previously been well engaged with this service, but her attendance at appointments has recently been sporadic and she has not collected her latest medication prescription. The team are concerned that she maybe in a state of crisis.

Jane has a son, Alex (14). Alex has been referred to CAMHS by his GP because of ongoing and increasingly challenging and aggressive behaviour at home, with violence towards his mother. Alex has been suspended from school as a result of his behaviour on more than one occasion and school are considering permanent exclusion.

Questions to consider:

- What are the key issues affecting this family?
- What would a 'Think Family' approach by professionals look like in response to these issues?
- What might the barriers be to working with a 'Think Family' approach?

Looked After Children

A looked after child is defined as any child that is removed from their home by the local authority for more than 24 hours. Most children become looked after as a result of abuse and neglect. The most recent figures in 2018 state that there were 75,420 looked after children in England, a 4% increase since the previous year. Although they have many of the same health issues as their peers, the extent of these is often greater because of their past experiences. Almost half of children in care have a diagnosable mental health disorder and two-thirds have special educational needs. Delays in identifying and meeting the emotional well-being and mental health needs of looked after children can have far-reaching effects on all aspects of their lives, including their chances of reaching their potential and leading happy and healthy lives as adults (Department for Education and Department of Health, 2015).

Looked after children and young people have particular physical, emotional and behavioural needs related to their earlier experiences before they became looked after (NICE, 2013). Looked After children are four to five times more likely to have a mental health disorder than those children who are living with their birth families (Bazalgette et al., 2015). Those leaving care are particularly vulnerable and may need continued support from specialist services (NICE, 2013). In addition to reports of a lack of attention to their emotional needs within their family environment, some children and young people have reported that they have been let down by a system that did not recognise their behaviours as a sign of distress and as a reaction to the adversity they have experienced. These system failures have further affected the development of secure attachments and as a result, multiple foster care placement breakdowns have ensued, leading to further loss and trauma.

Children's experiences of transitions in both health and other agencies are unacceptably poor (CQC, 2016). Changes and a lack of permanence in the professional arrangements for many looked after children are unsettling and can hamper effective work by professionals. Looked after children in care and those subject to child protection processes often feel powerless. They report feeling uninvolved in their care planning processes and often, they are not informed of the outcome of assessments. Children's rights include the right to participation in decisions made about them. For looked after children, this right is enshrined in the Children Act, 1989. In a review by Munro (2011), the main areas of criticism by looked after children themselves were frequent changes of social worker, lack of an effective voice at reviews, lack of confidentiality and, linked to this, the lack of a confidante.

Case Study (2): Abi

Abi is 13 years old. She has been living in a foster care placement for two years, but her carers are beginning to express concern that they cannot continue to look after her because she has started to self-harm. Her carers do not have the knowledge or skill to help her with this, and they are worried about how her behaviour might impact on their biological son, who is six years old. Abi's social worker told her that she would be better off in a residential children's home where the staff would have more experience and would be there overnight (when Abi's self-harming tends to be more severe).

Abi really does not want to move. Her current foster care placement is the first place where she has felt settled, and she feels that moving would make things much worse. She has so far resisted seeking treatment for the self-harming behaviour but now would agree to go to CAMHS if it meant she could stay with her carers. On that basis, Abi's social worker thought it was worth asking the foster carers if they would reconsider and suggested a package of support for them to help give them the confidence to support Abi if she continued to struggle.

The foster carers were happy to commit to another six months of looking after Abi on the condition that she engages with CAMHS and that they receive support.

Abi was fortunate to be offered an early appointment with CAMHS, and although it took some time for her to feel confident to open up to and trust the service, she gradually felt more able to manage her emotions and to use the support now available from her carers when she began to feel like self-harming.

Abi felt that she benefitted from building a relationship with just one CAMHS practitioner so that she did not need to explain her story over and over again. She felt able to trust the support and advice that CAMHS had given her over time.

Questions to consider:

- How did the services involved work together to support continuity for Abi in this scenario?
- Was this a child-focused approach? If yes/no, how?
- How can CAMHS practitioners tailor their practice to suit the additional emotional needs of a looked after child?

Child and adolescent mental health service practitioners have a key role to play in helping children and young people rebuild their lives following difficult early experiences, such as abuse and neglect. Organisational and operational challenges can result in many vulnerable young people not receiving the help they need when they need it. As professionals, as multi-agency partners and as a wider system, it is important that we work smartly in order to minimise the adverse effects that can be associated with this.

Key Safeguarding Issues

All practitioners, when working with children, should consider:

- **Listen to and collaborate with young people**, their verbal and non-verbal cues and their feedback on their experiences as service users. Use these to make changes and keep children and young people informed.

- **Work with families** to gain context as to what a child's world is like to live in, use a 'Think Family' approach and where safe and appropriate to do so, involve the child/young person in care and support planning. Consider the other issues that are present in the family. Can you link with the other professionals involved to adopt a joined-up approach to supporting this family? How do the other issues within the family impact on the child you are working with? Consider information sharing across agencies to prevent working in silos.
- **Manage transitions.** Ensure children and young people are informed and prepared for upcoming, unavoidable changes with regards to their care. For looked after children, ensure that foster carers understand the impact of repeated losses on looked after children and know how to support them.

Key References

Bazalgette, L., Rahilly, T. and Trevelyan, G., (2015). *Achieving Emotional Well-Being for Looked After Children – A Whole System Approach.* London: NSPCC.

HM Government, (2018). *Working Together to Safeguard Children. A Guide to Inter-Agency Working to Safeguard and Promote the Welfare of Children.* London: HM Govt.

Social Care Institute for Excellence, (2009). *Think Child, Think Parent, Think Family: A Guide to Parental Mental Health and Child Welfare.* London: SCIE.

5 Policy and Practice in Children and Young People's Mental Health

Pathiba Chitsabesan and Bernidka Dubicka

KEY CONCEPTS

- Delivering good outcomes for children and young people's mental health benefits from a systems-wide approach working collaboratively across agencies.
- Delivering evidence-based interventions requires a workforce with the relevant skills and competencies.
- Data and outcome metrics can contribute to improving transparency and accountability across the system.

Introduction

This chapter provides a summary of key policy initiatives in relation to children and young people's mental health in England, although many of the challenges and learning will be relevant to other nations.

Recent research indicates that 12.8% of 5- to 19-year olds and 5.5% of 2- to 4-year olds have a mental health disorder, with higher rates for older adolescents (NHS Digital, 2018). It was of particular concern that 24% of girls aged 17–19 years old had a mental health disorder, of which one in two are self-harming. There has been a significant increase in the number of children and young people referred to children and young people's mental health (CYPMH) services over the last five years. This is likely to be the consequence of a number of different factors, including an increase in the mental health needs of children and young people, in addition to increased awareness amongst the public and professionals. In England, the Care Quality Commission (CQC) regulates health care services to ensure that they meet safety and quality standards. The commission has published two thematic reports on mental health services for children and young people in 2017 and 2018. This raised concerns that complexity and fragmentation in mental health services were contributing to challenges for some individuals in accessing the support they needed.

Delivering good outcomes for young people will require co-ordinated action across different parts of government including health, education, local government and criminal justice. There are opportunities through increased investment and more collaborative commissioning and service delivery arrangements to deliver a systems-wide approach to providing care for children and young people.

This includes universal health promotion and prevention programmes to services provided in education and community settings, including targeted provision for vulnerable groups of young people, e.g. those in local authority care or in contact with the criminal justice system.

Universal services such as SureStart Children's Centres, schools, colleges, primary care and youth services can play an important role in both preventing mental health problems and in early identification when they arise, i.e. by supporting children and young people's mental health through a focus on health and well-being within an educational curriculum, tackling bullying and by ensuring environments support CYP who may be particularly vulnerable to mental health needs, including those with disabilities, looked after children, those in contact with the criminal justice system and CYP who identify themselves as lesbian, gay, bisexual or transgender (LGBT).

Following the Health and Social Care Act (2012), there has been an increased focus on mental health services and a commitment to providing 'parity of esteem' for mental and physical health services. Parity of esteem means that mental health is valued as much as physical health, emphasising equal access to care and the allocation of resources proportionate to need.

In 2015, the government set out its vision for children and young people's mental health services in its *Future in Mind* strategy (Department of Health, 2015). The strategy identified challenges within the current system from fragmentation to lack of investment, and collaborative working across agencies. It set out a broad vision of how children's and young people's services should be improved and included themes such as resilience and early intervention, and workforce development. The strategy identified a range of stakeholders (the NHS, public health, local authorities, social care, schools and youth justice services), as having an important role to play in supporting children and young people's mental health. Each of these has distinct and different accountability mechanisms.

Recent government initiatives in England for improving CYPMH services include:

- ***Five Year Forward View for Mental Health* (2016)** which covers all NHS mental health services in England, with specific objectives to improve children and young people's mental health services. Through local transformation plans (LTP), each CCG working alongside other stakeholders is expected to set out the local offer for children and young people, including how the needs of the most complex and vulnerable groups would be met.
- ***Transforming Children and Young People's Mental Health Provision: A Green Paper* (2017)**, jointly published by the Department for Health and Social Care and the Department for Education (2017) and due to be implemented from the end of 2019. Its focus is on developing the links between schools and health services.

  The Green Paper sets out plans for two new roles linked to education: mental health leads in schools and mental health support teams. The former will be responsible for overseeing the use of the 'whole school approach to mental health and well-being' and helping to identify children at risk of, or showing signs of, mental ill health. The mental health support teams will provide interventions to support CYP with mild to moderate mental health needs, supervised by local specialist CYPMH teams.
- ***NHS Health Long Term Plan* (2019)** continues investment in CYPMH services including expansion of services in schools, crisis care and eating disorder services and improving services for CYP with autism and learning disability, and young adults.

Local transformation plans contribute to larger scale regional Sustainability and Transformation Plans (STPs). Both STPs and integrated care systems (ICS) provide an opportunity to change how care is delivered by greater collaborative working across a number of health and local authority partners, including aligning commissioning and outcomes reporting.

Various other initiatives contribute to the delivery of *Future in Mind*. As Future in Mind is a cross-government strategy, some of these sit outside the remit of the NHS England. Some initiatives aim to support children and young people's mental health, rather than it being their primary focus, e.g. the Troubled Families programme run by the Ministry of Housing, Communities and Local Government.

As noted by the National Audit Office (2018), there has been a historic under-investment in mental health services for children and young people and, although recent initiatives are an important step towards parity between physical and mental health, substantial progress has yet to be made with regards to the vision set out in Future in Mind.

Service Delivery

The most well-known framework describing children and young people mental health services was a model dividing service provision into four tiers. This model helped differentiate between the different forms of services that might be available to children and young people. More recent models, including THRIVE, focus on the needs of children and young people and include a systems-wide framework in considering how support can be delivered by a range of different practitioners and agencies, including the role of parents and carers.

The THRIVE categories are needs-based groupings (Wolpert et al., 2015). The THRIVE framework conceptualises five needs-based groupings for young people with mental health difficulties and their families:

- Thriving
- Being offered advice
- Receiving help
- And more help
- Being offered risk support

Each of the five groupings is distinct in terms of the needs and/or choices of the individuals within each group, the skill mix required to meet these needs, the dominant metaphor used to describe needs, e.g. wellbeing, ill health, support and the resources required to meet the needs and/or choices of people in that group. The groups are not distinguished by the severity of need or type of problem. Rather, groupings are primarily organised around different supportive activities provided by children and young people mental health services in response to mental health needs and influenced by client choice.

Choice and Partnership Approach (CAPA) is a clinical service transformation model that brings together collaborative practice, goal-setting with regular reviews and demand and capacity management including lean thinking. It is an approach based on the key principles of shared decision-making and clarity of choice. CAPA focuses on helping people make explicit choices about what may most benefit them and links this with evidence-based packages of care. One of CAPA's key components is to change language to one that promotes strengths-based collaborative work and thinking about which skills are needed, rather than access to a particular professional discipline. In particular, CAPA segments work so that skills and capacity can be considered within a job-planning process.

The majority of CYPMH services have been commissioned to provide services for young people aged 5 to 18. This potentially under-estimates the importance of early-years provision and transition from 18 years.

The early years play a large role in determining mental health through childhood and beyond. In the early years, infants make emotional attachments and form relationships that lay the foundation for future mental health. The positive mental health and wellbeing of children and their parents during the first few months and years of a child's life enable their future health and attainment.

There is good evidence for a range of interventions that can promote mental health and well-being. Estimates suggest that up to one in seven mothers will experience a mental health problem in the antenatal or postnatal period. Anything that diminishes the ability of parents to communicate with and bond with babies and young children may affect their development of speech, communication and social abilities and contribute to emotional and behavioural problems in later life. Subsequently, policy initiatives focussing on supporting parents, particularly mothers with mental health needs, and infant mental health are increasingly common (*Five Year Forward View*, 2016; *NHS Long Term Plan*, 2019). Targeted support for vulnerable parents, e.g. the Family Nurse Partnership programme and positive parenting programmes, can improve outcomes for this group. In addition, good-quality nursery and pre-school education can help prepare children for school by supporting them with their cognitive and social development and ensuring school readiness.

For older adolescents, the transition to adult mental health services (AMHS) can be challenging, with many young adults failing to access services. More recently, services for young people up to 25 years of age have been developed in some areas, bringing together CYPMHS, AMHS and youth services to try to address some of the challenges of fragmented commissioning and differences in culture between CYP and adult services. NICE (2016) transition guidance emphasises the need for transition to be multiagency and to involve service users in the design and development of services. Further development and implementation nationally will be supported through the *NHS Long Term Plan* (2019 – see https://www.longtermplan.nhs.uk/).

The needs of other groups of vulnerable children and young people, e.g. looked after children and those with intellectual disability and autism, have often fallen through service gaps. As part of the NHS Long Term Plan, NHS England will work with the Department for Education and local authorities to improve their awareness of, and support for, children and young people with learning disabilities, autism or both. Over the next three years, autism diagnosis will be included alongside work with children and young people's mental health services to test and implement the most effective ways to reduce waiting times for specialist services. There will be a continuing expansion of Stopping Over-Medication of People with a learning disability, autism or both and Supporting Treatment and Appropriate Medication in Paediatrics (STOMP-STAMP) programmes. By 2023/24, children and young people with a learning disability, autism or both and those with the most complex needs, including those who face multiple vulnerabilities such as looked after and adopted children and children and young people in transition between services, will be given a designated keyworker.

Workforce Development and Data

Transforming the mental health workforce is fundamental to creating sufficient capacity to deliver accessible, quality services and good outcomes for children and young people. Developing new care models means building flexible teams working across organisational boundaries and ensuring they have the full range of skills and expertise to respond to service user needs in different settings.

Professionals supporting children with mental health needs may work in a variety of different settings and come from a variety of different backgrounds. Consideration must be given to the training of the wider workforce within communities, in addition to those working in specialist mental health settings. Access to regular supervision and consultation for staff is essential in providing effective services. Managers working within services should ensure that the well-being of staff is a primary concern and that staff are provided with the necessary training and support to deliver evidence-based quality care.

MindEd is a free educational resource developed for professionals working across community and specialist settings. It provides information on a range of mental health needs in CYP and key principles in providing assessment and support. Staff support and development is crucial for recruitment and retention which have been challenging across children and young people's mental health services (National Audit Office, 2018).

The children and young people's Improving Access to Psychological Therapy (IAPT) programme provides an important opportunity for training the workforce. It seeks to combine evidence-based practice with user involvement and outcome evaluation to embed best practice in child mental health. It includes five key principles underlying transformation: participation, increasing mental health awareness and reducing stigma, improving access and engagement, delivering evidence-based therapy and demonstrating outcomes and accountability through data collection. Ensuring services are delivering evidence-based treatments is essential for providing quality care and good outcomes for CYP. Packages of care that have been evaluated, including demonstrating cost-effectiveness, are subsequently recommended by, e.g. NICE guidance.

Data are important in providing transparency within the system with regard to commissioning and service delivery. Within England, NHS-commissioned services provide anonymised patient-level data through the Mental Health Services Data Set (MHSDS). MHSDS brings together key information including activity and access data from community and hospital-based services for children and young people in contact with mental health services. The NHS as a whole aims to prioritise the recording and use of data based on outcomes. There is a range of patient and clinician rated outcome measures (PROMs and CROMs) and patient rated experience of services measures (PREMs) that can be used in routine clinical practice. Commonly used measures include the Strengths and Difficulties Questionnaire (SDQ), Health of the Nation Outcomes Scales for Children and Adolescents (HONOSCA) and Revised Children's Anxiety and Depression Scale (RCADS).

The Child Outcomes Research Consortium (CORC) learning collaboration aims to aid alignment and integration of data and outcomes across agencies and organisations.

Summary

In recent years, there has been an unprecedented focus on mental health within the NHS, providing greater transparency regarding the needs of children and young people and the commissioning and service delivery required to meet those needs. Important principles in delivering effective CYPMH services include the need to build resilience, consider prevention and early intervention and develop a clear joined-up approach, linking services through care pathways. Delivering evidence-based interventions for CYP with mental health needs requires a sustainable, well-supported workforce with the relevant skills and competencies working across the system.

Multiple-Choice Questions

See answers on page 666.

1. What is the prevalence of mental health needs in children and young people aged 5 to 19 years of age?
   a. 12.8%
   b. 10%
   c. 5.5%
   d. 24%

2. What are the important systems and agencies for delivering good outcomes for children and young people with mental health needs?
   a. Health
   b. Children's social care/council
   c. Education providers
   d. Regulators
   e. Criminal justice system
   f. All of the above
3. What is the needs-led approach replacing Tiers for delivering children's mental health?
   a. CAPA
   b. IAPT
   c. THRIVE
4. Which policy guidance is jointly published and monitored by the Department for Health and Social Care and Department for Education?
   a. Five Year Forward View for Mental Health
   b. Transforming Children and Young People's Mental Health Provision: A Green Paper
   c. NHS Health Long Term Plan

Key References

Department of Health, (2015). *Future in Mind, 2015.* London

Department for Health and Social care and Education, (2017). *Transforming Children and Young People's Mental Health Provision: A Green Paper.* London.

NHS England, (2016). *Five Year Forward View for Mental Health.* London.

Helpful Websites (at Time of Publication)

MindEd, www.minded.org.uk.
The Child Outcomes Research Consortium (CORC), www.corc.uk.net.
Thrive, www.thriveapproach.com.
Choice and Partnership Approach (CAPA), www.capa.co.uk.
Values Based Practice, www.valuesbasedpractice.org.

6 Commissioning Services

Stephanie Ramsey

KEY CONCEPTS

- Commissioning is the continual process of planning, agreeing and monitoring services.
- It involves taking a strategic approach to how local needs can best be met with the resources available.
- Commissioning is not one action but many, ranging from the health-needs assessment for a population, through the clinically based design of patient pathways, to service specification and contract negotiation or procurement, with continuous quality assessment.
- Commissioning drives the transformation agenda through evidence about what works, what is required and then sourcing it innovatively and competitively.

Introduction

Commissioning is about assessing needs, available resources and priorities, and using this information to plan, buy and review services to ensure they meet the needs of customers, deliver and improve agreed health and social outcomes and provide value for money. Commissioning is more about 'what is needed' whilst procurement is 'how do we get it?' Procurement is a route through which the commissioning organisation can appoint a provider, or providers, to deliver the commissioning strategy for a given service. Not all commissioning will be done via procurement. Commissioning is practised on different scales or 'levels', from national commissioning of some NHS services, to regional commissioning of residential places, to a complex, individualised plan for a young disabled person. Strategic commissioning looks at intentions for populations, whilst individual (or micro) commissioning is focussed on specific arrangements for individuals achieved through assessment, support planning and the development of tailored care packages. It can refer to the sourcing and purchasing by individuals with personal budgets or self-funders of services, who will be their own 'commissioners'. Commissioning may occur at multiple levels, dependent on the population being served and the service being provided.

Process of Commissioning

Effective commissioning is a continuous process of action and improvement following a plan, do, review and analyse cycle. Each stage builds on the previous one from the identification of

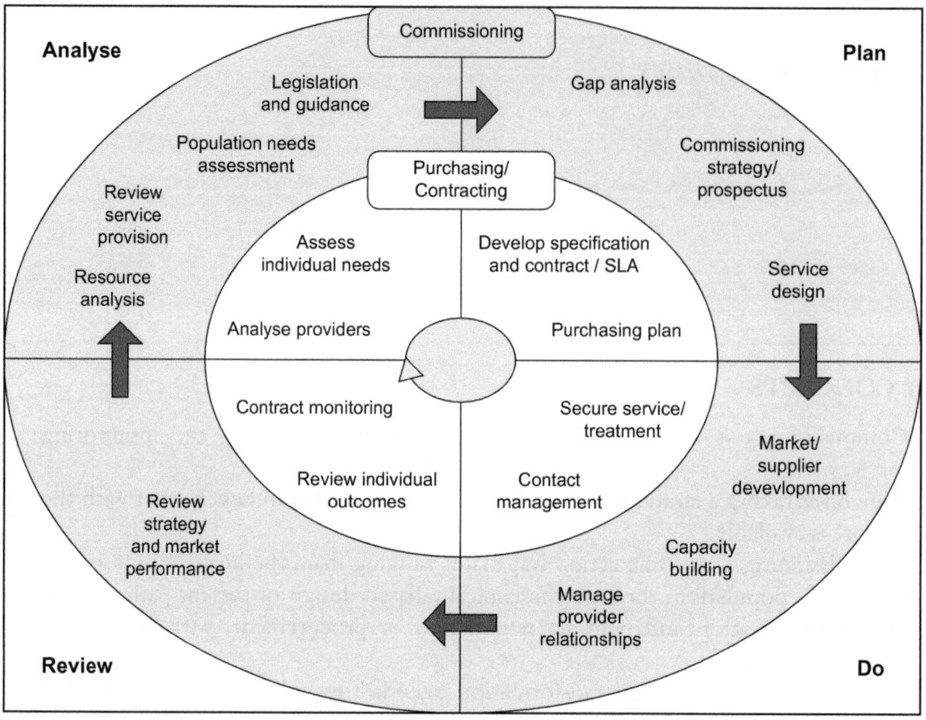

Figure 6.1 The process and interconnectedness with procurement and contracting.

needs through to review of delivery and achievement of outcomes and includes commissioning, procurement and contract management activity.

Analysis/Needs Assessment

It is important to identify local needs, resources and priorities and agree what the desired end product should be and to understand the needs and aspirations of whole populations and how the varying needs of individuals influence them. It is necessary to consider what is currently being provided and whether it is delivering the required outcomes and value for money, along with how requirements may change in the future. The role of a commissioner is to challenge existing models and review alternatives.

The local Joint Strategic Needs Assessment (JSNA) is a good starting point. This will provide an assessment of the current and future health and social care needs. Areas are free to undertake JSNAs in a way best suited to their local circumstances, and these will vary, but all will be based on Department of Health JSNA Guidance (2007). A needs assessment is 'a systematic method for reviewing the health and wellbeing needs of a population, leading to agreed commissioning priorities that will improve health and wellbeing outcomes and reduce inequalities' (DH, 2007; P7). The joint strategic needs assessment process provides a mechanism for gathering and analysing relevant data at a high level. This will usually be accessed via local authority websites.

Commissioners can draw on national and local research to guide commissioning decisions along with examples of best practice, comparative data and an understanding of legislative and regulatory requirements. Understanding current levels of provision, spend and patterns of demand and use over time is vital for deciding what services should be delivered in the future. Often commissioners will want to test the quality of a service by obtaining direct, independent feedback from customers by, for instance, asking young people, including those who choose not to use the service, for their views of services and how they contribute to better outcomes. The practitioners, clinicians and other stakeholders will have a significant amount of understanding, evidence and expertise to contribute.

Procurement data, such as market analysis or provider costs, will provide insight into the effectiveness of current service provision and the opportunity and stability of the market.

Pathway analysis is a helpful approach for understanding users' experiences of life or services and highlighting where the most efficient and effective points are for identifying and addressing needs and moving resources. This will help to identify the strategy for early intervention or prevention.

Plan

Planning will need to consider different ways of meeting the outcomes identified through the needs assessment. This will need to be done within the context of resources available. This is a challenge given ongoing financial pressures across the health and local authority system.

Commissioning strategies should reflect the full use of resources, not just financial aspects. This will include the workforce and what shape, skills or training might be needed, and facilities and what needs to be in place and where. This may include the co-location of services or resources, bringing together universal and acute services where appropriate or making use of existing community buildings. To promote efficiency, it is regarded as essential for commissioners to make the best of the resources in the system. It is outlined in *Good Commissioning Principles and Practice* (2010) that this is achieved through:

- Optimising the use of the money that commissioners control, and more importantly, influencing the money across the system that is not directly controlled, such as benefits and schools grants.
- Supporting parents to improve outcomes for their own children through co-production.
- Making best use of community provision and volunteers.
- Making effective links with housing providers and adult health and social care.
- Ensuring that facilities are in the right place, the right condition and that their use is maximised.
- Pooling resources.
- Developing and managing a specific market.
- Designing the right balance between workforce skills, capacity and people's location.

Do: Secure the Service or Model to Meet Outcomes

When it comes either to commissioning or, in some cases, de-commissioning services, there are many different mechanisms and tools to employ. These range from competition, service redesign and individual commissioning to influencing and working with local communities. Different mechanisms will have different results, and it is important to choose the right one for a particular service, market, population or group of needs, for example, spot purchasing is generally inefficient, but may be appropriate for small or one-off purchases in a competitive market.

The best service delivery model has to be considered. For a local authority this may mean outsourcing services to independent providers or 'externalising' by setting up an independent trust. In some cases, these changes in governance have been forced on the local authority in response to what was seen as a failure of in-house delivery. There is some concern about the use of outsourcing in children's services, particularly when it involves the use of for-profit providers. It is a challenging undertaking to do well. Yet evidence suggests that when used correctly outsourcing has the potential to help local authorities deal with the pressures they face, drive up standards and ultimately secure better outcomes for vulnerable children and young people.

Some existing services may need to be decommissioned to release resources for new developments. Improved commissioning and procurement require a good understanding of what the market can offer. Effective commissioning involves working towards being best able to meet the needs of service users, especially specific and diverse needs that are less apparent. There should be sustainable partnerships between commissioners and the 'suppliers' whether in the public, private, social enterprise or voluntary sectors, to design innovative services and understand risks and achievable outcomes.

Review

Commissioning influences how services are shaped and provided, either in-house or externally through partnership, but this needs to be accompanied by regular evaluation to ensure the services are still fulfilling the original needs or adapting to changing ones.

Principles Underlying Commissioning

Whether commissioning is a single or whole-system approach there must be clarity in the approaches and principles to be used. This will include factors such as:

- Improving outcomes for the local population will be at the heart of the commissioning process with commissioners taking shared responsibility for outcomes.
- Commissioning should seek to meet needs in an evidence-based way and contribute to the development of the local evidence base for effective practice.
- The commissioning process will integrate services around the needs of individuals and families, recognise local diversity and support greater personalisation and choice so that people are empowered to take personal responsibility and shape their own lives and the services they use. The market will be developed to reflect the needs of a diverse local population.
- Residents will be active participants in the commissioning process, i.e. in planning, design, monitoring and evaluation.
- There will be an increasing focus on prevention and early intervention and on tackling long-standing inequalities in outcomes.
- Resource allocation and commissioning decisions will be transparent, contestable and locally accountable and driven by the goal to achieve optimum quality, value for money and outcomes. Investment in the local community is a priority.
- The commissioning process should aim to ensure that the same approach, e.g. service specification and performance monitoring, is applied to all commissioned activity to ensure fairness and that no delivery vehicle is given or gains unfair advantage. This will require a clear distinction between commissioning and provider functions and responsibilities regardless of whether they co-exist within a single organisation.

- Commissioning arrangements will be sufficiently flexible and fluid to support a variety of different partnership approaches, e.g. with education, housing, other local authorities, the voluntary sector or other health partners, depending on the best way of delivering the required outcomes.

Good commissioning places the individual at the heart of the process. To ensure this, a commissioning approach should actively seek to involve service users at each stage so that they become co-designers and co-producers. This approach ensures that people are engaged throughout the whole process and acknowledges that those with 'lived experience' are often best placed to advise on what will make a difference. (see NHS England Coalition for Collaborative Care – http://coalitionforcollaborativecare.org.uk/).

The approaches taken need to be different for children, young people and their parents/carers. This is because, and it is important that we remember it when commissioning, children are not just smaller versions of adults. They are all growing and progressing, at different rates, through a range of physical, emotional, psychological, cognitive, social, psycho-sexual and neurodevelopmental stages of development as they age towards adulthood.

This simple fact is something that any adult would recognise, but the implications of this journey for each child are profound. They are the same child, but very different after each year of their childhood and adolescence. Different children of the same age are often at very different stages of development. In most adult services, unless an adult has a specific physical or learning disability, or has developed an infirmity or other recognised loss of faculty, we can usually treat them as sufficiently similar, self-sufficient, independent, responsible and accountable for their choices.

When professionals, e.g. teachers, youth workers, social workers, paediatricians, school nurses, health visitors, child psychologists, CAMHS nurses, are assessing the needs of a child for a service, they first have to determine at some level where that child/young person is at in their development in terms of what is normal for them. Because child development into adulthood is a slow transitional process, albeit with step changes in how children interact with and understand the world, most adults cannot remember their transition through these stages of development. Understanding them sufficiently well to relate to which stage a child is in and whether they have additional needs from others at their particular development stage is something that requires specialist training. In commissioning children's services well, commissioners must be mindful of these differences, and of what children and young people need of those professionals that work with them.

Children and young people are still developing, whereas adults are in a steadier state, and typically it is adults that make the assessment. This makes assessing children and young people more complicated. It makes commissioning for them more sensitive to ensuring the details are right. We need to think differently when designing services for children and young people. They are not economically independent and cannot access services in the same way. Provision should be made available in the school that they encounter every day. We must remember, as we do in commissioning for children and young people, that commissioners of adult or all-age services should recognise that for many aspects of services for children and young people, there are specific, dedicated workforces that have no direct equivalent once patients reach adulthood.

Outcomes-Based Commissioning

In commissioning it is important to focus on the impact on the service 'end user' and what has been achieved, rather than only on how time and money have been spent. Commissioning for outcomes is not about how many children have taken part in an activity course, but rather whether it has had the intended impact of increasing confidence and social skills. Rather than focussing on delivering activity-based contracts, it is crucial to agree tangible outcomes, identifying who benefits from these outcomes and what is the value of such outcomes. This allows for flexibility in the approaches to be used to meet that outcome and is more conducive to delivering early intervention and preventative programmes. It enables commissioners to focus on setting direction.

Legislative Context

Good commissioning will mean that purchasing power is used to promote the public sector equality duty and to promote sustainable and responsible procurement. *The Public Sector Equality Duty* (2010) requires public bodies to have due regard to the need to eliminate discrimination, advance equality of opportunity and foster good relations between different people when carrying out their activities. The duty applies to the public sector and to anyone carrying out public functions. The duty applies to all nine areas of discrimination listed in the *Equality Act* (2010).

The *Public Services (Social Value) Act* came into force on 31 January 2013. It requires people who commission public services to think about how they can secure wider social, economic and environmental benefits. Before they begin the procurement process, commissioners should think about whether the services they are going to buy, or the way they are going to buy them, could secure these benefits for their area or stakeholders. The Act is a tool to help commissioners gain more value for money out of procurement. It encourages commissioners to talk to their local provider market or community to design better services, often finding new and innovative solutions to difficult problems.

Integrated Commissioning

Commissioning may well be single agency, such as a local authority or a school, but increasingly it is identified that greater efficiency gains should be achieved through a partnership approach. Optimal use can then be made of available resources regardless of who invests them and it can be ensured that budgets from different sectors are aligned and are mutually reinforcing. Joint commissioning is an important means by which local agencies can ensure an integrated approach to service design and effective use of the total resources available across different funding streams.

Differing approaches to commissioning across organisations can lead to limited whole-system solutions, duplications and inefficiencies. This then leads to inconsistencies in the 'holistic environment for the customer' if organisations commission separate elements of service that do not fit together to support an overall aim or outcome.

Accountability and responsibility within joint working agreements are crucial to account for and reconcile different legislative and commissioning frameworks, accountability structures and expectations. Pooled budgets are a key enabler of effective integrated commissioning as resources are used to meet desired outcomes regardless of funding route with underpinning partnership arrangements within a clear legal agreement. This is most usually achieved through the use of an agreement made under Section 75 of *National Health Services Act* (2006) between a local authority and an NHS body in England. Section 75 agreements can include arrangements for pooling resources and delegating certain NHS and local authority health-related functions to the other partner(s) if it would lead to an improvement in the way those functions are exercised. This does encourage organisations to focus on shared outcomes and identify more efficient ways of working.

Partners that have successfully implemented pooled budgets tend to have effective relationships and a shared vision with a focus on outcomes. Effective, integrated commissioning can be challenging, particularly against a backdrop of changing governance structures in the health sector.

Changes in Health and Care Commissioning

In 2012 the *Health and Social Care Act* split responsibilities for health commissioning across clinical commissioning groups, councils and NHS England. This led to the concept of a 'purchaser–provider' split, but since 2016 this has been changing with the development of sustainability and transformation partnerships (STPs) bringing together the NHS and local authorities into larger areas to run services in a more co-ordinated way, to agree system-wide priorities and to plan collectively how to improve residents' day-to-day health. STPs are now evolving to become integrated care systems.

The *NHS Long Term Plan* set out the ambition that every part of England will be covered by an integrated care system by 2021, replacing STPs but building on their good work to date. Integrated care systems will take the lead in planning and commissioning care for their populations and providing system leadership. Commissioners will need to work more closely together, aligning their objectives with providers and taking a more strategic, place-based approach to commissioning. The focus now is on collaboration rather than competition

Whatever the landscape though, commissioning functions, as described in the commissioning cycle, will continue. Every system needs people to assess local needs and then plan, develop and monitor services.

Key Reference

Department for Education, (2010). *Good Commissioning Principles and Practice*. London: DfE.

Part II

The Physical and Psychological Development of Children and Young People

Margaret J.J. Thompson

An understanding of the psychological development of children and young people is important for all professionals working with them. The chapters on attachment, social development and emotional development will be useful here.

This section also outlines presentations of problems in children which require knowledge of paediatric development and conditions which might be important to understand when assessing a child presenting at the CAMH or paediatric services. This will be particularly true if working with young children and especially with children with learning difficulties.

Chapters by a speech and language specialist and a clinical psychologist remind us of the importance of looking at those profiles in children.

Many children and young people presenting to CAMHS will have other symptoms as well as the presenting behaviour problem, and these should be taken into consideration, while working on a formulation to account for their difficulties.

Part II

The Physical and Psychological Development of Children and Young People

[illegible]

7 Attachment Theory

Christopher Gale

Introduction

> We are, all of us, molded and remolded by those who have loved us, and though that love may pass, we remain nonetheless their work – a work that very likely they do not recognize, and which is never exactly what they intended.
>
> (Francois Mauriac, 1952)

Attachment theory refers to a constellation of ideas about emotional development that emphasise the importance of the relationship between an infant and their primary caregiver. This theoretical framework has proved susceptible to empirical experimentation, and this has permitted its development within mainstream scientific parameters. It has illuminated several aspects of early emotional development, namely, how emotions are socialised, how they are expressed and how communication of emotions is made acceptable.

KEY CONCEPTS

- Central to attachment theory is the concept of the 'secure base' provided for a child by their primary caregiver, usually the mother. This enables a child to explore the world with confidence knowing that they can seek comfort and safety in times of perceived danger or anxiety.
- There are four broad patterns of attachment in infants and children: secure, insecure/avoidant, insecure/ambivalent and disorganised/disorientated. They correspond to attachment representations in adolescence and adulthood and can be seen to increase or decrease the risk of a child/young person developing mental health problems.

The main premise of attachment theory is that the bond between mother and infant is biologically determined and forms the psychological 'umbilical cord' by which children develop, both physically and psychologically. It proposes that the quality of this relationship and its subsequent influence on the social and emotional development of the child is determined by:

- Temperamental factors in the child
- The mother/primary caregiver's own experience of attachment
- The circumstances in which it develops

John Bowlby is generally credited as the father of attachment theory. His work during the 1950s and 1960s and his collaborations with Mary Ainsworth and other authors form the founding premise of what has come to be known as attachment theory. His ideas build on some fundamental insights provided by experimental observations carried out before him (Harlow, 1959; Lorenz, 1965).

Harlow's Monkeys (Harlow, 1959)

One of such experiments was performed by Harry Harlow in Wisconsin. Harlow set out to disprove that infant behaviour was the product of learning. He isolated infant monkeys from their mothers at 6 to 12 hours after birth and placed them with substitute or 'surrogate' mothers, made of either heavy wire or of wood covered with soft terry cloth. In the most famous experiment, both types of surrogates were present in the cage but only one was equipped with a nipple from which the infant could feed. Even when the wire mother was the source of nourishment, the infant monkeys spent more time clinging to the cloth surrogate, proving that infant behaviour is instinctive.

The most interesting finding was to happen a few years later when surrogate-raised monkeys became bizarre later in life. They engaged in stereotyped behaviour patterns, e.g. clutching themselves and rocking constantly back and forth. They exhibited excessive and misdirected aggression and were incapable of caring for their own infants. This illustrated that maternal behaviour is not instinctive but learned in early infancy.

Lorenz's Filial Geese (Lorenz, 1979)

The second of these experiments was Konrad Lorenz's demonstration of filial imprinting in geese, at the turn of the century. He demonstrated that there was a short period, 35 hours, after hatching, when chick geese bred in an incubator would select an object and follow it around. The importance of this experiment for Bowlby was that it emphasised the idea of critical periods in development and a biologically determined proximity-seeking behaviour.

Key Concepts from Bowlby's Attachment Theory

- **Attachment behaviour**: any behaviour by the infant that had the effect of increasing the proximity to his/her carer.
- **The attachment behaviour system**: the repertoire of attachment behaviours and the decision-making process that identified which behaviour was more effective in different circumstances. This decision-making process involves some level of cognition and some degree of representation of the external world. Bowlby named this the 'internal working model'.
- **The emotional bond**: entails a representation in the internal organisation of the individual that is persistent, specific, significant and where there is distress and a wish for contact when separated.
- **The attachment bond**: is the emotional bond that is activated when the infant is in distress or under threat. A child's attachment figure is that person to whom he/she runs, when under threat.

Bowlby proceeded to describe the stages of separation, i.e. protest, despair and denial and set the ground for Mary Ainsworth's experiments in the 'strange situation' (Ainsworth et al., 1978). It produced the empirical foundation for one of attachment's most powerful concepts: secure and insecure attachment.

The Strange Situation and Categories of Infant Attachment

Mary Ainsworth and colleagues (Ainsworth et al., 1978) described three main patterns of attachment in their observations of infant children in the 'strange situation test'. They were:

- **Secure Attachment**
  When a child is securely attached, the mother provides a safe base from which the child can explore and the child is readily comforted, if distressed. When reunited with his mother, the distressed child will immediately seek and maintain comfort.
- **Insecure/Avoidant Attachment**
  A child with this pattern of attachment has no confidence that his caregiver will respond helpfully and in fact, the child expects to be rebuffed. He will happily explore away from his mother and is unduly friendly with strangers. When reunited with his mother, the child will ignore or avoid her.
- **Insecure/Resistant Attachment**
  The child who shows this pattern of attachment is unsure whether his mother's response will be available or helpful and he is uncertain about exploring and wary of new situations and people. He will be prone to separation anxiety and appear clingy. When reunited after separation he may be aggressive, angry and refuse to be comforted.
  A further pattern has subsequently been recognised (Bretherton, 1985):
- **Disorganised/Disorientated Attachment**
  These children seem confused and show stereotypies. When reunited with their mothers they seem to show conflicting feelings of fear, anger and a wish to be with her. Children in this category may display behaviours that would fit within the other two categories of disordered attachment, i.e. avoidant and resistant.

Attachment Disorders

The ICD-10 (WHO, 1992) outlines the diagnostic criteria for only two specific disorders of attachment that have not changed for the new ICD-11 (see Table 7.1).

The DSM-5 (APA, 2013) similarly delineates two clinical problems related to attachment; the previously inhibited form becomes 'reactive attachment disorder' (RAD) and the disinhibited becomes 'disinhibited social engagement disorder' (DSED). The latter is no longer considered a disorder of attachment (Zeanah and Gleason, 2014)The DSM-5 posits that less than

Table 7.1 ICD-10 Definition of Attachment Disorders (WHO, 1992)

Reactive Attachment Disorders with Inhibition of Attachment Behaviour (F94.1)	*Reactive Attachment Disorders with Disinhibition of Attachment (F94.2)*
• The capacity of these children to attach with adults is described as very inhibited. • They react with ambivalence and fear to the attachment figure. • They exhibit an emotional disorder with withdrawal, over-caution and impairment in their capacity for social play.	• Children show a diffuse, non-selectively focused attachment behaviour: attention-seeking and indiscriminately friendly behaviour: poorly modulated peer interactions; depending on circumstances there may also be emotional or behavioural disturbance. • Children with a disinhibited propensity seek contact without boundaries with the most varied caregivers.

Table 7.2 Brisch (2002) Defined Attachment Disorders That Supplement Those Described in the Diagnostic Manuals

Type I:	Little or no overt attachment – no protest on separation, even in very threatening situations.
Type IIa:	Undifferentiated – similar to F94.2 – lack of preference for a particular attachment figure.
Type IIb:	Risky behaviour – seeks out dangerous situations to force others into care-giving behaviours.
Type III:	Excessive clinging – fear of separation or loss of attachment figure is generalised, with a constant need for closeness and physical contact.
Type IV:	Inhibited attachment behaviour – similar to F94.1 – manifests in over-conforming behaviour, frequently as a result of domestic violence. Children more fearful of exploring their surroundings.
Type V:	Aggressive form of attachment behaviour – aggression a result of frequent rejection by attachment figure.
Type VI:	Role reversal – child serves as a secure emotional base for their parents, so receives little or no useful help in threatening situations.
Type VII:	Attachment disorder with psychosomatic symptoms – i.e. bed-wetting, eating problems or sleep disorder.

10% of severely neglected children develop it, usually only if they have experienced prolonged institutionalisation.

Brisch (2002) describes other types of attachment disorders that supplement those described in the diagnostic manuals (see Table 7.2).

Attachment in Children with a Learning Disability or High on the Autistic Spectrum

Attachment relationships are likely to be more challenging in children and young people with autism or a learning disability, not least because of the social communication and interaction difficulties they may have (Teague et al., 2018). Autistic children can show little interest in other people and will often demonstrate an apparent attachment to an inanimate, usually non-cuddly, object or collection of objects. A similar picture may present in children with severe learning difficulties.

Attachment Representations in Older Adolescence and Adulthood

The last important research tool that should be mentioned is the Adult Attachment Interview (AAI) (Main et al., 2002). This tool asks adults to make a list of the characteristics of important figures in their childhood and examines their capacity to construct a narrative around the details they give.

The adult attachment status elicited from the AAI can be useful when working with older adolescents and the categories respond to those identified by the strange situation test:

Autonomous (Secure)

Here the narrative is coherent and collaborative. The individual is neither derogatory nor angry towards parents, understanding the value of attachment relationships in the past and their influence on the present relationships. Within close relationships, they experience relative ease in becoming close to others and being dependent and depended upon. They are less worried about abandonment or someone becoming too emotionally close to them.

Dismissive (Anxious/Avoidant)

Here there are minimal explanations and no narrative is constructed. These individuals will most likely have been emotionally and/or physically rejected and/or neglected during childhood, but they work hard to present an idealised view of parents/carers. They dismiss the value of childhood attachment relationships and avoid discussion of a range of strong emotions, e.g. fear, anger, disappointment, hurt and loneliness. They will minimise the importance of any current difficulties and present as invulnerable. Within relationships they are uncomfortable being close to others and being interdependent. Partners will often want them to be more intimate.

Preoccupied (Anxious/Ambivalent)

These individuals are driven by their memories. They are often angry and confused about their childhood relationships with parents/carers. They value the importance of attachments, but narrating the past can be painful and involving. Anger within close relationships is seen as the least painful, most self-protective way to cope. However, they often want to emotionally merge completely with others, but find that those others are reluctant to become as close to them as they would like and will sometimes be scared away. The preoccupied adolescent/adult will often worry that their partner does not love them or will not want to stay with them.

Unresolved (Disorganised/Disorientated)

Here there is grief for the loss and trauma of childhood. It is not yet 'in the past'. Those individuals who have been subjected to significant levels of abuse and/or neglect at the hands of parents/carers will often feel unreasonably responsible in some way for their experiences. For the unresolved individual, there is no consistent pattern for dealing with stress, arising from a failure to integrate thoughts and feelings. Essentially, they have no 'internal working model'.

As a result, they can be aggressive or violent within any close relationships they manage to form, being extremely sensitive to criticism or implied humiliation, but insensitive to other people's feelings. Having no trust or respect for the feelings of others and systems of authority, the unresolved individual is likely to become involved in the criminal justice system.

Status in the AAI and 'strange situation' gives an indication of the nature of the person's 'internal working model'. This is significant when considering the risk and resilience around the development of mental health problems in later life.

- **Secure/autonomous** attachments indicate a perception of the main carer, and later close others, as responsive and assume that expressing emotions elicits a helpful response.
- **Anxious, avoidant and ambivalent** indicates a perception of the main carer as unresponsive and an assumption that expressing emotions does not necessarily bring comfort or help. Therefore, emotions are best dealt with internally and that may increase the risk of internalising mental health issues, e.g. depression, anxiety, deliberate self-harm and eating disorders.
- **Unresolved** indicates an absence of an internal working model, as the main carer did not give a consistent response. As there can be no underlying assumption about the

response to expressed emotions, there is no consistent way to deal with emotions. This may increase the risk of the development of anxiety, substance misuse and emerging personality disorders.

It is important to highlight that, whilst attachment representations may increase or decrease the risk of developing mental health problems, it is by no means the only contributory factor and should not be the sole basis for a diagnosis of mental health disorder.

Intergenerational Transmission of Attachment

The research literature around the transmission of attachment representations appears to indicate that if there is at least one autonomous parent/carer in the family unit, they will nurture securely attached children. With insecurely attached adults the transmissional pattern can be more complex and not necessarily corresponding (Crittenden, 2015; Shah et al., 2010). A dismissive parent/carer may evoke an intense ambivalent response in the child in order to increase the probability of caregiver response or reduce caregiver control. Conversely, a preoccupied parent/carer may employ angry or helpless demands, so the child might employ a strategy of caring for or complying with the caregiver, i.e. avoidant.

Attachment Theory and Cultural Contexts

Criticism has been directed towards Bowlby's conceptualisation of attachment, suggesting that it did not necessarily translate to non-westernised cultures (Rothbaum et al., 2000). This has been challenged, specifically when conceptualising the 'secure base' relationship (Posada and Jacobs, 2001), a term coined by Ainsworth when undertaking longitudinal observations of infant development in rural Uganda (Ainsworth, 1967).

She noted that infants 'do not always stay close to the mothers but rather make little excursions away from her, exploring other objects and interacting with other people, but returning to the mother from time to time' (Ainsworth, 1967, p. 345), the defining behaviour of a securely attached child. Posada and Jacobs (2001) propose that attachment relationships provide a broad context for early learning and acquisition of cultural norms, but culture and family shape how communication takes place between children and their caregivers.

Summary of Attachment

Attachment theory has contributed greatly to our understanding of emotional development, providing important conceptual tools that have made, and hopefully will continue to make, the study of emotional phenomena accessible to empirical research. It has placed the understanding of emotions by themselves on the research agenda.

Case Study: Michael

Michael (16) has a history of drug-related offences and was referred to CAMHS by his Youth Offending Team worker, because of acute episodes of anxiety and 'hearing voices'.

Michael attended the assessment with his YOT worker. He reported his experience of physical abuse and neglect under the care of his mother. She had recently asked him to leave home. Michael is the eldest of four siblings and considered them to have been treated better than he was. Michael reported a history of difficulties with his peer group and had no close friends. He attributed that to his outbursts of anger.

His education history was sporadic, with a number of exclusions from secondary school and attendance at a Pupil Referral Unit.

Michael's 'voices' were attributed to his acute anxiety about being out of the house. He was fearful that he might be assaulted by other young people. He moved about, staying on floors in 'safe' places that included wider family members and casual friends.

At the assessment, Michael presented as hostile and demanding, stating that medication would be the only way he could be helped. He was mistrusting of those conducting the assessment, asking why they were asking the questions they were and whom would the information be shared with.

From an attachment perspective, Michael would appear to fit within the unresolved, disorganised/disorientated category of adult attachment representation with some evidence of ambivalent/preoccupied representation, for the following reasons:

- Reported physical abuse and neglect by his mother
- History of difficulties within peer relationships, due to anger/aggression
- Poor engagement in education
- Involvement in the criminal justice system
- Mistrustful, hostile and demanding in the assessment session

Michael wants to 'feel safe' and that would be afforded him within a close and trusting relationship, but his behaviours resulting from an inability to form an internal working model mean that he often alienates others.

From a transference/countertransference perspective, Michael may display his intense anger/hostility with the CAMHS clinicians, and others before them, as a way of projecting the anger/distress he has experienced at the hands of adults throughout his life. For any CAMHS clinician, it may be very hard to 'like' Michael, when he is presenting in this hostile and demanding way. It would be important to recognise the countertransference that takes place here as that will give the clinician an insight into how others respond to Michael and how he feels about himself.

When trying to engage therapeutically with a young person like Michael, the following would be important to consider:

- It may take a long time to properly engage with the young person before any formal therapeutic work can take place. Michael will most likely anticipate, consciously or not, that the clinician/therapist will abandon and/or reject him at some stage. Therefore, his behaviour may be very hostile and dismissive regarding the work being done within sessions and towards the clinician's competence.
- Michael's basic needs will need to be met first in order to increase his sense of safety, i.e. securing permanent accommodation.
- It is important from the beginning to set the boundaries around where, when and how often sessions will take place, to provide a sense of containment within the relationship.
- Any future sessions missed through clinician annual leave or training would need to be discussed well in advance, so that Michael can grasp that this is not abandonment or rejection.
- If any sessions *are* cancelled by the clinician due to unforeseen circumstances, they should expect a level of hostility or lack of engagement by Michael in response, i.e. his punishment.
- As Michael's contact with the Youth Offending Team is likely to be time-limited if he does not commit any further petty crime, the clinician may become the 'secure base' for Michael. As long as professional boundaries are maintained, this can be healthy within

the therapeutic relationship. In the longer term, it would be the launch pad from which Michael could test out alternative, more positive approaches within his social relationships.

- The ending of any work with Michael should be planned well in advance, for these same reasons.

Multiple-Choice Questions

See answers on page 666.

1. Which of the following is NOT an attachment pattern/representation?
   a. Secure/autonomous
   b. Insecure avoidant/dismissive
   c. Role reversal/rescuer
   d. Disorganised/unresolved
2. Which of the following statements is true of children and young people with a diagnostic label of reactive attachment disorders with inhibition of attachment behaviour?
   a. They exhibit an emotional disorder with withdrawal, over-caution and impairment in their capacity for social play.
   b. They have a propensity to seek contact without boundaries with the most varied caregivers.
   c. They would meet the diagnostic requirements for an autistic spectrum disorder.

Key References

Bruce, M., Young, D., Turnbull, S., Rooksby, M., Chadwick, G., Oates, C., Nelson, R., Young-Southward, G., Haig, C., Minnis, H., Young-Southwards, G., Haig, C. and Minnis, H., (2019). Reactive Attachment Disorder in Maltreated Young Children in Foster Care. *Attachment and Human Development*, 21(2): 152–169.

Cassidy, J. and Shaver, P.R. (Eds), (2018). *Handbook of Attachment: Theory, Research, and Clinical Applications* (3rd edition). New York: The Guilford Press.

Crittenden, P., (2015). *Raising Parents: Attachment, Parenting and Child Safety* (2nd edition). Abingdon: Routledge.

8 Piaget's Stages of Cognitive Development and Erikson's Stages of Psychosocial Development

Margaret J.J. Thompson

KEY CONCEPTS

- Jean Piaget (1896–1980) was an influential researcher in the field of developmental psychology. His work is summarised in a paper by Huitt and Hummel (2003).
  - He believed that what distinguished human beings from other animal species was 'abstract symbolic reasoning'.
  - He was part of a group of writers whose literature formed the basis of the Constructivist theory of learning and instruction.
  - He noticed that younger children thought differently from older children.
- Erik Erikson (1902–1994) was a developmental psychologist and psychoanalyst who believed that personality develops in a series of stages, of psychosocial development, the experience of social experience over the whole life span. His work is summarised in a paper by Cherry (2011).
  - One of the main elements of Erikson's psychosocial stage theory is the development of ego identity. Ego identity is the conscious sense of self that we develop through social interaction.
  - Erikson suggests that our ego identity is constantly changing due to new experiences and information we acquire in our daily interactions with others, with each new experience developing or hindering the development. This will continue throughout life.
  - The development of a sense of competence by a person is important, and this will motivate behaviour and actions. This is sometimes referred to as ego strength or ego quality.

Process of Cognitive Development

Piaget was interested in how an organism adapts to its environment (its intelligence and behaviour). Behaviour is controlled through mental organisations called 'schemes' that the individual uses to represent the world and to designate action. This adaption is driven by a biological drive to obtain balance between schemes and the environment ('equilibration'). He hypothesised that babies are born with schemes operating at birth that he called 'reflexes'. Animals continue to use reflexes to control behaviour throughout life. At first, infants use reflexes to control their environment. These are gradually replaced throughout life with constructed schemes.

Piaget described two processes that an individual will use in its attempt to adapt to the environment

- **Assimilation**: the process of using or transforming the environment so that it can be placed into pre-existing cognitive structures.
- **Accommodation**: the process of changing cognitive structures to accept something from the environment. Both processes are used simultaneously and alternately throughout life. As schemes become more complex, they are termed 'structures', and they become organised in a hierarchical manner from general to specific.

Summary of Piaget's Theory (Sylva and Lunt, 1982)

Sensorimotor Stage: Birth to Two Years Old

By handling objects, the child learns about shape and texture in addition to permanence. The child is 'assimilating' new objects and 'accommodating' the new information into his 'action schema'. The child lives for the present and has not yet learned the capacity to reflect on the world, but has begun to learn cause and effect, e.g. crying will bring a parent and often produce food. The breast has a nipple and if the child sucks, milk will appear.

Preoperational Stage: Ages Two to Seven

Over this time, the child will

- Move from playing symbolically, e.g. copying car noises or having tea parties with cups, to playing made-up games and becoming creative, sometimes using magical thinking.
- Begin to have a conception of time, 'yesterdays and tomorrows'.
- Attribute life to inanimate objects, 'animism'.
- See rules as absolute.
- Believe that the world rotates around him. He is 'egocentric'.

If something should happen to a parent, e.g. the parent becomes ill or disappears unexpectedly, perhaps, say, because of a car accident, the child might believe it was their fault.

'Moral realism' is present in this stage. If two children make a mess while trying to be helpful to a parent, the one who makes the larger mess will be perceived as the naughtier.

Operational Stage: Ages 7 to 14

During this phase children develop an understanding of 'conservation', e.g. a spherical piece of plasticine is the same as the same amount of plasticine rolled out.

Formal Operations: Ages 14 to Adulthood

This is characterised by the ability of the young person to hold more than one concept in his mind at once, to be reflective, to argue from more than one point of view and to become idealistic. It is important to note that some adults may never attain this phase.

Stages of Psychosocial Development

Erik Erikson was an ego psychologist who developed one of the most popular and influential theories of development. Whilst his theory was influenced by psychoanalyst Sigmund

Freud's work, Erikson's theory centred on psychosocial development rather than psychosexual development.

In each stage, Erikson believed people experience a conflict that serves as a turning point in development. In Erikson's view, these conflicts are centred on either developing a psychological quality or failing to develop that quality. During these times, the potential for personal growth is high, but so is the potential for failure. If people successfully deal with the conflict, they emerge from the stage with psychological strengths that will serve them well for the rest of their life. If they fail to deal effectively with these conflicts, they may not develop the essential skills needed for a strong sense of identity and self.

Psychosocial Stage 1: Trust vs. Mistrust

The first stage of Erikson's theory of psychosocial development occurs between birth and one year of age and is the most fundamental stage in life. Because an infant is utterly dependent, the development of trust is based on the dependability and quality of the child's caregivers. At this point in development, the child depends utterly on adult caregivers for everything (i.e. food, love, warmth, safety, nurturing). If a caregiver fails to provide adequate care and love, the child will come to feel that he or she cannot trust or depend upon the adults in his or her life.

If a child successfully develops trust, he or she will feel safe and secure in the world. Caregivers who are inconsistent, emotionally unavailable or rejecting contribute to feelings of mistrust in the children they care for. Failure to develop trust will result in fear and a belief that the world is inconsistent and unpredictable. Of course, no child is going to develop a sense of 100% trust or 100% doubt. Erikson believed that successful development was all about striking a balance between the two opposing sides. When this happens, children acquire hope, which Erikson described as openness to experience tempered by some wariness that danger may be present.

Psychosocial Stage 2: Autonomy vs. Shame and Doubt

The second stage of Erikson's theory of psychosocial development takes place during early childhood and is focused on children developing a greater sense of personal control. At this point in development, children are just beginning to gain a little independence. They can perform basic actions on their own and make simple decisions about what they prefer. By allowing children to make choices and gain control, parents and caregivers can help them to develop a sense of autonomy.

Like Freud, Erikson believed that toilet training was a vital part of this process. However, Erikson's reasoning was quite different than that of Freud's. Erikson believed that learning to control one's bodily functions leads to a feeling of control and a sense of independence. Other important events include gaining more control over food choices, toy preferences and clothing selection.

Children who successfully complete this stage feel secure and confident, whilst those who do not are left with a sense of inadequacy and self-doubt. Erikson believed that achieving a balance between autonomy and shame and doubt would lead to will, which is the belief that children can act with intention, within reason and limits.

Psychosocial Stage 3: Initiative vs. Guilt

During the pre-school years, children begin to assert their power and control over the world through directing play and other social interactions. Children who are successful at this stage feel capable and able to lead others. Those who fail to acquire these skills are left with a sense of guilt, self-doubt and lack of initiative. When an ideal balance of individual initiative and a willingness to work with others is achieved, the ego quality known as purpose emerges.

Psychosocial Stage 4: Industry vs. Inferiority

This stage covers the early school years from approximately age 5 to age 11. Through social interactions, children begin to develop a sense of pride in their accomplishments and abilities. Children who are encouraged and commended by parents and teachers develop a feeling of competence and belief in their skills. Those who receive little or no encouragement from parents, teachers or peers will doubt their ability to be successful. Successfully finding a balance at this stage of psychosocial development leads to the strength known as competence or a belief in our own ability to handle the tasks set before us.

Psychosocial Stage 5: Identity vs. Confusion

During adolescence, young people explore their independence and develop a sense of self. Those who receive proper encouragement and reinforcement through personal exploration will emerge from this stage with a strong sense of self and a feeling of independence and control. Those who remain unsure of their beliefs and desires will feel insecure and confused about themselves and the future. Completing this stage successfully leads to fidelity, which Erikson described as an ability to live by society's standards and expectations.

Psychosocial Stage 6: Intimacy vs. Isolation

This stage covers the period of early adulthood when people are exploring personal relationships. Erikson believed it was vital that people develop close, committed relationships with other people. Those who are successful at this step will form relationships that are committed and secure.

Remember that each step builds on skills learned in previous steps. Erikson believed that a strong sense of personal identity was important for developing intimate relationships. Studies have demonstrated that those with a poor sense of self tend to have less committed relationships and are more likely to suffer emotional isolation, loneliness and depression. Successful resolution of this stage results in the virtue known as love. It is marked by the ability to form lasting, meaningful relationships with other people.

Psychosocial Stage 7: Generativity vs. Stagnation

During adulthood, we continue to build our lives, focusing on our career and family. Those who are successful during this phase will feel that they are contributing to the world by being active in their home and community. Those who fail to attain this skill will feel unproductive and uninvolved in the world. Care is the virtue achieved when this stage is handled successfully. Being proud of your accomplishments, watching your children grow into adults and developing a sense of unity with your life partner are important accomplishments of this stage.

Psychosocial Stage 8: Integrity vs. Despair

This phase occurs during old age and is focused on reflecting back on life. Those who are unsuccessful during this stage will feel that their life has been wasted and will experience many regrets. The individual will be left with feelings of bitterness and despair. Those who feel proud of their accomplishments will feel a sense of integrity. Successfully completing this phase means looking back with few regrets and a general feeling of satisfaction. These individuals will attain wisdom, even when confronting death.

Key References

Cherry, K., (2011). *Background and Key Concepts of Piaget's Theory.* Psychology - Complete Guide to Psychology for Students, Educators & Enthusiasts. Web. 02. Feb. http://psychology.about.com/od/piagetstheory/a/keyconcepts.htm retrieved on 10 retrieved on 16 January 2020.

Erikson, E.H., (1994). *Identity and the Life Cycle.* London: W.W Norton & Company.

Huitt, W. and Hummel, J., (2003). *Piaget's Theory of Cognitive Development: Educational Psychology Interactive.* Valdosta, GA: Valdosta State University.

Sylva, K. and Lunt, I., (1982). *Child Development: A First Course Publisher.* Oxford: Wiley-Blackwell.

9 Emotion Processing in Child and Adolescent Psychopathology

Georgia Chronaki

KEY CONCEPTS

- Emotion processing is an important concept in understanding social adjustment and mental health in children and adolescents.
- Research and clinical practice have shown that individual differences in emotion processing are closely related to children's social adjustment.
- Emotion processing is influenced by environmental factors, alongside neurobiological factors throughout developments.
- There are different emotion processing profiles associated with externalising and internalising disorders.
- Children with autism spectrum disorders often have difficulties recognising other people's emotions.

Emotion Processing

Emotion processing refers to a range of processes in the understanding and recognition of emotions in other people. Emotion processing is used to refer to the ability to process stress and other intense feelings. Children gradually develop an understanding of the causes of emotions and the way they recognise emotions in themselves and others.

The ability to 'read' non-verbal cues of emotion in others, e.g. facial expressions, gestures, postures and tone of voice, is fundamental to children's social competence (Rothman and Nowicki, 2004). Children who are better able to understand nonverbal emotional cues in social interactions develop better social skills and form positive interpersonal relationships over time (Trentacosta and Fine, 2010; Saarni, 1999). Empathy, defined as accurate detection of others' emotional signals (Hoffman, 1991), has been linked to lower levels of aggressive and challenging behaviour in children (Zahn-Waxler, Cole, Welsh and Fox, 1995).

Psychological Assessment

Although many clinical tools exist to assess children's socio-emotional development more broadly (Carter et al., 2004), fewer clinical tools exist to assess the recognition and understanding of emotions.

There are many batteries assessing emotion recognition in children and adolescents, although these measures are not diagnostic, e.g. the Cambridge Mindreading Face-Voice

Battery for children (Golan, Baron-Cohen and Hill, 2006), the Diagnostic Analysis of Nonverbal Accuracy (DANVA; Nowicki and Carton, 1993) and the Profile of Nonverbal Sensitivity (PONS, Rosenthal, 1979), using video-clips with faces, voices and body images. The Emotion Recognition Task in the CANTAB battery (Cambridge Cognition Ltd) has been used to assess emotion recognition in clinical populations.

Emotion understating and children's situational knowledge of emotion are often assessed with stories and vignettes; examples of measures include the Emotion Recognition Questionnaire (Bierman et al., 2014), that uses stories describing characters in emotionally evocative situations, the Schultz Test of Emotion Processing-Preliminary Version (STEP-P, Schultz et al., 2010), a video-based assessment tool of socio-cognitive functioning in pre-schoolers, and the Affect Knowledge Test, that assesses pre-school children's receptive and expressive knowledge of emotion by asking children to identify happy, sad, angry and afraid puppet faces (Denham, 1986).

Neurobiological Influences on Emotion Processing

Recent research has examined neural mechanisms underlying altered emotional processing in children and adolescents with psychopathology. Event-related potentials (ERP) measure changes in the electrical activity of the brain in response to emotional stimuli. ERPs can be a useful tool for understanding sensory, perceptual and cognitive mechanisms underlying emotion processing (Chronaki, 2016). Such methods can reveal emotion processing deficits or biases that may not be evident in children's observable behaviour, for example, altered brain responses to facial emotional expressions have been found in children with autism (Baron-Cohen, 1999; Dawson et al., 2004), psychopathic tendencies (Blair et al., 2009) and depression (Pine, 2009).

Individual differences in children's and adolescents' neural responses to emotional stimuli can serve as one of multiple markers that help early identification of individuals at risk for developing psychiatric conditions (De Haan and Gunnar, 2009). In addition, developing emotion regulation strategies during a time when the brain reaches heightened 'plasticity', i.e. the ability to change and adapt as a result of experience, may be a useful preventative target for psychopathology.

Environmental Influences on Emotion Processing

It is important to consider environmental factors, alongside neurobiological factors, when examining emotion processing in children and adolescents. Early emotional experiences can have a major influence on emotional development. Parenting environments and parental psychopathology have been related to emotion processing difficulties in children. Children who have experienced abnormal parenting environments, such as physical abuse, show faster recognition of anger and delayed disengagement from angry faces (Pollak and Tolley-Schell, 2003; Pollak et al., 2009). Similarly, children of mothers at elevated risk for depression selectively attend to sad facial expressions whereas children of never-disordered mothers attend to positive happy facial expressions (Joorman et al., 2007). High levels of maternal anger have been related to lower emotional knowledge in pre-schoolers (Halberstadt et al., 1999).

Early emotional experiences can influence the brain mechanisms underlying emotion processing in children, e.g. maltreated children display greater frontal brain activation in response to threatening, i.e. angry, facial expressions compared to non-maltreated children (Cicchetti and Curtis, 2005). Parents who are very controlling when interacting with their infants may increase the likelihood that their infants' brain responds more sharply to threatening, i.e. angry, voices (Zhao, Chronaki, Schiessl, Wai Wan and Abel, 2019).

Emotion Processing Profiles in Child Psychopathology

Although internalising and externalising disorders often co-occur in children, there are different types of emotion processing mechanisms underlying each disorder type. Children with externalising problems tend to be more prone to anger and impulsivity, whereas children with internalising symptoms are more prone to sadness (Eisenberg et al., 2001; Ellis et al., 1997). In addition, children who present both externalising and internalising problems are more impaired in emotion processing, compared to children who present either condition alone (Manassis et al., 2007).

Emotion Processing in Externalising Disorders

A range of externalising behaviour problems in children and adolescents are linked to inaccurate understanding of emotions. Emotion processing deficits, i.e. lower accuracy in perceiving emotions in others, and hostile attribution biases to others' intentions, i.e. a higher tendency to attribute hostility and anger to others, can place children at risk for heightened aggressive behaviour (Schultz, Izard and Bear, 2004). Children with inattention and hyperactivity show difficulties in recognising emotions from others' facial and vocal expressions, often because of inattentive and impulsive processing of emotion signals (Kats-Gold, Besser and Priel 2007; Norvilitis et al., 2000). Research has shown that difficulties in identifying emotions from faces and voices in children with hyperactivity are already present from the pre-school years (Chronaki et al., 2012). More recent research has identified atypical neural responses to vocal anger in children with attention deficit/hyperactivity disorder compared to typically developing children (Chronaki et al., 2015).

Emotion Processing in Internalising Disorders

In general, children with internalising symptoms find it difficult to control negative emotionality, as indicated by rumination, sadness and elevated worry. Children with anxiety disorders are more likely to present avoidant behaviours (Barrett, Rapee, Dadds and Sharon, 1996) because of a bias towards negative or threatening emotional information (Bar-Haim et al., 2007). Research has shown that larger neural responses to angry faces are associated with elevated symptoms of anxiety in children (Chronaki et al., 2018). Similar research has shown that increased neural responses to angry, versus happy, faces in young children predicted the development of anxiety symptoms two years later (O'Toole et al., 2013). Depression has been found to be associated with reduced neural responses to angry faces in children, suggesting a blunted emotional response and disengagement from emotional stimuli more generally in depression (Kujawa et al., 2015, Proudfit et al., 2015).

Emotion Processing in Autism Spectrum Disorders

Children with autism spectrum disorders often have difficulties in social interaction and communication and in recognising other people's emotions (Uljarevic and Hamilton, 2012). Some of these difficulties may be secondary to domain-general processing abnormalities, such as attention and sensory-perceptual processing (Nuske, Vivanti and Dissanayake, 2012). Some infants at high risk for autism spectrum disorders have been found to present atypical neural responses to emotional vocalisations (Blazi et al., 2015). Compared to typically developing children, children with autism spectrum disorders find it difficult to differentiate between emotional and neutral facial expressions (Dawson et al., 2004, Wagner et al., 2013). It is likely that impaired discrimination of facial and vocal emotional expressions may be a candidate marker of the social impairments observed in children with autism spectrum disorders.

In summary, emotions can provide a window offering a comprehensive view into children's mental health and adjustment. Future practitioners are encouraged to carefully consider children's understanding of emotion to better understand children's social behaviour.

Case Study: Jason

Jason is (four) lives at home with both his parents. Jason is a planned first child with a younger sister, Emily. When Jason was two years old, he was difficult to soothe when distressed and had frequent temper tantrums. He is often lonely and has few friends. During play with his sister, Jason often complains that his sister is angry and hostile towards him. As a result, he becomes oppositional and hits his sister.

Jason's mother asked the health visitor for help. After listening carefully to the problems and observing Jason and Emily playing together, the health visitor explained that Jason tends to perceive Emily as angry and as a result, he is likely to be aggressive towards her. Emily is more 'laidback' and finds Jason's behaviour confusing. She feels sad when Jason hits her and starts crying. That escalates the problem.

The health visitor gave Jason's mother some information and explained how she can help him to better recognise Emily's feelings. When his mother explained to Jason that Emily feels sad, Jason was more likely to show empathy and soothe Emily. With support from his mother and teacher, Jason has started to pay attention to other people's feelings at home and at school. His aggressive outbursts have reduced, and he has started making friends.

Multiple-Choice Questions

See answers on page 666.

1. Which statement is correct about emotion processing in children?
   a. Parental depression is bound to cause emotion processing abnormalities in children.
   b. Children with internalising and externalising symptoms show identical impairments in emotion processing.
   c. Children at higher risk for aggressive behaviour often tend to perceive others as hostile.
   d. Empathy is not related to children's pro-social behaviour.
   e. Mental health problems in children are a direct consequence of negative emotionality.
2. Which statement is correct about the neuroscience of emotion processing?
   a. Neuroscientific methods could help identify children at risk for developing emotion processing abnormalities and behaviour problems.
   b. Children's brain activity patterns can be easily observed in children's behavioural performance during various emotion tasks.
   c. Clinicians should use only neuroscientific methods to assess emotion processing in children.
   d. Difficulty in reading others' emotions in children with autism is due to small brain size.
   e. We can remedy children's negative emotionality by looking at how the brain works.

Key References

De Haan, M. and Gunnar, M.R., (2009). *Handbook of Developmental Social Neuroscience.* New York: The Guilford Press.

Feldman Barret, L., Lewis, M. and Haviland-Jones, J.M., (2018). *Handbook of Emotions* (4th edition). New York: The Guilford Press.

LoBue, V., Pérez-Edgar, K. and Buss, K., (2019). *Handbook of Emotional Development.* Springer.

Saarni, C., (1999). *The Development of Emotional Competence.* New York: The Guilford Press.

Trentacosta, C.J. and Fine, S.E., (2010). Emotion Knowledge, Social Competence, and Behavior Problems in Childhood and Adolescence: A Meta-Analytic Review. *Social Development*, 19(1): 1–29.

10 Emotional Literacy in the Education Context

Helena Hoyos

> We have gone too far in emphasising the value and import of the purely rational – what IQ measures – Intelligence can come to nothing when emotions hold sway.
>
> (Goleman, 1996)

KEY CONCEPTS

- Emotional health and well-being are now recognised as being of primary importance within schools and in the wider community.
- Indeed, when visiting schools, OFSTED considers 'the extent to which pupils know and understand factors which impact on their physical, mental and emotional health'.
- Emotional literacy is the descriptive term used in schools and is actively promoted.

When Goleman wrote about emotional intelligence in 1996, he was one of the first to publicly champion the importance of meeting children's emotional needs in order to enable them to learn effectively. Although the work of Goleman and his predecessors, such as Howard Gardner, Peter Salovey and Jack Mayer, uses the term 'emotional intelligence', the term 'emotional literacy', first introduced by Claude Steiner in 1984, has now been adopted by schools and is widely used by them. It is likely that one reason for this is to present a challenge to the idea of a fixed and unchanging state usually associated with the concept of 'intelligence', whilst we are familiar with the idea that 'literacy' can be taught and learned.

The following definition of emotional literacy was first given for emotional intelligence by Mayer and Salovey in 1997.

- The ability to perceive accurately, appraise and express emotion
- The ability to access and/or generate feelings that facilitate thought
- The ability to understand emotion and emotional knowledge

Emotional literacy is about learning to understand and talk about how we feel, to reflect on our emotions and how they are affecting our thinking and behaviour and to manage our emotions and those of other people in a productive way.

Emotional literacy is now actively promoted in many schools. This can take the form of a whole-school curriculum aimed at enabling staff and pupils to become more emotionally literate, e.g. through the use of the Government's Social and Emotional Aspects of Learning

(SEAL) materials. It can involve training specific individuals among the staff to work with children who are experiencing difficulty in recognising and managing their emotions. These staff members are often trained and supervised by educational psychologists.

Why Focus on Emotional Literacy?

The field of psychology has contributed greatly to our understanding of why emotional literacy is important. As early as 1943, Abraham Maslow was beginning to develop his theory of a hierarchy of basic needs, that motivate us as human beings.

Maslow's Hierarchy of Needs

This is usually shown as a pyramid in descending order with the 'top' of the pyramid first.

Self-Fulfilment Needs

- Self-actualisation

Psychological Needs

- Esteem
- Belongingness and love

Basic Needs

- Safety
- Physiological

Maslow suggests that all human beings must have the four lower levels of needs met before they can focus on the personal growth, development and learning characterised by the higher layers. Sadly, many of the children in our schools are struggling to have their basic needs met and are not, therefore, emotionally open to the learning opportunities which schools present. By introducing emotional literacy into schools, adults are helped to recognise these needs in children and to respond appropriately.

A child who feels unsafe or unheard due to an unstable home environment or bullying in the playground can be helped at school by the creation of a calm, ordered learning environment, with access to adults who listen and respond effectively. A child who feels unwanted at home and isolated at school can be helped to develop by interventions at school that foster a sense of belonging and being valued. Once this sense of belonging and being accepted is in place, increased self-esteem can follow and then the child will be ready to learn.

Howard Gardner's (1983) theory outlines **seven intelligences**:

- Linguistic
- Logical-mathematical
- Musical
- Bodily-kinaesthetic
- Spatial
- Interpersonal intelligence
- Intrapersonal intelligence

The concept of emotional literacy draws strongly on this idea of intrapersonal intelligence (the ability to understand oneself) and interpersonal intelligence (the ability to understand and interact effectively with other people). Goleman (1996) highlighted these two areas, which he characterised as personal and social competence. He suggested that if people could be helped to develop their ability to manage themselves and their interactions with other people, they would become much more successful in all areas of their lives.

What Does Emotional Literacy Include?

Emotionally literate people are able to understand and talk about their feelings and manage those feelings effectively, so that they do not overwhelm their capacity to think. They tune in to the feelings of other people and work co-operatively and sensitively with them. There are several components to emotional literacy that make this possible:

Conscious awareness and communication skills that enable us to identify how we are feeling and to develop a vocabulary that allows us to reflect on these feelings and communicate them to other people. This is often the first step for those working with children to help them develop their emotional literacy, exemplified within Case Study 1.

Case Study (1): Mary

Mary usually feels very strong emotions that she labels as 'good' or 'bad'. She does not yet have the understanding or vocabulary to break these categories down into smaller categories such as happy/excited or angry/sad. She tends to show the same 'good' or 'bad' behaviour in response to her feelings. One day, Mary refuses to do what her teacher asks her in class. She is rude to the teacher and is sent out of class. That morning, Mary's mother was ill and Mary feels worried about her, but because she is unable to recognise or talk about that feeling she is only able to show that she feels 'bad' by misbehaving. Her teacher reacts to the behaviour, not knowing the reason behind it, and so the situation worsens for Mary.

Understanding thoughts, feelings and actions so that behaviour is guided by informed choices, rather than being based on impulse, as seen in Case Study 2.

Case Study (2): Daniel

Daniel hits his friend when he asks to borrow Daniel's pen. Earlier in the day, Daniel's teacher told him off and Daniel feels angry because he thinks this was unfair. Instead of understanding that he feels angry with his teacher, Daniel just feels generally angry and takes this out on his friend. As a result, Daniel falls into more trouble, has difficulty with his friendship and feels increasingly angry. Had he been helped to understand the source of his anger he might have been able to control his response to his friend and the following difficulties would have been avoided.

Managing feelings so that we are able to control our responses and have our needs met, without our feelings overwhelming us and standing in the way (Case Study 3).

Case Study (3): Susan

Susan is often in trouble at school because she shouts out answers to questions, rather than putting up her hand and waiting her turn. Following some emotional literacy work, Susan becomes more able to manage her feelings of frustration and anxiety and is able to wait her turn. She begins to receive praise from her teacher and to feel much happier at school and better about herself. Learning to manage her feelings has promoted her self-esteem.

Managing Conflict

With increasing emotional awareness, we are more able to manage conflict effectively. We begin to recognise the triggers that make us angry and the signs that our anger is building, often felt in the body's reactions. This increased awareness gives us the choice to avoid the conflict before it escalates beyond our control. The benefits for all of us will be obvious and will have particular relevance for those working with children and young people at school.

Understanding Groups

As we become more aware of our own feelings and reactions and those of other people, we become more able to share attention and recognise the strengths and needs that both we and others bring to any situation. This helps us co-operate and communicate much more effectively in groups.

So Why Is Emotional Literacy Important?

As a responsible society, we have a duty to help children develop and reach their potential as well-rounded, emotionally healthy individuals who can play a full and active part in the society of their future. The development of emotional literacy is at the heart of how we can do this, in our homes, schools and all aspects of our lives.

Multiple-Choice Questions

See answers on page 666.

1. Which of the following statements is correct?
   a. Emotional literacy is about reading and writing.
   b. Emotional literacy is a fixed and unchanging state.
   c. Emotional literacy helps children's development.
   d. Emotional literacy is not taught in schools.
2. Which of the following is not one of the seven intelligences proposed by Gardner?
   a. Visual/spatial
   b. Emotional/feelings
   c. Logical/mathematical
   d. Verbal/linguistic
3. Which of the following is not a feature of Maslow's hierarchy of needs?
   a. All people need to have their physical needs met.
   b. All people need to feel a sense of belonging.
   d. All people need to feel safe.
   e. All people need to be formally educated.
4. Which of the following is not a key component of emotional literacy?
   a. The ability to communicate feelings effectively
   b. The ability to share attention with other people in groups
   c. The ability to explain the principles of emotional literacy
   d. The ability to understand links between feelings, thoughts and actions

Key References

Coughlan, B.J., (2010). *Critical Issues in the Emotional Wellbeing of Students with Special Educational Needs.* https://www.ssatrust.org.uk/pedagogy/networks/specialschools/CLDD/Pages/ThinkPiece6.aspx.

Department for Education and Skills/Department of Health, (2005). *National Healthy Schools Status: A Guide for Schools*. London: DH Publications.

Goleman, D., (1996). *Emotional Intelligence: Why It Can Matter More than IQ*. London: Bloomsbury.

11 Assessing Paediatric Development in Psychiatry

Catherine Thompson

Introduction

This chapter gives a framework for studying the development of children whilst understanding why certain skills develop in the order that they do and the neuro-anatomical, -physiological and -psychological principles behind these processes. The neuro-cognitive processes are explained in terms of the developing brain and the physiological and anatomical methods by which cognitive abilities evolve. Understanding them in this way will feel more valid in the context of the general assessment of a child and help explain why many psychiatric problems present the way they do.

Fascinatingly, this pattern of development occurs not only in western children, but, given adequate circumstance, in all humans across the world, with only small cultural variation. This demonstrates that cognitive maturation cannot, in the minds of most modern scientists, be purely a learned behaviour phenomenon but is based on pre-existing brain networks present at birth.

KEY CONCEPTS

- The neuro-cognitive processes required for normal development.
- The relevant anatomical, physiological and psychological elements of those areas.
- A comparison of these factors with the traditional task test/observational markers that are used, with validated tools, to screen for developmental delay.

The developmental milestones will be listed in table format with explanations tying the cognitive processes that work in parallel to allow success in the undertaken task.

Cognitive Functions: Anatomical, Physiological and Psychological Evolution in the First Five Years of Life

The relative sizes of different parts of a new-born baby or infant's brain are different to those of the older, more cognitively aware, child (eight, nine or ten years of age). The brain continues to evolve beyond infancy, mainly in executive functioning, emotion and other empathic/relationship-based abilities. Different sub-divisions of the cerebral cortex and brainstem are relatively more developed than others at birth. The cerebellum, medulla and pons (brainstem areas) are roughly equivalent in volume to those of the older child.

The majority of the higher cortical areas, however, are less well developed. Additionally, although these areas undergo a relatively large degree of functional maturation and specialisation after birth, the number of neurones we are born with is, for the most part, all we will ever have or need.

Functional ability and diversity are achieved via several mechanisms. The addition of new synapses between neurones is the first stage of maturation. The creation of synaptic linking of different neuronal pathways by bridging/inter-neurones allows regulation, co-ordination and feedback of information, e.g. the retina, amacrine and horizontal cells collate information from several cone/rod cells and interact with bipolar and retinal ganglia cells in the eye.

The myelination of neurones improves conduction velocity, allowing sensory or receptor neurones that carry information from the periphery towards the central nervous system, i.e. afferent neurones, to produce an appropriate and timely reaction in the motor or body systems via efferent neurones. For example, a stimulus caused by stepping on a sharp object carries the signal to the brain and is felt as pain. This results in efferent neurones stimulating the relevant muscles that retract the foot away from the offending object.

Pruning of unwanted and redundant neural cells occurs throughout ongoing cognitive maturation. This process is thought to be complete by about 25 years of age. If areas of the brain are damaged due to any cause, the supporting cells of the central nervous system, variants of the glial cells from which neurones have specialised, can re-differentiate and aid the recovery of some or all of the functions rendered deficient following the insult. This is called 'plasticity' of the brain and is more effective and dramatic if an injury occurs in infancy or early childhood. It is thought to be responsible for recovery after acute brain injury occurring in the later years of one's life. In adulthood the majority of compensation for injury results in re-specialisation of other areas of the brain rather than recovery of the primary functional area.

The parts of the central nervous system mentioned above, the cerebellum, medulla and pons, all contain areas with a high concentration of neural cell bodies, or nuclei. These constitute the basic relay systems required for basic body functions, awareness and the innate reflex responses which aid the survival of the new-born child. These basic functions include sleeping and waking mechanisms, eye movements, 'startle' responses, sucking and rooting, along with swallowing, breathing and prevention of aspiration. Development postpartum during the neonatal period and early infancy is predominantly noticeable in the motor and sensory systems. Fine and gross motor development occurs in a cephalic (head) to caudal (spine/tail) direction and with the proximal musculature before the distal.

Motor System

Development of the motor system occurs initially in the head and neck muscles followed by those in the trunk. Distinct collections of neurones are involved in carrying information from the cerebral cortex, the cerebellum and the brain stem to the different muscle groups in the peripheries. The origins, routes and resulting effects produced by the neurones in these fibre tracts tend to be relatively specific and well circumscribed. Patterns of sensory and motor loss following spinal injury can be used to identify the level of the injury, e.g. damage to the front or back of the spinal column, left versus right and different levels of injury (lumbar, thoracic or cervical) produce different patterns of sensation and motor loss in different limbs. Some neurones stay on the same side as the area they are receiving/sending information to, whereas some cross over (decussate) at or somewhere above or below the level they serve.

Initially head and neck movements, followed by the axial musculature, strengthen, presumably due to their importance and regular use in the goal-directed behaviours of early infancy. Increase in muscle bulk and improved co-ordination of synergistic groups acting together, via spinal cord sensory and motor feedback loops, facilitate improved head, neck and truncal control.

The development of other cognitive areas, i.e. co-ordination, procedural memory, visuo-spatial awareness, executive function, emotion and reward, is required and gradually, with adequate support, exposure, play and experimentation, the fine muscles of the hands and fingers come under co-ordinated, strong, conscious control over the first three to four years of life.

The Basal Ganglia

This is a collective term for a group of grey matter areas located inferior to the lateral ventricles and occupying the deep cortical areas around the internal capsule and the third ventricle. The basal ganglia can be split functionally into the thalamus, the striatum (caudate nucleus and the putamen) the lateral segment of the globus pallidus and the substantia nigra together and lastly, the medial segment of the globus pallidus.

The basal ganglia nuclei are essential partners of the motor system. As a unit they are responsible for preventing unwanted movements from being instigated, along with allowing the current constellation of motor signals, already occurring between the cortex and the spine, to continue to be relayed, unimpeded. The indirect pathway is responsible for the former, the direct pathway, the latter.

The neurones that inter-connect the nuclei are either excitatory (glutaminergic) or inhibitory (GABAergic) in nature, and signals are facilitated by different neurotransmitters, as indicated in the parentheses. A third set of neurones, thought to have both excitatory and inhibitory functions, depending on circumstances, originate in the substantia nigra and utilise dopamine as a chemical messenger. It is these neurones that degrade in Parkinson's disease and lead to the gradual onset of paucity of movement seen in these patients. L-DOPA, one of the drugs used to treat Parkinson's, is one of the breakdown products of dopamine that is metabolically active, i.e. binds to the receptors on the postsynaptic membrane of dopaminergic synapses and so exerts the same effects as dopamine.

The basal ganglia are thought to be involved in some common paediatric psychiatric conditions, e.g. anxiety, depression, ADHD and dyspraxia.

Cerebellum

The cerebellum is relatively well developed at birth when compared to the higher cerebral cortex. It receives information from various sensory organs and cognitive areas: the auditory system (vestibular nuclei and the superior olivary nucleus), the optic pathway (inferior olivary nucleus), proprioceptive feedback (spinocerebellar tract), basic autonomic information (from cranial nerve and brainstem nuclei) and higher cortical information (the planning, execution, adjustment in approach and emotional reactions to on-going tasks). The cerebellum, in turn, sends efferents back to all those areas, creating essential feedback loops. This allows the instigation, co-ordination and regulation of both reflex-based movements and higher motor pathways and combines these functions with information from vital sensory systems.

Three 'cerebellar syndromes' are regularly described and can be correlated with the lesion/damage site: unilateral cerebellar damage, i.e. ipsilateral: ataxia, dysmetria (inability to judge distance or scale), dysdiadochokinesia (inability to produce rapid alternating movements, past pointing, intention tremor and hypotonia); medial cerebellar damage (truncal ataxia, broad unco-ordinated gait but associated with intact limb co-ordination) and the posterior cerebellar syndrome (nystagmus that is greatest when the subject is looking in the direction of the lesion).

This occurs along with symptoms of brainstem compression: headaches, nausea and vomiting and dizziness, but with the absence of raised intracranial pressure with papilledema.

The cerebellum is thought to be important in dysmetria, dyscalculia, dyspraxia and poor time perception, all of which are seen with more frequency in children with ADHD in addition to occurring in other isolated conditions.

The Visual System

The visual system can be split into three sections: the anterior visual system, the primary visual cortex and the associative visual processing streams (the ventral/parietal and the dorsal/temporal streams). The anterior visual system incorporates the optic globe, the retina and its histological components (rod and cone receptor cells), amacrine and horizontal cells, bipolar cells and the retinal glial cells, and up to the formation of the optic nerve.

Systemic conditions with a psychological component often have associated eye signs which can be observed with a hand-held ophthalmoscope: Kayser–Fleischer rings in Wilson's disease and retinal haemartoma in tuberous sclerosis (TS) are two examples. Both these disorders have insidious onsets, and early discovery can either allow treatment to be instigated early, preventing further severe morbidity (e.g. in the case of Wilson's) or allow screening of other family members who may in time display a more severe phenotype than the index case (TS).

In the initial period of visual development, the brain develops, utilising synaptogenesis (formation of synapses), the creation of inter-neurones (connector neurones) and myelination resulting in the co-ordination of eye movements. This is synchronised via the cerebellum, using information from both gravity and head position, ensuring that the basic visual information streamed to the primary visual cortex is organised in such a way that the visual array can be reproduced accurately to perceive a single image.

Information from the temporal portion of the visual field of each eye, which is projected onto the medial aspect of the retina, decussates at the optic chiasm, whereas the nasal field input remains ipsilateral when it projects to the occipital lobe. The information of the right visual field (from the centre of the nose to the extremes of the right temporal field) is therefore projected to, and ultimately represented as, an inverted, spatially accurate map in the left occipital lobe. The anatomy of this is important so that if a detected developmental delay can be explained exclusively by, or is found to be associated with, defects in the visual fields, this will allow a potential unifying lesion or disease process to be identified.

Finally, two long-fibre cortical pathways link the primary visual areas of the occipital lobe with the parietal and the temporal lobes. The former evaluates the visual information with regards to the spatial organisation of objects. These cells do not receive information pertaining to certain aspects of the visual array, colour vision for example, or information from the fovea. This information is obsolete for their task. The cells instead are able to undertake the following: utilise binocular information and thus judge perspective and depth; evaluate the speed at which an object is moving; assess the relative relationship of separate parts of an object to the object as a whole; and analyse the interaction of multiple objects within the visual array, allowing them to be separated and their semantic category to be identified.

The temporal lobe is thought to be involved in this process of identifying objects in relation to semantic class (meaning of the word) and the young child's developing language lexicon (the internal filing system, allowing quick recall of an object's identity and vague function), incorporating this with declarative memory (explicit or factual memory) and emotional responses associated with previous encounters with such objects or situations. This facilitates further development/learning of language and other higher cerebral functions and allows quick, reflex responses to visual stimuli that might be associated with danger or approached with caution.

The Auditory System

The auditory system can be split into three components: the external auditory apparatus, the primary auditory cortices (I and II) and the higher cortical projections.

The fibres carrying information on the tone, pitch and frequency of incoming sound waves, detected by the ear, once coded, make up the cochlear nerve. Hair cells, i.e. the histological sensory unit, are located within the central core of the cochlear apparatus, a coiled structure located in the inner ear. The direction and degree of distortion of fluid surrounding the hair cells are dependent on the frequency and the intensity of the incoming sound wave, which causes the hair cells to fluctuate. This produces a responsive action potential.

Receptive hair cells located in the centre of the coiled cochlear apparatus are sensitive to sounds of low frequency, whereas the proximal hair cells detect sounds of higher frequencies. This information is relayed to the two primary cortical areas responsible for analysis of basic sound information, auditory I and II, via the inferior colliculus and the medial geniculate nucleus of thalamus. Cells within both the thalamus and the cortical areas associated with hearing organise these inputs in such a way that they have an accurate spatial representation of the location from which the sound originated.

The vestibular nerve (the other portion of the eighth cranial nerve) carries information on gravitational movement, vibration and linear/angular acceleration of the head relative to gravity. Sensory information is again detected by a hair cell apparatus activated by fluid shifts. These shifts occur within various sub-divisions of three, contiguous, semi-circular canals, which are located in the inner ear, superior to the cochlear apparatus. Each of these canals is orientated in a different three-dimensional plane, allowing a complete evaluation of relative orientation of the head and body.

This basic phonological information is projected to three main areas within the brainstem, to either the inferior colliculus (fibres of the cochlear portion of CN VIII) or one of the four vestibular nuclei (information for the vestibular apparatus), to the cerebellum or to the auditory cortex via the thalamus.

Higher cortical areas receive this information for further processing via two large trans-cortical bundles: the superior longitudinal fasciculus linking receptive and productive speech areas and the left uncinate fasciculus which is thought to facilitate auditory verbal memory specifically of the declarative type.

The Reticular Activating System

The reticular activating system is the underlying constellation of basic cortical nuclei and a series of diffuse fibre networks that link these nuclei with key midline subcortical structures and the whole of the higher cortex. The neuronal processes involved in keeping a subject awake and alert utilise, in general, the neurotransmitter noradrenaline. Its counterpart, which is inhibitory in nature and sleep-inducing, is the anticholinergic pathway. Other associative neurotransmitter pathways exist and are further involved in this sleep/wake balance. These pathways vary in degrees of activation and inhibition during rapid eye movement (REM) sleep versus non-REM sleep. The hypothalamus and the pineal gland are involved in further regulating the sleep/wake cycle. This involves the release of cortisol and melatonin in diurnal patterns.

The sleep/wake cycle of adults is actually 25 hours long. This adult pattern of sleep is not fully established until the age of five to seven years and involves the cyclical variation of cortisol levels throughout the day. It is the lack of this diurnal variation in cortisol levels that results in an infant sleeping for a much larger proportion of the day than adults and waking roughly every four hours for feeding. This is because the blood cortisol levels regulate the conversion of glucose into glycogen via the release of insulin and its breakdown, facilitated by glucagon.

If an infant, prior to transition towards a more mature diurnal rhythm, is not regularly fed, hypoglycaemia can ensue.

This can occur in infants that do not have an underlying metabolic disorder if it is associated with other stressors on the metabolic system, e.g. illness or failure, for whatever reason, to effectively establish feeding. Practically, a sleep/wake cycle 25 hours in length would not lead to good sleep hygiene. The sleep/wake cycle is regulated to the 24-hour mark due to the sensitivity of cortisol release to daylight and hours of darkness.

More recent examination of the diffuse cortical pathways involved in the reticular activating system has led to a distinction between fibres that project directly from the brainstem nuclei to the cortex and the fibres that project to the cerebral cortex via the thalamus. It appears that, although these two pathways operate separately, malfunctioning of either one of them renders the function of the other impossible.

Gross Motor Development

Table 11.1 shows the age at which the majority of children, with no known disability, will achieve a task/developmental stage.

Table 11.1 Motor Assessment

6 weeks	**Ventral suspension**: head level with body
3 months	**Ventral suspension**: head at 90°
	Prone: rests on forearms
	Standing: sags at knees
6 months	**Prone**: on straight forearms
	Standing: takes weight on legs
	Sitting: with support
	Extras: can roll
9 months	**Prone**: crawls
	Sitting: steadily for 10 min without support
	Standing: held standing bounces or stomps
12 months	**Stands**: pulls to stand and stands alone for a few seconds
	Walking: cruises
15 months	**Walking**: walks well
18 months	**Walking**: picks up toy and carries it whilst walking
2 years	**Walking**: runs
	Stairs: goes upstairs using two feet per step
	Ball play: kicks ball
	Extras: climbs furniture
2 ½ years	No gross motor milestones
3 years	**Walking** (1): stands briefly on one foot
	Walking (2): pedals
	Walking (3): jumps
	Stairs: goes upstairs using one foot per step
	Ball play: throws a ball over arm
4 years	**Walking** (1): hops
	Walking (2): stands on foot for four seconds
	Stairs: goes upstairs and downstairs using one foot per step
5 years	**Walking** (1): stands on one foot with his arms crossed
	Walking (2): tip toe walks well
	Walking (3): skips
	Ball play: bounces and catches ball

The first muscles to develop in the new-born are the muscles of the face, as they are needed for survival, followed by the muscles of the neck and shoulders.

The spinal pathways assist in the co-ordination of these with feedback loops and the myelination of the nerve sheaths. The muscles then become strong. The proximal muscles in the limbs develop earlier than the distal muscles. This is probably to the effect of gravity and postural actions. There is a larger muscle bulk proximally.

The ability to carry out more complex tasks, such as throwing a ball or riding a tricycle, is limited by both motor factors, such as co-ordination and voluntary control, and by other areas: the ability to see an object effectively so it can be identified; deciding why the object is to be used and in what context it should be used; the ability to track an object visually at long distances and to establish, in the visuo-spatial context, what the relationship of that object is to the person, e.g. the depth, location and orientation.

This has all to be assimilated before executing the motor functions that are required. These motor functions are constantly evaluated and adjusted following feedback. This requires working memory, selective attention and procedural memory, to name but a few skills, and is only seen in children beyond the age of three years or so.

The child has to be motivated to go through trial and error to try out different movements to improve and to develop further skills. This will result in improvement and progressive development in the ability to carry out more than one task both simultaneously and in series. This is complex and will occur in the later pre-school years.

Fine Motor and Vision

Initially this area of development is limited before the development of binocular vision and the ability to focus on objects. From there, spatial skills, such as depth perception, can begin to be established, with the maturation of parietal cells that process basic information from the visual array (the angle of lines, intersecting lines, shadows and overlapping objects, rotation of objects) and of temporal cells (mapping: identifying objects within the visual array and linking these with nominal verbal information).

The techniques used to develop visual spatial information processing, along with the co-ordination and use of the fine muscles of the hands, will depend on the infant's ability to see and follow objects and the development of type and strength of grip.

The ability to draw a vertical line can only occur once an infant has developed a strong and reliable pincer grip with which he can exert continuous pressure downwards onto the drawing paper. Due to the infant's ability to follow objects at first only through 90°, an infant can vertically scribble before he can produce a horizontal line.

The co-ordination and visuo-spatial ability of a toddler from eight months onwards limit the ability of that child to copy shapes on paper. Shape matching requires less mechanical skill and, because of the option of trial and error, less visuo-spatial prowess. The complexity of the shape becomes the rate-limiting factor. With the development of links between the cells involved in visual spatial processing, the young child can learn to differentiate between the angles of lines and shapes. As a result, a circle can be matched before a square, which can in turn be matched before a triangle. As the strength and precise nature of the pincer grip are developed, a child can learn to draw these objects in the same consecutive sequence.

Blocks are used initially in assessment as a judgement of fine motor ability along with the co-ordination and basic problem-solving of an infant/young child. Once a child is able to identify and orientate shapes within the visual array, he can use this and his improving cognition to build various shapes out of the blocks as demonstrated to him by the examiner. These tests can increase in complexity depending on the age of the child. A useful assessment tool in an older child is the 'Draw a man' test. (See Table 11.2.)

Table 11.2 Fine Motor and Vision

Age	*Fine Motor and Vision*
6 weeks	Fixation: fixates on a brightly coloured object through 90° (i.e. does not cross the midline)
3 months	Fixation: fixates on a brightly coloured object through 180° (i.e. can follow the object from one extremity of lateral vision to the other across the midline) Grip: has a palmar grip of a large object, e.g. a rattle
6 months	Grip (1): palmar grasp Grip (2): puts to mouth Grip (3): transfers Vision: watches rolling ball two metres away if the object is in same horizontal plane of vision (i.e. when baby is on the floor and ball is rolled away from him)
9 months	Grip: elementary pincer grip Vision: looks for dropped toys (object permanence) Blocks: bangs two blocks together
12 months	Vision: casting Blocks: puts a block in a cup
15 months	Grip: perfected pincer grip
18 months	Grip/drawing: scribbles Blocks: builds a tower of three to four blocks Shape matching: shape matches a circle Extras: turns pages of a book, given the book has thick, cardboard pages
2 years	Grip/drawing (1): copies a vertical line Grip/drawing (2): circular scribble Blocks: builds a tower of six to seven blocks once the principle is introduced Shape matching: shape matches a circle and a square Extras: can thread large beads (normally sewing thread stools) onto string
2 ½ years	Grip/drawing: copies a horizontal line Blocks: copies a 'train' model using blocks after it is demonstrated
3 years	Grip/drawing: copies a circle Blocks: builds a tower of eight blocks once the principle is introduced Shape matching: shape matches a circle, square and a triangle Colour matching: matches two colours (this can be done using a specific colour matching board as with shape matching or combined with language assessment by identifying, NB NOT NAMING as will be explained later, colours from a book or using the blocks available) Extras: able to use scissors independently
4 years	Grip/drawing (1): copies a cross Grip/drawing (2): draws a man with three distinct parts Blocks: copies a 'gate' model using blocks after it is demonstrated
5 years	Grip/drawing (1): copies a square Grip/drawing (1): copies a triangle Grip/drawing (2): draws a man with six distinct parts Grip/drawing (1): writes his name on request Blocks: copies a 'three-tiered step' model using blocks after it is demonstrated Extras: can thread tiny beads onto cotton thread

Speech and Language

Language acquisition can be functionally separated into receptive and declarative language received via the auditory route versus the written word. There are two main schools of thought with regard to how children develop language and then how the 'language explosion', the transition from knowledge of only a few words of an 18-month-old toddler into the language ability expressed by the first-day pre-schooler, occurs. Protagonists of the empirical train of thought such as Locke, Hume and, to a degree, Piaget, based their theories on the principle that children gain language purely by behaviourist techniques (reward-based with external stimulation). This view was radically challenged in the 1960s by Chomsky's extensive publications on language theory. He reframed the idea of language acquisition and presented the evidence found up to that point in support of his ideas. This was based on the theory that an innate framework seems to be present at birth with regard to the phonetics (sounds of human speech), semantics (study of meaning) and syntactics (principles and rules) of language. This work was further expanded and discussed by others pertaining to this rationalistic view (Pinker, Skinner and Piaget).

There is a pattern to developing language in the first few years, independently of the precise theory by which a child might learn language. Prior to the onset of babbling, during the first four months of life, an infant develops phonological distinctions, attempting to extract specific components of language from the overall cacophony of noise.

There are various theories as to how a child acquires language, and this seems to occur in all infants no matter what their language of origin. Examples of these techniques include: location of syntactic boundaries (rules of grammar), 'bootstrapping' (which involves isolating words according to their common first stem, so allowing even more words to be identified from the background noise), clustering, i.e. screening for phonological sounds that tend to occur together in different words and development of sensitivity to the prosody of language (the rhythm, intonation and related attributes of speech).

This wealth of knowledge with regard to the auditory structure of words is followed by the onset of babbling. It has not been established whether babbling plays a vital role in developing speech and therefore whether the structure of babbling should be more carefully examined. Evidence for the role of babbling in language development comes from the observation that babbling is seen in deaf children who have been exposed to sign language in infancy. Supporters of the view that babbling is essential would agree that, for this theory to be fully substantiated, babbling should include all the common phonological stems that are required for an infant to develop language in any culture. This has not been found to be the case. Other reasons for a child babbling may be to improve motor co-ordination of the fine muscles in the face, larynx and pharynx or to help develop the prosody of language. After a period of babbling and then a time with paucity of sound, the infant begins to use other new sounds and then begins by trial and error to form words.

During this production of early speech, infants and toddlers seem to make errors, and these errors can be seen to occur very regularly, both within a single child's speech development and between subjects. A further issue now is the semantic development of language. This has been extensively investigated, and the methods by which the young child links the sound of the word to its underlying meaning, shape and use are generally grouped under 'mapping'.

A child will use different techniques to overcome the mapping problem: a mixture of using the grammatical (in the linguistic sense, not in the educational sense) rules of language, grouping objects according to different factors and using non-verbal social cues to understand how his carer is using language in an interaction so that he can learn to assign meaning. Once the rules of semantic association (how a child builds a cognitive template with which he can combine his limited knowledge of language into a limitless productive method of communication and description) have been overcome, the language explosion follows at around two years of age.

The next stage of language development is syntactic development (the rules of language), and this depends on the following factors: a child's underlying cognitive ability and exposure to language, a child's emotional development and the development of theory of mind (the understanding that others exist independently of oneself and that actions have consequences on others' emotions and actions) and the ability to problem-solve and function executively. (See Table 11.3.)

Table 11.3 Speech and Language

Age	*Speech and Language*
6 weeks	Response to sound: stills to sound
3 months	Response to sound: turns if on level with ear
6 months	Response to sound: looks to parent's voice
	Vocalisation: babbles (consonants)
9 months	Response to sound: distraction test
	Language use: two syllable babble
	Language comprehension: 'no'
12 months	Words: has one to two words
	Extras: object recognition – uses brush to brush
15 months	Words (1): has several words
	Language use (1): jabbering
	Language use (2): echolalia
18 months	Words (1): has 10–20 words
	Words (2): understands up to 50 words
	Words (3): picture card: IDs one (where is the…)
	Body parts: two body parts
	Commands: one-step commands
2 years	Words (1): understands up to 50 words
	Words (2): picture card: IDs five (where is the…)
	Words (3): names three (what is this)
	Language use (1): two-word sentences
	Language use (2): understands fx of verbs
	Body parts: five to six body parts
	Commands: two-step commands
2 ½ years	Words (1): picture card: IDs seven (where is the…)
	Words (2): names five (what is this)
3 years	Words: names eight (what is this)
	Language use (1): talks in sentences three to four words
	Language use (2): name, age, sex on request
	Language use (3): pronouns and plurals
	Colours: knows some colours
4 years	Language use (1): counts to ten
	Language use (2): tells stories
	Language use (3): past tense
	Colours: IDs several colours
5 years	Language use (1): prepositions
	Language use (2): opposites
	Language use (3): definitions, e.g. banana
	Language use (4): size adjectives
	Commands: three-step commands
	Language comprehension: what do you do if cold, hungry, thirsty

Emotional and Social Development

The development of emotional capacity and self-regulation of emotions/behavioural responses is inherently linked to the need to make relationships and to survive in the society we (choose) to live in. Table 11.4 gives you some ideas of the developmental framework that an infant, child and adult will go through. Thinking in terms of developmental 'milestones' in this area is not ideal. It is important to develop your own intuitive sense of whether the child in front of you is able to use and apply emotions and social rules in order to function adequately at the current time.

The main things to think about are:

- Is a child's emotional and social functioning adaptive enough to maintain motivation and communication with those around them, including aspects such as their innate temperament and self-regulation capacity?
- The child's general capacity for using internal and external feedback to develop a complex framework of emotional processes around how their own physiology and facial gestures of others, for example, link to different feelings/emotions and how peoples' behaviours affect these in return.
- Whether a child is able to apply their current emotional framework to different people and situational contexts in life. This involves complex understanding of one's own goals and those of others and using natural consequences along with long- and short-term rewards to change how they apply their understanding. This is fundamental in building friendships and romantic relationships and maintaining them long-term.

There are several cognitive processes that need to be developed during the early years, before an identifiable, organised and consistent emotional self-profile can be established. Such processes are: the development of the autonomic system to produce physiological response to emotional states, long-term declarative, mainly episodic, memory, an understanding that one is a separate being from others and that one's actions have consequences on the other ('theory of mind' and key executive function abilities), along with selective attention and inhibition, allowing a child to make informed consistent judgements.

We know that damage to the limbic system (head of the caudate nucleus, anterior cingulate gyrus, the amygdala and ventral and dorsolateral aspects of the frontal lobe) and to some long fibre bundles linking areas of basic and higher cognitive functions can result in symptoms such as hallucinations, hypersexuality and general disinhibition. Depending on the exact location of damage to the limbic or other midline subcortical regions, emotional disturbance can take the form of two opposite syndromes of abnormal emotional response. First, a syndrome of complete absence of emotion and second, higher autonomic and higher emotional responses in certain situations than would be expected. This latter overstimulated emotional system, seemingly without awareness of the consequences, is seen in some congenital disorders, and the underlying pathology is presumably similar in some psychiatric diseases in which patients show similar extremes of positive emotional behaviour. Examples include William's syndrome, Noonan syndrome, tuberous sclerosis, early childhood autism before more diagnostic features, such as failure to acquire language, become apparent, storage diseases such as abnormal glycogen metabolism or heavy metal poisoning, temporal or frontal lobe epilepsy, mood disorders, ADHD, foetal alcohol syndrome, post-radiotherapy effects and substance abuse.

The alternate mood state that can be induced by acquired or inherited disease is a flat, unresponsive, unemotive affect. This can occur in Beckwith–Wiedemann syndrome, hypothyroidism or severe depression from primary or secondary causes.

Table 11.4 Social and Emotional

Age	*Social and Emotional*	
	Child	*Parent*
6 weeks	**Communication**: infant is able to express emotional (and physical) needs using sounds, facial and body movements adequately. IMPORTANT: level of alertness, motor tone and reflexes, visual development, hearing, e.g. problems with premature babies or drug withdrawal.	**Availability**: parent has the emotional and physical capacity/skills to notice when child is expressing emotional/physical needs. **Responsiveness**: Parent is able to acknowledge those needs often enough and consistently enough for infant to 'know' they are being heard/seen.
2 months	**Adaptive functions of emotions**: infant begins to associate their emotional experiences as pleasurable or unpleasurable. This guides activity in terms of approach or withdrawal from objects or people and begins to guide their facial expressions/cry-types and intensity. **Emotional regulation**: mainly at this early stage: **Emotionality**: child is able to react emotionality to relevant stimuli BUT also is able to be soothed when distressed/in need. AND **Reactivity**: child reacts to things you would expect them to react to BUT does not over-react to the degree that parent is surprised/cannot understand their needs.	**Effectiveness**: parent begins to 'learn' what facial expressions/cry-types link to different needs. IMPORTANT: joint attention between parent and child: both being aware of when they need and/or are trying to help, and getting positive feedback from this. **Self-regulation and emotional capacity**: parent is able to notice child's needs and respond to them effectively, especially in terms of reassurance, soothing and acceptance of the child. IMPORTANT: depression, anxiety, adult ADHD and social support are amongst the things that can affect parent–child emotional interaction at this stage.
3 months	**Communication and motivation**: The infants 'social smile' – begins to develop, aided by the child being more alert, having longer periods of wakefulness and development of focussed eye contact. **Self-regulation**: Infant begins to associate certain effective behaviours the parent uses to regulate their emotional states and begins to internalise these: distraction, hand to mouth, rocking, self-soothing their externalised emotions over time without parental input.	**Communication and motivation**: the parent responds to the child's increased social communication (presumably their own 'reward' for positive interaction) with increased interaction. This corresponds to the parent's increased sleep which leads to them taking the baby out more/increasing their social support and feelings of self.

(*Continued*)

Table 11.4 (Continued)

Age	*Social and Emotional*	
	Child	*Parent*
	Cognitive assimilation: an expression referring to a process described by Piaget; the infant explores the environment around them in order to discover what is new and make it familiar. This is sometimes referred to the beginning of 'mastery motivation' and 'mastery pleasure': the innate self-directed tendency of the infant to 'get it right'.	
6 months	**Social referencing**: infant begins to look at the facial expressions of others for 'clues' when they cannot make sense of what's happening around them (mainly with the primary attachment figure at first). This is typified by their reaction to the approach of a stranger/separation anxiety. This is also associated with the development of: **Object permanency** including remembering their goals/wants still exist when they are put out of sight, e.g. bottles, food, toys and caregivers.	**Shared goals and shared meaning**: with the increasing awareness of positive feedback and emotional states, the parent and child start anticipating the emotions their actions will induce in each other and encouraging these, e.g. peak-a-boo. IMPORTANT: the parent requires self-reflection and self-regulation in order to be able to 'see' the child as a 'psychological entity': because the child does not understand why they are feeling something, the parent needs to contain the child's emotions, anticipate their needs, work out what they think the child is experiencing and adapt the environment to 'fit' the child's understanding. 'Attunement'.
12 months	**Relational experiences and context of emotions**: in late infancy the infant adapts their emotions and subsequent behaviour to individual caregivers/ family members. This incorporates them into the family unit. **Attachment to primary caregiver**: due to separation anxiety the relationship of the infant with substitute caregivers can be difficult: the adult(s) needs to adapt their behaviour to accommodate this in a positive way. IMPORTANT: by nine months infants are able to 'know' when the way they are feeling inside does not match with the emotional signals they receive back, e.g. facial expressions. They also begin to be aware of others' moods and begin to understand the *intentions* of others from their behaviour, e.g. watching as the bottle is heated in the microwave and waiting without distress.	**Parent–child relationship**: the success of a relationship is reflected in the pleasure and mutual interest expressed by both parties, the range of positive and negative emotions the child shows and the child (and parent's) ability to moderate the behavioural expressions of these appropriately. IMPORTANT: aspects of parental/ caregiver **engagement** can be affected by their mental health either primary (e.g. post-natal depression, learning difficulties, lack of empathy, poor parental role model) or secondary (e.g. due to failure to attach and not receiving positive feedback from the child).

(*Continued*)

Table 11.4 (Continued)

Age	*Social and Emotional*	
	Child	*Parent*
18 months	**Motivation and emotions around success/failure**: with the onset of walking a child should now be expressing emotions like elation and pride and wants to share these socially with others. **Autonomy and rule setting/enforcing**: as a young toddler this is the first time restrictions need to be used. This is combined with the child pushing the distance limits which affects their attachment relationship and the feedback signals they need to interpret. This manifests as distress on being restrained or forced to stay in one place, e.g. dressing and bed time.	**Sensitivity vs. over-intrusiveness**: this is when a parent needs to strike the balance between: (a) allowing a child to explore the world and discover their limits/consequences of actions, while still (b) being sensitive to when they need help and how to give this without 'taking over'. IMPORTANT: things like anxiety can result in over-intrusiveness due to fears of what might go wrong. Other things, such as adult ADHD, can cause a parent to 'take over' because it is quicker and easier to do it themselves. Depression or absenteeism for other reasons can result in a lax parenting style, resulting in the child not getting boundaries to apply socially in later life.
24 months	**Self-reflection and empathy**: the child is more aware of times they do not 'get it right' in the world and begin to internalise this into a network of 'psychological causality': adding the intentions of self and others to the behaviour shown, emotions felt and the consequences that occur. This is the difference between the infant simply experiencing emotions and the older child's understanding of why they feel the way they do. This is aided by the child's growing awareness of how others are feeling, their interest in learning why they feel the way they do and how this is expressed. **Social referencing and cognitive assimilation**: toddlers use self-reflection and empathy along with development of language, ability to remember the timeline of events, drive for autonomy and experience of challenges to further organise and adapt their emotional understanding to 'fit' the world they live in. Self-speech begins during this second year, possibly reflecting the child beginning to reflect on experiences.	**Attachment, reactive control and child's emotional/social development**: the aim of the parent/caregiver in this period is to encourage the child to use positive strategies to alleviate distress or confusion (e.g. self-soothing, distraction or, if need be, proximity/closeness with them) and to minimise their need to use negative coping methods to manage/lower their emotions (avoidance, ignoring/freezing in place, harming others or themselves). This again requires the parent to have a good sense of self, be aware of what the child might be experiencing and adapt the environment/their methods of managing their child's expectations (e.g. '*beliefs*' about how the world 'should' work) and goals/*desires* accordingly. Consistency and congruity of response and management of their child's emotional needs are paramount. Finally, the emergence of speech and cognitive understanding of events allows the parent to start to explain the child's experiences and others' reactions to these.

(*Continued*)

Table 11.4 (Continued)

Age	*Social and Emotional*	
	Child	*Parent*
36 months	**Theory of mind**: when fully developed, this is a person's ability to understand the full range of mental states as occurring in their own mind and that these occur in others and may be different from their own. These include but are not limited to (different labelled) emotions, (and the physiological) feelings these produce, beliefs, desires, intentions and imagination. Theory of mind is only beginning to establish itself at this point. However, at three, children should be able to distinguish between a person having a physical experience vs. a mental one. **Social relationships**: at about 24 months, children begin to play in parallel with other children versus 'solitary play' that occurs in the second year. Over the third year this gradually moves from parallel play with little interaction to shared play with mutual interest, sharing toys and joint communication. By three, the motivation of making 'friendships' and getting positive self-belief from others encourages things such as turn taking and empathy when things go wrong.	**Play and social/emotional development**: play is important for physical and emotional development. Play occurs naturally in a parent–child dyad if the parent and child have all the skills and joint experiences outlined so far. Over time play changes in character: **Sensorimotor play** (0–12 months): motor actions and co-ordination along with understanding of the function of objects and practical skills and intelligence. **Constructive play** (12–24 months): language development, social relationship building and fine motor skills. BUT objects are only used for their true purpose. **Symbolic play** (24–36 months): beginning of the child's ***imagination*** emerging, e.g. using a block as a car and driving it along the table while making car noises. This is the foundation for 'role play': knowing that one object can represent another if it looks like, sounds like or acts like it in a realistic enough way.
3–5 years	**Narrative representation of emotional experiences and social understanding**: the development of language should allow a child to talk to 'safe' others about their emotional experiences and means the child can resolve conflicts between their understanding and actual reality much more effectively. This allows the child to incorporate the separate elements of mental states (e.g. emotions, feelings, beliefs, desires, intentions) together with the consequences of situations to adapt their emotional and behavioural reactions in the future.	**IMPORTANT**: the following are important reasons why children struggle to gain emotional and behavioural self-regulation and in turn have the skills and motivation to pursue social competency: **Personality aspects**: mainly temperament (i.e. emotionality and reactive control), effortful control (i.e. impulsivity and learned strategies for self-regulation) and innate tendencies around mood and affect (i.e. positivity vs. negativity.

(*Continued*)

Table 11.4 (Continued)

Age	*Social and Emotional*	
	Child	*Parent*
	Role play: the taking on of other 'roles' in combination with peers allows higher order processes essential for long-term social and emotional competence to develop. For example, altruism (caring or doing something for someone else at some cost to yourself), personalities within the group and how to tailor these for social inclusion (extroverts vs. introverts), risk taking vs. '(watching and waiting'). Imaginary friends are common at this age group and may be used to resolve issues around a child's success in managing their social/emotional self, for example: (a) in different contexts/situations (b) with different people and (c) when they are feeling different inside, e.g. when tired.	**Modelling self-regulation and the social rules/boundaries a child is brought up with**: parents and other significant others need to consistently model positive strategies of 'right and wrong' responses in emotive scenarios. What is 'right and wrong' is individual to the family and wider society and involves beliefs (e.g. moral or religious), family rules (e.g. the use of corporal punishment), society variations (e.g. educational expectations vs. achievement) and externally applied restrictions (e.g. a country's legal stance towards crime and punishment). **The child's internalising of a good enough sense of self**: overall a child needs to feel that they are loved/liked enough by significant others, would be missed if they were not there, have a safe base from which to experiment, know what they want from life and that they can achieve this realistically if they try hard enough.

Memory

Memory and attention along with executive functioning are heavily dependent on one another. The two fasciculi shown in parentheses on the flowchart in Figure 11.1 are further examples of long fibre tracts that allow assimilation of information between distant higher cortical areas, that may or may not be able to be anatomically located, carrying out different functions. As our knowledge of their physiology and neuropsychology increases, many more of these tracks are being implicated in the higher cortical functions that are unique to humans.

The function and neuropsychological testing of memory hypotheses are twofold: is memory capacity finite or non-finite, and is it domain or non-domain specific? This is often investigated in normal subjects, or those with common deficits in memory, using dual task methods. This involves the presentation of auditory or visual stimuli to one side of the brain or the other in isolation, often using either the left or the right visual fields. Distracter stimuli of different modalities are added to limit the capacity of primary/short/working memory or long-term memory depending on which aspect is being explored. Work has been undertaken in patients with split-brain syndromes (a technique that was used as a treatment for intractable epilepsy in the past) and those with certain anatomical abnormalities in areas considered to be fundamental to normal memory function. Long-term memory is thought to be more a diffuse function that has been covered within the relevant sections: language, emotion, attention and executive functioning.

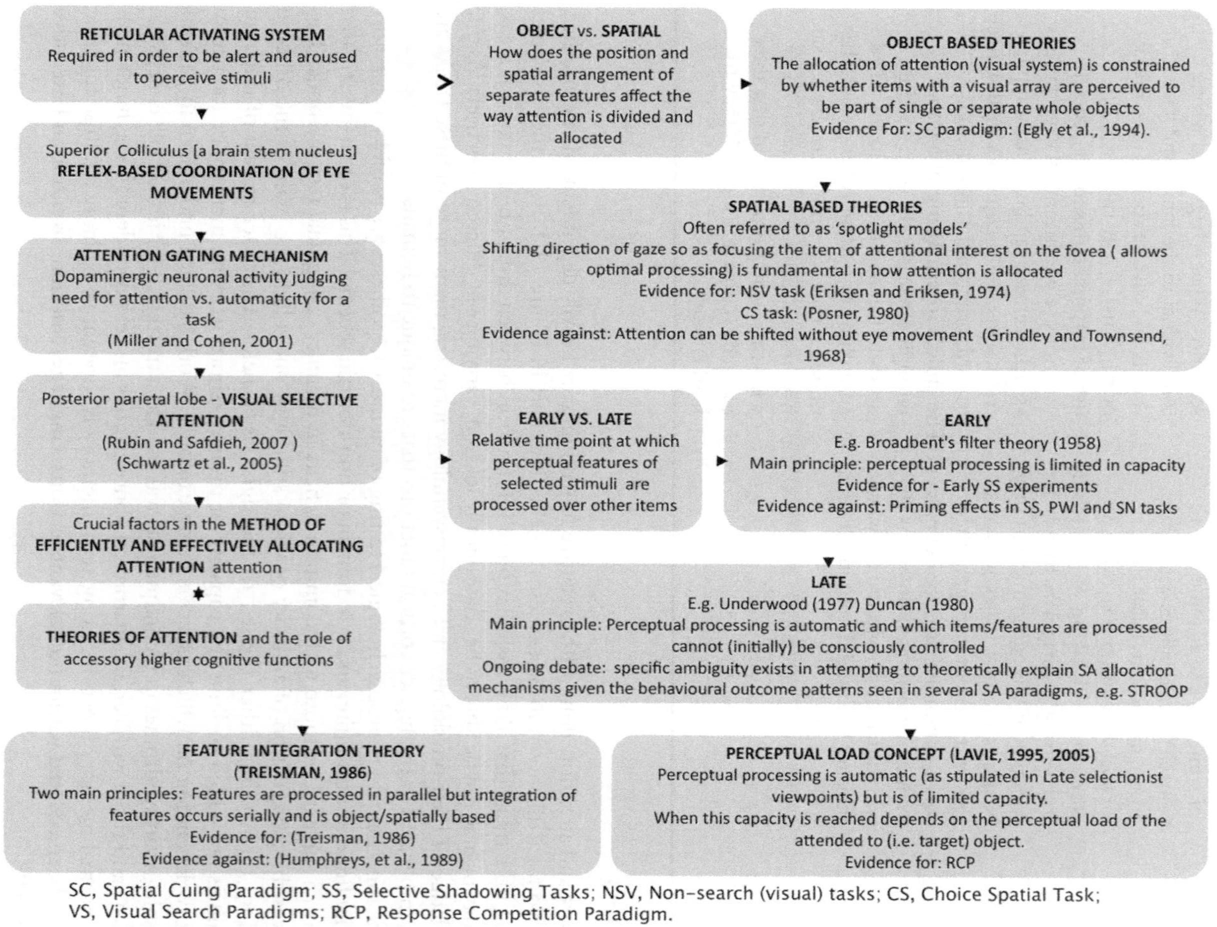
RETICULAR ACTIVATING SYSTEM
Required in order to be alert and aroused to perceive stimuli
Superior Colliculus [a brain stem nucleus] REFLEX-BASED COORDINATION OF EYE MOVEMENTS
ATTENTION GATING MECHANISM
Dopaminergic neuronal activity judging need for attention vs. automaticity for a task
(Miller and Cohen, 2001)
Posterior parietal lobe - VISUAL SELECTIVE ATTENTION
(Rubin and Safdieh, 2007)
(Schwartz et al., 2005)
Crucial factors in the METHOD OF EFFICIENTLY AND EFFECTIVELY ALLOCATING ATTENTION attention
THEORIES OF ATTENTION and the role of accessory higher cognitive functions
OBJECT vs. SPATIAL
How does the position and spatial arrangement of separate features affect the way attention is divided and allocated
OBJECT BASED THEORIES
The allocation of attention (visual system) is constrained by whether items with a visual array are perceived to be part of single or separate whole objects
Evidence For: SC paradigm: (Egly et al., 1994).
SPATIAL BASED THEORIES
Often referred to as 'spotlight models'
Shifting direction of gaze so as focusing the item of attentional interest on the fovea (allows optimal processing) is fundamental in how attention is allocated
Evidence for: NSV task (Eriksen and Eriksen, 1974)
CS task: (Posner, 1980)
Evidence against: Attention can be shifted without eye movement (Grindley and Townsend, 1968)
EARLY VS. LATE
Relative time point at which perceptual features of selected stimuli are processed over other items
EARLY
E.g. Broadbent's filter theory (1958)
Main principle: perceptual processing is limited in capacity
Evidence for - Early SS experiments
Evidence against: Priming effects in SS, PWI and SN tasks
LATE
E.g. Underwood (1977) Duncan (1980)
Main principle: Perceptual processing is automatic and which items/features are processed cannot (initially) be consciously controlled
Ongoing debate: specific ambiguity exists in attempting to theoretically explain SA allocation mechanisms given the behavioural outcome patterns seen in several SA paradigms, e.g. STROOP
FEATURE INTEGRATION THEORY
(TREISMAN, 1986)
Two main principles: Features are processed in parallel but integration of features occurs serially and is object/spatially based
Evidence for: (Treisman, 1986)
Evidence against: (Humphreys, et al., 1989)
PERCEPTUAL LOAD CONCEPT (LAVIE, 1995, 2005)
Perceptual processing is automatic (as stipulated in Late selectionist viewpoints) but is of limited capacity.
When this capacity is reached depends on the perceptual load of the attended to (i.e. target) object.
Evidence for: RCP
SC, Spatial Cuing Paradigm; SS, Selective Shadowing Tasks; NSV, Non-search (visual) tasks; CS, Choice Spatial Task; VS, Visual Search Paradigms; RCP, Response Competition Paradigm.

Figure 11.1 The field of attention.

Executive Functioning

Executive functioning has been studied extensively and was one of the first interests of neurologists, anatomists, surgeons and psychiatrists. Early work was mainly based on patients with acquired anatomical lesions secondary to injury and the resultant symptoms and disability that were found.

As a result of this research, many of the functions that were initially believed to be controlled by the frontal lobe, including problem-solving, planning and organisation, selective attention, working memory and ability to set shift, are now thought to be the product of the assimilation and organisation of projected information to the frontal lobe from associated centres of cognitive function. It is likely that the frontal lobe *does* play a significant role in facilitating these so-called higher cognitive functions.

Attention

The flowchart in Figure 11.1 outlines the main points of investigations and debate within the field of attention and related cortical processes.

Key References

Beattie, M., (2006). *Essential Revision Notes in Paediatrics for the MRCPCH* (2nd edition). Cheshire: PASTEST Ltd.

Bee, H.L., (1994). *Lifespan Development.* New York: HarperCollins College Publishers.

Gazzaniga, M., Ivry, R.B. and Magnum, G.R., (1998). *Cognitive Neuroscience: The Biology of the Mind.* New York: W.W. Norton.

Harley, T., (2001). *The Psychology of Language: From Data to Theory.* Taylor & Francis Group.

12 Genetics

Joanne Doherty and Anita Thapar

Introduction

Over the past two decades, knowledge about genetic risk factors that contribute to risk for different psychiatric disorders has advanced rapidly. Technological advances and very large-scale international collaborative efforts have led to the identification of novel genetic loci. The next step is to consider what these genetic discoveries mean for clinical practice.

KEY CONCEPTS

- Psychiatric disorders run in families and are heritable.
- Psychiatric disorders have a complex aetiology and are explained by the combination of multiple genetic and environmental risk factors.
- No single gene is either necessary or sufficient.
- Genetic risk factors are not specific to a single psychiatric disorder but rather show cross-disorder effects.
- Both common, small effect size, gene variants and rare, large effect size, gene variants contribute risk.
- Environmental risks are not independent of genetic liability; gene–environment correlation and interaction need to be considered.

Genetic Variation

Deoxyribonucleic acid (DNA) is located in the nucleus and mitochondria of the cell. It consists of a sugar-phosphate backbone and four different types of nitrogenous base: adenine, cytosine, thymine and guanine. Each base partner with a complementary base to form base pairs. The DNA molecule itself forms a double helix structure, which is tightly coiled. Nuclear DNA contains approximately 21,000 genes in humans and has been more extensively studied than mitochondrial DNA.

The human nuclear genome is arranged as 23 separate pairs of chromosomes, one set inherited from each parent. Only about 1% of the nuclear genome is protein coding, and this is known as the 'exome'. The remainder of the genome consists of other DNA elements such as regulatory regions that control gene expression. In order to produce a protein, DNA within the cell nucleus is transcribed into messenger ribonucleic acid (mRNA), which is then transported out of the nucleus for protein synthesis (translation) in the ribosome. The sequences

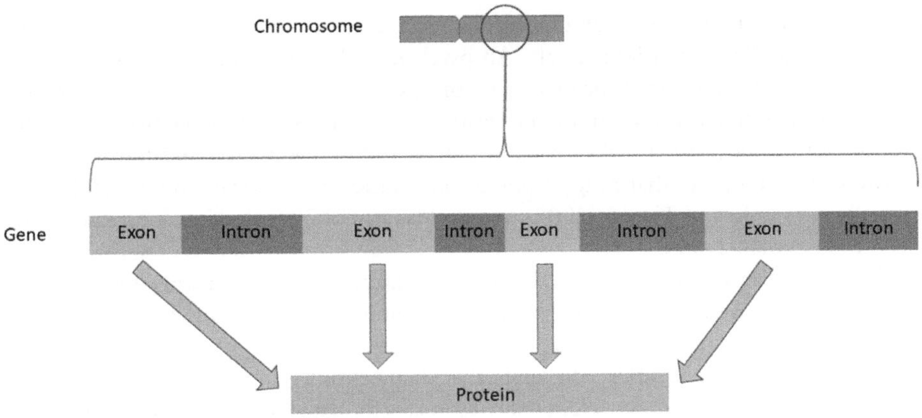

Figure 12.1 Genes consist of protein-coding regions (known as exons) and non-coding regions (known as introns). Exons and introns are nucleotide sequences within the DNA molecule; however only exon sequences are present in the mature mRNA molecule and translated in proteins. In whole-genome sequencing, the entire genome (exons and introns) is sequenced, whereas whole-exome sequencing focuses on the protein-coding regions (exons).

of bases, known as nucleotides, in the DNA and mRNA molecules determine the resulting protein. (See Figure 12.1).

In recent years there have been growing efforts to identify genetic variation and relate this variation to human disease and traits. There are many sources of genetic variation which occur at different rates in the population including variation in the total number of chromosomes (aneuploidy), structural variation of large DNA segments resulting in the deletion or duplication of DNA segments (copy number variation; CNVs) and variation of single nucleotides (single nucleotide polymorphisms; SNPS) that include common and intermediate frequency variants (>1% population frequency) and rare mutations (<1% population frequency). In each case, variation can be inherited or occur spontaneously (*de novo*), e.g. during gamete formation.

There are a number of different laboratory methods for identifying genetic variation. Karyotyping is used for the identification of chromosomal abnormalities such as trisomies (e.g. Down's syndrome). Large copy number variants can be identified using fluorescent in-situ hybridisation (FISH), in which specially designed probes can be designed to target specific known DNA sequences. However, this approach requires variation in specific chromosomal regions to be suspected.

More recently, agnostic approaches, such as array comparative genomic hybridisation (aCGH) or genotyping microarrays, have been used to identify structural variants across the whole genome. Genotyping microarrays can be used to identify single nucleotide polymorphisms. This technology allows millions of SNPs to be assayed simultaneously at relatively low cost. Next-generation sequencing (whole-genome or exome) is now available and can be used to decipher an individual's genetic code at the level of single base pairs.

Until recently the cost of sequencing techniques precluded their use in large-scale studies. However, technological advances in recent years have made such studies more feasible. As costs have declined, whole-genome sequencing is beginning to be used for diagnostic and treatment purposes in clinical practice for other areas of medicine, including neonatology.

Genetic Epidemiology

In addition to investigating genetics at a molecular level, genetic contribution can be inferred by assessing biologically related individuals. All psychiatric disorders cluster in families, and these early family studies suggested the possibility of a genetic contribution to these disorders. Family studies have been used to examine the relative risks of a first-degree relative having the same disorder as the index case, i.e. the proband. These studies report variable familial risks for different psychiatric disorders that range from an odds ratio of 2–4 for child and adolescent depression (Rice, Harold and Thapar, 2002) to an odds ratio of 30 for autism spectrum disorder (ASD) (Miller et al., 2019).

As family members share both genetic and environmental risk factors, twin and adoption studies and newer designs have been used to separate genetic and environmental influences. Overall, findings from twin studies provide evidence for high heritability (around 70–90%) of attention deficit hyperactivity disorder (ADHD), ASD and other child neurodevelopmental disorders as well as schizophrenia and bipolar disorder. Heritability estimates for depression and anxiety are lower, and conduct disorder and related behavioural problems show strong shared environmental effects. (See Figure 12.2.)

Family and twin studies have shown that familial and genetic liability confers risk across diagnostic boundaries, that may help to explain co-morbidity across disorders (Lahey, Van Hulle, Singh, Waldman and Rathouz, 2011; Miller et al., 2019). More importantly, it means that relatives of an index child in clinic will be at elevated risk not only of the same disorder as the index child, but of other psychiatric disorders, for instance, a child with autism with a sibling with ADHD and whose mother has recurrent depression. Studies of adopted children and other genetically informative designs, such as children-of-twins and assisted conception design (Thapar and Rutter, 2019), strengthen the evidence that there is a strong genetic contribution to ADHD, schizophrenia and bipolar disorder and highlight the importance of environmental contributions for depression, anxiety and conduct problems or for antisocial behaviour.

Molecular Genetics

Genetic epidemiological studies have provided strong evidence for the role of genetic risk factors in many psychiatric disorders. There have been intense efforts to identify specific genetic

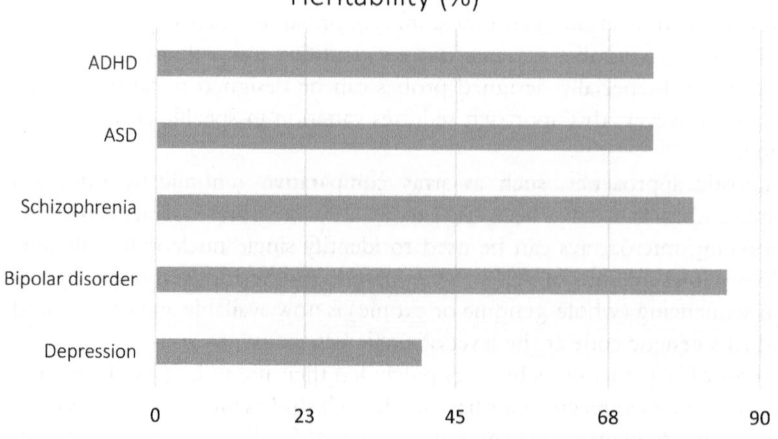

Figure 12.2 Heritability of ADHD, ASD, schizophrenia, bipolar disorder and depression.

variants associated with increased risk, as this could provide a window to the underlying biology of these disorders and in the future have important potential implications for both diagnosis and treatment.

Early molecular genetic approaches were mainly hypothesis-driven, selecting genes of interest *a priori* based on existing knowledge of biological pathways and investigating their association with disorders in either case-control or family-based association designs. These candidate-gene approaches have yielded few clear replicated findings and are, by their nature, less suitable for gene discovery than genome-wide approaches because of a high risk of false-positive discoveries.

Genome-wide studies do not rely upon prior hypotheses about which genes may be involved in a given disorder but consider all genes/genetic variation to be potential candidates. Genome-wide association studies (GWAS) have been employed to compare common genetic variants (>1%) between samples of patients and controls. Because each of these variants typically only exerts small individual effects, sample sizes for these studies need to be very large to detect such loci.

More than 100 reliable and reproducible genetic risk loci have been identified in adult samples for schizophrenia (Pardiñas et al., 2018) and depression (Howard et al., 2019), and around 30 for bipolar disorder (Stahl et al., 2019). Until recently, studies of children have been hampered by the paucity of large, adequately phenotyped samples. However, recent GWAS has identified 12 loci for ADHD (Demontis et al., 2019) and 5 loci for ASD (Grove et al., 2019a). GWAS loci only provide initial clues about the location of potential causal genes. Much more follow-up work is needed to elucidate the causal variant and underlying pathogenesis of these disorders.

An alternative approach to using GWAS findings involves investigating the summative risk from combinations of common variants, e.g. polygenic score analysis. Although each individual genetic variant exerts only a small effect, individuals with multiple risk variants are at increased risk of developing psychiatric disorders. At present, polygenic risk scores are only weakly predictive for psychiatric disorder and cannot be used for clinical testing. Nevertheless, studies that utilise composite measures of genetic risk have yielded important insights about the nature of psychiatric disorder. For example, it has been shown that many psychiatric disorders lie at the end of a population continuum, rather like hypertension lying at the extreme of blood pressure (Taylor et al., 2019).

Whole-genome approaches have been used to identify rare structural variants (copy number variants; CNVs). These studies have identified several segmental deletions and duplications that increase risk of psychiatric phenotypes (Kirov, 2015), particularly neurodevelopmental disorders, including ASD (Sanders et al., 2015), ADHD (Thapar, 2018), Tourette's syndrome (Willsey et al., 2017) and schizophrenia (O'Donovan and Owen, 2016; Sullivan et al., 2018). Recent studies have observed rare CNVs associated with mood disorder (Green et al., 2016; Kendall et al., 2019). Pathogenic CNVs tend to be large (>100 kilobases; kB) thereby disrupting more genes and rare (<1%). There is greater confidence about their causality when they occur *de novo* (i.e. are not inherited from a parent), which may reflect natural selection pressures.

Exome sequencing studies have been used to identify individual genetic variants in the protein-coding regions of the genome (approximately 1%) in both case-control cohorts and in families (to identify *de novo* mutations). Whole-genome sequencing is more time-consuming and expensive than whole-exome sequencing since both the protein-coding and non-coding regions are sequenced. Work is currently underway through the Whole Genome Sequencing for Psychiatric Disorders Consortium to integrate sequencing data across disorders in large cohorts of patients and controls that should yield some interesting insights into biological mechanisms underlying cross-disorder risk (Sanders et al., 2017).

The Genetic Architecture of Psychiatric Disorders

The genetic architecture of psychiatric disorders, like other common medical conditions, is extremely complex. Unlike Mendelian disorders, in which disorders are inherited in a dominant, recessive or X-linked manner, for common multi-factorial disorders like ASD, ADHD, schizophrenia and depression, no single gene is either necessary or sufficient for the psychiatric phenotype. Both common and rare genetic variants appear to contribute to these disorders, and these encompass chromosomal structural and DNA sequence variants.

Studies to date suggest that rather than acting deterministically, genetic risk variants for psychiatric disorders act probabilistically, increasing risk of psychiatric disorders with variable penetrance. These variants appear mainly to act additively, i.e. the more risk variants carried by an individual, the higher their chance of developing disorder. Although they may interact with other risk variants or indeed with other regions of the genome, this has not yet been shown. While genetic risk factors are important in the aetiology of psychiatric disorders, their incomplete penetrance highlights that the environment plays a key role.

Gene–Environment Interplay

The environment in which children grow and develop can have a profound influence on their mental health. These influences are not distinct from genetic liability. Accumulating evidence suggests that genetic risks influence environmental factors and environmental exposures can impact on gene expression. Gene–environment correlation occurs when exposure to environmental conditions depends on an individual's genotype or that of their parents, i.e. environmental risks are shaped by genetically influenced behaviours. Gene–environment interaction, on the other hand, occurs when the effect of a genetic risk factor is altered by the presence of environmental factors. Both gene–environment correlation and gene–environment interaction are likely to be important in contributing to psychiatric risk. To date, there is strong evidence that many environmental exposures, e.g. nicotine exposure *in utero*, life events and parent–child hostility, are correlated with genetic liability for different psychiatric disorders (Thapar and Rutter, 2019).

Genetic Discoveries for Specific Psychiatric Disorders

The field of psychiatric genetics has expanded hugely in recent years, and it is not possible to cover discoveries for each disorder. Here we focus on a few disorders to illustrate some of the most important findings.

Attention Deficit Hyperactivity Disorder (ADHD)

ADHD affects about 5% of children worldwide (Faraone et al., 2015) and is familial and highly heritable (Faraone and Doyle, 2000; Thapar, 2018). Twin studies consistently have observed that the heritability of ADHD is about 70–80% (Faraone and Larsson, 2019) and that clinically diagnosed ADHD represents one end of a continuous heritable spectrum (Larsson, Anckarsater, Råstam, Chang and Lichtenstein, 2012). Family and twin studies have demonstrated strong genetic overlap between ADHD and other child neurodevelopmental disorders including intellectual disability (Faraone, Ghirardi, Kuja-Halkola, Lichtenstein and Larsson, 2017), autism (Ghirardi et al., 2018; Miller et al., 2019), communication disorders and specific learning and motor disorders (Lichtenstein, Carlström, Råstam, Gillberg and Anckarsäter, 2010).

This genetic overlap extends beyond child neurodevelopmental disorders to include conduct disorder (Faraone, Biederman and Monuteaux, 2000), schizophrenia (Larsson et al., 2013), bipolar disorder (Faraone, Biederman and Wozniak, 2012; Larsson et al., 2013) and depression (Cole, Ball, Martin, Scourfield and Mcguffin, 2009). Familial and genetic loading for ADHD appears to be higher when ADHD persists into late adolescence and adult life (Faraone et al., 2000; Pingault et al., 2015).

ADHD is more common in children with aneuploidy, i.e. an abnormal number of chromosomes, than in the general population. This includes children with sex chromosome aneuploidy, e.g. Klinefelter's syndrome and those with autosomal aneuploidy, such as Down's syndrome.

ADHD is more common in copy number variant syndromes such as 22q11.2 deletion syndrome (Niarchou et al., 2015). Children with ADHD appear to have an excess burden of copy number variants compared to children without ADHD (Elia et al., 2012; Williams et al., 2010). The identified CNVs overlap with those associated with ASD and schizophrenia. A recent whole-exome sequencing study observed that rare mutations in ADHD strongly overlapped with those found in autism (Satterstrom et al., 2018).

Until recently, genome-wide association studies have failed to identify common genetic variants contributing to ADHD risk, most likely due to small sample sizes and subsequent low power to detect small effects. The first genome-wide significant common variants for ADHD were identified in 2018 using a combined sample of >20,000 individuals with ADHD. This study found 12 genetic loci and provided further evidence for ADHD diagnosis lying at the extreme of a continuous heritable trait (Demontis et al., 2019). ADHD shows genetic correlation with other psychiatric disorders, especially depression. ADHD polygenic risk scores have been observed to predict ADHD persistence into late adolescence (Riglin et al., 2016). Interestingly there was specificity as schizophrenia genetic risk scores did not predict ADHD persistence.

Autistic Spectrum Disorder (ASD)

ASD affects approximately 1% of children (Baxter et al., 2015) and can profoundly affect social and educational functioning. The heritability of ASD is estimated to be between 64 and 91% (Tick, Bolton, Happé, Rutter and Rijsdijk, 2016). As with ADHD, ASD is prevalent in children with chromosomal abnormalities, including Down's syndrome and CNV syndromes, such as 22q11.2 and 16p11.2 deletions and duplications. Children with ASD have a higher CNV burden than population controls with a particular excess of *de novo* mutations (Iossifov et al., 2014; Sanders et al., 2015). In addition, mutations in single genes have been found to be associated with ASD, such as the mutations that result in Rett syndrome, tuberous sclerosis and Fragile X syndrome. These CNVs and rare mutations are pleiotropic, that is, they are associated with risk for disorders other than autism, including ADHD and intellectual disability.

Recent whole-exome sequencing studies have found that more than a quarter of people with ASD have an identifiable protein-disrupting rare genetic mutation (Geschwind and State, 2015) and that many of the rare variants associated with ASD affect genes involved in neuronal communication or the regulation of gene expression (Satterstrom et al., 2018). Whilst much of the genetic research in ASD has been focused on the study of rare variants, common variants are likely to play a key role in the aetiology of the disorder (Gaugler et al., 2014).

Five genome-wide significant loci have recently been identified in the largest ASD GWAS to date involving more than 18,000 individuals with ASD (Grove et al., 2019a). This study found differences in the polygenic architecture of different clinical subtypes of ASD, shedding light on the biological basis of the clinical heterogeneity of ASD.

Depression

Major depressive disorder is uncommon in children (Kessler et al., 2001) but the prevalence increases after puberty to 4–5% in mid- to late adolescence (Costello et al., 2005). It is a major risk factor for suicide and can lead to social and educational impairments. Offspring of parents with depression are three to four times more likely than offspring without affected parents to develop depression (Rice et al., 2002). Both genetic and non-inherited factors, e.g. psychosocial adversity, are thought to contribute to this increase in risk. Twin studies of depressive disorders in children and adolescents find that heritability is low in childhood, but increases in adolescence (Thapar and Rice, 2006). The heritability of adolescent depression is estimated to be approximately 40% (Glowinski et al., 2003), which is similar to that reported in adults (Sullivan et al., 2000). Adoption, children-of-twin and assisted conception studies suggest that much or all of the parent–offspring transmission of depression risk in children and adolescents is environmental (Eley et al., 1998; Lewis et al., 2011; McAdams et al., 2015; Tully et al., 2008).

Genetic factors seem to contribute to adolescent depression not only directly but indirectly through gene–environment interplay (Thapar et al., 2012), for example, by increasing sensitivity to adversity (gene–environment interaction) and by increasing the probability of exposure to risky environments (gene–environment correlation). It has been suggested that the increasing heritability of depression with age may be at least in part due to gene–environment correlation, which increases around adolescence when young people begin to exert more influence on their environment (Rice, 2010). Copy number variants and rare deleterious mutations have not been observed to contribute to depression risk in the way that they do for neurodevelopmental disorders. A recent study using UK Biobank observed an increased burden of pathogenic CNVs in those with depression (Kendall et al., 2019).

It is intriguing as to whether these individuals have a typical form of depression or whether they have co-morbid neurodevelopmental problems. Genome-wide association studies of depression have required very large samples to identify genome-wide significant loci. Recent collaborative endeavours have resulted in the identification of more than 100 common variants (Howard et al., 2019) and suggest that depression lies at the extreme of a continuum of mood-related symptoms in the population. A genome-wide association study of adults with clinical depression found age effects in that depression with early age at onset (<27 years) was associated with genetic liability to schizophrenia and later depression was more strongly associated with depression genetic risk (Power et al., 2017).

A similar age-related association was seen with emotional problems in childhood, adolescence and adult life (Riglin et al., 2018). A recent population-based investigation of adolescent depression trajectories found that depression starting in late adolescence was associated with genetic risk for depression, whilst depression starting in early adolescence was associated with genetic risk for ADHD and schizophrenia (Rice et al., 2019). This suggests that depression, including in children and adolescents, is heterogeneous and that early-onset cases are more likely to involve a neurodevelopmental component.

Schizophrenia

Schizophrenia affects approximately 1% of the population and is associated with considerable morbidity and excess mortality (Owen, Sawa and Mortensen, 2016). Psychotic symptoms are extremely rare in pre-pubertal children, with an estimated incidence of 0.04% (Driver et al., 2013). As with depression, its prevalence increases rapidly during adolescence (Thomsen, 1996). Childhood-onset schizophrenia, identified as an onset of psychosis before the age of

12 years old, is defined in the same way as later-onset disorder, but is associated with more severe symptoms, more commonly associated with premorbid neurodevelopmental disorders, brain abnormalities and higher genetic loading (Rapoport and Gogtay, 2011).

Genetic studies of children and adolescents with psychosis are sparse. Findings from studies of adults can be informative given there is no reason for considering the disorder to be genetically different in younger people. Family, adoption and twin studies have all shown that schizophrenia is highly heritable with an estimated heritability of about 80% (Hilker et al., 2018). There is marked familial and genetic overlap with bipolar disorder and with other psychiatric disorders. Genome-wide association studies have identified more than a hundred common gene variants associated with schizophrenia risk. These common gene variants are associated not only with risk for schizophrenia. There is strong genetic overlap with bipolar disorder and more intriguingly, schizophrenia polygenic risk scores are associated with anxiety, depression and child neurodevelopmental problems, especially ASD and autistic traits (Cross-Disorder Group of the Psychiatric Genomics Consortium, 2013; Jones et al., 2016; Riglin et al., 2017; St Pourcain et al., 2018).

Individuals with psychosis show an elevated burden of rare structural variants, and exome sequencing studies have highlighted potentially causal deleterious rare sequence mutations. Those with earlier onset have been found to be more likely to carry a rare structural variant (CNV) than those with adult-onset schizophrenia (Walsh et al., 2008). Both common and rare structural and sequence variants contribute to schizophrenia risk. These variants have been found to predominantly affect genes involved in synaptic transmission and immune function (Hall et al., 2015; Owen et al., 2016).

Bipolar Disorder

Epidemiological studies find the lifetime prevalence of bipolar disorder to be between 1 and 2% (Ferrari et al., 2016). The age at first onset is typically in late adolescence and early adulthood, but a bimodal distribution has been suggested with peaks at 15–24 years and 45–54 years (Kroon et al., 2013). Pre-pubertal onset is less common and is associated with poor prognosis (Leverich et al., 2007). As with schizophrenia, there are few genetic studies of children and adolescents with bipolar disorder, but findings from the adult literature can be informative.

Bipolar disorder has a heritability of about 85% (McGuffin et al., 2003). To date, 30 common variants have been associated with bipolar risk (Stahl et al., 2019). These variants affect ion channels, neurotransmitter transporters, synaptic, metabolic and immune components. There are significant genetic correlations with schizophrenia, depression, traits of ASD and anorexia nervosa. Interestingly, cases with a bipolar I diagnosis have higher schizophrenia polygenic risk scores than cases with bipolar II. Bipolar II cases have higher depression polygenic risk scores than bipolar I cases. Fewer CNVs have been associated with bipolar disorder than with schizophrenia or neurodevelopmental disorders (Green et al., 2016), and increased CNV burden may be limited to schizoaffective cases (Charney et al., 2018). This may provide a biological basis for clinical subtypes of bipolar disorder.

Implications of Genetic Findings

One of the most striking findings from recent psychiatric genetic research is that, far from confirming the validity of current diagnostic categories, studies highlight the overlaps between disorders. The same genetic variants seem to increase risk across several disorders rather than mapping onto individual disorders on a 1:1 basis (Demontis et al., 2019; Doherty and Owen,

2014; Grove et al., 2019; Lichtenstein et al., 2010). This is also the case for some environmental risk factors, e.g. maltreatment. This finding emphasises the limitations of our current systems of psychiatric classification at least in terms of mapping onto aetiology and calls for alternative approaches. It is worth noting that genetic and environmental risk factors cross diagnostic boundaries for physical health disorders.

An important clinical implication for recent genetic findings concerns genetic counselling. Until recently, estimating the recurrence of disorders within families has been based on data from family studies. However, for rare, highly penetrant mutations (e.g. CNVs such as the 22q11.2 deletion), it is possible to test family members to find out if they carry the same mutation as the proband. Understanding that their disorder may have arisen due to an underlying genetic cause could help affected individuals and their families to make sense of their symptoms (Curtis, Adlington and Bhui, 2019). Confirmation of a risk CNV would enable affected families to access appropriate support, treatment and monitoring for any associated conditions. On the other hand, accurately estimating risk based on mutations with variable penetrance and which are highly pleiotropic is problematic, and genetic testing may lead to anxiety, family conflict and potentially increase stigma and discrimination (Demkow and Wolańczyk, 2017). As yet, genetic testing for psychiatric disorders is not part of routine clinical practice in most child and adolescent psychiatry clinics.

However, in the UK increasingly, children with intellectual disability are being offered microarray testing with a relatively high yield (Bass and Skuse, 2018). In some countries, this is recommended for children with autism. Consideration should be given to the use of genetic testing for children with complex presentations of ADHD and schizophrenia and those with multiple affected family members, co-morbid physical health problems, e.g. congenital cardiac or palatal abnormalities, and/or facial dysmorphology. Clinicians should refer to both local and national guidelines regarding genetic testing and contact their local clinical genetics service for advice since recommendations for testing and resources available vary. Polygenic risk scores are too weakly predictive at present to provide clinical utility. It is plausible that as prediction strength increases these risk scores coupled with clinical variables could be used to aid clinical decision-making and tailor intervention.

While precision medicine based on pharmacogenomics remains some way off, in the future, pharmacogenetic investigations may not only lead to the identification of novel treatment targets, but may help to identify individual patients most likely to respond to, or have side effects from, particular drug treatments, based on knowledge of their genetic background. This would be a tremendous advance in a field in which treatment options are currently very limited.

Multiple-Choice Questions

See answers on page 666.

1. The protein-coding part of the genome is known as the:
   a. DNA
   b. Chromosomes
   c. Exome
   d. Copy number variant
   e. mRNA
2. Deletion or duplication of chromosomal segments is known as:
   a. Single nucleotide polymorphism
   b. Aneuploidy
   c. Single nucleotide variation

   d. Meiosis
   e. Copy number variation
3. Which type(s) of studies can be used to dissociate the contributions of genes and the environment?
   a. Candidate gene studies
   b. Twin and adoption studies
   c. Gene-environment interaction
   d. Family studies
   e. All of the above
4. The heritability of which disorder is estimated to be about 40%?
   a. Depression
   b. ASD
   c. ADHD
   d. Schizophrenia
   e. Bipolar disorder
5. The effects of common variants:
   a. Are typically small
   b. Can be investigated using genome-wide association studies
   c. Can be summed to give a polygenic risk score
   d. All of the above
   e. None of the above

Key References

Doherty, J.L. and Owen, M.J., (2014). Genomic Insights into the Overlap Between Psychiatric Disorders: Implications for Research and Clinical Practice. *Genome Medicine*, 6(4): 29.

O'Donovan, M.C. and Owen, M.J., (2016). The Implications of Shared Genetics of Psychiatric Disorders. *Nature Medicine*, 22(11): 1214–1219.

Thapar, A., (2018). Discoveries on the Genetics of ADHD in the 21st Century: New Findings and their Implications. *American Journal of Psychiatry*, 175(10): 943–950.

13 Cognitive Assessment in Children and Young People

Anastasia Sedikides

Introduction

Cognitive assessments or intelligence tests are used to determine a young person's overall learning ability and to identify their strengths and weaknesses in areas of cognitive capacity such as verbal reasoning, memory, visual processing and speed of processing. Emotional and/or behavioural difficulties can impact a young person's cognitive abilities, for instance, making it harder to concentrate or to process what is being said.

Conversely, weak cognitive abilities in the form of a learning disability or some more specific form of developmental delay can be the primary issue that underpins emotional and behavioural difficulties, e.g. anxiety, low mood, poor concentration, oppositional behaviour, frustration and anger outbursts. Understanding such difficulties and knowing whether they underlie or exacerbate the young person's emotional and/or behavioural problems can be difficult but useful when it comes to providing support for them.

KEY CONCEPTS

- For some young people referred to mental health services, cognitive difficulties are the primary concern, underlying the emotional/or behavioural difficulties they present with.
- Cognitive assessments can measure a range of cognitive abilities including general ability (IQ), verbal and non-verbal skills, memory, attention and educational attainment.
- Findings from cognitive assessments are considered together with information obtained from other sources to produce a comprehensive understanding of a young person's strengths and difficulties.
- Understanding where a young person's primary difficulties lie can help with diagnosis and with focusing support appropriately.
- Information obtained from a cognitive assessment can help tailor intervention and treatment strategies to maximise their effectiveness.

How Can Cognitive Assessments Help?

Cognitive difficulties can be subtle and not easily identifiable in face-to-face conversations alone. Cognitive assessments (IQ tests) are the tools to measure these difficulties. IQ tests provide information about a young person's abilities in a range of areas, including verbal and non-verbal skills, memory and processing speed. They can be used to gain an estimation of a young person's general abilities, i.e. an intelligence quotient (IQ), in addition to a profile of their strengths and weaknesses. Extra measures, such as those assessing educational attainment or specific cognitive domains such as memory, attention or executive function, can be administered, if this is clinically indicated.

Combined with information from other sources, cognitive assessments can add to our understanding of why the young person thinks, feels and behaves as they do. In turn, this information can be used to help inform decision-making regarding educational planning and clinical intervention. Understanding a young person's ability to attend to, comprehend and reason can help ensure that the interventions are pitched at the appropriate level.

Who Can Carry out Cognitive Assessments?

Cognitive assessments can only be carried out by psychologists (clinical psychologists, educational psychologists and assistant or trainee psychologists under supervision).

When to Consider a Cognitive Assessment

Completing assessments can, on occasions, be anxiety-provoking or stressful for young people. The process of administering, scoring, interpreting and writing up an assessment can be lengthy and time-consuming. The added value of understanding a young person's difficulties and planning interventions or support merits careful consideration. Other indicators of cognitive ability may be available from different sources and provide equally useful information about a young person's abilities. One example would be the cognitive attainment tests (CATS) that are carried out in school.

Points to Consider in Relation to Cognitive Assessments

During administration of a cognitive assessment, observations are made of the young person's characteristics, e.g. their problem-solving approach, language, mood, ability to follow instructions, desire to perform, interest in certain tasks, reaction to difficult tasks, attention, concentration and activity level. For young children, it is important to note whether they can cope with separation from the caregiver. These observations help to determine the validity of the results obtained. For instance, a child who finds it difficult to focus or gives up easily will not be able to demonstrate what they can do, and the assessment result could underestimate their true ability.

The data obtained from cognitive assessments should be considered alongside information obtained from other sources, including school reports and discussions with parents/carers. A comprehensive picture can then be formed about a young person's cognitive abilities and how these relate to his or her day-to-day functioning and manifest problems.

Cognitive is a highly individualised process. The purpose of the assessment needs to be clear. When considering whether a young person might benefit from a cognitive assessment, it is important to identify what question it would help to answer. Examples of such questions include:

- Could this young person's anxiety be due to developmental delay and ensuing inability to meet other people's expectations?
- Could this young person's behavioural difficulties be due to his lack of understanding of what is being said to him?

Specifying the reasons for referring a young person for a cognitive assessment can help the psychologist to tailor the assessment and focus on particular areas of concern.

Cognitive development follows a well-defined trajectory. It becomes stable around the age of seven years and is not expected to change dramatically over time. Exceptions to this are events such as brain injury that may cause cognitive impairments. When making a referral for a cognitive assessment, it is advisable to check whether or not an assessment has been carried out previously.

Case Study: Jamie

Jamie (nine) was referred to CAMHS due to destructive temper outbursts and self-harm, i.e. repeatedly banging his head against the wall when distressed. Initial assessment revealed that Jamie was having a daily outburst, during which he would shout, throw things, hit and kick. Self-injury followed these behaviours. Jamie was noted to have difficulty in retaining information and with attention and concentration, although not with hyperactivity.

Developmentally, he appeared to have met his milestones within the timeframe expected, but he was found to be struggling with some aspects of language when he started school. He received a short programme of speech and language therapy.

A referral for cognitive therapy was made to help ascertain whether any cognitive difficulties could be underlying or exacerbating his frustration, distress and behavioural outbursts.

Cognitive assessment revealed that Jamie was of average cognitive ability, but that he had significant difficulties in terms of his verbal reasoning skills. These were considerably weaker than expected and at a level more typical of a six-year old than of a nine-year old.

Jamie's many strengths in other areas meant that his verbal difficulties were not always apparent to those talking to him. He was often able to comply with instructions by copying those around him, and his cheeky and endearing manner meant that he was generally able to cope socially, even if he did not understand what was being said. His weakness in verbal skills was a source of considerable frustration for him. It meant that he struggled academically and made mistakes due to misunderstanding.

This was a significant contributing factor to Jamie's outbursts and self-harming. His verbal difficulties were an important factor in terms of his attention difficulties as he 'switched off' when he did not understand what was being said.

Intervention would need to include those communicating with Jamie pitching their language at the right level for him to understand. Supporting verbal information with non-verbal information, e.g. pictures and diagrams, would help him to understand what was being asked.

Multiple-Choice Questions

See answers on page 667.

1. Which of these statements is not true? Cognitive difficulties can…
   a. Always be recognised easily
   b. Be exacerbated by emotional or behavioural difficulties
   c. Lead to emotional/behavioural difficulties
   d. Be subtle and difficult to pin down and quantify
2. Which of these statements about cognitive assessments is correct?
   a. Cognitive assessments are quick and easy to undertake.
   b. Data from cognitive assessments can be used in isolation to draw conclusions about young people.
   c. Cognitive assessments simply measure IQ.
   d. Cognitive assessments can only be carried out by psychologists.

3. Which of these abilities do cognitive assessments not measure?
   a. Processing speed
   b. Non-verbal skills
   c. Sensory abilities
   d. Working memory
4. Which of the following is not true?
   a. Findings from cognitive assessments can help with knowing how a young person's difficulties started.
   b. Findings from cognitive assessments can help with knowing where to focus support for a young person.
   c. Findings from cognitive assessments can help with knowing what level a young person is functioning at.
   d. Findings from cognitive assessments can help with knowing what level to pitch interventions at.

Key References

Flanagan, D.P. and Alfonso, V.C., (2017). *Essentials of WISC-V Assessment.* Hoboken, NJ: Wiley.

Wechsler, D., (2013). *The Wechsler Preschool and Primary Scale of Intelligence* (4th UK Edition (WPPSI-V UK)). Pearson Assessment UK.

Wechsler, D., (2016). *The Wechsler Intelligence Scale for Children* (5th UK Edition (WISC-V UK)). Pearson Assessment UK.

14 Mental Health and Behavioural Issues in Children and Young People with a Learning Disability

Chris Hardie, Chantal Holman, Becky Sparks and Catherine Thompson

Research has consistently demonstrated that children and young people with learning disabilities are at increased risk of developing mental health problems.

KEY CONCEPTS

- Children and young people with a learning disability (LD) are at an increased risk of developing mental health problems when compared to their typically developing peers.
- Challenging behaviour is often associated with mental health problems and is the most common reason for children and young people with learning disabilities to be referred to the child and adolescent mental health services (CAMHS).
- Assessing the mental health needs of children and young people with learning disabilities requires a highly specialist set of skills involving an understanding of the relationship of genetic, neurological and social pre-dispositions of this client group to mental health problems.
- Children with challenging behaviour, especially those with self-injurious behaviour (SIB), may have an underlying physical health problem. Remember diagnostic overshadowing.
- Children and young people with LD are more at risk from abuse that may in turn manifest in challenging behaviour.

Introduction

Rutter et al.'s (1976) Isle of Wight Study was one of the first to identify the increased prevalence rate of mental health issues in children and young people with a learning disability, highlighting that they are three to four times more likely to develop mental health problems than their typically developing peers. Many studies have reached similar conclusions, and it is now well accepted that approximately 35–40% of children and young people with learning disabilities will develop mental health problems (Emerson and Hatton, 2007), including conduct disorder, anxiety disorders, attention deficit hyperactivity disorder (ADHD) and autism spectrum disorders (ASD). For many families, it is the challenging behaviour that can be associated with mental health problems that poses the greatest challenge. This can impact not only on the child/young person's health and well-being, but that of the family as a whole.

This chapter will give an overview of the factors relevant to the mental health of children and young people with learning disabilities, moving on to consider the assessment of need and interventions suited to the client group.

Definition of Learning Disability

Learning disability, as defined by Valuing People (Department of Health, 2001), includes the presence of:

- A significantly reduced ability to understand new or complex information or to learn new skills, i.e. impaired intelligence
- With reduced ability to cope independently, i.e. impaired social functioning
- And which started before adulthood, with a lasting effect on development

A diagnosis of learning disability is traditionally applied in practice when an individual's IQ score falls below 70 on a psychometric assessment. The level of learning disability is defined based on an individual's overall score. A child may have a very unequal profile of strengths and weaknesses, and a full-scale IQ may not be especially helpful or a child may not have had a previous psychometric assessment. A diagnosis of learning disability may therefore be applied based on an individual's level of impairment in social or adaptive skills. (See Table 14.1.)

Aetiology

The aetiology of learning disabilities is a combination of genetic, organic and psychosocial factors that impact upon development at the prenatal, perinatal and postnatal stages. The most common causes at each stage are highlighted in Table 14.2.

Definition of Challenging Behaviour

The most widely accepted definition of challenging behaviour is:

> Culturally abnormal behaviour of such intensity, frequency or duration that the physical safety of the person or others is likely to be placed in serious jeopardy, or behaviour that is likely to seriously limit use of, or result in the person being denied access to, ordinary community facilities.
>
> (Emerson, 1995)

The most common challenging behaviours reported in children and young people with learning disabilities include:

- Verbal and/or physical aggression
- Damage to property

Table 14.1 Levels of Learning Disability (IQ)

Levels of Learning Disability (IQ)				
	Mild	Moderate	Severe	Profound
ICD-10	69–50	49–35	34–20	Less than 20

Table 14.2 Common causes of learning disability

Prenatal	*Perinatal*	*Postnatal*
Chromosome disorders, e.g. Down syndrome	Premature birth and its complications	Environmental deprivation, e.g. psychosocial disadvantage, child abuse and neglect, chronic social and sensory deprivation.
Autosomal deletion disorders, e.g. cri du chat syndrome, 22q11.2	Lack of oxygen causing asphyxia	Injury (accidental and non-accidental)
Triplet Repeat Expansion Disorder, e.g. Fragile X	Complications through abnormal labour and/or delivery, e.g. haemorrhaging in the brain	Infection, e.g. meningitis, encephalitis
Gene mutation, e.g. tuberous sclerosis (autosomal dominant, AD)	Hypoglycaemia	
Smith–Lemli–Opitz (autosomal recessive, AR)		
Prenatal insults, e.g. infection, CMV, rubella		
Alcohol and substance misuse, e.g. fetal alcohol syndrome		

- Self-injurious behaviour
- Non-compliance
- Stereotypical/ritualised behaviours
- Inappropriate urinating/defecating, including smearing
- Inappropriate sexualised behaviours

Challenging behaviour is the most common reason for children and young people with learning disabilities to be referred to CAMHS. Emerson et al. (1999) offered two suggestions as possible ways in which challenging behaviours may be associated with mental health problems:

- Challenging behaviours may be an atypical presentation of an underlying mental health problem.
- Challenging behaviours may be a secondary feature of mental health problems or underlying psychiatric symptoms may establish and maintain challenging behaviours.

In addition, the authors would propose that the presence of challenging behaviour indicates a level of emotional distress within the child/young person that needs to be recognised.

Risk Factors

Children and young people with learning disabilities face a multitude of biological, psychological and social risk factors affecting their mental health.

Psychological Risk Factors Include

- Fewer coping strategies.
- Low self-esteem.
- Awareness of disability and difference from their typically developing peers.
- Physical ill health in parents.

- Mental ill health in parents. Emerson and Hatton (2007) found that 44% of children with learning disabilities are cared for by a mother with mental health difficulties, compared to 24% of the typically developing population.

Social Risk Factors Include

- Abuse.
- Bullying.
- Isolation.
- Living in residential/institutional care.
- Living in poverty. Approximately 55% of families of children with disabilities have a low income compared to 30% in the typically developing population, and the cost of bringing up a child with a disability is three times greater (Emerson and Hatton, 2007). There are more children with learning disabilities living within single parent families.

Biological Risk Factors Include

- Physical disability
- GI problems, e.g. reflux and constipation
- Sensory impairments
- Epilepsy
- Specific genetic syndromes, e.g. velocardiofacial syndrome

Behavioural Phenotypes

The term behavioural phenotype refers to behaviours that are believed to be an integral part of certain genetic disorders. William Nyhan (1972) first formally introduced the concept in connection with the self-harming behaviours that characterise Lesch–Nyhan syndrome. Flint and Yule (1993) have since provided a more thorough definition:

> The behavioural phenotype is a characteristic pattern of motor, cognitive, linguistic and social abnormalities which is consistently associated with a biological disorder. In some cases, the behavioural phenotype may constitute a psychiatric disorder; in others, behaviours which are not normally regarded as symptoms of psychiatric diagnosis may occur.

Table 14.3 provides a brief overview of the behavioural phenotypes, the genotype, medical conditions associated with them and associated psychiatric disorders for some of the more common syndromes. Not all children and young people will display all aspects of the behavioural phenotype. For a more comprehensive overview, the reader should refer to specific genetic texts or to the Society for the Study of Behavioural Phenotypes (www.ssbp.org.uk).

Assessment

Assessing the mental health needs of children and young people with learning disabilities, who often present with behavioural challenges, is a complex task. The child's ability to communicate their thoughts, feelings and experiences may be significantly impaired or altogether absent. Assessment is comprised of information pulled together from a variety of sources, including:

Table 14.3 Overview of the Behavioural Phenotypes, the Genotype, Medical Conditions Associated with Them and Associated Psychiatric Disorders for Some of the More Common Syndromes

Condition	*Comment*	*Physical Findings*	*Behaviour/Mental Health*
22q11.2 Interstitial deletion	1:4,000 Includes velocardiofacial syndrome and Di-George syndrome	Cleft palate Congenital heart defects Renal disorders Lack of or underdeveloped thymus and parathyroid glands Immunological dysfunction	Attention deficit disorder/attention deficit hyperactivity disorder Exaggerated response to threatening stimuli Fearfulness of painful situations Autism spectrum disorder In adolescence/early adulthood can develop- Schizophrenia/ schizoaffective disorder Manic depressive illness/psychosis Rapid or ultra-rapid cycling of mood Mood disorder, depression
Angelman Autosomal deletion 68–75% (mother) Uniparental disomy 2–7% (father) Imprinting centre defects 2–5% Mutation in UBE3A gene (8–11%) Some not found	1:4,000 live births Also known as happy puppet syndrome 15q11-13	Hypopigmented hair, skin and eyes compared to other family members Ataxic movements Initial hypotonia to hypertonia Over 80% develop seizures with a characteristic EEG appearance	Sleep difficulties Increased levels of smiling, laughing and being happy Excessive sociability Hyperactivity and poor attention Aggression
Cornelia de Lange Gene mutation	1:50,000 20–50% NIP-BL gene on chromosome 5 SMC3 on chromosome 10 and X linked SMC 1–5% and milder phenotype	Low birth weight Short stature Distinctive facies Gastrointestinal disorders especially reflux and aspiration Vision and hearing problems Cardiac problems Genitourinary problems	Shy and socially anxious Selective mutism Autism spectrum disorder (ASD) Compulsive behaviour – tidying up, lining things up Self-injurious behaviour (SIB)

(*Continued*)

Table 14.3 (Continued)

Condition	*Comment*	*Physical Findings*	*Behaviour/Mental Health*
Cri du chat Autosomal deletion	Deletion of the short arm of chromosome 5 (5p-) One of the most common deletion syndromes Incidence 1/20,000 to 1/50,000 births 85% de novo	Cat-like cry Feeding difficulties and failure to thrive in infancy Microcephaly Growth retardation Gastro-oesophageal reflux Respiratory tract infections Ear infections	Sleep difficulties Aggression (SIB) Hyperactivity
Down syndrome Trisomy 21 (95%) Translocation (2%) Mosaicism (2%) Chromosome rearrangements (1%)	Incidence: 1:7,300	Visual problems Hearing difficulties – 38–78% individuals Endocrine-hypo/hyperthyroidism -diabetes Congenital heart disease – incidence around 50% Growth delay Obstructive sleep apnoea – incidence: 30–75% Gastrointestinal Occur in about 5% Cervical spine disorders – X-ray **not** predictive	Stubborn Obsessional Dislike of conflict *Under 20 years* 17.6% psychiatric disorder ADHD Anxiety ASD Conduct/ oppositional Aggression
Fragile X Xq27.3 Triplet repeat – CGG >200 Fragile X 55–100 pre-mutation	1:4,000–1:6,000 Most common inherited form of LD 80% of males have LD	Can be difficult to detect Clinically large head, long face and prominent ears Connective tissue dysplasia leading to joint laxity and heart valve problems Vision problems Hearing problems Problems with numeracy and visual spatial skills Issues for both male and females with a pre-mutation	Social anxiety and aversion to eye contact Anxiety Hand flapping ADHD Aggression ASD – 30% (SIB especially hand biting) Those without autism said to be socially more responsive and affectionate

(Continued)

Table 14.3 (Continued)

Condition	*Comment*	*Physical Findings*	*Behaviour/Mental Health*
Prader–Willi Autosomal deletion 70% (father) Uniparental disomy 25% (mother) Rest-imprinting centre defects and unbalanced translocations	Incidence: 1:29,000 15q11-13	Severe hypotonia at birth Growth/nutrition – FTT in infancy and obesity due to excessive appetite and hyperphagia develops between 1 and 6 years of age Hypogonadism	Changes in routine leading to temper tantrums leading to aggression and severe behavioural problems SIB – skin picking Obsessional traits Impulsivity ASD
Rett 95% due to MECP2 gene on the X chromosome	1:10,000–1:23,000	Breathing irregularities Repetitive hand movements Epilepsy (about 50%) with EEG abnormalities Unsteady gait (about 50% become independently mobile), scoliosis Muscles more rigid as age leading to joint deformity Feeding difficulties and growth retardation Gut-reflux and constipation	Self-injurious behaviour Sleep difficulties Anxiety Mood changes Teeth grinding
Rubinstein–Taybi	1:125,000 55% due to deletion in 16p13 5% due to changes in 22q13 Rest not known as yet	Feeding difficulties Gastro-oesophageal reflux CHD Vision problems Constipation High pain threshold Dislike loud noises	Sleep problems (? secondary to breathing difficulties) Happy and friendly Dislike change in routine Short concentration span Rock, spin and flap
Smith–Lemli–Opitz Gene mutation – autosomal recessive	Incidence: 1:20,000 to 30,000 Mutations in DHCR 7 gene on 11q13 Inborn error of cholesterol synthesis	Webbing of toes Dysmorphic facial features Microcephaly CHD	Sleep difficulties SIB ASD

(*Continued*)

Table 14.3 (Continued)

Condition	*Comment*	*Physical Findings*	*Behaviour/Mental Health*
Smith Magenis ? due to a single gene defect	Birth prevalence of 1:25,000 Deletion of 17p11	Infantile hypotonia Failure to thrive (FTT) as an infant Congenital heart disease (CHD) Vision and hearing problems 75% peripheral neuropathy resulting in insensitivity to pain	Severe sleep problems-settling, wakening and shortened length Severe challenging behaviour, temper tantrums and severe aggression Features of ADHD Self-mutilation
Tuberous sclerosis complex Gene mutation	1:6,000 Spontaneous mutation in 70% Autosomal dominant in 30% Two genes – TSC1 (9q34) TSC2 (16p13.3)	Multi-system disorder Brain, kidneys, heart, eyes, skin, teeth, bone, lung and others 50–60% LD	Sleep difficulties 25% ASD ADHD SIB Adolescents/adults-anxiety and depression
Williams syndrome Autosomal deletion	Incidence 1:7,500–1:20,000 Deletion of 7q11.23	Hypercalcemia in infancy (15%) FTT, feeding difficulties and short stature Congenital heart disease – supravalvular problems Kidney problems Constipation Hyperacusis Cocktail chatter Dental caries	Abnormal attachment behaviours as infants Sleep difficulties Anxiety and fears Preoccupations and obsessions Highly sociable/overly friendly particularly with adults Overactivity, poor concentration and distractible

- Medical assessment and investigations to ensure that there are no underlying physical health problems that may be impacting on the child's behaviour, particularly if there is self-injury
- Observations across environments
- Interview with child/young person, when possible
- Parental knowledge
- Interviews with other professionals
- Use of standardised behavioural measures where applicable, e.g. The Developmental Behaviour Checklist (Einfeld and Tonge, 1992)
- Information gathering from previous assessments
- Are there any child protection concerns?

The professional will need to employ a range of strategies to engage the child/young person as much as possible in the assessment, taking into consideration factors such as any additional special needs of the child, e.g. sensory difficulties, communication style and ability.

The environment in which such assessments are undertaken should be afforded careful consideration. Often simply accessing unfamiliar environments, e.g. the CAMHS clinic or GP surgery, can be anxiety-provoking for children and young people with learning disabilities. A more suitable environment may be the child's home or school environment where they are familiar with the surroundings and the people supporting them.

A highly specialist set of skills is required to carry out such assessments. Alongside a thorough understanding of the needs of children and young people with learning disabilities, those involved in the assessment process should understand the genetic, neurological and social predispositions of this client group to mental health problems. A sound knowledge base of developmental disorders, particularly ADHD and ASD, due to their high co-morbidity in children and young people with learning disabilities, is required (McDougall, 2006).

Diagnostic Overshadowing

This is where a child's presenting symptom(s) may be attributed to their learning disability, rather than to a potentially treatable cause. If the child develops a new, troubling behaviour or a behaviour he already has becomes worse, consider:

- **Physical**: pain from a tooth, ear infection, reflux, constipation or a deterioration in vision or hearing
- **Psychological**: depression, anxiety, psychosis
- **Social**: abuse, bereavement, change in carers

Interventions

Whilst the evidence relating to the mental health needs of children and young people with learning disabilities is growing, it remains in its infancy. At present, there is no significant body of evidence relating to the effectiveness of interventions for treating the mental health problems of children and young people with learning disabilities. There is no reason to suggest that children and young people with learning disabilities will respond any differently to the biological, psychological, educational and social interventions currently employed for children and young people without learning disabilities.

Such interventions rarely refer to the age of the child. A CAMHS service working with children and young people between the ages of 5 and 16 is likely to cover a 'developmental range' from the 4-year level to the 20-year level. Most young people with learning disabilities, despite their chronological age, are likely to fall within this developmental range: the exception being children and young people with severe and profound levels of learning disability.

Interventions can be made accessible in two ways:

- Age-appropriate intervention is chosen and modified to make it developmentally appropriate.
- Developmentally appropriate intervention is chosen and then modified to make it age appropriate.

In addition, many CAMHS interventions, e.g. parental training and family therapy, are directed towards parents and carers, rather than the child. Such interventions are not dependent on the child's ability to engage.

Treatment Options for Medical Conditions Associated with Behavioural Difficulties and Learning Disability (Tables 14.4 and 14.5)

Table 14.4 Treatment Options for Medical Conditions Associated with Behavioural Difficulties and Learning Disability

Condition	*Interventions Considered Effective*	*Consideration for Children and Young People with Learning Disabilities*
Anxiety disorder	• Behavioural interventions and CBT are first-line treatment (see Cognitive Behaviour Therapy) • Involvement of parents is recommended • Psycho educational approaches for managing anxiety	There is strong evidence for behavioural interventions with children and young people with learning disabilities, and they are often the intervention of choice. Cognitive approaches will be affected by the child's ability but cognitive approaches can be used with children under ten years of age.
ADHD	• Behaviourally based parent management training • Behavioural interventions across settings • Alterations to environment • Medication • Teaching of coping strategies to the child	Parent management training is dependent upon engagement of parents, as with typically developing peers. There is no evidence to suggest response to medication is any different for children with learning disabilities, although consideration would need to be given to its interaction with any other medication the child may be taking.

Table 14.5 Treatment Options

Condition	*Investigation*	*Treatment*	
Reflux	pH probe Barium swallow and follow through Endoscopy	Environmental Drugs	Raise head off bed 6–8 inches Gaviscon, H2 blocker Domperidone/omeprazole Surgery
Unsafe swallow	Videofluoroscopy	Thicken liquids/mash food Gastrostomy	Dietetic involvement Surgery
Constipation	History Rarely X-ray	Fluids and dietary manipulation Laxatives	NICE guidelines
Pain	Dependent where?	Pain relief	
Dental pain	Dentist	Pain relief Dental treatment	Preventative-fluoride
Sleep problems	History Investigations undertaken at home/overnight stay	Good sleep hygiene Medication Sleep clinic	Straightforward Vallergan/melatonin More complex Use of sedatives/atypical antipsychotics (i.e. risperidone) can be considered but under specialist supervision, high risk of side effects and possible worsening of the symptoms
Epilepsy	Eye-witness account of the episode(s) Electro encephalogram (ECG)	Medication Vagus nerve stimulation (VNS) Diet	
Visual difficulties	Ophthalmological opinion	Glasses	Special teacher advisor for children with visual impairment Special classroom aids
Hearing difficulties	Audiology opinion	Refer to ear nose and throat specialist	Hearing aids STA children with hearing impairment
Sensory difficulties	Occupational therapy sensory assessment	Sensory diet/ programme	
Hyperacusis	Audiology/ENT assessment	Acoustic training	

Case Study (1): Amy

Amy (ten) has a mild learning disability, autism and epilepsy. She lives at home with her mother and younger sister and attends a mainstream school with additional support. Amy was referred to the local CAMHS team by her GP due to a high level of challenging behaviour that was placing her at risk of exclusion from her school placement. Amy's behaviour had a considerable impact upon her family. Her mother had given up work to provide additional care for Amy, placing extra financial stress upon the family, and she had been prescribed antidepressants by her GP. Amy's sister's sleep and education were affected by her behaviour. She experienced many sleepless nights and was falling asleep in her lessons at school.

A detailed assessment and functional analysis led to the development of a behaviour programme that was implemented across environments. Changes to Amy's environment, the introduction of communication systems, the use of scheduling, teaching of relaxation skills and the introduction of reward systems were some of the techniques used.

The interventions brought about positive changes in Amy's behaviour that both prevented an exclusion from school and increased the opportunities available to her, because she was able to start accessing after-school activities. A more settled education placement meant that Amy's mother was able to seek part-time employment. Reduction in challenging behaviours at home meant that Amy's sister was able to settle into a healthy sleep routine, improving her alertness at school. A considerable increase in her academic achievement was noted. The all-round reduction of stress and anxiety meant that Amy's mother was able to speak with her GP about no longer needing antidepressants.

Case Study (2): Joe

Joe (four) has autism and a severe learning disability (SLD). Joe has historically presented with self-injurious behaviour in the form of head-banging. He does not have any words and only situational understanding. A detailed history was taken from his mother and it appears that Joe has lost his appetite recently and when examined, had not gained any weight. Although he has been opening his bowels every other day, his stools are 'like rabbit droppings' (Bristol Stool Chart Type 1). He has faecal masses when his abdomen is palpated.

A dietary sheet and advice about fluid intake are given to his mother. Copies are given to his special school and his respite carer. Laxatives were started, as per NICE guidelines, and a bowel chart instituted. On review, Joe is now opening his bowels regularly, his self-injurious behaviour has greatly reduced and he is putting on weight. His diet remains restricted, but with the intervention of a learning disability nurse, occupational therapist and speech and language therapy, he has begun to extend the range of food he eats.

Conclusion

Children and young people with learning disabilities are exposed to higher risk factors impacting upon their mental health than their typically developing peers. Awareness of this and an understanding of the epidemiology and aetiology of learning disability are crucial when considering the mental health and/or behavioural challenges of this population group. A thorough assessment of need requires a specialist skill set and input from many disciplines if an appropriate understanding of the difficulties is to be reached and an effective care plan developed.

Multiple-Choice Questions

See answers on page 667.

1. A diagnosis of learning disability is traditionally applied in practice when an individual's IQ score falls below:
    a. 90
    b. 80
    c. 70

2. Approximately how many children and young people with learning disabilities will develop mental health problems?
   a. 40%
   b. 30%
   c. 10%
3. Which mental health problem is more prevalent amongst children and young people with learning disabilities?
   a. Psychosis
   b. Anorexia nervosa
   c. Anxiety disorder
4. Which intervention is often the treatment of choice when managing challenging behaviour in children and young people with learning disabilities?
   a. Pharmacological interventions
   b. Family therapy
   c. Behavioural interventions

Key References and Weblink

Bernard, S., (2010). Epidemiology and aetiology. In R. Raghavan, S. Bernard and J. McCarthy (Eds.), *Mental Health Needs of Children and Young People with Learning Disabilities.* Brighton: Pavilion Publishing.

Department of Health, (2001). *Valuing People: A New Strategy for Learning Disability for the 21st Century.* London: The Stationary Office.

Emerson, E., (1995). *Challenging Behaviour: Analysis and Intervention in People with Learning Disabilities.* Cambridge: Cambridge University Press.

Emerson, E., (1998). Working with People with Challenging Behaviour. *Clinical Psychology and People with Intellectual Disabilities*, 127–153.

Emerson, E. and Bromley, J., (1995). The Form and Function of Challenging Behaviours. *Journal of Intellectual Disability Research: JIDR*, 39(5): 388–398.

Emerson, E., McGill, P. and Mansell, J., (2013). *Severe Learning Disabilities and Challenging Behaviours: Designing High Quality Services.* Springer.

Emmerson and Hatton 2007, Hatton, C. and Emerson, E., (1995). Staff in Services for People with Learning Disabilities: An Overview of Current Issues. *Mental Handicap Research*, 8(4): 215–219.

15 Speech and Language Disorders

Janet Stephens

Introduction

Language is not learned in a vacuum. It evolves through an interactive process incorporating significant adults and a responsive environment.

> **KEY CONCEPTS**
>
> - Communication is an interactive process.
> - Speech and language development is affected by several factors: medical, sensory, environmental, social, behavioural and/or emotional.
> - Speech and language development follows a chronology across six domains: attention and listening, play, understanding, spoken language, speech sounds, pragmatics.
> - Speech and language development can be delayed or disordered.
> - Research indicates a high level of co-occurrence of speech and language difficulties with emotional and behaviour problems in children.
> - Language disorder is a predictor of later psychiatric or mental health problems.

Speech and language concerns in children may be manifested through:

- Emotional and behavioural difficulties
- Dysfluency
- Selective mutism
- Pragmatic language disorders
- Poor receptive and expressive language skills

Research indicates that the neonate is motivated to communicate and is born 'hard-wired' to do so. Noam Chomsky, an American linguist, identified what he called a 'Language Acquisition Device' that he defined as an innate capacity to learn language, often despite adverse environmental, medical and social factors. Language acquisition takes place within the context of securely attached relationships, usually with one or two primary caregivers in the first instance. These adults will support, imitate and reciprocate the baby's early movements and vocalisations, to enable the child to move from pre-intentional communication at birth to intentional interaction within a few months of birth. At just 17 minutes old a child is able to imitate his father poking his tongue out (Social Baby DVD).

Recent progress in brain-imaging and scanning techniques has enabled us to observe the damaging effect of the lack of attachment on the size and capacity of the developing infant brain. Secure relationships help to promote the intentionality of communication, which means that it is vital for parents and care-givers to be made aware of the importance of talking with babies, even if the perception is that 'babies don't talk back'. There are thought to be several 'windows of opportunity' for speech and language development during the child's early years, but by three years of age, the critical window for speech development begins to close.

It is known that the time spent in carer–child joint attention predicts subsequent vocabulary growth. Research indicates that children from high-talking families have, at three years of age, at least three times more receptive vocabulary, i.e. words understood, than peers from low-talking families and consequently at least twice as many words in their own spoken vocabulary (Hart and Risley, 1995). From the beginning, 'communication, language and thinking are rooted in relationship' (EYFS, 2007).

Communication is fundamentally interactive in that it requires reciprocity by both communication partners. Communication does not happen when a child is playing a computer game or spends hours watching television programmes or DVDs alone. It involves the passing of verbal and non-verbal messages. It is believed that approximately 80% of human communication is non-verbal. Speech and language skills develop within this broader context of communication. The symbolic system known as 'language' comprises six specific components that combine to represent meaning within a culture.

These elements are:

- Phonology (sound system)
- Prosody (rhythm and intonation)
- Syntax (grammatical structures)
- Morphology (grammar)
- Semantics (meaning of words)
- Pragmatics (language in social context)

Bloom and Lahey devised a model to illustrate the relationship between the component parts of communication in children who are developing their language skills normally (Figure 15.1).

Language learning is a unique and individualised process. It follows a chronology from birth to approximately seven years of age, but there is a wide range of what would be considered 'normal' development (Learning to Talk ICAN DVD).

Significant language problems will be identified for approximately 7–10% of the pre-school population in England and Wales. Research has indicated several significant factors that may affect a child's language development.

Medical Factors

- Prematurity.
- Birth trauma, e.g. cerebral palsy.
- Epilepsy.
- Chromosomal disorders, e.g. Down's syndrome.
- Impaired sensory input should be considered, i.e. visual impairment and/or hearing impairment, from fluctuating or intermittent glue ear, to a more permanent sensory-neural loss.

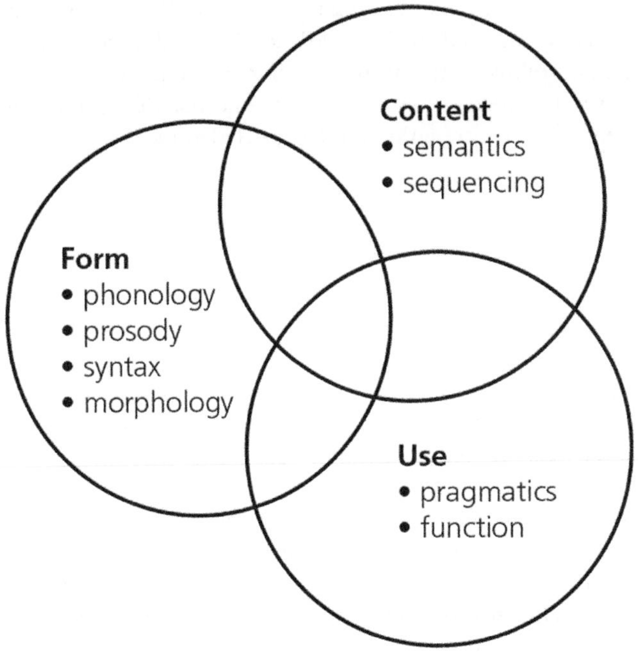

Figure 15.1 Content, form and use of speech.

Environmental and Social Factors

- Mother/carer–child interaction.
- Parenting style.
- Home environment and socio-economic status.
- Mother's level of education and her access to a support network.

Familial Factors

- Gender – boys are twice as likely to have speech and language problems as girls.
- Position within the family.
- Family history of speech and language difficulties.

Behavioural Factors

- Attachment difficulties.
- ADHD-type presentations.

Cultural Factors

- Learning language as a bi- or multi-lingual speaker.
- Cultural-specific attitudes to 'play'.

Language skills are assessed and monitored across six domains, and difficulties in one or more of these areas may result in a diagnosis of speech and/or language delay or disorder. Speech and language development is described as 'delayed' if the child's level of skill is below that expected for their chronological age, but following the normal developmental pattern.

Speech and language development is described as 'disordered' if the normal developmental pattern is not followed and an uneven profile of strengths and deficits is identified.

The **six domains** considered are:

- Attention and listening
- Play skills
- Understanding (receptive language)
- Spoken language (expressive language)
- Speech sounds
- Social use of language (pragmatic language)

Skills develop between birth and seven years of age, following a recognised chronology and pattern, in each of these areas.

A growing body of research evidence has linked language difficulties with a variety of emotional and behavioural problems. Poor receptive and expressive language skills are frequently present in the populations of excluded school children and among young offenders. There is a growing awareness of the occurrence of undetected communication difficulties among children with behavioural, emotional and social difficulties (BESD). Studies suggest the incidence of communication difficulties in this group to be between 55% and 100% (Giddan et al., 1996). Several longitudinal studies show that, in the absence of appropriate support, these children are more likely to develop associated behavioural difficulties than their peers.

A recent report by Stringer, Lozano and Dodd (2003) indicates that the rates of behaviour difficulties reported in children with speech and language disorders are around 50%, compared with 10% in the 'normally developing' population. As they grow older, these children are more at risk of poor emotional health and have a stronger likelihood of mental health problems in adulthood (Clegg et al., 1999). These young people may have difficulties in understanding complex instructions and expressing their emotions and feelings verbally. Intervention may focus on improving listening skills and on building self-esteem. In mainstream schools, the speech and language therapist may contribute to the behaviour programme delivered by the emotional literacy support assistants (ELSA).

All research indicates that language disorders are more closely associated with behaviour difficulties than speech disorders. Language disorder has been shown as a predictor of later psychiatric problems.

How Do Emotional and Behavioural Difficulties Manifest Themselves in Speech and Language Problems Assessed at Community Clinics and in Schools?

Dysfluency or stammering has a multi-factorial basis that considers environmental, linguistic, medical and psychological factors and examines how difficulties in some, or all, of these areas may trigger a stammer in particular individuals. It is a disorder principally of childhood. Approximately 5% of the population of three-year olds at any time are likely to develop a stammer. Of these, 2% will recover spontaneously, 2% will either recover or develop sufficient compensatory strategies to manage the stammer well and 1% will stammer into adulthood.

Therapeutic intervention will initially consider parent–child interaction strategies, often through the medium of video-footage and subsequent discussion between the parents and the speech and language therapist. The outcome of these discussions may lead to modifications to family routines or expectations that remove or reduce the environmental or psychological triggers to stammering. Other interventions will be designed to devise ways to enable the child to better balance emotional or linguistic demands with his current capacity and skill level.

Selective mutism is defined in the DSM-5 (2013) as 'a persistent failure to speak in specific social situations, despite being able to speak in other more familiar situations'. Intervention may consider a behavioural approach to reducing the child's anxiety, comprising a systematic, stepped progression, changing one variable at a time, simultaneously maintaining a consistent approach within the environment where the child is not talking and gradually enabling the child to become an active partner in the treatment process (see *The Selective Mutism Resource Manual*).

Pragmatic language disorder may co-occur with symptoms of autistic spectrum disorder (ASD) or may present as a discrete specific language impairment. Difficulties include problems with verbal reasoning, understanding and using higher level language skills, such as inference, e.g. the picture of a boy sitting in a bath wearing his clothes and the question 'Why is this funny?', and responding appropriately rather than literally, to idiomatic language, e.g. 'Pull your socks up'. Therapeutic intervention may work on social skills training, e.g. 'Talkabout', the use of visual prompts and timetables, to reinforce spoken instructions and reduce anxiety about routines and developing 'social stories' to prepare the child for change and transition or to modify a socially unacceptable behaviour.

A recent Education and Skills Committee report (2005–06) noted a high correlation between children with special educational needs and youth crime. In a recent study, 25% of young offenders had been identified as having special educational needs. More specifically, between 50 and 60% of the UK prison population has been identified as having literacy difficulties, compared with 17% of the general population. At least half of these offenders have speaking and listening skills at a basic level, but appropriate training and support to develop their oral communication skills have been shown to help reduce recidivism. Recent research indicates that approximately 40% of young offenders are likely to have difficulty with mediation involving spoken language (Bryan K., 2004).

Multiple-Choice Questions

See answers on page 667.

1. What are the optimal conditions for a baby to begin to develop his communication skills?
    a. Spending time in a room with noisy adults with the television on.
    b. Spending time with parents who make efforts to include their baby in all social interactions and talk to their baby about everyday events and routines.
    c. Spending time with a series of different adult carers who have no relationship with the baby.
    d. Mother has post-natal depression and has struggled to bond with her child.
    e. Spending hours in front of the television with no adult support.
2. What is meant by 'interactive' when describing communication?
    a. It just happens like all other aspects of development.
    b. If you leave the child alone, he will learn by himself.
    c. There is no point talking to a baby as he cannot talk back.
    d. Both communication partners are engaged in the conversation.
    e. A baby will learn by watching television.
    f. He will learn to talk at nursery.

3. What factors should we consider when speech and language development goes wrong?
    a. Prematurity, family history and glue ear.
    b. Parents cannot read or write well.
    c. Family has not engaged with any support services.
    d. He is lazy.
    e. Father has a strong Scottish accent.
4. What presentations might you see in a child with 'pragmatic language disorder'?
    a. Unable to say words beginning with 's'.
    b. Engages in long conversations with familiar adults.
    c. Responds appropriately to questions.
    d. Chooses not to speak at school.
    e. Stammers on the first word in the sentence.
    f. When told by his teacher to 'pull your socks up' with reference to working harder for his exams, he interprets this literally and does what he has been asked to do.
5. Which would be a valid therapeutic intervention for pre-school dysfluency?
    a. Practise saying words beginning with 't' daily.
    b. Take Calpol three times a day.
    c. Apply for the X-Factor.
    d. Parent–child interactions filmed and then discussed to change environmental behaviours at home.
    e. Wait for the child to 'grow out of it'.

Key References

Bryan, K., (2004). Preliminary Study of the Prevalence of Speech and Language Difficulties in Young Offenders. *International Journal of Communication and Language Disorders*, 39(3).

Davison, F. and Howlin, P., (1997). A Follow-Up Study of Children Attending A Primary Age Language Unit. *European Journal of Disorders of Communication: The Journal of the College of Speech and Language Therapists, London*, 32(1).

Law, J., (Ed), (1992). *The Early Identification of Language Impairment in Children*. London: Chapman and Hall.

16 Feeding/Eating Problems in Young Children

Liz McCaughey, Sue Evans and Margaret J.J. Thompson

KEY CONCEPTS

- Eating problems in children are fairly common.
- Children who have developmental delay, severe learning difficulties or neurological difficulties may have additional needs that require a more specialist approach.
- Here we consider children with normal or slightly delayed development.
- Support to the child and parent is essential when instigating a management plan.

Introduction

This is a common problem and may include:

- Refusal of solids, i.e. texture
- Poor appetite/disinterest, i.e. quantity
- Faddiness, i.e. limited range
- Immature oral motor skills
- Poor table behaviour
- Lack of age appropriate self-feeding, i.e. delayed development
- Eating of inappropriate objects, i.e. pica
- Failure to thrive

Over 30% of five-year olds are described as having mild or moderate eating or appetite problems (Butler and Golding (1986), 16% of three-year olds had a poor appetite and 12% were thought to be 'faddy' (Ridwan (1982).

Aetiology

Early Aversive Feeding Experience

- Organic, e.g. vomiting, gagging, choking, reflux or pain associated with eating or drinking
- Force fed or reprimanded while eating
- Parent anxious/angry while feeding the child
- Experience of sensitivity reaction or bowel change, e.g. diarrhoea or constipation

Distortion of Feeding Experiences

- Lack of early oral feeding experience due to alternative feeding methods, e.g. early use of nasogastric tube or gastrostomy feeding
- Immature oral motor skills or oral hypersensitivity
- Late introduction of solids, i.e. later than a year old
- Parents' refusal to let the child self-feed

Parental Emotional State

- Frustration
- Depression
- Loss of confidence
- Anxiety

Maintaining Factors

- Parental management
- Parent/child relationship, family/marital problems
- Child's learned avoidance or fear of food
- Child's general behaviour problems

Assessment

Physical Setting

- Seating arrangements
- Eating implements used.
- Type and quantity of food offered/taken. It is helpful to keep a food diary.
- Time taken for solids and drinks.

Child's Behaviour/Skills

- Symptoms
- Interest and anticipation
- Desire/ability to self-feed/drink
- Quantity, texture and range eaten
- Ability to concentrate and persevere with eating
- Oromotor skills
- Psychical parameters, e.g. growth, height and weight, and nutritional state should be assessed, e.g. iron levels

Parents' Behaviour

- Control
- Management methods used, e.g. force, passive attitude
- Encouragement, distraction
- Emotional state, e.g. frustration, anger
- Awareness of child's needs and demands

Eating Management

- Dietary advice
- Enhancing oral motor skills
- Eating arrangements, i.e. seating, implements, social setting
- Eating management methods

Behavioural Management

Graded Approaches

- Introduce new foods. Variety, then increase textures.
- Introduce solids. NB Stage 2 foods, e.g. coarse puree, liquids plus lumps and mixed textures are more complicated to take/cope with.
- May be better to use mashed home food to give uniform texture. Otherwise, lumps will be spat out.
- Increase quantity.
- Improve concentration and sitting.
- Encourage self-feeding.
- Monitor oral motor control.
- Reduce oral hypersensitivity.

Setting the Scene

- Establish regular mealtimes. No snacks or not within two hours of the meal. Some children need snacks, and they can be useful for weight gain or developing oral skills. Expect the child to sit at the table to eat.
- Family should eat together, whenever possible.
- Appropriate portion size.
- Remove distractions. Orientate child's attention to food, i.e. no TV.

Reinforcement

Positive praise and rewards for:

- Finishing
- Trying a new food
- Sitting down
- Eating solids
- Self-feeding

Extinction

- Ignore non-eating
- Ignore demands for different foods or presentation
- Ignore disruption
- Time limits on length of meal, e.g. 30 minutes maximum
- Avoid aversive situations

Pica

It is normal for infants and young children to mouth, and occasionally eat, strange things, but pica is when a child regularly and excessively eats inappropriate substances, e.g. soil, paper, wood, cloth or paint. Pica has many causes, including adverse environmental circumstances and emotional distress. It may be associated with distorted developmental patterns and learning difficulty. Iron-deficiency anaemia may result, and lead levels may be elevated. This used to be associated with lead-containing paints, but fortunately this is seen much less frequently now. Lead levels should be measured to exclude lead poisoning and its sequelae. Management of pica will depend on the nature of the problems but should **never** be ignored

Feeding Difficulties and Failure to Thrive

Child Factors

Organic disorders including:

- Metabolic disorders
- Neuro-muscular disorders
- Immunological disorders
- Medical factors, e.g. cardiac or renal
- Developmental level
- Health status
- Growth, height and weight

Feeding Problems

- Neglect and abuse
- Parental management
- Lack of knowledge
- Lack of oromotor skills
- Lack of experience
- Anxiety
- Early feeding experience
- Family discord
- Depression

Mealtime Observations Check List

Environment

- Which room is used?
- Are there distractions, e.g. TV, noise, room temperature too hot or too cold?
- Behaviour of others, e.g. sibling 'playing up', mother cooking other food, other distractions?

Child's Seating (Posture, Support, Head Control)

- Is the child sitting in a high chair, on a booster seat on an adult upright chair, on a cushion on an upright adult chair, adult upright chair, easy chair or sofa, child's low chair?

- Are the child's feet resting on the floor or a foot-rest?
- Is the child's plate on a table or food tray? If not, where is it?
- How high is the table surface? Below waist/waist level/above waist?
- Does the child have to hold his/her arms up high to reach the plate?

Child's Implements

- Is the drink in a bottle, feeder cup or open cup? Is there a straw? Does the child hold the container or is it held by the person feeding the child?
- Does the child have a bowl or a plate, an adult bowl or plate, teaspoon, child's knife, fork and spoon or adult cutlery?
- Does the parent/carer cut/mash/feed the food?
- Is there a non-slip mat, child's own placemat, keep-warm plate, finger food?

Position of Child

- Is the child fed or does he/she eat on their own?
- Are other family members also eating?
- Where are those other people sitting, around the same table? In the same room?
- Is the parent/carer sitting next to/opposite/behind the child?

Food and Drink Given

- Is the child's meal the same as the rest of the family? (Record what is offered and the amount.)
- Is the texture mashed or whole?
- How long is the child given to eat?
- How long do the rest of the family spend eating?
- How much food does the child actually eat, e.g. mouthful/half the plateful?
- Does the child feed him/herself or is he/she fed? No/a little/a lot?

Child's Behaviour

- Does the child refuse or delay coming to the meal?
- Does the child seem uninterested in the food?
- Is the child physically awkward feeding him/herself in that situation? Is he/she interested in feeding themselves?
- Is the child easily distracted or finding it hard to concentrate?
- Is the child fidgety?
- Does the child refuse to eat when fed, e.g. keeps mouth closed, pushes spoon away?
- In what way?

Parents' Behaviour

- Does the parent offer encouragement? Positive or negative?
- Is the parent tolerant/patient? Too much/adequately/too little?
- Is there some opportunity for the child to eat independently? Too much/ appropriately/ too little?
- Is the parent aware of the child's needs and demands? Too much/appropriately/too little?

- How does the parent try to intervene, e.g. feeding the child, forcing, distracting, playing games, e.g. 'airplane', encouraging, shouting, any other ways?
- Who is controlling the situation? Mostly the child/equally/mostly the parent?

Multiple-Choice Questions

See answers on page 667.

1. When helping a family whose child has an eating problem, what routines may help?
   a. Allow the child to eat alone.
   b. Establish a routine, eat together, ensure appropriate portion size and remove distractions.
   c. Encourage them to sit still whilst eating.
   d. Offer small amounts frequently.
2. What should you observe during a mealtime observation?
   a. The environment, the implements
   b. The child's sitting position and the food and drink offered
   c. The parents' and child's behaviour
   d. All of the above
3. What factors may contribute to a child developing a feeding or eating problem?
   a. Organic difficulties
   b. Parental anxiety
   c. Abuse or neglect
   d. All of the above

Key Reference

Nicholls, D.E., Lynn, R. and Russell, M., (2011). Viner Childhood Eating Disorder: British National Surveillance Study. *The British Journal of Psychiatry*, 198, 295–301.

17 Constipation and Soiling

Melissa Bracewell (updated by Margaret J.J. Thompson)

KEY CONCEPTS

- Soiling is usually caused by constipation and overflow but can result from fast bowel transit time with resulting loose stools and urgency of defecation, or poor wiping after bowels are opened.
- Medical treatment of the above conditions should always be started before, or alongside, behavioural treatments. Treatments include education, improvement in diet and toileting, in addition to laxatives when constipation is present.
- Long-term soiling has a significant impact on self-esteem, behaviour and social isolation.

Definition

Constipation is generally defined as passing a stool fewer than three times a week. Stools are usually hard, dry and difficult to pass.

The ROME III consensus (2006); Rasquin et al. (2006) gives a more detailed definition of constipation based on the presence of two or more of the following criteria in the previous two months in a child with a developmental age of at least four years:

- Two or fewer defecations in the toilet a week
- More than one episode of faecal incontinence, i.e. 'soiling', a week
- A history of retentive posturing or excessive volitional stool retention
- A history of painful or hard bowel movements
- A history of large-diameter stools that may obstruct the toilet
- Presence of large faecal mass in rectum

Soiling is the involuntary passage of small amounts of stools, resulting in staining of underwear.

Encopresis is the active passage of stools in inappropriate places after the age when bowel control is normally expected. In older children, encopresis can be associated with oppositional defiant disorder, conduct disorder or sexual abuse. Constipation, soiling and encopresis must be assessed and treated in primary care and/or secondary paediatric services for constipation and soiling before referral to child mental health services (CAMHS).

Incidence/Prevalence

Worldwide prevalence of childhood constipation in the general population ranges from 0.7 to 29.6%, in both boys and girls (Van Den Berg et al., 2006). It becomes chronic in over one-third of children (Bardisa-Ezcurra et al., 2010).

Causes

In 95% of children with constipation no pathological cause is found. The following underlying causes should be considered, but rarely need to lead to investigations.

- **Anatomical**, e.g. imperforate anus, anal stenosis, Hirsprung's disease
- **Metabolic**, e.g. hypothyroid, hypercalcaemia, hypokalaemia, cystic fibrosis, poorly controlled insulin dependent diabetes mellitus (IDDM)
- **Gastroenterological**, e.g. coeliac disease, inflammatory bowel disease
- **Neurological**, e.g. abnormal spinal or lower limb neurology, muscle weakness/wasting disorders
- **Drugs**, including iron, anticholinergics, opioid analgesics, some antihistamines and anticonvulsants

Soiling is rarely a psychological problem and should always be assessed for these causes before referring to psychology services.

- Constipation and stool holding with leakage of runny stools around impacted faecal mass. Soiling is involuntary, and the child is often unaware of it. Stool is often very offensive smelling to everyone but the child.
- Fast bowel transit time leading to loose stools per rectum and urgency toileting, with stool leakage before toilet is reached.
- Poor wiping after defecation.

Assessment

History

- Age of onset of problem. If constipation started at one month old or less and any delay in passage of meconium >48 hours needs referral to a hospital paediatric service.
- How long has the child had a problem with stools?
- Stool pattern: <three per week, type 1–2 stools on Bristol Stool Chart suggests constipation. The child may have soiling with type 6–7 stools.

  Two or more stools per 24 hours with type 5–6 stools suggest fast bowel transit time.
- Ask about defecation, any pain, straining, blood on paper. Ribbon-like stools suggest possible bowel pathology.
- Ask about fluid intake and diet.
- Drug history is very important. Medications can cause constipation.
- Is there a history of any problems with toilet training?
- Any recent change in family circumstances, e.g. a change of school/nursery, move of house, parental separation.
- A family history of similar problems.

Examination

- All children must have height and weight measured and plotted on growth charts. Any faltering growth suggests possibility, for instance, of inflammatory bowel disease, celiac disease, hypothyroid, cystic fibrosis.
- Abdominal examination is important, particularly for palpable faeces.
- An inspection of the anus, if the child is happy to be examined and child/parent gives informed consent, but digital rectal examination should only be performed by those professionals who can interpret the findings (Bardisa-Ezcurra et al., 2010).
- Inspection of spine, sacral area, gait and lower limb neurology.
- A general examination of other systems.

Investigations

- These are rarely needed, but may include blood tests: full blood count, U+E, LFT, ESR, TFT, celiac screen, immunoglobulins.
- Abdominal X-rays should not be performed in constipation.
- Marker transit study X-rays should not be performed, except in specialist centres.
- If there is any suggestion of infective cause for loose stools, send stool for culture.

Management

- Soiling and constipation will only resolve with treatment of the constipation with laxatives.
- Movicol Paediatric Plain is the recommended first laxative to be used for all children, some needing disimpaction regimes before regular doses (Bardisa-Ezcurra et al., 2010).
- If not tolerated, stimulant laxatives, usually Senna, can be substituted or added into the Movicol if/when the highest doses are ineffective.
- Rectal preparations are not normally recommended in the treatment of constipation and should only be used by specialists.
- Diet and fluid management, i.e. increasing fruit and vegetables and good fluid intake, should be given once constipation is improving to help prevent the problem recurring, but should not be first-line management.
- The child must be encouraged to sit on the toilet regularly, at least daily, in correct posture, i.e. child toilet seat and foot stool. Praise and encouragement should be given for sitting to try to defecate.

To help the child to understand the difficulties they are experiencing, a narrative approach can be helpful, e.g. 'beating Sneaky Poo', designed to help children co-operate when establishing toileting routines.

Case Study (1): Leo

Leo (11) has mild learning difficulties and poor school attendance. He has had constipation and soiling since he was first toilet trained. He has been seen by three different services for his problem and has had an admission to an inpatient unit for two months when he was six years old, where he made good progress initially, but relapsed on discharge.

Leo's mother died when he was five years old, and he lives with his father and paternal grandmother. He has given up any hope of improvement. He is bullied at school and often refuses to attend. When Leo does attend the clinic, he is found to be taking Senna syrup intermittently and refuses to accept any advice or change in management. After several appointments where Leo has the cause of his soiling explained using diagrams and internet education programmes, he agrees to start filling in simple bowel charts and to take his Senna regularly.

Several sessions later, Leo has had his Senna dose adjusted to produce a soft daily stool each morning after breakfast. His school attendance improves. The school staff support Leo with dealing with any bullying. He starts to lead the clinic appointments, showing his charts and discussing his medication.

Sadly, Leo's grandmother, who has been attending clinic, becomes unwell, and attendance at the clinic declines. The family is contacted and Leo's father agrees to take over supporting Leo with his management. It is difficult for Leo's father to attend appointments, and on-going contact is made by telephone and Leo continues to improve.

Case Study (2): Brian

Brian (seven), a looked after child, moves into the area to join new foster parents. He has daily soiling. He refuses to undress or wash for the first four weeks in his new placement. He is seen regularly by a child psychologist and his looked after children (LAC) nurse and after four weeks is undressing and bathing daily. His soiling continues despite good drinking, diet and regular toileting.

Brian will not discuss how often he has his bowels open or his stool type. Constipation is suspected by his LAC nurse and, with advice from a consultant paediatrician, Senna and Movicol PP are started.

Brian is seen weekly by his LAC nurse and starts to make some progress with his soiling. Eventually, Brian allows the LAC nurse to palpate his abdomen, and he is found to have obvious faecal impaction. Treatment is started with a Movicol PP disimpaction regime. Brian finds it a difficult process, but he is well supported by his foster parents. Following disimpaction with regular Senna and Movicol PP, Brian stops soiling and starts to slowly wean off his laxatives.

Over the summer holidays when the LAC nurse is on annual leave, Brian begins soiling again. His foster mother makes telephone contact with the consultant paediatrician, who advises an increase in laxative doses. SSD arrange an appointment with a private child psychiatrist who believes Brian's soiling is behavioural and stops all of Brian's laxative medication.

Brian's soiling worsens markedly. His foster mother is confused by the conflicting advice, but feels that, as Brian's soiling had improved with laxative treatment, to contact his LAC nurse. The laxative treatment is restarted and Brian makes good progress. He is able to start school in the autumn and has continuing support for his constipation from his LAC nurse and from CAMHS, for his behavioural issues.

Multiple-Choice Questions

See answers on page 667.

1. Soiling is usually a behavioural problem.
   True or False
2. Soiling can result in low self-esteem and poor school attendance.
   True or False
3. Children are often not aware when they have soiled their underwear.
   True or False
4. NICE guidelines recommend treatment of constipation with Senna and Movicol Paediatric Plain.
   True or False
5. Suppositories are commonly used in children with faecal impaction.
   True or False

Key References and Sources of Further Information

Bardisa-Ezcurra, L., Ullman, R., Gordon, J. and Guideline Development Group, (2010). Diagnosis and Management of Idiopathic Childhood Constipation: Summary of NICE Guidance. *BMJ: British Medical Journal*, 340: c2585.

Black, T., Poo Go Home and Williams I with Illustrations by Wright,Y Sneaky Poo Published as One Cartoon Book by ERIC on HealthUnlocked.

Guiraldes, E., Hyams, J.S., Staiano, A., Walker, L.S., Hyams, J.S., Staiano, A. and Walker, L. S., (2006). Childhood Functional Gastrointestinal Disorders: Child/Adolescent. *Gastroenterology*, 130(5): 1527–1537.

International Children's Continence Society, www.i-c-c-s.org.

NICE, (2010). *Guidelines Constipation in Children and Young People May 2010.* London: NICE.

Van Den Berg, M.M., Benninga, M.A. and Di Lorenzo, C., (2006). Epidemiology of Childhood Constipation: A Systematic Review. *American Journal of Gastroenterology*, 101(10): 2401–2409.

18 Enuresis

Melissa Bracewell (updated by Margaret J.J. Thompson)

KEY CONCEPTS

- Enuresis is very rarely deliberate or caused by behavioural/psychological problems. All children with enuresis should be offered assessment and medical treatment before referral to/treatment by CAMHS.
- Children with enuresis commonly have low self-esteem, disturbed sleep that can worsen challenging behaviour, poor concentration in school/home, that can mimic ADHD and suffer bullying in school. Treatment of enuresis has been shown to improve all of these areas.
- NICE guidelines for the treatment of nocturnal enuresis (May 2010) recommend treatment with bed-wetting alarms and/or Desmopressin, both of which have good success rates and are well tolerated by children and their parents (O'Flynn, 2011).

Definition

Enuresis is the intermittent loss of urine at night or intermittent leakage of urine when asleep, in a child of at least five years of age. (Neveus et al., 2010). It is known as 'primary' when the child has never been dry at night, or 'secondary' when the child has previously been dry at night for a continuous period of at least six months.

It can be monosymptomatic, i.e. when there are no other urinary symptoms, or non-monosymptomatic, i.e. when there are other urinary symptoms, e.g. daytime urgency, i.e. the inability to hold on, or frequency, i.e. voiding more than 7 times in 24 hours.

There are NO differences in the incidence of behaviour problems in children with enuresis and those who are dry at night (Neveus et al., 2010; Hirasing et al., 1997), but children with enuresis have low self-esteem and suffer bullying and social isolation. Night wetting can affect performance in school, and a study of children in Hong Kong showed an improvement in IQ of 10 points with successful treatment of enuresis.

Prevalence

- 10% of 10-year olds, 5% of 10-year olds and 1% of 19 year olds.
- Spontaneous resolution is common between the ages of five and seven years, but research has shown that five-year olds who wet more than three nights a week and seven-year olds with any wet nights will need treatment (McGee et al., 1984).

Causes

All children with bed-wetting are unable to wake at night to urinate in the toilet when their bladders are full. This poor arousal at night has been shown to be secondary to chronic tiredness because enuresis disturbs sleep. Arousal, sleep and performance in school improve with treatment of the enuresis (Yeung 2008).

Most children actually achieve dry beds whilst sleeping through the night, because the amount of urine produced overnight is held in the bladder until the morning.

Enuresis occurs when the amount of urine produced overnight exceeds the amount the bladder can hold and the child is unable to wake and urinate in the toilet.

There are therefore two subgroups of night wetting:

1. **Nocturnal polyuria**, i.e. large nocturnal urine production
    - Normal bladder function but large volumes of urine overnight, usually have abnormal circadian rhythm of ADH production, but very occasionally have increased solute excretion. Approximately 70% of cases.
2. **Children with small nocturnal bladder capacity**
    - Due to various types of bladder dysfunction, either only after sleep at night, or both, i.e. during day and night time. Approximately 30% of cases.

There is a strong genetic predisposition with a positive family history in 63% (von Gontar A, 2001).

Assessment

History

- Determine whether primary or secondary.
- Record severity: how many wet nights a week?
- Time night wetting occurs, i.e. wetting prior to between midnight and 1 a.m. is usually due to nocturnal polyuria.
- Amount of wetting: a large wet patch is usually due to nocturnal polyuria; a small patch is usually due to small bladder capacity.
- Number of wetting accidents a night, i.e. >once usually due to small bladder capacity.
- Ask about drinking habits, especially in the evening.
- Ask about sleeping arrangements, e.g. bunk or cabin beds, toilet access at night, fear of the dark.
- What, if any, previous treatments tried.
- Family history, past medical history, drug history and allergies.
- Any developmental problems, special needs or behavioural problems that may influence treatment recommendations.

Examination

- Not required in primary monosymptomatic enuresis.
- In non-monosymptomatic enuresis, if day symptoms do not resolve in three months with bladder training (good drinking and regular toileting during day), examine spine, lower limb neurology, abdomen and if possible, genitalia.

Investigations

- None needed in primary nocturnal enuresis.
- In secondary nocturnal enuresis, do urinalysis to exclude diabetes mellitus, urinary tract infection and renal disease.

Management

- Chart pattern of wet nights for one to two weeks.
- Chart day drink volumes and day voided volumes, i.e. measure wee into a measuring jug for 24 hours.
- Measure nocturnal urine volumes by
  - Waking child every two to three hours and recording voids in jug, sum and add first morning void.
  - Put child in nappy or pull-up until morning and measure first morning void in a jug. Nocturnal urine volume = weight of wet nappy in grams, weight dry nappy in grams + first morning void in ml.

First-Line Treatment

- Remove nappy or pull-up at night and stop parents lifting child at night to use the toilet, when not spontaneously roused to full bladder.
- Ensure child is able to use toilet easily at night, e.g. not on top bunk, toilet nearby and not on different storey of house, light on between bedroom and toilet.
- Stop blackcurrant, fizzy and caffeine drinks.
- Stop any drinks for two hours before sleep time and improve day drinking habits. Child should drink two glasses of water at each meal and one in between.
- Promote regular toileting, 1½ –2 hourly during day. Child must void just before sleep.

Second-Line Treatment

NICE guidelines (2010) recommend treatment with Desmopressin or alarms.

Logically, Desmopressin should be used for children with nocturnal polyuria. It is an analogue of ADH and will, if taken at sufficient dose, reduce night urine volumes until they no longer exceed bladder capacity and the child will then be sleeping through dry. It comes in two formulations tablets, preferred by over 12-year olds, and melts which dissolve under the tongue. Desmopressin nasal spray is no longer licensed for use in night wetting, because of the variability in absorption from the nasal mucosa. Treatment is given every night for three months. Sixty percent of children remain dry long term when Desmopressin is stopped. The rest begin Desmopressin again for as long as it is required, having breaks off medication every three months to assess whether it is still needed. Every year 15% will achieve long-term dry nights.

Alarm treatment should be used in children with small nocturnal bladder capacity. Historically, it was assumed that alarm treatment worked by teaching the child to wake to the sound of the alarm, until gradually the child could wake before wetting and was then dry. Research showed that only 35% of children achieved dry beds by waking to the alarm ringing, the remaining 65% were dry and sleeping through the night without the alarm ringing.

Further research showed that bladder capacity increased in children using alarm treatment until large enough to hold a normal overnight urine volume, thereby achieving dry nights (O'Flynn, 2011). Alarm treatment at night can help those with day symptoms from small bladder capacity. Sixty percent of children respond to alarm treatment, but only half of them remain dry six months later.

The most important factor in deciding which treatment to use is parental and child preference. Even if a child has obvious night polyuria, there is no point in using Desmopressin if the child/family do not want medication. Likewise, alarm treatment will not be used unless the child and family are prepared to wake to the alarm ringing.

It is common to combine treatments where one alone has not achieved dry nights.

Other treatments can be used in specialist centres.

Case Study (1): Lucy

Lucy (14), attends clinic after referral from her school nurse. She has always wet the bed, having had only the occasional dry night. Her mother, who attends clinic with her, wet the bed until she was 15 years old and so had never asked for help with Lucy's wetting.

Lucy was seen by the school nurse, because school staff had become concerned by a change in Lucy's concentration, mood and attendance at school. When seen, Lucy tells her school nurse that she has her first boyfriend and is anxious that he would find out about her bed-wetting. She had told her best friend, who laughed and teased her, threatening to tell her classmates at school. Since then, Lucy has been trying to avoid school and finds it difficult to concentrate as she is so anxious her classmates will find out about her bed-wetting. Lucy had not told her mother about any of her concerns.

At clinic, Lucy was delighted to hear that she could receive treatment for her bed wetting. Her charts showed that she was following good drinking and toileting routines. She had measured her night urine volumes that demonstrated nocturnal polyuria. She was offered treatment with either Desmopressin or an alarm, but was unwilling to use a bed-wetting alarm, feeling 'too old' for it.

Lucy started treatment with Desmopressin and returned to clinic dry three months later. She was delighted to report that she was completely dry. Her school attendance and performance improved.

Lucy had a trial of stopping the Desmopressin, but her wetting returned immediately. She restarted the Desmopressin for a further three months. Lucy was told that the Desmopressin could continue for as long as it was needed, as long as she had breaks off Desmopressin every three to six months to see whether it was still necessary.

Lucy continued to respond well to her treatment and was able to stop her Desmopressin after one year and was discharged from clinic.

Case Study (2): Jim

Jim (seven) attends clinic. He has a history of night wetting for the last year, having previously been dry from age three years. He is now wearing a pull-up. He has good drinking and toileting routines and no other medical problems. Screening tests exclude diabetes, UTI and other renal problems.

His mother reports a pattern of a few months of Jim having dry nights and then a period of wet nights. For the last three months, he has been wet every night. She and Jim do not know the time that he wets at night, nor the amount of wetting.

Jim is started on treatment with a bed-wetting alarm and makes excellent progress and returns to clinic dry. His mother asks to be discharged.

Three months later, Jim is referred back to clinic with a return of his night wetting and requests alarm treatment again. Jim and his mother are told about Desmopressin, but prefer not to use medication. An alarm is issued. Jim again makes good progress with the alarm, sleeping through the night, but unfortunately relapses.

Both parents attend Jim's next appointment. During the consultation, Jim has to be taken out of the clinic room by nursing staff when his mother starts shouting and behaving aggressively towards his father. She admits to mental health issues and agrees to approach her GP. Jim's father agrees to take over the management of Jim's night wetting. Jim returns into the consultation room and is told very clearly that his mother is not angry with him or about his wetting, and that his wetting is not his fault and is not the cause of his mother's problems.

Jim returns to clinic with his father. A new start is made to Jim's treatment. Good information is provided by his father, that supports the use of a bed-wetting alarm. After detailed discussion, Jim and his father feel that they can manage alarm treatment again without worsening the family situation. Alarm treatment is well tolerated, and Jim achieves being dry this time without any recurrence. His mother responds well to treatment of her mental health problems.

Multiple-Choice Questions

See answers on page 667.

1. Night wetting 'enuresis' has a significant financial impact on families.
   True or False
2. Night wetting is only treated from age seven.
   True or False
3. Treatment of night wetting improves self-esteem.
   True or False
4. Treatment for night wetting always starts with bed-wetting alarms.
   True or False
5. Treatment with Desmopressin can continue long-term for many years and even into adulthood.
   True or False

References and Sources of Further Information

Hirasing, R.A., Van Leerdam, F.J.M., Bolk-Bennink, L.B. and Bosch, J.D., (1997). Bedwetting and Behavioural and/or Emotional Problems. *Acta Paediatrica*, 86(10): 1131–1134.

Neveus, T., Eggert, P., Evans, J., Macedo, A., Rittig, S., Tekgül, S., Robson, L., Yeung, C.K., Robson, L. and International Children's Continence Society, (2010). Evaluation of and Treatment for Monosymptomatic Enuresis: A Standardization Document from the International Children's Continence Society. *The Journal of Urology*, 183(2): 441–447.

NICE, (2010). *NICE Guidelines for Treatment of Nocturnal Enuresis May 2010.* London: NICE.

O'Flynn, N., (2011). Nocturnal Enuresis in Children and Young People: NICE Clinical Guideline. *British Journal of General Practice: The Journal of the Royal College of General Practitioners*, 61(586): 360–362.

von Gontar, A., Schaumburg, H., Hollmann, E., Eiberg, H. and RITTIG, S., (2001). The Genetics of Enuresis: A Review. *The Journal of Urology*, 166(6): 2438–2443. doi: 10.1097/00005392-200112000-00117. PMID: 11696807.

Yeung, C.K., Sreedhar, B.I.J.I., Sihoe, J.D., Sit, F.K. and Lau, J., (2006). Differences in Characteristics of Nocturnal Enuresis between Children and Adolescents: A Critical Appraisal from a Large Epidemiological Study. *BJU International*, 97(5): 1069–1073.

19 Behavioural Sleep Problems in Children and Adolescents

Catherine Hill

KEY POINTS

- Sleep is a learned behaviour. Babies need to learn to self-soothe to sleep at the start of the night.
- Waking up at night is a normal part of sleep. Crying for parental attention is a learned behaviour unless the child needs feeding or has a medical problem.
- Children need healthy sleep environments, appropriate diets, exercise in the day and a bedtime routine to experience optimal sleep.
- Twenty to thirty percent of parents and carers report that their child has difficulty falling asleep or staying asleep.
- Sleep problems can have a detrimental effect on children's day-time behaviour and mental health.
- As children do not always grow out of their sleep problems, these problems should be addressed.
- Careful assessment is required to identify the underlying cause of the sleep problem.

Introduction

Sleep problems are common with 20–30% of children having difficulties at some time during their childhood. As may be expected, sleep problems are most commonly reported in pre-schoolers with up to one-third having difficulties settling to sleep or waking at night. Contrary to popular belief, children do not always grow out of their sleep problems and, if they are ignored, they can continue into later childhood and adolescence. It is likely that sleep problems are overlooked in clinical practice as, by their very nature, they happen 'out of sight', during the night and are invisible to the clinician. Sleep has historically been a blind spot in clinical training programmes, leaving clinicians feeling unconfident in their management.

This chapter will focus on behavioural insomnia of childhood, the commonest cause of chronic insomnia in this age group. Chronic insomnia is defined by the International Classification of Sleep Disorders III as difficulties falling asleep or staying asleep for three or more nights a week over three or more months. While behavioural insomnias are common, practitioners need to be aware of the spectrum of sleep disorders that may present in childhood and, importantly, that behavioural insomnias may co-exist with other disorders, e.g. sleep apnoea or parasomnias.

In clinical practice children rarely present with an isolated sleep problem. More commonly, they will have behavioural and emotional difficulties during the day. There are several reasons why it may be appropriate to prioritise the management of the sleep problem. A growing body of research highlights the detrimental effect of sleep problems on children's day-time behaviour and ability to learn in addition to the effect on the mental health of their parents and carers. Put simply, exhausted parents will struggle to manage day-time behavioural problems in their child, and exhausted children are likely to have day-time cognitive and behavioural difficulties. Addressing the sleep problem makes sense.

To what extent are day-time behavioural difficulties associated with sleep problems? Research over the past decades in primary school-aged children has demonstrated significant associations between parental report of sleep problems and risk of behaviour difficulties in the day including conduct problems, hyperactivity, inattention and internalising symptoms. At the other poles of the age spectrum, both in younger pre-school children and adolescents, sleep problems have been associated with increased internalising and externalising problems. In adolescents insufficient sleep is associated with substance misuse, accidental injury, risky sexual activity and increased suicide risk.

Sleep problems in childhood may have long-lasting effects. Anxiety, depression and aggressive behaviour later in life have been associated with parental report of sleep problems during school years.

In summary, there are good reasons to actively manage behavioural sleep problems and a reasonable expectation that, for many children, improving their sleep quality will have positive knock-on effects on their day-time mental health.

Understanding Behavioural Sleep Problems

Sleep is an active process comprised of four stages, i.e. non-REM sleep stages I–III and REM sleep. Each sleep stage has quite distinct characteristics in terms of what is happening in both the brain and the body. Sleep stages occur in a predicable sequence during the night and are punctuated by brief awakenings. (See Figure 19.1.) Perfectly healthy and well-adjusted children, in satisfactory sleep environments, have routine wakeful moments every night. Few, if any, of these awakenings are remembered. A key concept in the management of behavioural insomnia of childhood is the notion that achieving a consolidated night's sleep is a learned process, i.e. a developmental task of early childhood is the learned ability to return to sleep independently after a spontaneous night waking.

Behavioural sleep problems fall into two categories that may be familiar to the practitioner:

Sleep-Onset Association Disorder

Sleep-onset association behavioural insomnia occurs where a child needs certain specific conditions to fall asleep independently at the start of the night and again following natural night-time awakenings, i.e. the child learns to associate falling asleep with certain conditions. The commonest condition is the presence of a parent/carer in the bedroom and, depending on the age of the child, may involve cuddling, stroking or rocking.

Other 'associations' may include musical toys, soothing lights, warm milk and so on. With these conditions the child may fall asleep easily at the beginning of the night, and so may not present with a settling problem. But when the child wakes up, they will need to recreate the conditions they enjoyed at the start of the night to fall back asleep (they cannot 'self-soothe' without these conditions). Invariably the child will awake fully and call on a parent/carer to help them again. Parents may not recognise settling as a problem, but will usually be troubled by the child waking at night.

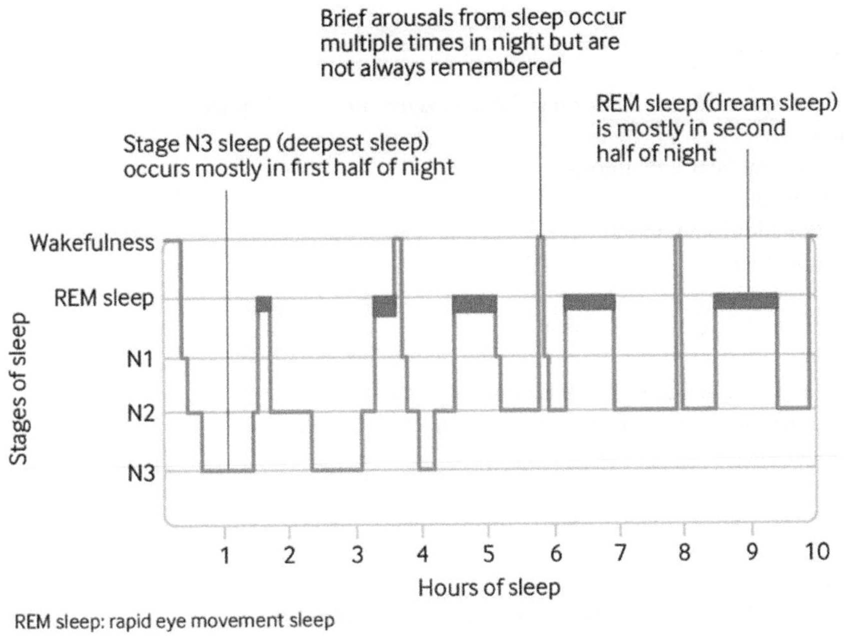

Figure 19.1 Hypnogram illustrating a typical sequence of sleep stages during a night.

Limit-Setting Disorder

Limit-setting behavioural insomnia is another common difficulty for young children and those with developmental disorders. The child resists settling to sleep independently. This can set up a pattern of behaviour where bedtime becomes a protracted battle. Exhausted parents, struggling to settle their child to sleep, may use inconsistent behavioural techniques. Sometimes, parents will have 'tried everything' to win this battle, causing high levels of stress at the end of the day and often giving in for a 'quiet life'.

An understanding of behavioural insomnia allows the practitioner to plan a logical approach to their management, but it should be recognised that the two disorders often overlap. For instance, when a child has battled at bedtime, the defeated and exhausted parent may 'give in' and sleep alongside the child. This 'sleep-onset association' then perpetuates signalling behaviour during natural night waking.

Assessment of Children with Sleep Problems

It can be tempting, as a professional, to give 'off-the-cuff' advice to a parent complaining that their child is not sleeping. Managing sleep difficulties needs to be specific to the sleep disorder, and effective treatment can only be achieved once a full assessment has been carried out and an accurate diagnosis made. It is important to gather information about the child's specific sleep problems and the psychosocial context within which they occur, to find out more about the individual child, his/her family, the environment and specific details relating to bedtime routines, night waking patterns and day-time sleeping habits.

The following important factors should be considered when assessing an individual family.

Child Factors

- Any medical diagnosis, e.g. check on asthma, eczema, nocturnal epilepsy
- Chronic illness
- Established mental health diagnosis
- Physical disabilities
- Description of additional needs
- Learning difficulties
- Means of communication
- Sensory impairments, e.g. vision/hearing
- Medication
- Equipment, e.g. sleep systems in children with cerebral palsy
- Feeding patterns/diet and caffeine consumption
- Child's temperament

Family Factors

- Family members. Who lives at home?
- Extended family/friends. Who else is supporting the family?
- Parental age. Young? Unsupported?
- Parental styles.
- Do parents agree how to manage the sleep problem?
- Attachment.
- Parental perception of sleep problem.
- Cultural beliefs.

Environmental Factors

- Housing/garden/space.
- Child's bedroom. Is it full of electronic toys? Is it dark? Is it shared?
- Income. Is this a source of stress? Does it impose practical limits on the family?
- Nursery/school. Sleep and behaviour pattern in other settings?
- Transport to school, particularly for children accessing special education, who can have long journeys and fall asleep.
- Respite care. How does the child sleep in other settings?
- Social activities and opportunities.
- Friendships.
- Appointments. Other demands on the family?
- Neighbours. Is there a supportive network available to family?
- Any safeguarding concerns?

Sleep Factors

- Sleep history.
- Activities carried out before bedtime.
- Bedtime routine.
- Settling procedure. Does child fall asleep by him/herself, without distractions, such as screen-based entertainment or music?

- Night waking. How often? What do parents do to resettle child?
- Morning routine. Does child need waking?
- Are there any other sleep-related behaviours?
- What effect is the sleep problem having on the family?

Other factors affect sleep in children, and it is important that these are explored during the assessment interview. The following list is not necessarily exclusive:

- Breathing difficulties and snoring
- Enuresis
- Sleep walking
- Sleep terrors
- Rhythmic movements (e.g. body rocking/head-banging)
- Restless sleep
- Nightmares

Information from assessment interviews can be supplemented with sleep diaries. It is useful for parents to keep a sleep diary throughout the course of assessment and treatment so that improvement or deterioration in sleep problems is continuously monitored.

It may be that further investigations are required before a behaviour management plan can be put in place. Home infra-red video recording is now widely available and can be useful when the interview alone yields confusing results (e.g. when it is unclear what is happening at bedtime). Actigraphy, where the child wears a small wristwatch-like accelerometer device, can be employed to objectively distinguish periods of sleep and wakefulness and measure how long it takes a child to fall asleep, how much sleep they have at night and what their sleep quality is like.

Formulation

Once the assessment is complete, the salient features should be drawn together into a formulation that highlights the central features of the sleep problems and links these to pre-disposing, precipitating and maintaining factors. The strength and vulnerabilities of the family must be considered, as these have implications for resolving the problem. Parents need to be emotionally robust to tackle a sleep problem. Treatment can fail if the timing is not right and may lead to a further erosion of parental esteem. It is helpful when professionals offer regular, structured support to the sleep programme that is drawn up in negotiation with the family.

Management of Behavioural Insomnia

Having identified that a child has a behavioural insomnia, there are a number of available therapeutic options. Choice will be influenced by multiple factors such as

- **Parent/carer's perspective**: what is acceptable to one family will not be acceptable to another.
- **The child's characteristics** including but not limited to, their developmental stage, temperament and complicating health problems.

A range of strategies are available to the practitioner, each with its own strengths and limitations. The most important principle is that these consider the unique situation of the child and are sensitively negotiated with the family.

The first priority is to ensure that the child has good 'sleep hygiene'. This concept underpins all behavioural management techniques. Sleep hygiene includes three dimensions that influence sleep:

The sleep environment: a child's sleeping space should be a safe, comfortable, quiet place with low light or ideally complete darkness, free from distractions. Many children in the developed world use their bedrooms as play spaces or study spaces in the day and their sleeping space can be stockpiled with toys and electronic media. Meta-analysis data from around the world have clearly shown that when school-aged children have access to and use of a media device around bedtime they sleep less, have poorer quality sleep and are tired in the day. Screen-based entertainment and learning are becoming the norm worldwide and are increasingly used by pre-school children. Our recent systematic review indicates that sleep in pre-schoolers is similarly adversely affected by screen exposure. Children need quiet time before they settle to sleep. The use of electronic media and stimulating activities should be avoided in the hour before bedtime.

Bedtime routines: promoting a consistent and calming bedtime routine exploits classical conditioning theory to teach a child to associate a predictable sequence of events, e.g. upstairs, bath, brush teeth, nightclothes, to bed, story time, etc., with bedtime and sleep onset. These routines can usefully be linked to positive reinforcement approaches or 'special time activities', including story-telling, lullabies and close physical contact. Evidence clearly shows that when children lack consistent bedtime routines they have a shorter night-time sleep, up to one hour less in school-aged children.

Day-time activities: exercise is known to improve sleep quality. Children who exercise more, fall asleep more rapidly and have the potential for a longer night's sleep. One study has shown that when adolescents exercise regularly for 8.5 hours per week, they have more deep sleep than those who only exercise for 2 hours per week. Our systematic review data show that this holds true for pre-school children where better sleep is associated with outdoor play.

Sleep is influenced by diet. Caffeine consumption within six hours of bedtime can make it more difficult for children to fall asleep. Later bedtimes typically result in a shorter night's sleep. Caffeine exerts its effects though blocking adenosine receptors in the brain that regulate sleep onset and affects sleep quality by suppressing deep sleep. The Sleep in America Poll reported that 27% of pre-schoolers and 41% of school-aged children consumed at least one caffeine-containing drink per day.[1] Children with sleep problems should avoid caffeine-containing food and drinks. It is important that children do not go to bed feeling too full or too hungry. The gut naturally slows down in sleep, and a full stomach at bedtime can cause discomfort.

Good Bedtime Routine

- Lively play calms to quiet play.
- Bedtime preparations in the same sequence each night.
- Use of clock to signal bedtime, even before the child can tell the time.
- Bedtime story, with clearly limited time, usually between 3 and 20 minutes, depending on age.
- Nursery tapes and lullabies, limited and same time each night.
- Hugs and kisses, between one and three minutes.
- Dimmed light, corridor light, if necessary and night lights that are orange/red, not white/blue or green.

- No use of electronic media for an hour before 'lights out' and no access to media after lights out.

There are several approaches to the management of behavioural insomnia that are supported by convincing research evidence for their effectiveness.

Unmodified Extinction – 'Cry It out Technique'

This technique was introduced over 50 years ago and aims to 'extinguish' a child's learned behaviour by the withdrawal of parental attention at bedtime. Parents are advised to completely ignore the child from 'lights out' to morning waking, other than safety checks if needed. This abrupt approach is likely to result in an 'extinction burst' (the child 'ups the stakes' and behaviours deteriorate in the short-term). This technique can be very effective for some children, but parents need considerable persistence and strength of resolve to follow it through.

Families need to understand that if they give in to the child's demands or cries, this will act as a powerful reinforcement that will maintain the behaviour. Parents need to know that this strategy is stressful, and they may need time to think about it. Not surprisingly, extinction is not a popular technique for millennial parents and is at odds with contemporary attachment parenting approaches. It is crucial to understand how families would feel about this approach before recommending it.

Controlled Comforting/Sleep Training

This modification was popularised in the 1980s through self-help books, e.g. Ferber (1985), and more recently thorough popular television shows such as *Supernanny*. The aim is to negatively reinforce the child's bedtime protests by ignoring their cries. Rather than do this indefinitely, the parent is instructed to return to the bedroom, provide brief and unrewarding reassurance at pre-set intervals. If the child attempts to leave the bedroom they are calmly returned to bed with minimal interaction. The parent is instructed to return the child to bed mechanically and unemotionally, with no kisses, refreshments, conversation or angry words.

It is crucial that the child is returned every time. Sometimes gates at the door are helpful to break a pattern. Interval checks can be evenly spaced or gradually extended. There is no absolute right or wrong about the timing of intervals between checks, or whether a fixed, e.g. every 10 minutes, or incremental, e.g. 5, then 10, then 15 minutes, etc., regime is preferable. In clinic, this is best negotiated with the parent depending on their tolerance limits.

Gradual Retreat/Camping out

This is another modification of the extinction approach, but the parent stays in the child's bedroom. It is useful when parents are in the habit of lying physically close to the child and allows a gradual 'distancing' programme.

The idea is to gradually increase the physical space between the parent and child whilst ignoring the child's requests for attention or physical contact. As with graduated extinction, if the child leaves the bed they should be returned calmly with minimal interaction. This technique may be particularly helpful in the school-aged anxious child or the child who does not tolerate rapid change, e.g. a child with autistic spectrum difficulties.

The key concept underlying all of these techniques is to promote the child's ability to fall asleep independently at the beginning of the night, so that when they experience natural night waking, they are able to use the same learned techniques to self-soothe back to sleep independently.

Stimulus Control Techniques/Bedtime Fading

Children with long-standing difficult behaviour at bedtime 'learn' that this is a time of conflict and stimulation, as do their parents. Extinction techniques may make this conflict worse in the short-term. An alternate 'stimulus control' technique can be used for a child who has become very oppositional. It works well in children with limited awareness of 'clock' time. Having established what time the child usually falls asleep, expectations are changed so that this becomes new bedtime for the start of the programme, i.e. the child who is put to bed at 7 o'clock, but won't fall asleep until 9 o'clock is, instead, settled into bed at the later time of 9 o'clock. If the child doesn't fall asleep within 20 minutes, they are removed from the bedroom and bedtime is delayed for a further agreed time, e.g. 30 minutes. Ideally, this removes the bedtime struggles and over-stimulation that goes along with these behaviours and reduces the level of conflict between parent and child.

Stimulus control programmes need to be carefully supervised by the practitioner to gauge the child's response, support the parent and ensure early 'bail out' if the child continues to employ resistant behaviours that progressively delay bedtime. It is critical that sleep hygiene is maintained and that the child's settling routine is adjusted to the delayed bedtime. Once the child has learned to achieve struggle-free settling, the bedtime is incrementally adjusted to be 15 minutes earlier every day, until a desirable bedtime is achieved. It is important that throughout the programme the child is woken at a regular time in the morning to avoid shifting their biological clock.

General Considerations

Reassuring Parents That Their Child Will Come to No Long-Term Harm

Bedtime can be a vulnerable time for families. It usually involves separation and takes place at the end of the day when parents are tired and least resilient. Many parents will worry that controlled comforting techniques will cause lasting psychological damage to their child or adversely affect their relationship.

Some helpful recent research has provided reassurance for parents. A large population of 326 infants with sleep problems at 8 months of age were randomised to either behavioural intervention (controlled comforting/bedtime fading and positive routines) or care as usual. Follow-up five years later showed no differences in parent reports of children's behaviour, psychosocial quality of life, parent–child relationship, attachment or parental mental health.

A subsequent study went one step further to compare controlled comforting, bedtime fading and control conditions, i.e. sleep education only. A total of 43 infants aged 6–16 months were randomised to controlled comforting (n = 14), bedtime fading (n = 15) or sleep education (n = 14). Based on parent report and infant actigraphy, children in the intervention groups fell asleep significantly more quickly and children in the controlled comforting group had fewer night wakings than the sleep education group.

Infant stress, measured through morning and afternoon salivary cortisol samples, interestingly, showed small-to-moderate decreases compared to controls, i.e. the infants in the intervention groups appeared to be less stressed. Similarly, mothers' stress showed small-to-moderate decreases over the first month for the intervention group. A year later, there were no differences in child emotional and behavioural problems or secure-insecure attachment styles as assessed using the 'strange situation' procedure. These data go some way to offer reassurance to parents that these tried-and-tested techniques do no psychological harm to either child or parent.

Co-Sleeping

For some families, co-sleeping, where the child shares the parental bed, is a positive choice and part of normal routine. It is not advised in infancy because of the risk of sudden infant death. In older children, co-sleeping is associated with sleep difficulties when it is used as a 'fall back', because the child will not sleep in their own bed. The parental bed is the greatest 'reward' of all for many children. Exhausted parents who relent and allow the child to co-sleep during the night have undone all the hard work they have put in earlier in the evening teaching a child to settle to sleep. When a child creeps in silently whilst parents are sleeping, practical measures, e.g. a bell on the door, can alert the parent so that they can return the child to their own bed.

Timing

Only begin a sleep programme when parents have the resources to see it through, e.g. when partner is about to be home for a long weekend, begin on a Friday evening.

Maximise Parents' Strengths

For example, if a father can cope more easily with crying than the mother, then perhaps the mother could go to a friend's house for four or five evenings, half an hour before the child's bedtime, to allow the father to make a start on the programme. Always acknowledge and resolve parental conflicts before the programme starts.

Take It a Step at a Time

Where there are several difficulties, it is a good idea to encourage the parents to work at part of the problem at first. Often, they will choose to work on 'settling' problems first, as they feel stronger in the evening rather than in the middle of the night. Success at one stage builds up parental confidence and leads to good results in the next phase.

Use Positive Reinforcement

When a child can understand what is expected of him/her, it is useful to reward small and achievable goals using a star chart or, say, a lucky-dip box in the morning; such rewards need to be fine-tuned to the interests and intellectual ability of the child, so that some success can be achieved early on.

Medication

Families are often prescribed medication for a child's sleep problem as parent and physician alike fail to recognise the behavioural nature of the difficulties. Whilst such a 'quick fix' may appeal to exhausted parents and to the busy physician, it fails to address the underlying problem and does no more than 'plaster over the cracks'. It is not logical to sedate a child that is expected to learn a new behaviour.

The British National Formulary for children advises 'The prescribing of hypnotics to children is not justified. There is a risk of habituation with prolonged use and problems settling children at night should be managed psychologically'.

A major limitation in the use of any medication for behavioural insomnia is the absence of good research data telling us exactly what can help, in what situation and at what dose. Most sleep clinics will use medication selectively. Crucially, it will always be used alongside sleep hygiene advice and behavioural management. For a helpful and full review of 'When to use drugs to help sleep', see Gringras (2008).

Prevention

As behavioural insomnia is so common, should more be done to educate parents when children are very young? Ideally, parents should understand some basic principles before a child reaches six months of age. From this time, children begin to learn to sleep through the night since they no longer need night feeds. Research shows that when parents receive appropriate education antenatally and when their babies are young, their infants have improved sleep.

Case Study (1): Reena

Reena (three) recently began to have problems settling to sleep after starting playschool. Her parents were exhausted, because it was becoming more and more difficult for her to settle. She seemed to need one or the other of them to stay with her until she fell asleep. They had a good routine established at the beginning of the evening, starting with a bath and then story time. But story time was becoming longer, and even after the stories had finished, Reena became distressed when they tried to leave her. This resulted in Reena settling to sleep later and later and not wanting to wake up in the morning. She often missed playschool although she enjoyed it.

Careful assessment showed Reena to be progressing well developmentally and to have no medical problems, which reassured her parents. Discussion with Reena's parents about her sleep routine discovered that they were allowing Reena several stories that could be exciting, and following these she was awake and wanting more. Both parents found it difficult to leave Reena to cry, and so a gradual retreat with parental presence approach was adopted, along with limiting story-time to short calm stories. One or the other of her parents would sit next to Reena whilst she fell asleep, gradually moving their position until she managed to fall asleep without their presence.

With this approach, Reena was woken at the same time each day so that she could attend morning playschool. Reena's father found it easier to set the limits on stories and routines, so he supported Reena's mother. Within three weeks Reena's bedtime routine was well established and she was settling to sleep without her parents' presence after only one story.

Case Study (2): David

David (12) had been having problems settling to sleep for several years, leading to increased conflict at bedtime that included shouting and banging doors. David was encouraged to settle to bed at 8 pm, but was not falling asleep until 10 pm. He was constantly requesting his iPad, which was confiscated at bedtime. His parents were desperate for him to go to sleep. Not only did they want some time to themselves but they were sure David's sleep problems were having a knock-on effect on his schooling. He was often late to school, because of the difficulties they had in waking him. Bedtime was dreaded by all. There was never a night without conflict.

David has moderate-severe learning difficulties and cannot yet tell the time. He is reported to be tired in school and occasionally naps in lessons after lunch.

Following assessment, David's parents chose to work on a bedtime fading technique. Screen-time on his iPad was limited to no later than 7 pm.

In this approach, David was kept up until 10 pm. The parents chose to start this approach during the half-term break so that David's schooling was affected as little as possible and his evening routine was adjusted to the new sleep time. David was still woken at his normal time for school, 7.30 am. At first, David did not settle even at 10 pm, and he was removed again from his bedroom for a further 20 minutes and then taken back to bed. This was repeated on the first night until 11 pm, when he finally went to sleep. During the time when he was brought back downstairs, no stimulus was given and no access allowed to electronic media. David was allowed quiet activities until he wanted to try to go to sleep again.

The second night the same pattern was repeated. David was kept up until 11 pm. He was tired and asked to go to bed at 10.30 pm. His parents agreed, and he settled quickly. The following night he went to sleep at the same time. Over the next few weeks, his parents gradually adjusted his bedtime by 15 minutes every 3 days, and within 2 months he was regularly settling to sleep by 9 pm. Both David and his parents were happy with his progress.

Multiple-Choice Questions

See answers on page 667.

1. Which statement about children's sleep problems is correct?
   a. Almost all children under the age of two years will have some kind of sleep problem.
   b. Sleep problems in children over five years are the result of inappropriate parenting strategies.
   c. All children will grow out of their sleep problem by the age of five.
   d. All sleep problems in childhood need further investigation.
   e. Child sleep problems are prevalent in up to 25% of the population.
2. Which statement about the consequences of sleep difficulties in children is true?
   a. All child behaviour problems are caused by child sleep difficulties.
   b. Poor sleep does not have a negative effect on cognitive functioning.
   c. All children with a sleep problem will also present with a behaviour problem.
   d. Both learning and behaviour may be affected in children with sleep problems.
   e. Sleep problems in childhood are not associated with emotional difficulties later in life.
3. Which of the following statements about behavioural insomnia is correct?
   a. Limit-setting behavioural insomnia is common in children with developmental disorders.
   b. Children with sleep-onset association do not always have problems settling at the start of the night.
   c. There may be overlap between limit-setting and sleep-onset association.
   d. Parental reports are important when assessing a child for behavioural insomnia.
   e. All of the above.
4. Which statement about infant sleeping is true?
   a. Infants should sleep through the night from birth.
   b. Infants are unable to sleep through the night until 12 months.
   c. Inappropriate parenting strategies are the cause of infant sleep problems.
   d. Unmodified extinction is the best method to treat behavioural insomnia.
   e. Controlled crying does not cause long-term emotional distress in the child.

5. Which of these statements regarding the treatment of childhood sleep problems is true?
   a. Medication is never appropriate for children under five years.
   b. Underlying physical problems should always be considered before embarking on behavioural management.
   c. Medication should always be considered for children over the age of two years.
   d. The use of positive reinforcement strategies is not effective.
   e. Treatment does not always require a full assessment.

Key References

Hill, C.M. and Everitt, H., (2018). Assessment and Initial Management of Suspected Behavioural Insomnia in Pre-Adolescent Children. *BMJ*, 363: k3797.

Mindell, J.A. and Owens, J.A., (2015). *Sleep in the Pediatric Practice in A Clinical Guide to Pediatric Sleep*. Southern Holland, the Netherlands: Wolters Kluwer.

Recommended Resources for Parents

For pre-school children:

Pediatric Sleep Council. Baby Sleep (https://www.babysleep.com/)
A website constructed by international sleep experts and researchers with advice for parents on common sleep problems in the early years.

For all ages:

Raising Children Network (Australia) (http://raisingchildren.net.au/) – Age-specific guidance for parents on common childhood and adolescent behavioural issues including sleep.

Royal College of Psychiatrists. Sleep problems in childhood and adolescence: for parents, carers and anyone who works with young people (www.rcpsych.ac.uk/healthadvice/parentsandyouthinfo/parentscarers/sleepproblems.aspx).

20 Epilepsy

Salvatore Rototendo and Margaret J.J. Thompson

It is important for child psychiatrists to know how children, who could have epilepsy, might present. This is important in making diagnostic decisions with children who present with unexpected symptoms. Keeping these symptoms in mind will help in identifying a child who is presenting for the first time with epilepsy, or to be able to recognise when the seizure control is not optimal.

KEY CONCEPTS

- Epilepsy symptoms may be misconstrued as psychiatric symptoms and vice versa.
- The symptoms might reflect the position of the underlying focus for the seizure.
- Children may have cognitive impairments.
- Medication for epilepsy may produce side effects.

Presentation

Children with seizures may present with physical symptoms or emotional symptoms before the seizures happen or afterwards. Equally, seizures could be confused with psychiatric symptoms. Early seizure symptoms may present with warnings that could be misconstrued as psychosomatic symptoms. The children may say that their thoughts are racing or that they have strange tingling feelings in their hands or butterfly feelings in their stomach. They might say they have an odd taste or smell a strange smell. They sometimes talk about hearing sounds or having a feeling that something has happened before or deny something has happened (déjà vu/jamais vu).

Children can be very apprehensive with all these feelings and can become alarmed. Sometimes they may report that the feelings are pleasant. They can present with physical symptoms of dizziness, headache, light-headedness, nausea and numbness in fingers or other places, e.g. the side of the face. Seizures can happen without warning. The presentation of seizures symptoms may depend on where the seizure originates.

Seizure Symptoms Presentation

Sensory

- Confusion
- Deafness/hearing sounds

- Smell
- Electric shock feeling
- Loss of consciousness
- Visual loss or blurring
- Spacing out
- Out of body experience

Emotional

- Fear or panic (especially in young children)

Physical

- Chewing movements
- Tonic-clonic movements
- Difficulty in talking
- Drooling
- Eyelid fluttering
- Eyes movements
- Drop attacks
- Apnoea

Children might have a memory loss after a seizure and that can be distressing. They might have difficulties in speech and gross and fine motor skills. They might be confused, fearful or embarrassed. They might be frustrated if they do not know what is happening to them. Children with epilepsy may feel different to other children, especially if the seizures happen in public, e.g. at school, and if the fear of seizures makes it difficult for parents or teachers to let the children do the same things as other children, e.g. go swimming or boating. This can lead to sadness or depression. It is always more difficult for children if the epilepsy occurs for the first time in adolescence when normally a young person would be becoming independent. Children may suffer physical sequelae after an epileptic attack, with bruising or injuries. They can feel nauseated, thirsty and weak, with headaches or painful muscles. Children may be very sleepy, exhausted and find talking difficult. Children may also have an urge to urinate or defecate.

Types of Seizures

Self-Limited Seizure Types

Generalised Seizures

- Tonic-clonic
- Clonic, i.e. shaking
- Absence seizures i.e. staring
- Myoclonic absence
- Tonic, i.e. stiffness
- Myoclonic, i.e. jerk movements
- Myoclonic atonic
- Atonic, i.e. drop
- Reflex seizures

Focal Seizures

- Focal motor seizures
- Gelastic seizures, i.e. laugh
- Hemiclonic seizures
- Secondarily generalised seizures

Continuous Seizures

- Generalised status epilepticus
- Focal status epilepticus

In generalised epilepsies, the epileptic activity affects the whole brain from the onset. Patients can present with problems of impulsive behaviour, poor frustration tolerance and short attention span, likely to be linked to frontal lobe dysfunction. Children with secondary generalised epilepsy have often significant cognitive impairments and are more likely to present with depressive, anxiety or attention deficit disorders.

During epilepsies of focal origin, the seizure activity starts from an identifiable cortical region. Reported psychiatric symptoms in these epilepsies depend on the area of the brain affected. Symptoms of depression and anxiety have been associated with seizures originating in the temporal lobe, frontal lobe or both.

Psychiatric symptoms can occur from 72 hours before a seizure occurring to 120 hours afterwards. They consist typically of irritability, poor frustration tolerance and impulsivity. Parents often can predict the occurrence of seizures as their child becomes more restless, impulsive and irritable. After the seizure the child may feel depressed, anxious or even experience psychotic episodes lasting several days. Psychiatric symptoms may present between seizures and include low mood, anxiety and be similar to behavioural disorders/attention deficit disorders. Differentiating these symptoms from psychiatric disorders in their own right may prove very difficult.

It is important to be able to differentiate epileptic seizure from non-epileptic seizure, a number of which are of psychogenic origin. These often mimic true epileptic attacks to a degree that is regularly misdiagnosed.

Alongside neurobiological reasons in determining psychiatric symptoms, other factors may be responsible for behavioural disturbances. Effects on self-esteem and confidence in social settings because of the possible occurrence of seizures in public places and parental overprotectiveness lead to social isolation and decrease involvement in academic activities. Other neurological disorders associated with the seizure disorder can affect many areas of the child's general functioning, i.e. cerebral palsy.

Anti-Epileptic Drugs (AED) and Their Side Effects

All AEDs have potentially behaviour-changing effects on children that are sometimes difficult to predict, as they may depend on individual genetic and environmental factors. Some of these effects, that may vary in intensity, may be opposite in quality, e.g. valproate, levetiracetam and vigabatrin may induce sedation in some individuals, but can cause irritability and anxiety in others.

Sedative AEDs (barbiturates, benzodiazepines, valproate, gabapentin, tiagabine and vigabatrin) affect energy levels, impact concentration and induce low mood. At the same time, they can be effective in controlling anxiety, mania and are hypnotics. Conversely, activating AEDs (e.g. felbamate and lamotrigine) can cause anxiety, insomnia and agitation, but possess antidepressant effects and improve attention. AEDs with both inhibitory and excitatory properties, e.g. topiramate, levetiracetam and zonisamide, can cause anxiety, irritability and depression. In children already in treatment, weaning off AEDs can trigger behavioural deterioration. This may happen because of the loss of the positive psychotropic effect of the pharmacological agent. The discontinuation of drugs that have mood-stabilising properties, e.g. carbamazepine, valproate and lamotrigine, can unmask an underlying mood affective disorder.

Partial treatment, e.g. 'outgrown dosage', poor compliance, pharmacological interaction, and response to treatment, 'difficult epilepsies', are determinant factors for poor control in epilepsies that are associated with, and sometimes preceded by, behavioural disturbances.

Diagnosis

The diagnosis of epilepsy remains a clinical one. A detailed and accurate history of presenting symptoms and past medical problems, together with a complete physical, including neurological, examination are often more valuable then subsequent investigations. Witnessing a suspected seizure, or viewing a video-recording of the episode by carers, may be very informative for a diagnostic formulation. A typical example are 'daydreaming' episodes of inattentive children that can often be confused with absence seizures and vice versa.

Electroencephalography

EEG may help in diagnosing epilepsy but only in limited circumstances. It is important to remember that 44% of children with epilepsy will have a normal first EEG. Sometimes a repeat EEG, with or without sleep, can increase the diagnostic yield. Conversely, misleading EEG abnormalities can be found on up to 10% of routine EEGs. Only careful clinical and EEG correlation will improve diagnostic accuracy.

Case Study (1): Anna

Anna (14) was referred for behaviour problems at school, especially not wanting to finish tasks and not appearing to pay attention. She had had epilepsy since she was five years of age, and it had always been reasonably well-controlled in the past. She had always been a good pupil.

Careful observation in class indicated that actually her times of inattention might well be evidence of seizures with confusion afterwards, leading to apparent non-compliance. An EEG indicated that her epilepsy was no longer well-controlled and when her medication was increased, her behaviour improved.

Case Study (2): Tom

Tom had just been diagnosed with temporal lobe epilepsy following a period of investigation for odd experiences of 'hearing voices' and experiencing odd tastes and smells. He then had a seizure at school.

Tom was embarrassed about the seizure at school, depressed that he would have to take medication and that he would not, at least for a while, be able to do the things he enjoyed, like swimming and kayaking. He and his parents met with the specialist epilepsy nurse who explained all the facts about epilepsy to them, and advised Tom about looking after himself. She gave Tom time by himself to talk through his feelings and anger about his situation.

Gradually he was able to discuss with his friends, family and teachers how to allow him to carry on with his hobbies safely with sensible safeguards built in.

Multiple-Choice Question

See answers on page 668.

1) Which symptoms may be experienced by a child who could have epilepsy?
   a. Painful stomach
   b. Headache
   c. Nausea
   d. Tingling in hands
   e. Fear or panic
   f. All of them

Key Reference

Beattie, M., (2006). *Essential Revision Notes in Paediatrics for the MRCPCH* (2ns edition). Cheshire: PASTEST Ltd.

Webpage

Epilepsy Action, www.epilepsy.org.uk.

21 Chronic Health Conditions and Mental Well-Being in Children and Young People

Julie Waine (updated by Christopher Gale)

Introduction

There is no universally agreed definition of chronic illness or health conditions. Van Der Lee et al.'s (2007) systematic review in this area found that most research definitions considered both the duration of symptoms and their impact on daily life. The prevalence of chronic illness in children in the developed world has increased partly because of the increase in survival rates from serious congenital and acquired illness (Zylke and DeAngelis, 2007).

KEY CONCEPTS

- A chronic health condition is a stressor that increases the risk to children of both developing a mental health disorder and of impeding their development trajectory.
- Family functioning is an important mediator of outcome for the child.
- Adolescence is characterised by thinking in the 'here and now' and risk-taking behaviour, both of which may interfere with treatment adherence.
- Education alone does not increase adherence.
- A multi-disciplinary paediatric liaison team can provide timely, evidence-based interventions to minimise the impact of a chronic health condition on a young person's mental health.

Studies have demonstrated that children and young people with a chronic physical health issue are disproportionately impacted by mental health difficulties compared to those without (Butler et al., 2018; Ferro, 2016). Parents of children with chronic illness report behavioural and emotional difficulties at least twice as often as do the parents of healthy controls (Mrazek, 2002). This incidence rises if the condition directly affects the brain.

The Office for National Statistics survey of the mental health of children and adolescents in Great Britain found that 4% of all 5–15-year olds sampled had an emotional disorder. The prevalence of any mental disorder was 37% in young people with epilepsy and one in six in children (17%) with a life-threatening illness (Meltzer et al., 2000). At follow up, three years later, physical illness was found to be a predictor of the persistence of an emotional disorder. Of the group who had a physical illness when originally sampled in 1999, 6% fulfilled criteria for an emotional disorder. This compared with only 2% of the group with no physical disorder (Meltzer, 2003).

Chronic illness can be viewed as a stressor that may prevent a child or young person reaching their developmental potential, but happily this is not the most common outcome (Eiser, 1993). Gannoni and Shute (2010) used focus groups to ask parents and children about adaptation to illness. They found parents and children taking positive steps to cope with their challenges by, e.g. using problem-focused coping strategies.

Possible Mental Health Consequences of a Chronic Health Condition in Children and Young People

The level of association between physical conditions and mental health difficulties is relatively homogenous (Reaume and Ferro, 2019); whether the illness is life-threatening or life-limiting, static or progressive, predictable or of uncertain prognosis, acquired, genetic or inherited, all will influence how the young person, and their family, views and lives with the illness or condition.

The most common psychiatric diagnosis made is that of an adjustment disorder, after a physical health diagnosis is made (Mitchell et al., 2011). An adjustment disorder is defined as emotional symptoms and/or behaviour that are temporarily linked to a life event and that subsequently resolve, within six months of the life event. This is without the presence of other diagnosable mental health conditions, such as major depressive disorder.

Young people with a physical health condition may develop depression that can be complicated by the misattribution of somatic symptoms, i.e. tiredness, weight loss and sleep disturbance, to the former. Equally, mental distress may influence a physical illness. Stress has been associated with acute exacerbation of asthma (Sandberg et al., 2000).

The mental effects of a physical illness may remain dormant for several years, until a later stress activates them, e.g. pre-school serious illness is thought to be a risk factor for later depressive symptoms at age 15.

Chronic Physical Health Conditions and Adjustment

Children and young people with chronic illness have the same developmental needs and health concerns as their healthy peers, including forming a sexual identity, considered by the World Health Organization to be a central aspect of being human (WHO, 2004). They have the same coping strategies (Abbott, 2003). Children will have their own temperamental characteristics that will influence how they and their family cope with the demands of the illness. In addition to factors within the child/young person, family functioning predicts adjustment to illness.

Chronic physical health conditions increase the burden of care for the child or young person on the family. In addition to responsibility for outpatient attendance and possible hospital admissions, care may be needed beyond that generally expected for a child of that age, e.g. needing to toilet a middle childhood child. This is alongside needing to administer or supervise medication and/or therapy. It is important to help the family find a workable balance between providing the care that is needed for the optimum health of the child/young person and fulfilling the family's ordinary everyday needs.

School/College

School/college attendance is an important measure of the impact of an illness or long-term condition. Children and young people with chronic conditions miss school through illness and planned hospital attendances, potentially limiting their academic potential. School phobia after time in hospital is recognised. School can have an important influence on the young person's successful adjustment to their condition, and schools within hospitals can be helpful in keeping them up to speed with schoolwork and liaising with the child/young person's school or college.

Conversely, if a child/young person's condition is poorly understood by teaching staff and peers, it can have a detrimental impact on the individual's psychosocial and cognitive development, e.g. teachers inappropriately lowering their expectations of the child/young person's academic performance or the child being subjected to bullying by other children/young people. A nurse specialist may have a role to play in visiting the school or college to educate staff about the needs and abilities of the child/young person. They can facilitate realistic discussions about the possible health and safety risks that require assessment and management. This is particularly important with conditions such as epilepsy, where a seizure can be unexpected and very public.

Chronic Illness at Different Stages of Childhood

There is some evidence to suggest that the diagnosis of a chronic illness before the age of five years is associated with a negative impact on later cognitive performance (Eiser and Lansdown, 1977). This finding was noted in survivors of childhood cancer, and has been shown in young people with early onset diabetes. It is thought to be due to the adverse effects of the illness process, e.g. the effect of hypoglycaemia in diabetes, the use of radiotherapy for brain tumours.

Early diagnosis of chronic illness can be associated with delayed developmental milestones. The impact of separation on attachment as demonstrated in Robertson's film 'A two-year-old goes to hospital' (1952) led to a change in policy so that parents were encouraged to stay with their child in hospital.

Chronic illness developing early may limit the opportunity of the child to socialise, and this can have an impact on the child's ability to benefit later from school. During middle childhood, time missed at school may set a pattern for later attendance. Children who are having kidney dialysis may have fantasies about what the dialysis 'monster' machine is doing. They may worry about the possibility of a kidney transplant and what kind of person may have donated them their kidney.

Adolescence

Case Study: Asha

Asha (14) was diagnosed with insulin-dependent diabetes two years ago after a short viral illness. Her diabetic control is sub-optimal, and she needed an emergency admission to hospital due to ketoacidosis in the past two months. The psychologist from the multi-disciplinary liaison team is working with Asha using a motivational interviewing approach to help her integrate diabetes into her self-image.

Adolescence is traditionally thought of as a time of emotional turbulence, as the young person grows emotionally and physically towards becoming a mature adult. Separation from the family, and increasing autonomy, are viewed as the tasks of adolescence, along with maturation into a sexual being. The opinion of friends and acceptance into a peer group increase in importance.

It is not difficult to imagine how a chronic illness could interfere with these important developmental changes. Integrating illness into a positive self-view may be difficult. Self-esteem could be affected if physical appearance is altered beyond the normal range of peers. Cystic fibrosis, for instance, may slow growth and delay puberty. Delayed puberty itself can lower self-esteem, particularly in boys, and result in the adolescent being treated in an inappropriately immature way (Suris et al., 2004).

Children and young people with cystic fibrosis may have questions and worries about their own mortality. This is especially true if they have serious lung disease and have limited social contact with other children with the same condition because of contamination. If they have developed flatulence and feel 'fat', this might inhibit their eating and lead to an eating disorder. Adherence to treatment may become more of a problem during the teenage years, although non-compliance with treatment plans is not solely the domain of young people. Many factors influence treatment adherence. Adherence can be viewed as on a spectrum rather than an all-or-nothing phenomenon (Lask, 1994).

Why Might an Adolescent Not Adhere to a Treatment Plan?

Most health care practitioners caring for adolescents would hope that the young person themselves would become increasingly responsible for completing their treatment, ideally with a gradual handover of responsibility from their parents. For this to be successful, both parent and child must negotiate the change at a pace they are both happy with and with a degree of acceptance as to the seriousness of the illness.

For a young person, the daily care necessary to treat their illness is a daily reminder of being different and unwell. Adolescence is a time of risk-taking and feelings of invincibility, all recognised aspects of normal adolescent thought processes. These might counteract adherence, and chronic illness is associated with an increase in risk-taking behaviour (Suris et al., 2008)

Non-conformity with a treatment regime may mirror non-conformity in other aspects of the adolescent's life. The young person may choose not to adhere, thereby taking back some control over their life. In assessing adherence, it is always important to exclude depression as a possible cause. A young person struggling with accepting a life-limiting illness may currently decide that rigid adherence to a strict treatment regime is not a priority for them, as they will die anyway, just a bit younger than some of their peers (Esmond, 2000).

Effect on Siblings

The research findings on the effects of chronic illness on siblings are mixed. An excess of somatic symptoms and attention-seeking behaviour has been found, as have increased rates of pro-social behaviour. Understandably, siblings have been found to be concerned about their brother or sister, but in addition, they can be worried about their own risk of illness and the effect of the illness on their parents. Siblings may suffer from the effects of social isolation, as the illness isolates the family (e.g. infection risk may deter parents from allowing their children to attend nursery or pre-school).

Long-Term Outcome

The long-term outcome for young people with chronic illness is difficult to assess. A significant volume of available research is based on young people treated at specialist centres. It may not be possible to generalise those findings to the outcomes of young people who receive care from less specialist centres (Gledhill et al., 2000). In general, most young people remain well-adjusted, although females who remain chronically ill seem at most risk of psychiatric sequelae.

What Can Be Helpful?

The following list gives some suggestions as to possible areas of intervention, to strengthen resilience factors in the child/young person and their family.

Family

- Have the parents themselves come to terms with the illness/condition?
- Are they ready to allow you to discuss it with the child or young person?
- Work out together what the parents are happy for you to say to the child or young person. Assess the parents'/carers' mental health and coping strategies.

Explain the Illness to the Child/Young Person

- Use age-appropriate language. Young children may view illness as a punishment. Older children and young people may understandably feel a sense of anger and injustice. It is useful to reassure them explicitly that the illness is not their fault and that it is normal to feel angry.

Talk to the Child/Young Person and Encourage Their Questions

- Asking questions is a step on the path to assuming responsibility for self-care. Prepare the child for specific procedures and the likely questions of others. Disease-specific websites, roleplay and literature from patient-support groups may be helpful.

Use of Art or Play Therapy

- If the child/young person experiences difficulties coping with procedures and pain, play therapists, art therapists or psychologists can be very helpful in talking through procedures and role playing. Social stories may be helpful.

Educate and Enable the Parents or Carers about the Illness/Condition

- Although there is no direct correlation between illness knowledge and subsequent adherence with treatment, it may provide the parent with realistic expectations of health care professionals and offer the child/young person an adult who can answer some of their illness-related questions.
- It is important that their child can talk to them without fear of them becoming overly upset or disproportionately negatively judgmental.

Encourage the Family to Lead as Normal a Life as Possible

- Setting age- and ability-appropriate limits and boundaries and allocating responsibility for household chores are all important for normal emotional development.

Encourage the Parents to Look after Themselves and Their Adult Relationships

- Facilitate this by encouraging the acceptance of offers of help.

Allow the Child/Young Person as Much Choice in Their Life as Possible

- Chronic illness removes choice in many aspects of life.

Model a Collaborative Relationship with Other Health Care Professionals

- Collaboration, particularly a shared therapeutic goal between the child/young person and their families and the medical team, has been shown to positively influence treatment adherence. The child mental health team have an important role in a paediatric hospital supporting the paediatric team working with children with chronic illness in assisting them to understand how children think and why they might react the way they do. Staff who have to make difficult medical decisions need the support of these colleagues, the child and the family. There needs to be discussion with the paediatric staff about the importance of the transition to adult teams, as children and their families will want to be reassured that they will be given the same level of support from the new team. Joint handovers are essential.

Multiple-Choice Questions

See answers on page 668.

1. A chronic health condition in childhood is…
   a. A well-defined entity.
   b. Less prevalent in the developing world.
   c. Invariably associated with behavioural or emotional disturbance.
   d. More likely to cause emotional disturbance if the condition directly affects the brain.
   e. Most often dealt with by parents and children using emotion-focused coping strategies.
2. Which of the following statements are true of mental health and a chronic health condition?
   a. The least common co-morbid mental health issue is an adjustment disorder.
   b. Symptoms of depression are easy to distinguish from symptoms of the physical illness.
   c. Usually persist into adulthood.
   d. The attachment between a parent and child can be affected by chronic illness.
3 Which of the following statements are true of chronic illness and school/college?
   a. Repeated absences are unlikely to be a major issue for a junior school-aged child.
   b. It is usually appropriate for staff to lower their expectations of the child's attainment.
   c. Intervention to improve social skills is rarely helpful.
   d. Chronic illness may be a vulnerability factor for bullying.
   e. School attendance is not a useful marker of the impact of an illness.
4 Which of the following statements are true of chronic health conditions in adolescence?
   a. They are unlikely to interfere with the adolescent's sense of self.
   b. They are unlikely to interfere with the developmental processes associated with adolescence.
   c. Are rarely associated with non-compliance with treatment.
   d. Usually adherence to a treatment regime is all or nothing.
5. Helpful suggestions for families dealing with chronic illness include…
   a. Not discussing the illness for fear of upsetting the young person.
   b. Advising against parental research on the internet.
   c. Telling the adolescent robustly what to do.
   d. Usually exempting the affected adolescent from household chores.
   e. Addressing necessary procedures with the adolescent.

Key References

Butler, A., Van Lieshout, R.J., Lipman, E.L., MacMillan, H.L., Gonzalez, A., Gorter, J.W. and Ferro, M.A. (2018). Mental Disorder in Children with Physical Conditions: A Pilot Study. *BMJ Open*, 8(1-10).

Eiser, C. (1993). *Growing Up with a Chronic Disease: The Impact on Children and Their Families.* London: Jessica Kingsley Pub.

Gannoni, A.F. and Shute, R.H. (2010). Parental and Child Perspectives on Adaptation to Childhood Chronic Illness: A Qualitative Study. *Clinical Child Psychology and Psychiatry*, 15(1): 39–53.

Wallander, J.L. and Varni, J.W. (1998). Effects of Pediatric Chronic Physical Disorders on Child and Family Adjustment. *Journal of Child Psychology & Psychiatry*, 39(1): 29–46.

Zylke, J.W. and DeAngelis, C.D. (2007). Paediatric Chronic Diseases-Stealing Childhood. *JAMA*, 24(297): 2765–2766.

22 Sexual Orientation

Charlotte Young (updated by Christopher Gale)

Introduction

It is well known that adolescence can be a turbulent period of identity formation. Part of this involves developing sexual identity and the consequent awareness of sexuality. It appears that young people are experiencing this at younger ages. Research has shown that the average age for 'coming out', i.e. when a person discloses their sexuality, is 15 years (Stonewall, 2010). This is a pertinent issue for CAMHS as evidence shows that those young people who are questioning their sexuality, or see themselves as not part of the 'expected' heterosexual group, have difficulties maintaining their mental health.

KEY CONCEPTS

- Research has shown that half of lesbian and bisexual women aged under 20 years have self-harmed compared with 1 in 15 of the general population.
- Young people who identify themselves as non-heterosexual are more likely to have attempted suicide than young people who identify as heterosexual (Fish, 2007).
- Exacerbating any existing mental health difficulties, young lesbian and bisexual females are more likely to smoke and drink alcohol to excess than their heterosexual counterparts.
- Young gay and bisexual males are more likely to misuse illegal substances (Fish, 2007).
- Research has not identified a causal relationship between being non-heterosexual and mental health problems, even though homosexuality was once, and in some cultures, still is, considered a mental health disorder. The development of mental health difficulties of this group of young people is more likely to be the consequence of living in a society that is predominantly heterosexual with the resultant isolation, prejudice, hostility and potential violence experienced (Kitts, 2005).

Young people who are questioning their gender identity often come to CAMHS presenting with gender dysphoria and may be diagnosed with gender identity disorder (GID). Although historically 'trans' and non-binary young people would mix with the LGB community and often use the same support groups, it is important to recognise that gender identity, how someone identifies in their own mind, and gender expression, how they portray gender to the world through communication, behaviour and appearance, differ from biological gender, i.e.

the genetic/physical characteristics assigned at birth, and sexual orientation, i.e. to whom one is emotionally, spiritually and physically attracted, based on their gender in relation to one's own.

Definitions in Relation to Sexual Orientation

It is important to recognise that definitions in the areas of sexual orientation and gender identity are continuously revisited and refined. The definitions below are considered currently accurate and based on information made available from the LGBT charity Stonewall:

- **'Bi' or 'bisexual'** is an umbrella term used to describe a romantic and/or sexual orientation towards more than one gender or person. It is often used interchangeably with the terms 'pan' or 'queer'.
- **Gay** refers to a male who has a romantic and/or sexual orientation towards males. It can be a generic term for lesbian and gay sexuality. Some females define themselves as gay, rather than as lesbian. Some non-binary people identify with this term.
- **Heterosexual/straight** refers to males who have a romantic and/or sexual orientation towards females or to females who have a romantic and/or sexual orientation towards males.
- **Homophobia** is the fear or dislike of someone, based on prejudice or negative attitudes, beliefs or views about lesbian, gay or bi people. Homophobic bullying may be targeted at people who are, or who are perceived to be, lesbian, gay or bisexual.
- **Lesbian** refers to a female who has a romantic and/or sexual orientation towards females. Some non-binary people identify with this term.
- **'Pan' or 'pansexual'** refers to a person whose romantic and/or sexual attraction towards others is not limited by sex or gender.
- **Queer** is a term used by those wanting to reject specific labels of romantic orientation, sexual orientation and/or gender identity. It can be a way of rejecting the perceived norms of the LGBT community, e.g. racism, sizeism, ableism. Although some LGBT people view the word as a slur, it was reclaimed and embraced in the late 1980s by the queer community.

For those young people questioning their sexuality, this has the potential to be a traumatic and difficult time. Large-scale research in UK secondary schools and colleges suggests that 55% of LGB young people experience homophobic bullying at some point (Guasp, 2012). As with other forms of bullying, this can increase the risk of low mood, anxiety, self-harming behaviours and attempts of, or death by, suicide. Caution is expressed at over-focusing on homophobic bullying and LGB young people being portrayed as victims in need of support, as this can deflect away from the importance of celebrating diversity and promoting inclusive attitudes and behaviours among young people (Formby, 2015).

Historically, CAMHS policy and guidance in relation to LGBT young people is clear. The National Service Framework (NSF) for Children Young People and Maternity Services (Department of Health, 2004) stated that services should be provided regardless of a young person's sexuality or gender. LGBT young people's rights are enshrined within the Equality Act (HM Government, 2010), protecting against discrimination on the grounds of sexuality in the provision of business and public services. This covers both schools and health care provision. Equality is further recognised with the age of consent for sexual intercourse being 16 for young people of all sexual orientations. It is recognised that LGBT people of all ages still face barriers and discrimination in their public life (Government Equalities Office, 2018).

For young people accessing CAMHS who are considering being open about their sexuality or have already 'come out', concerns expressed may include:

- They or their family holding beliefs that reject their sexuality as immoral.
- Living in an isolated setting where sources of support, such as other non-heterosexual young people or organised support groups, may not be available.
- Their family or social groups may not represent their sexuality (Morrow, 2004).
- They may perceive their family and friends to be homophobic and fear parental rejection (Morrow, 2004).
- Experiencing conflict around their sexuality leading to denial or living a 'double life', lying to friends and families about their relationships.

For those young people who have not yet disclosed their sexual orientation or gender dysphoria to family and peers, the response of the CAMHS practitioner, who may be the first person to be told, is important.

Case Study (1): Andreas

Andreas (16) was initially referred to CAMHS by his GP due to bulimic behaviours and emotional dysregulation. On assessment, it was clear that Andreas was coming to terms with his sexuality. He later identified himself as gay. Creating a setting where questions on sexuality were actually asked offered an environment in which Andreas could 'come out' (Meckler et al., 2006). This was in a non-judgemental way, and Andreas felt comfortable to open up to the practitioners (Kitts, 2005). A practitioner was assigned to work with him and a colleague to work with his mother.

Emerging sexuality issues can provoke uncomfortable emotions in practitioners, and clinical supervision is essential. It is important for both practitioner and supervisor to examine their attitudes/beliefs around sexuality and how this might impact on their practice (Dootson, 2000). In a positive and accepting environment, Andreas was able to express his worries about his sexuality (Morrow, 2004). Providing literature about local support groups for LGBT youth and posters advertising inclusivity enabled Andreas to be supported in his environment (Kitts, 2005).

Confidentially was key, as his family were initially unaware of his sexuality. The practitioner supported Andreas in developing coping strategies to respond to whatever reaction his parents had to his 'coming out'. His family had strong religious beliefs that viewed homosexuality as morally wrong. The practitioner did not challenge them on the issue but allowed them to explore their worries and fears. Part of this role was to prepare them for family therapy where the issue was further explored.

Case Study (2): Nicole

Nicole (15) was referred to CAMHS after an overdose that warranted admission to a local hospital. The practitioners who assessed her were careful to use inclusive language, and Nicole felt able to disclose the worries about her emerging sexuality that had precipitated the overdose (Kitts, 2005). It transpired that Nicole had been subject to homophobic bullying at school. It was important not to use the words 'lesbian' or 'gay' as Nicole was not yet ready to label herself. Her parents had begun to be aware of her sexuality and were supportive of Nicole. This improved her self-esteem and sense of well-being (Ryan et al., 2010).

A practitioner worked with Nicole to explore the association between her enduring low mood and coming to terms with her sexuality. Nicole self-harmed, and this was explored in relation to the anger at her sexuality and about not feeling 'normal'. A careful risk assessment was carried out because of the risk of further self-harm, arising from the psychosocial stressors associated with her sexuality (Morrow, 2004; Kitts, 2005). With her permission, the CAMHS team liaised with Nicole's school to highlight the homophobic bullying and ensure that it was addressed in a sensitive manner. Nicole was put in touch with local youth LGBT support groups.

Multiple-Choice Questions

See answers on page 668.

1. Sexual orientation refers to:
   a. How one identifies in their own mind in terms of gender
   b. How one portrays their gender to the world through communication, behaviour and appearance
   c. Genetic/physical characteristics assigned at birth
   d. To whom one is emotionally, spiritually and physically attracted, based on their sex/gender in relation to one's own
2. The percentage of LGB young people who have experienced homophobic bullying at some point during their school/college careers is:
   a. 15%
   b. 35%
   c. 55%
   d. 75%
3. What is the legal age of consent in the UK for adolescents to engage in sexual intercourse?
   a. 16 for both heterosexual and homosexual sex by males and females
   b. 18 for homosexual sex and 16 for heterosexual sex
   c. 16 for male homosexual and heterosexual sex, 18 for female homosexual sex and 16 for heterosexual sex
   d. 16 for both heterosexual sex and male homosexual sex. No age of consent for female homosexual sex

Key References

Busseri, M., Willoughby, T., Chalmers, H. and Bogaert, A.R. (2006). Same-Sex Attraction and Successful Adolescent Development. *Journal of Youth and Adolescence*, 35: 563–575.

Ryan, C., Russell, S.T. and Huebner, R. et al. (2010). Family Acceptance in Adolescence and the Health of LGBT Young Adults. *Journal of Child and Adolescent Psychiatric Nursing*, 23: 205–213.

Useful Resources

Gray, L. (2018). *LGBTQ+ Youth: A Guided Workbook to Support Sexual Orientation and Gender Identity.* Eau Claire, WI: PESI Publishing & Media, written for American health care professionals, but contains useful resource materials to engage and support LGBTQ+ young people.

www.fflag.org.uk, FFLAG are a national charity who are dedicated to supporting parents and their lesbian, gay, bisexual and trans children.

www.schools-out.org.uk, Schools Out is the UK's only national charity campaigning to make schools safe spaces for LGBT+ people as students, teaching and support staff, parents and carers and school leadership.

www.stonewall.org.uk, A charity that campaigns on behalf of LGB people. It has excellent guidance on working with young people who identify as LGB.

23 Gender Dysphoria in Children and Young People

Hannah Stynes, Martin McColl and Eilis Kennedy

Key Features of Gender Dysphoria (DSM-5, APA, 2013)

Children

- A strong desire to be of the other gender or an insistence that one is the other gender
- A strong preference for wearing clothes typical of the opposite gender
- A strong preference for cross-gender roles in make-believe play or fantasy play
- A strong preference for the toys, games or activities stereotypically used or engaged in by the other gender
- A strong preference for playmates of the other gender
- A strong rejection of toys, games and activities typical of one's assigned gender
- A strong dislike of one's sexual anatomy
- A strong desire for the physical sex characteristics that match one's experienced gender

Adolescents and Adults

- A marked incongruence between one's experienced/expressed gender and primary and/or secondary sex characteristics
- A strong desire to be rid of one's primary and/or secondary sex characteristics
- A strong desire for the primary and/or secondary sex characteristics of the other gender
- A strong desire to be of the other gender
- A strong desire to be treated as the other gender
- A strong conviction that one has the typical feelings and reactions of the other gender

Introduction

Gender identity is an integral component of human development, comprising the internal feelings and psychological understanding of one's own gender. At birth anatomical characteristics determine the sex an individual is assigned, and for most people, this will remain aligned with their gender for the duration of their lives. A minority of others will experience strong and persistent discomfort arising from a misalignment between their internal gender identity and biological sex characteristics.

Gender dysphoria, formerly known as gender identity disorder (GID), refers to a marked incongruence between an individual's experienced and assigned gender. This is accompanied by clinically significant and persistent distress, and impairment of functioning in key domains (APA, 2013). Classifications in the fifth edition of the Diagnostic and Statistical Manual of

Mental Disorders (DSM-5) separate the expression of gender dysphoria in younger childhood from those in adolescence.

For children, there is predominantly a focus on asserted beliefs and behaviours related to gender identity, e.g. displaying strong preferences for clothing, toys, gender roles, playmates of the other gender. In adolescents, the criteria chiefly reflect the expression of desires, e.g. to be of the other gender, to be treated as such, to be rid of sex characteristics in favour of those aligned to the experienced gender, recognising a more mature cognitive development in older children. This classification locates adolescent gender identity with adult gender identity, implicitly acknowledging the profound impact that the physical and emotional changes of puberty can have on the lives of children as they move into the years of evident sexual maturation.

The new international classification of diseases has reformulated what was previously 'gender identity disorder of childhood' to 'gender incongruence of childhood' (WHO, 2018). Other commonly used terms include 'gender variant' and 'gender diverse'. Unlike gender dysphoria, these categorisations do not presume that significant suffering and functional impairment need necessarily be present, though diagnostically, many may fulfil the criteria for gender dysphoria at some point in their lives. In ICD-11, gender identity has been moved from classification under mental health disorders to sexual health conditions. These shifts, sensitive to concerns about labelling and stigma, reflect advocacy for equality, in addition to a move away from a view of gender difference as a mental disorder, towards more positive perceptions of gender identity and expression. It follows the radical reassessment of the pathologisation of homosexuality in the 20th century (Drescher, 2015). Any terminology, including 'gender dysphoria' (DSM) and 'gender incongruence' (ICD), risks raising disputes about meaning, labelling and validation and is likely to evolve as time progresses and the knowledge base expands.

Transgender people are those whose gender identity does not align with their birth-assigned sex and include people who experience gender dysphoria (though this is not strictly necessary), those who identify as a gender other than that assigned to them at birth and those who identify outside of binary categories of male and female. The latter may identify as non-binary, gender queer, agender or gender fluid. Importantly, a transgender identity does not necessarily depend on a person having undergone medical intervention.

Sexual orientation is separate from gender identity and refers to a combination of a person's sexual attraction, sexual behaviour and self-identification as heterosexual/straight, homosexual/gay, bisexual, asexual or other.

Gender Dysphoria in Children and Young People

From around age three, children typically acquire an understanding of gender and the ability to label themselves and others as girls or boys. By age seven, they have a good understanding of gender constancy, i.e. the notion that gender is independent of external variables and is fixed.

Many children may exhibit gender-variant behaviours or 'do gender' in a way that is transgressive of stereotypical gender roles, but that does not necessarily challenge their gender identity. Others will express gender incongruence or dysphoria at a young age that ultimately resolves over time and through experiencing the puberty associated with their birth-assigned sex. A limited pool of longitudinal research has suggested that a proportion of these children grow up to be gay, lesbian or bisexual (Drummond et al., 2008; Steensma et al., 2013; Wallien and Cohen-Kettenis, 2008).

There are children who exhibit a strong and consistent certainty that their sex assigned at birth is fundamentally mismatched with their gender. These children often show the most severe dysphoria and cross-gender behaviour and appear to be the most likely to have a stable transgender identity that lasts into adulthood (Steensma et al., 2011; Steensma et al., 2013).

Presentation in early childhood features children from a range of backgrounds, with both typical and neuro-diverse development (deVries, Noens, Cohen-Kettenis, van Berckelaer-Onnes and Doreleijers, 2010; Hisle-Gorman et al., 2019; Yildirim et al., 2017). Parents may have noted their child's fascination with opposite-sex clothes and toys, and possibly with hair and make-up. Children may express the idea that they are a girl, rather than a boy, and vice versa and they may object to their penises and vaginas. They may say 'I want to be a girl', or 'I am a boy'. There may be no significant history of trauma or loss, but this can certainly be the case for some (Drescher and Byne, 2012; Ehrensaft, 2011).

Social development, school and family life may all be satisfactory, without major clinical concerns, and continue with little disruption. Nevertheless, disturbance can occur, as some families find disclosure and subsequent adaptation difficult and concerning, particularly coping with the uncertainty around future social implications for the child. Families may experience social isolation from extended networks, including family and friends (Riley et al., 2013). Some children's relationships with peers may be marked by caution, isolation and conflict (Kaltiala-Heino et al., 2015).

Increasingly, families attending clinic have begun to allow children to change their appearance and dress style, choose a preferred name and use new pronouns in a way that aligns with their experienced gender identity (Fast and Olson, 2018). Parents may initially restrict this to home, although clinical accounts would indicate that in many cases, this may extend beyond the home environment (Edwards-Leeper et al., 2016; Steensma and Cohen-Kettenis, 2011). Primary schools increasingly accommodate children who wish to make a social transition and who want to use the changing rooms and the toilets of the opposite gender. It is argued by some that social transition and affirmation of gender identity constitute active psychosocial treatments that may increase persistence rates of gender dysphoria relative to a 'wait-and-see' approach (Zucker, 2020; Zucker, 2018). Alternatively, there is evidence to suggest this type of early social transition may be associated with lower rates of depression and anxiety in pre-pubertal transgender children and that family acceptance of gender identity in young people may improve outcomes (Durwood et al., 2017; Ryan et al., 2010). Given this is a relatively recent focus of research, ongoing studies are likely to shed further light on the outcomes associated with early social transition in childhood.

For adolescents, puberty is a time of complex adjustment, not just to the individual's internal and external changes, but to the social expectations relating to their gender. Young people, their families and peers must navigate the passage to sexual maturation and the formation of intimate and romantic relationships. These challenges are daunting enough for straight and gay adolescents, but they are heightened by the impact of diverse gender identity on developing relationships in families, schools and communities. Those young people who present in adolescence with strong and persistent dysphoria appear more likely than younger children to have a transgender identity that continues into adulthood (Drescher and Byne, 2014).

Whilst one young person may be comfortable with the uncertainty about issues of gender and sexuality, another may be distressed by this lack of clarity. Young people may feel let down by people around them who are cautious about confirming their views or alternatively, they may feel pressurised by too strong an affirmation of their exploration of gender issues and insufficient acknowledgement of their hard-to-articulate doubts.

In recent years, there have been fluctuations in the patterns of referrals to gender services for children and young people. Amongst an overall increase in referral rates, a particular rise has been observed in adolescents presenting to clinics, and a shift in the sex ratio of these adolescents wherein birth-assigned females now make up the bulk of referrals for this age category (Kaltiala et al., 2020). The reasons for this are as yet under-explored.

Interestingly, the range of presentations of gender identities has shifted for this group (de Graaf and Carmichael, 2019). Whilst younger children will generally identify according to a binary model of gender and present in ways stereotypical of the opposite gender to that assigned them at birth, the adolescent position can be less fixed and unconditional. Their understanding of gender may be more dimensional, and preferred identities may include non-binary, gender queer or gender fluid.

Epidemiology

Little good information indicating prevalence rates for gender dysphoria in the general population exists for young people, but it is generally agreed that it is still a relatively rare condition. In a survey of school-aged children in the United States, 1.3% selected the response option of 'transgender' when asked 'what is your gender?' (Shields et al., 2013). Similarly for adolescents, 1.2% stated 'yes' when asked 'Are you transgender?' in a survey of New Zealand high school students, whilst 2.5% were unsure (Clark et al., 2014). Eisenberg et al. (2017) reported 2.7% of high school students overall identified as transgender or gender non-conforming (TGNC). This prevalence was much higher for birth-assigned females (3.6%) than for birth-assigned males (1.7%) (Eisenberg et al., 2017).

Parent endorsement of the gender identity item, 'wishes to be of the opposite sex', on the Child Behaviour Checklist (Achenbach, 2001) is around 1% for non-referred boys and 1.2% for non-referred girls (genders assigned at birth) aged 6 to 12 years. For clinic-referred children, the percentages are higher at around 2.7% and 4.7% respectively, with similar figures for clinic-referred adolescents, aged 12 to 18 (2% and 5% respectively) (Zucker, 2017).

For adults, the Arcelus et al. (2015) meta-analysis of prevalence for transsexualism indicated 4.6 in 100,000, 6.8 for transgender women and 2.6 for transgender men. They acknowledged that much of the prevalence estimates are derived from numbers attending gender identity clinics for assessment and medical treatment. Consequently, these figures inevitably underrepresent the true numbers of TG/NC people in the general population given that (a) not every person will want to attend or have access to a gender clinic and (b) not every person will want to pursue medical treatment.

Assessment and Intervention

Internationally, services to support children and adolescents with gender identity issues have been established and developed country by country over the last 30 years. These follow the innovative multi-disciplinary services pioneered in the second half of the 20th century for transgender adults. Services have experienced a significant and universal increase in referrals over time, with a particularly marked upsurge occurring in 2015 (Giovanardi, 2017).

The 'Dutch Approach', established by clinicians at the Centre of Expertise on Gender Dysphoria in Amsterdam (deVries and Cohen-Kettenis, 2012), laid the foundation for treatment models across such clinics, including services in the United Kingdom. Intervention, according to this framework, should consist of a psychosocial assessment, followed by physical and psychological treatment options working in tandem, where requested and appropriate.

The Dutch protocol argued that the use of puberty suppression in early adolescence, around Tanner stage 2, may facilitate a reduction in distress associated with pubertal development and provide time to reflect and explore the complexities of a developing gender identity (Cohen-Kettenis and van Goozen, 1998). A similar approach was adopted as part of the treatment recommendation outlined in both the World Professional Association for Transgender Health (WPATH) Standards of Care (Coleman et al., 2012) and, more recently, the Endocrine Society Guidelines for the Treatment of Transsexual Persons (Hembree et al., 2017). Both guidelines recognise the importance of offering hormonal suppression once adolescents meeting the criteria for gender dysphoria or gender incongruence first exhibit physical changes associated with puberty.

A comprehensive psychosocial assessment helps to establish several key pieces of information to guide treatment and care. These include the nature and characteristics of the young person's gender identity and level of dysphoria, the presence of any co-occurring conditions, their medical and family history, social and emotional functioning and their eligibility and readiness for particular interventions and treatments. Mental health professionals involved in this process are guided by the Standards of Care to provide psychoeducation for families about therapeutic options and their possibilities and limitations, in order to facilitate informed consent (Coleman et al., 2012).

Analogues of gonadotropin releasing hormones (GnRH) to suppress the development of primary and secondary sex characteristics have been used in paediatric practice in the treatment of precocious puberty (Mul and Hughes, 2008). For birth-assigned males, regular use delays the deepening of the voice and decreases the growth of body hair, whilst for birth-assigned females, use inhibits breast and hip development and delays or halts menstruation. Ceasing treatment with GnRH analogues resumes pubertal development, although clinic-based studies suggest that many adolescents starting GnRH have tended to move on to cross-sex hormones (Butler et al., 2018).

For young people seeking treatment with cross-sex hormones, the Endocrine Society Guidelines recommend a demonstration of sufficient mental capacity to give informed consent because of the partially irreversible effects of these drugs. In most cases, this is at 16 years. There may be compelling reasons to initiate treatment at a younger age (Hembree et al., 2017). Despite this, clinicians may be hesitant to facilitate earlier physical intervention given that there is limited evidence for this age group regarding safety, tolerability and physical and psychological outcomes (Olson-Kennedy et al., 2019). Longitudinal research is currently being carried out to map the use and longer-term physiological and psychological effects of both hormone blockers and gender-affirming hormones in gender-dysphoric youth (Allen et al., 2019).

In the United Kingdom, the nationally commissioned service for children and young people, the Gender Identity Service (GIDS), offers multi-disciplinary assessment and intervention according to best practice in line with international guidance from WPATH and the Endocrine Society Guidelines (Butler et al., 2018). In recent years, rates of annual referral to GIDS have increased substantially, rising from 77 in 2009/2010, to 2,590 in 2018/2019 (GIDS, 2020). This mirrors a trend observed internationally in the last decade across both child and adult gender services (de Graaf and Carmichael, 2019; Fielding and Bass, 2018; Wood et al., 2013).

Complexities and Controversies

On a personal level, individuals with gender dysphoria can experience ostracism and hostility from family and community at all ages. They are often at heightened risk for harassment, victimisation and abuse, both on- and off-line (Collier, Van Beusekom, Bos and Sandfort, 2013; Grossman, D'augelli and Frank, 2011; Kosciw, Greytak and Diaz, 2009; Ybarra, Mitchell, Palmer and Reisner, 2015). These external pressures may amplify any internal dissonance and distress. Personal experiences can be affirmed by loving and supportive family members, including peers, and flexible and accommodating institutions, particularly schools and colleges attended in childhood and adolescence. Children and young people remain vulnerable, and co-occurring issues arise even in those who do have good social support, including low self-esteem, low mood and self-harm (Becerra-Culqui et al., 2018; Poteat, Scheer and Mereish, 2014). A significant proportion of gender-dysphoric young people have autistic traits that may compound difficulties in social integration (Glidden et al., 2016).

For families, adjusting to a young person's diverse gender identity can be a slow and challenging process marked by the co-occurrence of both accepting and rejecting behaviours (Ryan et al., 2010). Parents, in particular, may experience a sense of grief and ambiguous loss when navigating their new family structure (Wahlig, 2015), and parental anxiety can increase with the level of gender non-conformity present in their child (Kuvalanka et al., 2017).

A small body of research has documented the perspective of parents with a more 'critical' view of gender identity affirmation. A study conducted by Littman (2018) collected reports from the parents of a group of primarily birth-assigned female adolescents, who had recently and unexpectedly disclosed their gender identity status. These families expressed concern about the sureness and apparent suddenness with which these young people had asserted their convictions and sought to pursue the process of transition. In particular, they raised the possibility of influence from peers, on-line communities and other social outlets, and insufficient clinical evaluation of the underlying causes of their child's dysphoria.

Despite controversy surrounding the conclusions and implications of this research, and critiques regarding biases in sampling and measurement (Restar, 2019), several clinicians in the field have advocated in favour of more carefully evaluating the aetiology and differential presentations of gender dysphoria based on their observations in working clinically with such patients (Hutchinson et al., 2019). Alternative viewpoints have been offered, i.e. the possibility that young people who have been grappling with their identity for a prolonged period but who anticipate an adverse reaction to such disclosure may delay expressing their gender identity openly, despite having been aware of their feelings for some time (Boivin et al., 2020).

Clinical services and professionals working with children and young people may experience pressures stemming from the recent rise in referrals, particularly of those presenting in adolescence, and birth-assigned females (Kaltiala et al., 2020). Established guidelines for assessment, use of GnRH and cross-sex hormones may be questioned by the appearance of this new and disproportionate number of a narrow group of patients. As individual trajectories for young people vary to such a degree, the clinical work with families often encourages and supports them to sit with a level of uncertainty and be open to multiple potential pathways in identity formation (Wren, 2019).

The prime age to administer hormone blockers has been a controversial topic. Those favouring earlier intervention believe that the prolonging of a puberty that does not align with a young person's experienced gender represents an unacceptably high level of risk to their wellbeing (De Vries et al., 2014; De Vries et al., 2011). Intervention prior to the development of secondary sex characteristics alongside social transition could, they argue, ultimately improve outcomes for the young person. It may reduce the need for later invasive surgeries and treatments to correct pubertal developments. In contrast, there is the argument that blocking puberty may compromise bone development (Vlot et al., 2017) and, in the longer term, impact on cardiovascular health (Prentice and Viner, 2013) and result in complications around genital confirmation surgery in adulthood (Butler et al., 2018; Milrod, 2014).

Careful consideration of fertility preservation needs to be incorporated into endocrine care given that long-term treatment with gender-affirming cross-sex hormones may impair gonadal function, impacting on reproductive functioning. A large proportion of young people progress from initial pubertal blockade to gender-affirming hormone therapy (Butler et al., 2018); thus it is important for informed discussions around the options for preserving reproductive options, i.e. cryopreservation in the form of sperm banking or oocyte retrieval, to take place prior to initiating GnRH (Johnson and Finlayson, 2016). Utilisation rates, however, are low (Nahata et al., 2017) perhaps due in part to the immaturity of the young people required to make such a significant decision. Amongst treatment-seeking transgender young people the potential to have biological children has been shown to rank lower in priority than being in good health, making money and having positive close relationships (Chiniara et al., 2019).

Finally, gender-diverse and dysphoric young people with a minority ethnic background remain a poorly understood and marginalised group. Their multiple minority status puts them at increased risk of experiencing cumulative effects of oppression and discrimination (de Graaf et al., 2019). In the UK, ethnic minority population groups are significantly underrepresented in gender services for young people relative to child and adolescent mental health services (CAMHS) and the general population (de Graaf et al., 2019).

Potential barriers to equitable access to specialised care at the individual level may include language barriers, both real and perceived stigma and fear of ostracism by their communities. At the service level, a lack of cultural awareness and ability to manage patients from diverse backgrounds on the part of clinicians may play a role in underrepresentation (de Graaf et al., 2019). Much of the existing research from which conclusions regarding transgender and gender non-conforming youth are derived has been carried out using predominantly Caucasian samples, and further work investigating the intersectionality of gender, age, race and ethnicity is warranted.

Multiple-Choice Questions

See answers on page 668.

1. The most recent World Health Organization ICD-11 classification for atypical gender development is:
   a. Gender identity disorder
   b. Gender dysphoria
   c. Gender variance
   d. Gender incongruence
2. The majority of referrals to gender clinics in recent years have been:
   a. Adolescent birth-assigned males
   b. Adolescent birth-assigned females
   c. An equal ratio of adolescents assigned male and female
   d. Children under 12 years of age
3. Social transition can involve:
   a. Changing name
   b. Changing pronouns
   c. Changing appearance or dress
   d. Any, or all, of the above
4. Prevalence estimates for gender dysphoria in children and young people lie between:
   a. 0.5 and 1.5%
   b. 1.2 and 2.5%
   c. 2.5 and 4.3%
   d. 4.5 and 6%
5. The WPATH Standards of Care guidelines for assessment and treatment were informed by:
   a. The Danish protocol
   b. The Dutch protocol
   c. The Swiss protocol
   d. The French protocol

6. Children and young people with gender dysphoria have a greater likelihood of experiencing:
   a. Bullying and victimisation
   b. Self-harm
   c. Traits of autism spectrum disorder
   d. All of the above
7. Uptake rates for fertility preservation amongst gender-dysphoric youth pursuing physical treatment are currently:
   a. High
   b. Moderate
   c. Low

Key References

Busseri, M., Willoughby, T., Chalmers, H. and Bogaert, A.R. (2006). Same-Sex Attraction and Successful Adolescent Development. *Journal of Youth and Adolescence*, 35: 563–575.

Ryan, C., Russell, S.T., Huebner, R. et al. (2010). Family Acceptance in Adolescence and the Health of LGBT Young Adults. *Journal of Child and Adolescent Psychiatric Nursing*, 23: 205–213.

Useful Resources

Gray, L. (2018). *LGBTQ+ Youth: A Guided Workbook to Support Sexual Orientation and Gender Identity.* Eau Claire, WI: PESI Publishing & Media, written for American health care professionals, but contains useful resource materials to engage and support LGBTQ+ young people.

www.fflag.org.uk, FFLAG are a national charity who are dedicated to supporting parents and their lesbian, gay, bisexual and trans children.

www.schools-out.org.uk, Schools Out is the UK's only national charity campaigning to make schools safe spaces for LGBT+ people as students, teaching and support staff, parents and carers and school leadership.

www.stonewall.org.uk, A charity that campaigns on behalf of LGB people. It has excellent guidance on working with young people who identify as LGB.

24 Cultural Competence in Working with Children, Young People and Families

Karen Davies (updated by Christopher Gale)

Introduction

Working with diversity in child and adolescent mental health requires that individuals understand difference and the need to develop the capacity to deliver culturally competent care. When we move beyond the limits of our own cultural experiences to incorporate the perspectives of other cultures, we begin the journey of cultural competence.

KEY CONCEPTS

- Cultural competence refers to the ability to interact effectively with people from different cultures and is essentially comprised of four components: awareness of one's own cultural worldview, our attitude towards cultural differences, knowledge of different cultural practices and worldviews and cross-cultural skills.
- Cultural competence is not an 'add-on' and must be integrated into effective, quality mental health service provision for children, young people and their families.

The term 'cultural competence' is now frequently encountered in many care services language and settings. It first appeared in social work and counselling psychology literature beginning in the early 1980s (Gallegos, 1982; Pedersen and Marshall, 1982). Although cultural competence has been referred to as a theory by some (Wuand Martinez, 2006; Lum, 2010), there has been on-going debate as to whether cultural competency meets the criteria for a theory or whether the description of cultural competence fits more comfortably as a model, framework, skillset or perspective (Gallegos et al., 2008).

The concept of cultural competence in health is based on the principles of **social justice**: (a) every person is entitled to fair and equal opportunities for health care and (b) **human rights**, every person has the right to access quality care, to participate in care decisions and to be assured of safe health care.

By practicing culturally competent care, health care professionals are contributing to a reduction in health disparities by empowering individuals and integrating their cultural beliefs into care interventions (Purnell, 2005). Dalrymple and Burke (1995) state that 'unless clients are considered as true partners, culturally sensitive care is not being achieved; equal partnership involves trust, acceptance and respect as well as facilitation and negotiation'.

The *Delivering Race Equality in Mental Health Care Action Plan* (Department of Health, 2005) delivered a vision for mental health services that focused on:

- Decreased fear of services
- Increased satisfaction and effective communication
- Better management of challenging situations
- A more balanced range of effective interventions
- A workforce that can deliver appropriate and responsive services to black and minority ethnic (BME) communities

The following legislation and guidance underline the clinical necessity of incorporating the cultural competence and equality agenda:

- *Equality Act* (HM Government, 2010). This sets out the public sector equality duty.
- *The NHS Constitution for England* (2015).
- *Every Child Matters* (Department for Education and Skills, 2003).
- *NICE's Objectives and Equality Programme 2016–2020* (NICE, 2016).
- *Future in Mind* (Department of Health, 2015).

These all identify the importance of appropriate and responsive services, engaged and more accessible communities, better information and communication and cultural competency training being made available to all staff. All children, young people and their families have their own individual identity, and each come with their own life experiences that inform their independent beliefs, attitudes and values regarding culture, faith and community. Some communities may have a different perception of mental health and fear the stigma of a diagnostic label, or have concerns around possible discrimination within services. Practitioners require training and skills development to implement culturally competent principles in all aspects of their work with culturally diverse clients, in addition to a thorough knowledge of the legislative requirements.

Cultural competence does more than provide a non-discriminatory service to clients, it includes a policy framework that supports a culturally sensitive response, a collaborative model with ethnic and minority communities and agencies to ensure that specific ethnic groups are understood, their needs addressed and partnerships developed. Assessment and intervention processes that take account of the culturally defined needs of young people, their families and community need to be implemented. Papadopoulos et al. (1998) devised a model for the development of transcultural nursing and cultural competence, later updated and expanded in 2016.

The PTT model consisted of four constructs: 'cultural awareness', 'cultural knowledge', 'cultural sensitivity' and finally 'cultural competence' (Papadopoulos et al., 2016):

Cultural awareness: the degree of awareness one has about one's own cultural background and cultural identity. By understanding the importance of our own cultural heritage and that of others, we are more able to recognise the dangers of ethnocentricity.

Cultural knowledge: this derives from several disciplines, e.g. anthropology, sociology, psychology, biology, nursing, medicine and the arts. Meaningful contact with people from different cultural groups can enhance our knowledge about their health beliefs and behaviours and identify any specific problems they face.

Cultural sensitivity: this implies the development of appropriate interpersonal relationships with people. An important element in achieving cultural sensitivity is how we as professionals view those in our care. In children and young people's services, unless individuals and families are considered as true partners, culturally sensitive care is not being achieved.

Cultural competence: this is the capacity to provide effective health care, taking into consideration people's cultural beliefs, behaviours and needs.

Multiple-Choice Questions

See answers on page 668.

1. What are the four guiding principles for culturally competent practice?
   a. Professionalism, beliefs, equality, knowledge
   b. Awareness, attitude, knowledge, skills
   c. Communication, challenge, anti-discriminatory practice, attitudes
   d. Respect, values, judgements, understanding
2. Which statement is correct about cultural competence?
   a. Cultural competence predicts behaviour.
   b. Cultural competency is providing resources in different languages.
   c. Cultural competence is a developmental process that evolves over an extended period.
   d. Cultural competence is treating everyone equally.
3. Who is responsible for implementing and delivering culturally competent practice within agencies/services?
   a. Managers and policy development team.
   b. It is for individuals to research if they have a BME client.
   c. It is part of professional training modules for different disciplines, e.g. nursing or social work.
   d. Every individual has a responsibility to continue to learn and develop their practice.

Key References

Lum, D. (2010). *Culturally Competent Practice: A Framework for Understanding Diverse Groups and Justice Issues* (4th edition). Pacific Grove, CA: Brooks/Cole.

Papadopoulos, I. (2006). The Papadopoulos, Tilki and Taylor Model of Developing Cultural Competence. In: Papadopoulos, I. (ed.), *Transcultural Health and Social Care: Developing Culturally Competent Practitioners.* Oxford: Elsevier.

Papadopoulos, I., Shea, S., Taylor, G., Pezzella, A. and Foley, L. (2016). Developing Tools to Promote Culturally Competent Compassion, Courage, and Intercultural Communication in Healthcare. *Journal of Compassionate Health Care*, 3(2); 1–10.

25 Young Carers

Charlotte Pyatt (updated by Christopher Gale)

Introduction to the Author

I qualified as a registered nurse (mental health) in 2007. I was a carer for my mother at times throughout my adolescent years during her episodes of depression. My contribution to this book uses both my personal and professional experiences of caring for an individual experiencing mental ill health.

> **KEY CONCEPTS**
>
> - Data from the 2001 and 2011 census suggest a 24% increase in young carers (5–24) in the UK, but a 67% proportionate increase in 5–9-year olds (Wayman et al., 2016). The official figure stood at 403,603.
> - Census data are likely to under-report numbers of young carers, because reporting is undertaken by parents of those under 18.
> - It is estimated that one in four of the adult UK population will experience mental ill health at some point in their lives (NHS England, 2019).
> - Many children will grow up with a parent who experiences ongoing mental health difficulties, with peaks of crisis.

When I was a caring for my mother, I never even realised I was a carer. Young carers are defined as 'a person under 18 who provides or intends to provide care for another person (of any age, except where that care is provided for payment, pursuant to a contract or as voluntary work)' (HM Govt, 2014). My mother experienced episodes of depression for some time. After my father and two older sisters left home, she found it increasingly difficult to cope. I helped much more around the house: small jobs like cooking, cleaning or looking after my little sister. I remember calling my mother's employer to report her off sick when she was too unwell to be there and I would go food shopping. I would sit and chat with my mother, giving emotional support. I enjoyed doing all of those things. It made me feel important and special to my mother and sister.

Caring can sometimes help cement bonds between parents and children, as children who care feel both valued and included (Aldridge and Becker, 2003). There is support available for children and young carers, and it is vital that young carers are identified. If a family is unsupported in this situation, they may struggle to cope and rely on children within the family to take on inappropriate caring responsibilities (Frank and McLarnon, 2008). Even if identified, the degree of their caring role and the impact it has on the young carer's own development may not be identified quickly or assessed thoroughly (The Children's Society Young Carers Initiative, 2006). It is not inevitable that children are at risk of significant harm because they care for a parent with a mental illness. For various reasons, young carers can remain hidden, and their needs and those of the person that they care for are only identified in a crisis.

There are many reasons why children and young carers may remain hidden. In my case, I did not view my situation as different or unusual. My mother's depression was undiagnosed and untreated largely due to her fear of the stigma associated with mental illness. Other young carers are so loyal that they do not want to ask for help or may fear their family will be split up. Children who are exposed to mental illness in the family may display the following:

- Social withdrawal or isolation.
- Anxiety.
- Find it difficult to concentrate on their schoolwork, leading to under-achievement in education and limited life opportunities.
- Low self-esteem and depressed mood.
- A fatalistic acceptance of their life situation.
- Behavioural difficulties, violent or self-destructive behaviour.
- Paranoid or suspicious behaviour if they believe their parents' delusions.
- Many children are teased or bullied because of their unwell family member.

Some children have periods of separation from their parents, who are admitted to hospital, which can be a confusing and stressful time. Health care professionals need to consider what arrangements are made for visiting and to identify and meet the needs of the child or young person arising from loss and separation (Barnardo's, 2007). Daily routines may be changed, education disrupted and siblings separated, all of which have an impact on the child.

Research has shown that many mental health professionals are unaware that their service users are parents (Aldridge and Becker, 2003). This in turn raises questions for adult mental health services to consider. Mental health professionals should find out if their patients are parents, documenting names and date of birth of children and enquiring about the impact their illness is having on other family members.

For the children themselves, the following needs should be addressed:

- Someone whom they trust to talk to, preferably one key worker who will respond promptly and positively when they ask for help. This is often a difficult step to take.
- Children and young people may have important information about the person with the mental illness; they need to know they will be listened to and their perspective considered in care plans.
- Help in recognising the behaviour signs that indicate their parent/sibling is becoming ill.
- They need to know what is not acceptable behaviour from an adult, and they will need to know who to contact at any time for help.
- Additional support at school, such as learning support, access to counselling or education welfare. They may wish to keep school and friends separate from their caring responsibilities, which must be respected.
- For pre-school age children, there are alternative options for support. When working with a child under five, the health visitor should be contacted as the first port of call for support and signposting: information about who this is can be found through the GP surgery. Referrals to children's social services may be beneficial for the assessment of the required level of support.

- Providing practical support to the family, such as shopping and domestic chores, can reduce the stress for the child or young person.
- Evidence suggests that what young carers often require most is recognition of their caring contribution, alongside practical support (Aldridge and Becker, 2003).

Case Study (1): Isabelle

Alice was experiencing an episode of psychotic depression. Her four-year-old daughter, Isabelle, was her carer at times. Alice was a single mother and while her ex-partner, Steve, was involved in the care of Isabelle and Alice, the couple did not live together. Working with the well parent and the extended family can help support the child or young carer. When appropriate, it is helpful to include children in discussions about their caring responsibilities and consult with them about their family's needs. When very young children are involved, they must be made to feel comfortable, relaxed and supported by professionals interacting with them at their level.

During a visit one day by the community mental health practitioner, Isabelle would not leave the room, intent on being present, despite her young age. Children and young carers' predominant feelings may be of fear or guilt regarding the ill person, while anger and embarrassment tend to be more common amongst adolescents (The Children's Society, 2008). It is likely that Isabelle was seeking reassurance by staying with Alice during the visit and by protecting her, as young carers do. She stood next to Alice, holding and stroking her hand. Alice was talking about her lack of sleep due to panic attacks when Isabelle said 'I climb into bed with mummy to make sure nothing bad happens to her, I wait until she goes to sleep and then I can go to sleep'. During the visit Isabelle fetched a glass of water for Alice saying 'Please drink this mummy, it's good for you'. The practitioner began to talk to Isabelle about what she likes to play with and Isabelle brought her favourite doll. This interaction was playful and caring and Isabelle responded very well. It is crucial that children can still be children despite the mature caring role they may have adopted. Importantly, the health visitor should be made aware of Isabelle's needs as a young carer, because children and young people need to be looked after themselves as well as the person they care for and will need 'time out' for themselves. A referral to social services would be appropriate for an assessment of Isabelle's needs.

Case Study (2): Tom

Children who observe a family member experiencing symptoms of mental illness may be confused about the illness. This can leave them feeling scared or angry and feeling powerless to change the situation. Tom was nine years old and could not understand what was happening to his mother, Rachel. He knew she was sometimes happy and sometimes sad and would ask the community mental health practitioner 'why is mummy sad sometimes?'

Rachel is diagnosed with bipolar affective disorder. Explaining the diagnosis to Tom in an age-appropriate manner may help him to understand her emotions and reduce any feelings of fear, guilt or anger. Research indicates that giving information to young carers helps them to cope (The Children's Society, 2008). An additional source of support with the caring role may be accessed through a young carers project group. Young carers can meet with other children and young people who have had similar experiences. The projects run various social activities and offer emotional support. Young carers projects have been found to be invaluable, appreciated by young carers their families and professionals (Aldridge and Sharpe, 2007).

Case Study (3): Oliver

Oliver (15) was beginning to fall behind in his schoolwork; he struggled to concentrate because he was worried about his father who had been admitted to hospital. Oliver was going out with his mates; he started smoking cannabis and stayed up late; as a result, his education was disrupted. It is imperative that schools are able to identify and support young carers.

> Schools might find it helpful to have one member of staff to act as a link between young carers, the education welfare service, social services and young carers projects. Their role would be one of liaison with the relevant services. This would be a proactive way of recognising the difficulties faced by young carers and getting help to them, both within and outside the school. Young carers may need the opportunity to talk to someone at school, perhaps their teacher or someone else with the right skills, in a way which is confidential and sensitive.
> (The Princess Royal Trust for Carers, 2005, p. 11)

Multiple-Choice Questions

See answers on page 668.

1. How can a young carer be defined?
   a. Children and young persons who visit a relative in a care home every week.
   b. Children and young persons under 18 years old who provide, or intend to provide, care, assistance or support to another family member.
   c. Children and young persons who walk to school with their parent to collect an older sibling.
2. What is the proportional increase of UK young carers between the ages of five and nine between the 2011 and 2011 census?
   a. 47%
   b. 67%
   c. 87%
3. What major issue has been identified for families who have a parent with a mental health problem?
   a. Lack of joint working between mental health teams and children's services.
   b. They don't want any support.
   c. There are no issues.
4. Young carers can remain hidden, which of these are possible reasons?
   a. There is no support available for young carers.
   b. Young carers aren't hidden.
   c. Loyalty, stigma, unaware the situation is unusual.
5. What can mental health professionals do to ensure young carers are identified?
   a. Look at the patient's notes.
   b. Find out if their patients are parents, documenting names and date of birth of children, enquiring about the impact their illness is having on the family.
   c. Assume other professionals have obtained this information.

Key References

Aldridge, J. and Becker, S. (2003). *Children Caring for Parents with Mental Illness. Perspectives of Young Carers, Parents and Professionals*. Bristol: Policy Press.

Frank, J. and McLarnon, J. (2008). *Young Carers, Parents and Their Families: Key Principles of Practice. Supportive Practice Guidance for Those Who Work Directly with, or Commission Services for, Young Carers and Their Families.* London: Young Carers Initiative, The Children's Society.

Social Care Institute for Excellence, (2009). *Think Child, Think Parent, Think Family: A Guide to Parental Mental Health and Child Welfare.* London: SCIE.

26 Young Carers from Black Asian Minority Ethnic (BAME) Communities

Julia Pelle

Introduction

A number of Department of Health reports in the UK have acknowledged the integral role young carers play in the recovery of parents and other family members with mental health problems (DH, 1999, 2003, 2004, 2005, 2007, 2009).

The term BAME (formerly BME) includes people from Black African, Afro-Caribbean, South Asian and Chinese heritage in addition to individuals from white communities who have a heritage different from that of the majority population, e.g. Irish, Gypsy and travelling communities and Eastern European migrants.

KEY CONCEPTS

- People from BAME communities are more likely to experience poverty, discrimination and unemployment.
- Individuals from the Black African and Black Caribbean communities are more likely to be given a diagnosis of schizophrenia and are less likely to be diagnosed with affective or mood disorder (Bhugra, 2002; Sharpley, 2001; Wordsworth, 2008).
- These individuals experience higher rates of admission to inpatient units and compulsory detention (DH, 2003, 2005; NBCCWN, 2002, 2008).
- Children and adolescents from BAME communities not only experience the impact of a parent, sibling or other family member with a mental health problem, but may have to endure the added stigma of perceived cultural stereotypes.
- Some young carers belong to first-generation migrant families who find themselves adapting to a very different way of life in the UK (Green et al., 2008). Other young carers are part of the second-generation migrant community and although they have acculturated to what is their birth place, they can be vulnerable to inequalities within education, social exclusion, racial discrimination, insecure housing and the criminal justice system (Fatimelehin, 2007).

For young carers, parental and sibling mental health problems can have a negative impact on their development, breakdown in family relationships, interrupted and incomplete education and risk of child abuse. Young carers can find it uncomfortable to discuss family matters with those people whom they perceive to be 'outsiders', e.g. teachers, mental health nurses or social workers. They may become more vulnerable as a result of poor communication between themselves and the adult mental health services (Grant et al., 2008; Green et al., 2008).

Case Study (1): Aisha and Her Brother, Khaleel

Aisha (nine) lives at home with her parents, Youssuf and Afsana, and five other siblings. Aisha's oldest brother Khaleel (16) has drug-induced psychosis and has recently been diagnosed with schizoaffective disorder. Aisha remembers when Khaleel used to look after her, play with her and protect her, but now he can be very angry over any little thing. She and her other siblings are scared of being around him. Aisha says she sometimes sees Khaleel talking to himself and wonders who he is talking to. Aisha knows that sometimes Khaleel has to go into hospital and her mother and father have to spend time with him. All the siblings in the family are bi-lingual, but neither of Khaleel's parents speaks very good English and they are reliant on their older daughter, Eiliyah (14), to be their interpreter.

Mark is Khaleel's key worker and is a community CAMHS nurse. He arranges to visit the family a week after Khaleel's discharge from the local mental health unit. Mark observes that both parents are very distressed and Aisha is hiding behind the door in the hallway. Khaleel is somewhat withdrawn. Both parents express their concern about the number of young black men they have seen in the mental health hospital when they visited Khaleel and are adamant that they do not want him to be re-admitted.

Assessment

- Explain to the parents the reason for the visit and explain the importance of finding out how Khaleel thinks he is managing since returning home.
- Explain and discuss the usefulness of first speaking to Khaleel by himself and then speaking to both parents.
- After speaking to Khaleel, discuss with his parents how the family care for Khaleel and find out how they are coping.
- What contact do the parents have with their local GP, when caring for their son? Identify what support they have from their GP.
- Explore with the parents what their everyday experience is of caring for their son.
- Complete carer assessment form with the family.
- Establish during conversation any cultural preferences that Khaleel's parents have.
- Review the discharge plan and establish whether both parents and Khaleel are still happy with the discharge plan.
- Discuss what support the community mental health services can give to the family and to Khaleel.
- Evaluate the relationship between (a) Khaleel and his siblings and (b) between Khaleel and his parents.

Possible Interventions

- Education for parents about drug-induced psychosis.
- Consider which education materials could be useful for both Khaleel and his siblings.
- Check with the family if they have computer access and 'signpost' them to user-friendly information that further explains mental health problems and could identify local carer support groups and service user groups.

- Identify how the parents can explain Khaleel's mental health problem to Aisha, as the youngest child, and to his other siblings.
- Discuss opportunities to have leisure time as a family, e.g. meeting with other families who care for a child with a similar mental health problem.
- Consider accessing the interpretation services for future meetings.
- Family-centred work.

Outcomes

- Carers often complain about the lack of information on mental health problems and the lack of support when caring for a family member with a mental health problem.
- By signposting the family to local community support networks, this can make it easier for them to meet with others experiencing the same difficulties and offer opportunities to share better ways of accessing information and managing issues around caring.
- By empowering parents with the information that they need about their son's mental health problem, they can then explain this to other family members.
- It is important to ensure that parents are aware of any local support networks, other than the statutory mental health services.

Case Study (2): Jade and Her Mother, Monique

Jade (12) has been caring for Monique since she was ten years old. Monique has been diagnosed with paranoid schizophrenia. Jade has an older sister, Joleesa (18). Joleesa found their mother 'too weird' and left to live with their grandparents. When Monique is very unwell, she 'sees' people who are not there and hears voices. She has been known to experience tactile hallucinations.

Jade does most of the cooking during these times and is able to cook a number of traditional Caribbean dishes. She helps her mother with the weekly shopping. Monique has accused Jade of trying to poison her when Jade tries to encourage her to take her medication. Often what follows then is that Monique threatens to throw Jade out, but Jade knows this is because she is unwell. Monique struggles with trusting health professionals, but she has agreed to meet with Sharon, her keyworker, although she worries that Jade will be taken away from her. During the meeting Jade speaks 'patois' to her mother and switches to English when speaking to Sharon.

Sharon meets with Jade and Monique and observes that their relationship is a very loving one. Both have a great sense of humour. Sharon observes that Jade looks very tired and appears to be under-weight. Sharon discusses the possibility of respite care for Jade, but Monique becomes noticeably upset.

Assessment

- Young carer assessment form.
- Identify what support Jade already has.
- Review how she manages schoolwork and home/housework and looking after Monique.
- Monitor how Jade takes care of herself each day. Review any barriers to her own self-care.
- Jade already cooks traditional Caribbean meals for her mother. Explore what other aspects of her culture are important to her.
- Assess what leisure activities Jade engages in (a) with Monique and (b) with others.
- Review the relationship between (a) Jade and her sister, Joleesa, and (b) Monique and Joleesa. Jade may feel like a 'go-between' or 'piggy in the middle' in that relationship.

- Discuss with Jade what her understanding of her mother's mental health problem is and ask if she would like more information. If she does, offer useful educational material appropriate for Jade's age that could help her recognise triggers with Monique and help her to build self-esteem around her caring skills.
- The change in Monique's mental state can have a negative impact on Jade's self-esteem, particularly when Jade tries to help Monique with taking her medication.

Intervention

- Continue to build up trust with Jade and Monique. Discussions about cultural identity can be initiated through asking about the Caribbean dishes that Jade cooks. Build on the aspects of Caribbean culture both individuals identify with.
- Provide information on respite care and types of respite care for Jade and her mother to read about together.
- Explain that some respite time for Jade would help Monique in the long term.
- Consider activities where Jade and Monique can have leisure time together.

Outcomes

It is important to build up a trusting relationship with both the carer and the person being cared for. Understanding their daily routine helps the mental health nurse to see where there may be barriers to the caring relationship and to consider what options are available to overcome those barriers.

Finding out about the cultural identity of the young carer, and their parent or relative, can help put them at their ease, demonstrate interest and may lead to information on how best to support the family.

Some parents are concerned about their children receiving respite care because:

- They may perceive this as an opportunity for their children to be taken away from them.
- Of concerns about how they will cope when the young carer is not around.
- They are unable to trust anyone else to give them the care they need and in the way they like to be cared for.
- Of concerns that the young carer may decide they no longer wish to care for their parent or relative.

The mental health nurse needs to reassure that parent or relative that respite is really for the short term and will be jointly discussed with them. It is important to reiterate the need for young people to have the opportunity to be 'young' and enjoy childhood. Explain that this is a chance for young carers to meet other carers going through similar experiences and that it is good for the physical and mental well-being of the young carer. This can only help the young carer to develop more confidence in their caring abilities and extend their scope for support.

Case Study (3): Evelina

Evelina (17) looks after her younger brother, Alexander (8), and their mother Viktorya. Alexander has attention deficit disorder (ADD) and Viktorya suffers with severe depression. Evelina's father left the parental home shortly after the family arrived in England from Russia, four years ago. Evelina and Alexander speak very good English, but Viktorya's English is very limited, so Evelina fills out any forms they need to complete and helps her brother and mother to be ready for each day.

Alexander attends a special school five days a week, but Evelina finds him difficult to manage at the weekends. Evelina says life is easier now that she is not at school, although she attends the local college where she is studying music and art. Viktorya, has been very well recently. She no longer wants to take medication and wants to do more around the house and look after her son herself. She feels guilty that Evelina has to do so much for her and is missing out on her youth.

Joan is Viktorya's key worker and meets with the family for a weekly visit. Evelina looks particularly tired and drawn and is pre-occupied with her brother, Alexander. Viktorya mentions to Joan that she wants to stop the medication she is currently prescribed, because she wants to be more in control and fulfil her role as a mother.

Assessment and Intervention Options

- Young carer assessment form.
- Identify what support Evelina already has.
- Discuss with Evelina how she manages her college work and home/housework in addition to looking after Viktorya and Alexander.
- Assess what leisure activities Evelina engages in, if any, or establish what she would like to do, if she had time to herself.
- Review the relationship between (a) Evelina and her brother and (b) her mother.
- Discuss with Evelina her understanding of Viktorya's mental health problems and ask if she would like more information. If she does, offer useful educational material for Evelina and maybe explore whether Evelina would like to have the information in her native Russian language or in English.
- Discuss with both Evelina and Viktorya the importance of not abruptly stopping medication.
- Family-centred work.

Outcomes

For some young carers, caring for a parent or relative can lead to dropping out of the educational system to become full-time carers and missing out on developing opportunities for themselves. For those young carers who do go on to further education, the challenge can be how they balance studying with caring and any other activities. The mental health worker should review how a young carer is currently managing to balance the various responsibilities and consider different support mechanisms.

Not all members of the BAME community necessarily want to have close links with others from their community. There may be a sense of shame about having to care for a relative with mental health problems and they may wish to keep this private. It is useful to explore who they would like to receive support from, both within the mental health services and within the community.

When young carers are caring for more than one member of the family, this brings an added burden to their everyday lives. Discussing the opportunities for respite care can be important as a way to help relieve some of the burden of care.

Multiple-Choice Questions

See answers on page 668.

1. Individuals from Black African and Caribbean communities are *more* likely to receive a diagnosis of...
    a. Schizophrenia

   b. Mood disorder
   c. ADHD
   d. Anorexia nervosa
   e. Emotionally unstable personality disorder
2. Individuals from Black African and Caribbean communities are *less* likely to receive a diagnosis of…
   a. Schizophrenia
   b. Mood disorder
   c. ADHD
   d. Anorexia nervosa
   e. Emotionally unstable personality disorder
3. Which of the following would *not* be considered a key intervention with young carers from a BME background?
   a. Completion of a young carer assessment form
   b. Contacting the family's heritage community for support
   c. Providing information to young carers around the illness
   d. Providing information around statutory and voluntary sources of support
   e. Offering family-centred work

Key References

Department of Health, (2009). *Delivering Race Equality in Mental Health Care: A Review*. London: HMSO.

Grant, G., Repper, J. and Nolan, M. (2008). Young People Supporting Parents with Mental Health Problems: Experiences of Assessment and Support. *Health and Social Care in the Community*, 16(3): 271–281.

Greene, R., Pugh, R. and Roberts, D. (2008). *Black and Minority Ethnic Parents with Mental Health Problems and their Children*, Research Paper. London: Social Care Institute for Excellence.

Part III
Trauma

Christopher Gale

This relatively short section addresses some of the key issues that adversely affect children, young people and their families – the experience of trauma. Trauma can come in different forms, be it the loss of a loved one or some other adverse event, being subject to abuse and neglect or the experience of migration and homelessness. The expression of significant trauma can be through a child or young person's interaction with their world (behaviour) or a diagnosed form of mental health crisis (such as post-traumatic stress disorder – PTSD). This section explores some of the helpful interventions that can be instigated by CAMHS practitioners.

27 Managing Grief, Loss and Bereavement

Sue Ricketts

KEY CONCEPTS

- CAMHS clinicians need to be aware of how an unresolved experience of loss can present in different ways and may include physical, psychological and behavioural symptoms.
- Certain states of mind form part of the experience of grief. They do not follow a neat consecutive path but may return repeatedly.
- Helping individuals feel contained enough to safely explore their loss through verbal or non-verbal means requires a consistent and reliable setting, but not necessarily a clinic base, if the setting can be protected from intrusion.
- The loss of a child is not a normal experience and places those affected under the most extraordinary emotional and psychological distress. Grief reactions in bereaved parents are often more extreme and may include suicidal thoughts and feelings.

Theoretical Underpinnings

We are living in a time where our knowledge of the experience of loss and how it affects us psychologically is increasingly sophisticated. The Western understanding of grief is that successful mourning implies that the bereaved must disengage from the deceased. Persisting in an attachment to the dead person can be perceived as denying the reality of the loss.

Freud believed the purpose of mourning was to relinquish and adjust to the reality of the loss. John Bowlby wrote about how understanding grief is intrinsically linked to what happens when attachments are broken and that the strong emotional reactions that ensue (distress, anger and withdrawal) all have a place in the process of grieving.

Bereavement is the loss of someone significant to you.

- Bereavement is what happens.
- Grief is what one feels in relation to the bereavement.
- Mourning is what one does to express grief.
- To be deprived of someone of value implies attachment. The level of attachment will determine the degree of loss experienced, that leads to grief.

Colin Murray-Parks developed the idea that grief consists of a predictable set of behaviours to be gone through in phases before the final acceptance of the loss. Dorothy Judd (1995) and Darien Leader (2009) have helped deepen our understanding of grief reactions and the importance of helping the bereaved to mourn their loss. Leader suggested that clinical depression and low mood may result unless this 'work of mourning' is carried out adequately. Thanks to the work of Judd (1995) we know more about the workings of the mind of a child facing their own death and how best those around them can support both the individual child and the family.

The Four Phases of Grief

- **Denial**: shock, disbelief, sense of unreality
- **Pain/distress**: hurt, anger, guilt, worthlessness, searching
- **Realisation**: apathy, fantasy
- **Adjustment**: readiness to engage in new activities and relationships

The experience of loss is a normal part of the human experience. The grief we feel because of the loss is expressed in many different ways by adults and by children. Services, such as CAMHS, become involved in the process when mourning a loss has, in some way, become unhelpfully altered or suspended. In the day-to-day work of CAMHS, clinicians are often faced with a range of symptoms that, once explored, can be seen as linked to the experience of loss. These symptoms may present, often much later, as sleeplessness, angry outbursts, headaches and various anxiety states. The CAMHS clinician needs to be alert in the initial assessment to the losses that the individual may have experienced, but which have been overlooked or unavailable to attend to until now.

We encounter many forms of loss during our work, for instance, the loss parents feel during pregnancy when they are told that their unborn child may have a disability. The process of mourning the healthy longed-for child must be adjusted to, both psychologically and emotionally. Children may have suffered birth trauma that limited their abilities and their parents will need to make huge adjustments, emotionally and in addition, practically, in caring for a child with special needs. Siblings may be living with knowing that their sister or brother may not live on with them. All these scenarios can be encountered daily in the work of a CAMHS clinician. Although some referrals may arrive as clearly needing bereavement work, sometimes it may only emerge after a while that it is the experience of loss that is at the root of the difficulties.

Our views of grief and bereavement have changed over time. The cultural practices ascribed to them range from Queen Victoria remaining in black after the loss of her beloved husband to the introduction of jazz bands and colour at funerals. Dora Black (1978) writes 'the combination of a heavy death toll by the end of World War 2 and medical treatment breakthroughs led to a taboo on talking about death, for doctors consider death a failure'.

More recently there has been renewed interest in the processes surrounding loss and bereavement and fortunately, bereavement counselling is far more available. Psychologically, death which occurs naturally in old age, at its right time and place, however painful, is different from the death of a child or the unexpected death of a parent that shocks us to the core and tests all of our emotional and psychological resilience.

Through the work of people such as Colin Murray-Parks, we began to think about a recognised emotional process connected with loss and bereavement. There are five or six main identified reactions:

- **Numbness** at the news of the death, denial that it has happened.
- **Regression.** Earlier patterns of behaviour are often brought to the fore in relation to the loss. Returning to an earlier stage of development is quite common in children experiencing loss.

- **Depression.** It is appropriate to have depressed feelings. However, as Donald Winnicott says, 'depression at the normal end is a common, almost universal, phenomenon and relates to mourning'. The CAMHS clinician needs to be able to distinguish between what we would term a 'normal' experience of depression and clinical depression that requires psychiatric treatment.
- **Bargaining.** Kubler-Ross (2008) interprets this stage as an attempt to postpone the death. Superstition and ritualised or obsessional behaviour can often occur in this theological state.
- **Acceptance.** With some acceptance of death, it may be possible to maximise the remaining time before death, and following death, the person who has died can be remembered, commemorated and treasured in both concrete and emotional ways.

These outline the major states of mind that individuals travel through when coming to terms with loss and bereavement. Whereas previously we thought these followed a rather neat consecutive path, it has become evident latterly that different states of mind such as these are visited and re-visited in the process of coming to terms with loss.

Far more is now known about how differently children think about death and loss depending on their age group. Work by Brooklyn in 1959 and 1967 found that children between the ages of 5 and 8 years, and later between the ages of 13 and 16 years have a more emotional response to death. Children in the middle years of 9 to 12 years are generally more defended and less able to access the raw emotion that may be connected with loss. Brooklyn believes children know about death 'as the extinction of all life from early on, but then a range of defences are used psychologically in order to not be fully aware of its implications'. Likewise, Dorothy Judd (Judd, 1995) notes that children 'can both know and deny the existence of death'.

Case Study (1): Jenny

Jenny (four) was referred into CAMHS by a pre-school nursery worker. She had missed several play sessions and her mother was concerned about her complaints of stomach aches. These had already been investigated physically. Jenny's mother thought they might have an emotional root. The clinic team met with the parents to gain a more comprehensive understanding of the family, including Jenny's early history. It emerged that Jenny's paternal grandmother, who had lived with the family during different times in Jenny's young life, had died suddenly nine months before.

The parents were invited to discuss their own experience of this bereavement, for instance, had the grandmother been talked about in the family since her death? Was she remembered through photographs? And so on. Jenny's father had been taking time off work with unexplained back problems. The parents had believed that Jenny was too young to be spoken to about this loss, but through discussion with the nursery staff, it emerged that Jenny had been playing a repetitive game in the dolls' house at the nursery, centred on people suddenly disappearing.

With the parents' permission, we invited the nursery worker to join the session to think about what Jenny might be expressing in her play and how it linked with the death of her grandmother. The nursery worker offered Jenny some individual play time. She then met with the team to discuss what she observed.

The parents began to mention grandmother's name at home and observe how Jenny reacted. The nursery worker offered Jenny six weekly sessions of play in the dolls' house. She then liaised with CAMHS to relay her observations and receive supervision. After several weeks, Jenny was attending play school regularly and no longer complaining of stomach pains. Talking with Jenny about the figures in the dolls' house disappearing and having permission from the parents to link this to the disappearance of her grandmother seemed to have brought about the relief for Jenny.

Case Study (2): Stephen

Stephen (nine) was referred to CAMHS by his GP for increasingly aggressive outbursts at home and at school, an inability to concentrate and complaints of headaches. He was listless at home. Stephen was a keen footballer in a local team but had recently made excuses not to attend training sessions. His mother and the school staff were becoming increasingly worried.

Stephen's parents lived apart but were both invited to the first appointment. Stephen's mother, the main carer, gave CAMHS permission to have a discussion with the school to gain a fuller picture prior to the first appointment.

A full family history established that the relationship between Stephen's parents had broken down two years after the birth of Stephen's younger sister, who had been diagnosed with a rare genetic disorder. Over the years this had required intensive hospital visits and the parents were now faced with a decision about major surgery that could either enhance or endanger her life.

Stephen's father had left home when Stephen was four years old, but football remained a genuine shared father–son interest. His parents had tried to protect Stephen from the medical discussions about his sister, but a scarcity of childcare meant this was not always possible. He was thus acutely aware of the life and death issues around her and of the real possibility that she may not live much longer.

The nurse therapist who led these initial appointments thought that Stephen may have signs of ADHD, but firstly wanted to explore these other issues, i.e. the impact of the separation of his parents and the very significant knowledge and experience of living with a sibling with a life-limiting illness.

The team's child psychotherapist met with the family and then with Stephen on his own. Over four individual sessions, Stephen gradually began to relax and play with the cars and with a football game and then to talk about his life at home, the heavy worries he carried in relation to his sister and his concern about his mother's ability to cope. He expressed powerful angry feelings towards his father for having left him at home with so many difficult issues to deal with.

Through a little boy in his imaginative play, clearly recognisable as himself, Stephen was able to say, 'I just don't think I can do anything to help'. In addition, he showed through play that he believed his sister's illness could be infectious and, despite having been told repeatedly and clearly that this was not the case, he had a morbid fear that he carried the same life-limiting illness. Gradually, Stephen began to understand that his anger was an attempt to hide his sadness and act as 'the man of the family' by trying to take control of a situation that was completely out of his control. In parallel, the Nurse Therapist met with the parents to talk with them about appropriate boundaries regarding information for Stephen with regard to his sister and how important it was that his father was in consistent contact with him, making time to listen to his worries.

The teamwork with Stephen ended after three school terms, but his mother continues to be seen by CAMHS to help her cope with the issues surrounding the anticipated grief for her daughter. Stephen had not only suffered the loss of his father but was living with a sister who was likely to die within the next two years. He continues to be monitored by the school and may need further support in the future.

Case Study (3): Sakiya

Sakiya (15) has muscular dystrophy and is increasingly becoming multiply disabled. She was referred to CAMHS by a community nurse because of vomiting, for which no physical cause had been found. The family were known to the community services because Sakiya already received home visits following her various operations.

At the first CAMHS appointment, it soon became evident that both of Sakiya's parents were experiencing mental health difficulties, Sakiya's mother with anxiety and her father with intermittent clinical depression. They indicated that they were not robust enough to undergo family sessions but supported individual work for Sakiya.

With their permission, the CAMHS clinician consulted with both Sakiya's paediatrician and her consultant in the acute services to ascertain the likely prognosis for her and whether any further medical interventions might be needed within the next year.

Despite Sakiya's limited mobility, it was clear that she was well able to convey her thoughts verbally. She talked animatedly about her love of 'soap operas' and was completely absorbed in the adult issues they addressed. Indeed, it seemed that Sakiya was almost 'overdosing' psychologically and emotionally on the content of infidelity, abortion, murder and so on. She was often left highly stimulated by what she had watched, with no-one to speak to about it.

The clinic staff were worried that Sakiya may be unable to process much of what she was watching on the television. The vomiting was a response to her inability to 'digest' these adult issues emotionally. Crucially, there were many other underlying questions for Sakiya about the shortening of her life and her hope to live long enough to experience some of the issues she was witnessing on screen.

Sakiya was offered individual work and the vomiting ceased, but it was clear that she needed some safe psychological space to explore her thoughts and feelings about her illness. Although Sakiya's parents appreciated the potential consequences for Sakiya of watching these programmes, they were caught, as many parents of children with a life-limiting illness are, in wanting to allow their child every 'apparent' enjoyment.

Multiple-Choice Questions

See answers on page 669.

1. What is essential information to gather in the assessment period?
   a. Number of siblings
   b. Quality of attachment to significant adults
   c. Losses the child or young person may have suffered in their life
2. Is supporting the bereaved person best carried out by:
   a. Teacher
   b. Nurse
   c. Professional who knows the individual well and who can access skilled supervision in this area of work
   d. Professional bereavement counsellor
3. What does the author claim is crucial in bringing about the best possible outcome for the patient?
   a. Timing of the intervention
   b. Setting
   c. Training
   d. Both (a) and (c)
4. How many of these are true in what we know about the stages of grief? They
   a. Follow in sequence
   b. Cannot occur without assistance
   c. Do not follow a set sequence
   d. Are completed in a set period

Key References

Black, D. (1978). The Bereaved Child. *Journal of Child Psychology and Psychiatry*, 19(3): 287–282.
Judd, D. (1995). *Give Sorrow Words.* Oxford: Haworth Press.
Kubler-Ross, E. (2008). On Death and Dying. (40th Anniversary edition). London: Routledge.
Leader, D. (2009). *The New Black, Mourning, Melancholia and Depression.* London: Hamish Hamilton.

28 Developmental Trauma

Val Forster

Introduction

The term developmental trauma was first used in 2005 by Dr Bessel van der Kolk, an American psychiatrist. He said that, not only do traumatised children develop a range of unhealthy coping strategies that they believe will help them survive, they do not develop essential daily living skills.

KEY CONCEPTS

- Developmental trauma is the term used to describe the impact of early, repeated adverse childhood experiences (ACE) that happen within a child's important relationships.
- It is a means of capturing the complex psychological, biological and interpersonal sequelae of the experiences of neglect and abuse, such as physical, emotional or sexual abuse and any type of household dysfunction such as violence in the home, alcoholism, drug abuse and mental health issues.
- Any kind of trauma that repeatedly occurs during infancy and childhood impacts brain development. What happens in the first months of life, both prenatal and postnatal, has lifelong effects.
- Developmental trauma has remained a description of a cluster of symptoms and behaviours rather than a diagnosis.

Researchers continue to gather evidence to increase understanding, and clinicians strive to find better ways to help children and families whose lives are affected.

The Impact on Brain Development

The idea that trauma has an indelible impact on developing personality has a long history in psychology. Furthermore, the perpetrator of neglect or abuse is most often one of the primary caregivers. Such developmental trauma is relational, not a single event but cumulative, a characteristic feature of an impaired attachment relationship (Schore, 2015). The ongoing repetitive relational stressors embedded in a severely mis-attuned attachment relationship mean that the infant is experiencing not acute but chronic stress in the first two years of life. In this critical period, the human brain grows faster than at any other stage in the life cycle. This interval exactly overlaps the period of attachment so intensely studied by contemporary developmental psychology. A fundamental tenet of Bowlby's model is that, for better or worse, the infant's 'capacity to cope with stress' is correlated with certain maternal behaviours. Thus, the early social environment, mediated by the primary caregiver, directly influences the final wiring of the circuits of the infant brain responsible for the future social and emotional capacities of the individual.

The ultimate product of this social-emotional development is a particular system in the prefrontal area of the right brain that is capable of regulating emotions, including positive emotions such as joy and interest, as well as negative emotions such as fear and aggression. Experience not only affects the structure of the brain but the way the system of chemicals in the human body works. Chemicals, such as hormones (released from an endocrine gland into the bloodstream) and neurotransmitters (released by nerve terminals), send signals between neurons and other bodily systems. Some commonly known ones include serotonin, dopamine, adrenaline and oxytocin. High levels of stress in pregnancy lead to the production of the stress hormone cortisol, which crosses the placenta and can affect the developing foetus. Experiences of neglect or trauma, even when not consciously remembered, can affect both behaviours and hormonal systems.

The early years are vital. We are biologically predisposed to respond to potential danger by flight, flight or freeze, and quick surges of adrenalin and the release of cortisol are essential and lifesaving when a predator such as a man-eating tiger appears. Generally, after such shocks the body quickly goes back to normal, with blood pressure and heart rate reducing as we relax. The psychiatrist and neuroscientist Bruce Perry has described how traumatised children can barely relax, are constantly on the move and are in a desperately anxious and hyper-vigilant state. Such heightened physiological responses are a sign of a highly activated sympathetic nervous system. There is another response to the nervous system to stress and trauma, an activation of the parasympathetic nervous system. Here the body closes down, rather like a creature 'playing dead' in front of a predator. Blood pressure and heart rate drop and parts of the brain that specialise in logical thought often shut down, while primitive survival mechanisms take over. This can give rise to the phenomenon of dissociation, in which an individual can seem to be cut off from their own experience. This may be part of the explanation why many children from highly stressful backgrounds often do not achieve well academically. They have learned to cope by being hyper-alert to danger, which impedes ordinary relaxed concentration, or they may go into a shut-down dissociative mode in which the thinking part of the brain shuts down.

Severe neglect has been shown to lead to atrophy in parts of the brain and to developmental delay, as well as to serious deficits in the ability to empathise, regulate emotion and manage intimacy and ordinary social interaction. Studies of severely neglected children adopted from Romanian orphanages have shown that areas of the brain primed for emotional understanding and expressiveness have shockingly little activity.

The Seven Pieces of the Developmental Trauma Puzzle

The seven areas of developmental trauma can be mapped onto the order in which the brain develops from the brainstem to the cortical brain.

Sensory Development

Infants and toddlers have not yet developed language to make sense of their experiences. All their memories are therefore sensory memories, and the baby operates mainly out of their brainstem, the bottom part of the brain responsible for basic functions such as heart rate, temperature and behaviours which aim to keep them alive. Memories before language are known as implicit, which means that, while the child cannot later recall and talk about them, their body has stored the memories in its sensory systems. Because traumatised children are stuck in fear mode as they grow up, their hyper-vigilance to signs of danger reduces their ability to filter out irrelevant sensory experiences, such as background sights, sounds and textures. This can mean that the child's sensory system becomes overloaded and they feel danger to be imminent, even when they are completely safe.

When a traumatised child is feeling stressed, they may have sensory flashbacks which means that they re-experience the bodily feeling of immediate danger, with no way to make sense of it or to communicate verbally, since the memory has no language attached to it. Children will either over-respond or under-respond to incoming sensory information because their brain cannot find the middle ground of working out which information is necessary and which information means danger. They may struggle to know how much force to press on things, find it difficult to recognise the nature of textures (e.g. rough, smooth, heavy or light), and they may struggle to find good balance and co-ordination.

Dissociation

Dissociation is a survival mechanism and one that is often over-looked in traumatised children. When a child is subjected to physical abuse, in the moment of violence they cannot physically escape, but they can escape in their mind. All humans have a natural ability to 'leave the room' when their trauma is utterly unbearable. Babies and toddlers dissociate when they are in danger or when their experience is intolerable. It is vital for infants who are suffering frightening things. It enables them to keep going in the face of overwhelming fear. Dissociation is a separation or disconnection between thoughts, feelings *and* behaviours and a separation between the mind and the body. It is the mind's way of putting unbearable experiences and memories into different compartments, e.g. a child may remember a traumatic event but have no feelings attached to the memory or may show challenging behaviour, but have no memory behind the behaviour. These different parts of the child's experience are connected, but they learn to survive by becoming unaware of the connection.

In developmental trauma, the child often continues to dissociate, even when they are no longer in danger. Their brain cannot turn it off. Because memories are fragmented into many little pieces by dissociation, children often have a flashback to a memory, a feeling, a behaviour or a physical pain, with no understanding of why or what triggered it. This can feel disorienting and confusing, as the child believes they are in immediate danger. The more frightening the child's traumas were, the more likely they are to dissociate and the more sophisticated the ways they develop to dissociate. Children are usually unaware that they dissociate or 'zone out' and they cannot put into words what is happening. Dissociation leads to a range of behaviours that can often be understood by adults as challenging, naughty or lazy.

Attachment Development

Children who start life in a frightening or neglectful environment adapt to their environment. Children learn from as early as a few months old that certain behaviours keep danger at bay and other behaviours increase the chances of danger. They develop a range of attachment strategies. These are there both to prevent harm and to keep a parent/carer as close as possible. Traumatised children tend to develop one main attachment style, which could be either insecure avoidant or insecure pre-occupied (anxious). These terms are a better way of understanding what is happening than the more general disorganised style.

Avoidant children learn early on that showing their feelings and having needs bring danger and make their parent/carer withdraw. They learn to hide their feelings and act as if everything is fine. Inside they feel frightened, vulnerable, worthless and hopeless, but on the outside, they often seem bright and competent. These children are often not a concern for parents and teachers until later childhood, because they do not show behaviour problems until these are triggered by something stressful.

Pre-occupied children learn that showing feelings and extravagant behaviours is the only way to be noticed and keep parents/carers close by. They learn to exaggerate behaviour and emotions and to be angry and upset for long periods. Inside they feel petrified, anxious and unlovable. On the outside they appear angry, aggressive, disruptive and rude. To have an adult solve the crisis would be frightening, as it might mean the adult goes away. Some children swing between these strategies. It appears disorganised, but is in fact highly adaptive. It explains why school staff often see one part of the child and the parents/carers another.

Emotional Regulation

Emotional regulation is a skill that children learn in early childhood. It means that, by the time they are six or seven, they know how to notice that they are having an emotional reaction, know what the emotion is, express it in a healthy and clear way and finally manage the emotion well, so that they can become calm. Babies and toddlers cannot regulate their emotions. They rely on their parent to co-regulate. This means that the way the parent responds to the child's emotions regulates the emotions for them, which trains their brain how to respond to emotions in the future. Through this co-regulation babies learn that their feelings are acceptable and manageable and will not kill them or push others away. A baby or toddler whose crying is repeatedly met with being hit, ignored, mocked or by panic in the parent, learns that their feelings are dangerous, hurt others and hurt themselves. This becomes an internal working model.

In children who have moved frequently between carers or who have harmful parents, the part of the brain responsible for emotional regulation does not develop as it should. It becomes stuck in the toddler phase of emotional regulation where they cannot do it for themselves and need an adult to co-regulate for them. In children with developmental trauma, their brain's ability to regulate their emotions is the same as a 3-year old, even though they might be 14. The child cries, shouts, sulks, stomps their feet, slams doors, bites, hits, runs away, explodes with no warning, over-reacts to small things and so on. This explains why these children are often described as naughty or attention-seeking. The toddler-like behaviour is seen but the emotional need is hidden. If adults can respond to the child's emotional age rather than their actual age, then the child can be helped by co-regulation and begin to learn that skill. Children who have poor emotional regulation often turn to unhealthy regulation coping strategies as they grow into adolescence, such as drug and alcohol abuse, self-harming and sexual encounters. These strategies function to either enliven them from feeling dead inside or relax them from high levels of anxiety.

Behavioural Regulation

Each individual has a 'window of tolerance', i.e. a state of physical and emotional arousal that is tolerable and bearable. In this state, a child can think, learn, love and relax. For traumatised children, small everyday things, like a request to brush their teeth or a change of classroom, spirals them out of this calm relaxed state. They become hyper-aroused (overly aroused) or hypo-aroused (under-aroused). Traumatised children will be over- or under-aroused most of the time and, in either state, their behaviour is out of their hands. They cannot control it as they are in automatic survival mode and they cannot think, reason or rationalise when feeling under threat. Children who are overly aroused are in fight/flight. Their brain tells them they are in danger and their body responds. They can run, hit, scream, shout, squirm and disrupt. Under-aroused children shut down. They go numb, zone out and cannot connect or think. In both states the child's heart rate is very fast. They might sweat or shake and they are hyper-vigilant to every detail in their environment. It is worth remembering that, at the core of a trauma experience, there is a loss of control. Traumatised children become experts at regaining control, and these behaviours cause significant challenges for adults.

Cognition

Developmentally traumatised children often struggle with under-developed cognitive skills, meaning their ability to do things like plan ahead, problem-solve, organise themselves and learn from mistakes. This is because they are often 'stuck' in their limbic system and brainstem and are exhausting all their reserves trying to stay safe and to work out whether adults can be trusted or not. This leaves few resources for the higher brain skills which are needed for good cognitive functioning.

Self-Concept and Identity Development

Our self-concept starts forming from the very first messages we receive about ourselves from the adults in our lives. If children receive the message that they are not worth keeping safe, that they are disposable or that their crying pushes others away, their self-concept will reflect this. Those who have suffered early trauma often live with a very deep sense of being bad and unwanted. This becomes their template for how they see themselves and for how they think others see them. Accepting that they are lovable and worth keeping safe can take a very long time. Chronically traumatised children often feel confused and lost. They do not feel as though they belong with anyone or anywhere and are often in search of validation from others. This can make them very vulnerable to being exploited in relationships or present as flitting between friends and groups to try to fit in.

Mental Health Symptoms

Developmental trauma is an umbrella term for these seven areas of impact. In addition to these developmental difficulties, a child can experience discrete mental health difficulties, such as episodes of depression, anxiety and specific trauma symptoms. Often these symptoms are understood and treated in isolation. However, for chronically traumatised children, seeing mental health symptoms as part of the overall picture of developmental trauma is key. Dr Allan Schore, Dr Bruce Perry and Dr Bessel van de Kolk, and many other clinicians and researchers, are clear that developmental trauma can be repaired over a long enough period. Children are resilient and adaptable, and neuroscience is showing us all the time that the brain is flexible and open to being re-wired, if given the opportunity.

Case Study: Mary

Mary was seven when she was referred by her school who were having trouble managing her behaviour, as were her adoptive parents. Both Mary and her older full sister were taken into care following interventions begun prior to Mary's birth. They lived in separate foster homes.

Her birth parents used drugs and alcohol and had a violent relationship. They were not able to recognise that this had a negative impact on the children's development both in pregnancy and after and failed to alter their behaviour. Both parents had poor childhood experiences.

Mary moved to her adoptive home when she was three and a half. She had one foster family but also spent periods of time with her birth mother until she was one and a half while assessments were carried out. She has not seen her foster carers since. It was reported that Mary struggled with developing friendships. She needed 1:1 support in the classroom and was indiscriminate about hugging and kissing both staff and pupils. Her behaviour was at times described as sexualised. Her parents feel she functions much younger than her chronological age. She is disruptive and controlling and destructive with toys. She screams, tantrums and stamps her feet. She can be aggressive to other children and has been excluded from school for this.

The initial assessment was able to conclude that Mary's early life fulfilled the description for developmental trauma. Mary's parents were invited to attend a group for parents and carers that offered information and strategies about developmental trauma. They began to feel that they understood that Mary's early experiences had affected her and became more creative in dealing with the difficult behaviour by bearing her attachment style in mind and by responding to her emotional age rather than her chronological one. Mary was offered an assessment and then weekly work in a creative therapy to carefully explore her thoughts and feelings in a way that was attachment focused with sensory elements. She began to explore themes of abandonment, belonging and control. The work continues.

Multiple-Choice Questions

See answers on page 669.

1. What is an ACE?
   a. Average childhood experience
   b. Acrimonious childhood experience
   c. Adverse childhood experience
   d. Anxious childhood experience
2. Explain why traumatised children continue to dissociate when they are no longer in danger.
   a. They were never taught to dissociate by their caregivers.
   b. Memories become fragmented.
   c. Memories merge and become overwhelming.
   d. It is linked to their temperament and not any traumatic experience.
3. What are the two types of attachment style most seen in traumatised children?
   a. Avoidant and pre-occupied (anxious)
   b. Avoidant and secure
   c. Avoidant and disorganised
   d. Disorganised and secure
   e. Pre-occupied (anxious) and disorganised

Key References

Music, G. (2011). *Nurturing Natures - Attachment and Children's Emotional, Sociocultural and Brain Development.* East Sussex: Psychology Press.

Schore, A.N. (2015). *Affect Regulation and the Origin of the Self.* London: Routledge.

van der Kolk, B.A. (2004). *The Body Keeps the Score.* London: Allen Lane.

29 The Effect of Childhood Maltreatment on Brain Development

Dennis Golm and Jana Kreppner

KEY CONCEPTS

- Childhood maltreatment can be defined as 'any acts of commission or omission by a parent or other caregiver that results in harm, potential for harm, or threat of harm to a child' (Child Maltreatment Surveillance, 2008).
- These acts do not have to be intentional in order to be classed as maltreatment. Acts of commission include various forms of abuse: physical, emotional or sexual abuse (Leeb, 2008).
- **Physical abuse** refers to the cause of a physical injury by nonaccidental means, i.e. bruises caused by spanking. **Sexual abuse** refers to attempted or actual sexual contact or exposure to sexual stimuli, i.e. exposure to pornographic films, rape. **Emotional maltreatment** refers to when a child's emotional needs are not met, i.e. witnessing violence between caregivers, constant screaming or cursing at the child, or when a caregiver is insensitive to a child's developmental level and needs, i.e. a school-aged child is not allowed to play with friends (English & the LONGSCAN Investigators, 1997).
- Acts of omission include various forms of neglect that result in failure to provide for a child's emotional, physical, medical or educational needs or a lack of adequate supervision of a child (Leeb, 2008). Examples of neglect include having children not attend school (i.e. educational neglect) or leaving the child with an intoxicated caregiver, i.e. lack of adequate supervision (English & the LONGSCAN Investigators, 1997).
- Children often experience multiple types of maltreatment (Herrenkohl and Herrenkohl, 2009). One exception might be the institutional deprivation experienced by Romanian children in orphanages under the Ceausescu regime that marks an especially severe case of global, i.e. social, physical and emotional, neglect.

We will explore the consequences of these adverse early experiences later.

Prevalence of Maltreatment

A large study conducted in the US which used data from the National Child Abuse and Neglect Data System Child files, 2004 to 2011, estimated the cumulative prevalence of maltreatment before the age of 18 years from confirmed reports of abuse and neglect (Wildeman et al., 2014). The study reported a cumulative prevalence of 12.5% (5,689,900) children, with almost half of the reports occurring before a child's fifth birthday. Most reports were of neglect (80%).

This cumulative prevalence is important, as the majority of studies looking at informant-reported maltreatment, e.g. maltreatment reported by health professionals, doctors or the concerned public, focus on prevalence within a one-year period (Stoltenborgh et al., 2015). For the study above, the 1-year prevalence was 0.9%, a rate almost 14 times lower (Wildeman et al., 2014).

The majority of studies rely on retrospective self-report asking participants whether they experienced any maltreatment before the age of 18 years (Stoltenborgh et al., 2015). A meta-analysis of self-report studies reported prevalence rates of up to 36% for various maltreatment types: sexual abuse 7.6% for boys, 18% for girls; physical abuse 22.3%; emotional abuse 36.3%; physical neglect 16.3%; emotional neglect 18.4%.

While studies relying on self-report seem to report higher prevalence rates of maltreatment in general, documented cases of maltreatment are largely based on neglect rather than abuse. A recent meta-analysis (Baldwin et al., 2019) compared the overlap between maltreatment identified prospectively during childhood, <18 years of age, mostly parent-report and child protective services records and subsequent retrospective self-reports, mostly during adulthood, within the same samples, and found the agreement between the two assessment types to be poor. The authors suggested that retrospectively and prospectively identified at-risk individuals might represent two different populations, with it being unclear whether the same risk mechanisms would be involved (e.g. regarding mental health).

The Situation of National and International Adoptees

In the UK, a documented history of childhood maltreatment is the most common reason for children to enter the care system. From the 75,420 looked after children in England, 63% were looked after due to abuse or neglect. Of these, 2,230 were placed for adoption with the majority of those being between 1 and 4 years of age.

For international adoptees, the situation is different, as many of these children will have experienced institutional care prior to adoption (Hellerstedt et al., 2008). While care conditions in institutions vary, the care provided is often characterised by low staff to child ratios and a lack of individualised care (IJzendoorn et al., 2011). In addition, experiences of abuse are common in institutions (Sherr et al., 2017).

World-wide, 2.7 million children under the age of 18 years are estimated to be living in institutional care (Petrowski et al., 2017). The global deprivation experienced by children in Romanian orphanages under the Ceausescu regime during the 1980s constitutes one of the most severe examples of institutional maltreatment in recent history (Kumsta et al., 2015).

Maltreatment and the Risk for the Development of Mental Health Problems

Experiences of childhood maltreatment and neglect have been linked to a range of adverse physical and mental health outcomes (Norman et al., 2012), though the majority of studies are based on retrospective reports. A meta-analysis by Norman and colleagues in 2012 across 124 mainly retrospective studies compared children with and without a history of non-sexual abuse and neglect. The authors reported a higher risk for emotional problems, e.g. anxiety and depression, child behavioural problems and conduct disorder for children with a history of maltreatment. Another meta-analysis by Li and colleagues (2016) that only included prospective longitudinal studies confirmed a higher risk for emotional problems in children with a history of maltreatment, but did not include other psychiatric problems as outcomes. One important question is how these adverse experiences lead to an increased risk for mental health problems. A multitude of biological systems have recently become the focus of this discussion, amongst them structural and functional brain abnormalities (Berens et al., 2017).

How Do Maltreatment Experiences Get under the Skin?

During brain development there are time windows during which brain areas are especially susceptible to certain environmental experiences (Knudsen, 2004). If key experiences are missing during such sensitive periods, developmental trajectories are likely to change. The formation of a secure attachment bond to a caregiver during infancy marks such a period (Nelson, Zeanah and Fox, 2019). Sensitive periods, where development can still be redirected, have to be distinguished from critical periods where the change is irreparable (Knudsen, 2004).

A growing evidence base suggests that changes to the brain following maltreatment reflect an adaptation of the brain to the abusive and/or neglectful environment (McCrory et al., 2017; Teicher et al., 2016). For instance, Hein and Monk's (2017) meta-analysis across 20 studies with 1,733 participants showed that a history of maltreatment is associated with abnormal threat processing in the amygdala. In a threatening environment, i.e. being at risk of physical abuse by a caregiver, the early detection of threat followed by successful avoidance can secure survival (Teicher et al., 2016).

When the environmental context changes, however, for instance from a threatening to a secure and nurturing environment via adoption, those changes relating to heightened vigilance to threat may no longer be adaptive and may be in the way of developing rewarding social relationships or attending and focussing on tasks in the classroom. As such, these 'cognitive adaptions or maladaptations' represent a form of latent vulnerability for later life mental health problems (McCrory et al., 2017).

For instance, the degree to which amygdala reactivity in response to negative faces exceeded the reaction to positive faces was related to increased anxiety symptoms in adolescents with a history of early deprivation in orphanages, but not in adolescents who grew up in their biological families (Silvers et al., 2017). Whether or not a child with a history of adversity and a form of latent vulnerability will develop such symptoms may depend on the presence of later life stressors or protective factors (McCrory et al., 2017).

Functional Changes

A history of maltreatment has been associated with altered processing in brain networks linked to the processing of (a) threat, (b) reward and (c) emotion regulation (McCrory et al., 2017).

(a) In addition to an increased amygdala activation in response to threat, the meta-analysis by Hein and Monk (2017) reported hyperactivation of the superior temporal gyrus, the parahippocampal gyrus and the insula. In line with the theory of latent vulnerability, hyperactivation of the amygdala (Ohman, 2005) and superior temporal gyrus (Hein and Monk, 2017) might aid the early detection of threat and thus reflect an adaptation to a threatening environment. This may increase the risk for later psychopathology (Hein and Monk, 2017) as hyperactivation of the amygdala has been demonstrated in patients with anxiety disorders (Etkin and Wager, 2007).

(b) This hyperactivation to threat in limbic and temporal areas is contrasted by hypoactivation of a key structure of the reward system (the ventral striatum) Teicher et al., 2016) that shows a decreased response to received or anticipated reward. Hypoactivation of the striatum has been linked to depression (Keren et al., 2018).

(c) Emotion regulation studies show an altered activation pattern in the ventral anterior cingulate cortex and the medial prefrontal cortex (Gerin et al., 2019), regions implicated in implicit emotion regulation (Etkin et al., 2015), and the latero-prefrontal cortex (Gerin et al., 2019), a region implicated in explicit emotion regulation (Etkin et al., 2015). Altered emotion regulation is in turn associated with a heightened risk for anxiety and depression (Young et al., 2019).

Structural Changes

Some of the functional correlates are reflected in structural network changes particularly in affect regulation and processing networks. A meta-analysis across 12 data sets across children, adolescents and adults reported smaller grey matter volumes of a ventrolateral prefrontal-limbic temporal network spanning the right orbitofrontal/superior temporal gyrus, amygdala, insula, parahippocampal, middle temporal, left inferior frontal and postcentral gyri (Lim et al., 2015).

A meta-analysis across 38 studies on adults with a history of maltreatment reported reduced grey matter volume in a prefrontal-limbic network, namely in the right dorsolateral prefrontal cortex, right hippocampus and right postcentral gyrus across 19 whole brain voxel-based morphometry studies and reduced hippocampal and amygdala volume across 17 respectively 13 region-of-interest studies (Paquola et al., 2016). Though the regions only partially overlap, both meta-analyses report smaller grey matter volumes in networks associated with emotional processing and affect regulation. Reduced grey matter volume within the dorsolateral prefrontal cortex, amygdala and parahippocampal gyrus have been linked to depression (Bora et al., 2012).

The meta-analyses included studies across the maltreatment spectrum, and the vast majority of evidence comes from retrospective reports. Given the poor overlap between retrospective and prospective reports of maltreatment, it is difficult to determine the extent to which these associations are due to bias. We will focus on prospective longitudinal studies focussing on a specific type of maltreatment, i.e. institutional deprivation.

Evidence from Prospective Longitudinal Studies of Romanian Orphans

The English and Romanian Adoptees Study (ERA) and the Bucharest Early Intervention Study (BEIP) are the two most prominent longitudinal studies on the impact of neglect in the form of institutional deprivation on development. The studies differ with regard to study design and type of sample. The ERA study (Rutter, 1998) was launched by Professor Sir Michael Rutter in the early 1990s and follows a group of 165 Romanian children adopted from the severely depriving conditions of the Ceausescu orphanages into nurturing UK families and a comparison group of 52 children adopted within the UK as young infants and without a history of early deprivation. The ERA study therefore utilises a natural experiment design (Rutter, Kumsta, Schlotz and Sonuga-Barke, 2012). Children were assessed at ages 4, 6, 11 and 15 years and twice in young adulthood. Brain imaging data was only collected during the last assessment point in young adulthood, though a small subsample had brain imaging data collected at age 16 years.

The BEIP is a randomised controlled trial (Zeanah et al., 2003) which began in 2000, a decade after the fall of the Ceausescu regime. Out of a sampling pool of 136 children living in institutions, children were randomised to either one of 57 available foster care placements or care as usual, i.e. remaining in the institutions. In addition, the study assessed a comparison group of 72 never institutionalised children living in Romania with their biological parents.

The children were followed up at 42 months, 54 months, 8 years, 12 years (Nelson, Fox and Zeanah, 2014) and most recently at 16 years (Wade et al., 2019). Brain imaging data were collected between the ages of 8 and 11 years and at 16 years (NB not yet published). The two studies differ in some important points: first, the type of research design, natural experiment vs randomised controlled trial, second, their selection of comparison groups, i.e. the development of post-institution reared, adopted children in the ERA study is compared to that of within-UK non-deprived adoptees while the development of post-institution reared, fostered children in the BEIP is compared to (a) children who remained in care as usual, e.g., for most, institutional care, and (b) never institutionalised Romanian children growing up in their biological families and third, the timing of removal from institutional care. The children in the ERA study experienced institutional deprivation typical in pre-revolution Romania, prior to, and during the fall of the Ceausescu regime, whilst the children in the BEIP trial experienced institutional deprivation in post-revolution Romania after the fall of the Ceausescu regime. It is difficult to tell how conditions improved in the orphanages after the fall of the regime and to what extent the deprivation experiences are comparable with regard to severity.

Findings from the Bucharest Early Intervention Project

Children with any history of institutionalisation, a combined foster-care and care-as-usual group, showed more symptoms of inappropriate friendliness towards strangers, i.e. disinhibited social engagement and withdrawn attachment behaviour at baseline (Bos et al., 2011) prior to being randomised into foster care or care-as-usual. At age 54 months (Bos et al., 2011) and age 12 years (Humphreys et al., 2015) children with any history of institutionalisation showed higher rates of emotional problems and externalising problems, including ADHD.

In the BEIP, good-quality MRI data were collected from 74 children between 8 and 11 years of age, 29 in the care-as-usual group, 25 children in the foster-care group and 20 never institutionalised children (Sheridan, Fox, Zeanah, McLaughlin and Nelson, 2012). After adjustment for effects of age and sex, children with any history of institutionalisation, care-as-usual and foster-care children combined, displayed significantly smaller total grey matter brain volume in comparison to never institutionalised children. Brain volume did not differ between the two groups with a history of institutionalisation. Only children in the care-as-usual group had lower white matter volume in comparison to never institutionalised children and did not differ from children in the foster-care group. No mentionable effects were found for subcortical brain structures.

Another BEIP study (McLaughlin et al., 2014) assessed cortical thickness. In comparison to the never institutionalised children, cortical thickness within the combined groups of never institutionalised children was reduced across various prefrontal, parietal and temporal regions. Importantly, reduced cortical thickness was related to symptoms of ADHD. Moreover, the association between a history of institutionalisation and symptoms of ADHD was mediated by cortical thinning across frontal, parietal, temporal and limbic regions.

Findings from the English and Romanian Adoptees Study

Romanian adoptees who spent more than six months in the orphanages showed higher rates of neurodevelopmental symptoms (Sonuga-Barke et al., 2017), symptoms of ADHD, autism and disinhibited social engagement, from age six into young adulthood and a late emergent pattern of emotional problems (Sonuga-Barke et al., 2017). The effect of institutionalisation on emotional problems in adulthood was mediated by neurodevelopmental problems at age six years (Golm et al., in press). Cognitive functioning was severely impaired in childhood and showed remarkable catch-up into young adulthood.

The ERA study collected brain imaging data in young adulthood and, for a small subgroup, in early adolescence. The study in early adolescence, age 16 years, was conducted as a pilot study and compared 12 Romanian adoptees, 14 for the structural study, with a history of severe institutionalisation, with 11 UK adoptees.

For the functional task, a monetary incentive delay task to activate the reward system, the study confirmed the results of meta-analyses on general forms of maltreatment and reported a hypoactivity of the striatum during the anticipation of reward (Mehta et al., 2010). The structural component of the study found that, relative to the comparison group and consistent with findings from the BEIP, the Romanian adoptees had smaller total white and grey matter volume. The study examined the volume of the amygdala, corpus callosum and hippocampus. Effects were only found for the amygdala.

In contrast to meta-analyses of studies on maltreatment, amygdala volume was larger for the previously institutionalised group.

In young adulthood, 67 Romanian adoptees who had experienced between 3 and 41 months of deprivation were compared to 21 UK adoptees (Mackes, Golm, Sarkar, Kumsta, Rutter, Fairchild, Mehta and Sonuga-Barke, 2020). In comparison to UK adoptees, Romanian adoptees displayed an 8.57% reduction in total brain volume. (Similar reductions were observed when examining grey and white matter volume separately). Importantly, total brain volume correlated negatively ($r = -0.41$, $p < 0.001$) with duration of deprivation, measured as the age of placement with UK families. Each additional month spent in the orphanages was associated with a 3.00-cm^3 (0.27%) reduction in brain volume. These results remained significant after controlling for potential confounding factors such as overall height, birth weight and subnutrition measured as a weight 1.5 standard deviations below the UK weight norms at time of entry to the UK. In contrast to meta-analyses on general forms of maltreatment (Lim et al., 2014; Paquola et al., 2016), there were no differences in limbic areas.

An important question regarding structural brain abnormalities is how they relate to clinical symptoms or functional impairments. In our study of young adults, the reduction in total brain volume statistically mediated the relationship between deprivation experience and ADHD symptoms in addition to general cognitive ability (IQ; Mackes et al., 2020). Specifically, those individuals within the institutionalised group who presented with more ADHD symptoms and a lower IQ had a smaller total brain volume. Even though the ERA study did not find mediation effects of cortical thinning between a history of institutionalisation and ADHD symptoms as reported by the BEIP (McLaughlin et al., 2014), this pattern seems to be in line with the link between total brain volume and ADHD observed in the ERA study (Mackes et al., 2020).

Summary and Discussion

Functional brain imaging studies on the effects of maltreatment have mainly focussed on the processing of threat and reward in addition to emotion regulation and generally report activation changes in limbic and frontal brain regions (McCrory et al., 2017). Changes in a prefrontal-limbic network have been reported in studies on structural changes in people with a history of maltreatment (Lim et al., 2014; Paquola et al., 2016). A significant limitation of this work is that most of the evidence stems from retrospective reports. Prospective studies starting in childhood and imaging studies on children with a history of maltreatment in general are lacking. Considering data from two well-controlled prospective studies on institutional deprivation, a specific form of extreme neglect, findings suggest that early institutional rearing is associated with an overall reduction in brain volume.

In the ERA study's young adults, ADHD symptoms and impairments in IQ are associated with concurrently measured brain volume and reduction in brain volume mediated the effects of institutionalisation on ADHD symptoms and IQ. Although the ERA study did not find any cortical-thinning effects in adulthood, the BEIP study reported cortical thinning in frontal, parietal and temporal regions in childhood which mediated the effects of institutional deprivation on ADHD symptoms (McLaughlin et al., 2014). Taken together, institutionalisation appears to be associated with structural changes in the brain linked to the development of ADHD symptoms.

Neither the ERA study nor the BEIP reported any structural effects in limbic brain regions, apart from the small-scale pilot study in adolescence. The effect found in the pilot study was in the opposite direction to the effect reported in meta-analyses of maltreatment, i.e. larger, as opposed to reduced, amygdala volume (Mehta et al., 2009). There are several possible explanations (Mackes et al., 2020). First, institutional deprivation experienced by the ERA sample is a particularly severe form of neglect and more 'common' forms of neglect might not be comparable in nature. Second, experience of adversity in both studies of Romanian institution-reared children took place particularly early in life. Third, studies on maltreated children where maltreatment occurs within families are genetically confounded. That is not the case for the ERA study where maltreatment occurred in institutions followed by adoption into UK families. Fourth, several previous studies focussed on regions of interest rather than the whole brain (Paquola et al., 2016), and it is possible that at least some of them did not control for the effect of overall brain volume (Mackes et al., 2020), e.g. if total brain volume is reduced, the amygdala would be smaller as well, thus regional analysis would need to control for total brain volume. In general, more prospective longitudinal studies and studies in children are needed.

Case Study: Andrei

Andrei was born in Romania in June 1988. When he was three months old, he was abandoned by his parents and brought to a local orphanage. Conditions in the orphanage were appalling. Bathrooms were dirty with excrement. Food was of low nutritional value and generally scarce. Andrei spent most of his time in his crib in a room with 20 other boys and girls. There were no toys available, and interactions with staff members were few, which resulted in Andrei often laying in his own urine or excrement for several hours. To clean him up, he was hosed down with cold water. In summer 1991, after two years in the orphanage and shortly after his third birthday, Andrei was adopted by a UK-based family.

At the time of adoption, his height, weight and head circumference were 1–1.5 standard deviations below the Romanian norms for his age and sex. He had not developed any language. He was unable to form a secure attachment to his adoptive parents, and his attachment behaviour was categorised as disorganised. His cognitive functioning, with an IQ of 72, was almost 2 standard deviations below the average.

After entering school, the teachers complained about Andrei not paying attention in class. At this point, his weight was in the normal range for his height. His height had improved but was still 0.7 standard deviations below the Romanian norms for his age and sex. His head circumference remained 1 standard deviation below the norm and did not show signs of catch-up.

A neuropsychological and clinical assessment revealed that his cognitive skills had caught up somewhat by about half a standard deviation (80). He no longer showed an impairment in language development and was fluent in English. The Strength and Difficulties questionnaire was completed by his mother and teacher. Both questionnaires showed elevated scores on the hyperactivity scale in the abnormal range (mother: 7, teacher: 8, out of a maximum of 10). A diagnostic interview (DAWBA) did not confirm a diagnosis of ADHD. All other scores were within normal range, as were his social communication skills measured with a parent-reported Social Communication Questionnaire. A neuropsychological test battery further revealed problems with executive functioning, regarding working memory.

Outcome Measures

Modified Maltreatment Classification System (rating of case records for prospective studies):

English, D.J., Bangdiwala, S.I. and Runyan, D.K. (2005). The Dimensions of Maltreatment: Introduction. *Child Abuse & Neglect, 29*(5): 441–460. https://doi.org/10.1016/j.chiabu.2003.09.023

Childhood Experience of Care and Abuse (CECA; retrospective measure): https://lifespantraining.org.uk/types-of-training/childhood-experience-of-care-abuse-ceca/ceca-introduction-and-background/

Multiple-Choice Questions

See answers on page 669.

1. How would you categorise institutional deprivation?
   a. Physical abuse
   b. Emotional abuse
   c. Sexual abuse
   d. Neglect
2. Is the following statement true or false? Prospective and retrospective measures of maltreatment can be used interchangeably.
   a. True, retrospectively and prospectively assessed cohorts vastly overlap.
   b. False, retrospectively and prospectively assessed cohorts hardly overlap.
   c. True, as long as interviews are used as the retrospective measure.
   d. False, prospective measures are better.
   e. False, retrospective measures are better.
3. How many children are estimated to live in institutions world-wide?
   a. Roughly 3 million
   b. Roughly 75,000
   c. Roughly 5 million
   d. Roughly 500,000
4. Which of these functional brain alterations has not been frequently associated with childhood maltreatment?
   a. Threat processing
   b. Reward processing
   c. Motor processing
   d. Emotion regulation
   e. Emotional processing

Key References

Mackes, N., Golm, D., Sarkar, S., Kumsta, R., Rutter, M., Fairchild, G., ... Sonuga-Barke, E. (2019). Early Childhood Deprivation Is Associated with Alterations in Adult Brain Structure

Despite Subsequent Environmental Enrichment. *Proceedings of the National Academy of Sciences of the United States of America* (PNAS).

McCrory, E.J., Gerin, M.I. and Viding, E. (2017). Annual Research Review: Childhood Maltreatment, Latent Vulnerability and the Shift to Preventative Psychiatry–The Contribution of Functional Brain Imaging. *Journal of Child Psychology and Psychiatry*, 58(4): 338–357.

Nelson, C.A., Zeanah, C.H. and Fox, N.A. (2019). How Early Experience Shapes Human Development: The Case of Psychosocial Deprivation. *Neural Plasticity*, 2019.

Teicher, M.H. (2018). Childhood Trauma and the Enduring Consequences of Forcibly Separating Children from Parents at the United States Border. *BMC Medicine*, 16(1): 146.

30 Asylum Seekers, Refugees and Homeless Young People

Pam Campbell, Ann Spooner and Sarah Gale

Introduction

For both young asylum seekers and homeless young people, the common theme is that they have lost their home. It may be, particularly in the case of young homeless people or those originating from countries experiencing long-running violent conflict, that they never had anywhere that was stable, warm and loving to call home.

KEY CONCEPTS

- Asylum seekers can be defined as people who have moved to a country to seek asylum.
- A refugee is someone who has arrived in another country, sought asylum and been granted either a fixed or indefinite period of leave to remain.
- Definitions of homelessness vary considerably, but include having no security of tenure in rented accommodation, living in bed and breakfast housing, hostels or refuge houses for people fleeing from domestic violence.
- In working with both asylum-seeking and homeless children and young people, the most important factor is to build trust by being caring and honest.
- Professionals should seek to understand mental health issues in the context of the young person's whole life and not in isolation.

Asylum Seekers and Refugees

For young asylum seekers home is another country, often literally a whole world away. It is important to recognise that this is the only factor that asylum seekers and refugees have in common. They are a diverse group. Asylum seekers can be defined as people who have moved to a country to seek asylum. They are offered accommodation, sometimes in detention, whilst awaiting the outcome of their claim. If it is rejected, they are deemed to be in the UK unlawfully and will have to leave. The alternative to this is destitution and a life below the radar of authorities and all that this implies. If their asylum claim is successful, they will be allowed to remain in the UK, sometimes for a fixed length of time. At this point, they assume the status of a refugee. A refugee is a person who is living outside of their country of nationality and who cannot return because of fear of persecution. Both asylum seekers and refugees are fully entitled to NHS services.

For asylum seekers the seeds of their mental distress have usually been sown in their own countries. They have had, or are fearful of having, experiences that mean they must leave home, extended family and everything they know In extreme cases, both adults and children may experience depression and/or post-traumatic stress disorder, or even symptoms of psychosis (Hodes and Vostanis, 2018). In all cases, there will be a sadness and pain at who and what has been left behind. The circumstances of their travel usually mean that asylum seekers are not able to take many possessions with them. The journey itself can often be hazardous.

Once here in the UK there are other difficulties and issues that can cause or exacerbate mental health issues.

- Asylum seekers find themselves dispersed to a place that may not be of their choosing and placed in accommodation that may be quite poor.
- Often the key issues for the clients are homesickness, social anxiety and managing the difficulties of living in the system here (Cavill, 2000).
- There is a considerable uncertainty inherent in being an asylum seeker. People do not know when their asylum claim will be heard and are anxious about its outcome.
- Families must get used to a new culture, learn a new language and navigate the local school and health care systems, all of which can be extremely daunting.
- Children may feel the burden of responsibility to act as a support and interpreter for their parents when dealing with statutory bodies, such as the Home Office, local authority or the NHS (Woodhead, 2000). This is often an additional burden on a young person who is trying to integrate into a new culture, a new school and make new friends.

Many asylum-seeking children come to the UK as part of a family unit, but some young people are unaccompanied. Hodes (2008) highlights that 'Lone asylum-seeking children are at much greater risk of mental health problems, such as post-traumatic stress symptoms, than their accompanied peers'. Unaccompanied asylum seekers are more likely to be suffering from the aftereffects of extreme experiences in their home countries, e.g. being involved in combat or being tortured, sexually assaulted, witnessing physical and sexual violence towards loved ones or possibly being the one individual elected to leave the home and escape death or imprisonment (Hodes and Vostanis, 2018). On arrival in the UK they are often placed in temporary accommodation rather than a more supportive environment, such as foster care.

Homeless Young People and Families

One study has demonstrated that homeless children and their mothers have a high level of mental health problems (Vostanis et al., 1998). There are many reasons for this. Vostanis (2002) found that 'the majority of families become homeless because of domestic violence'. Witnessing domestic violence can cause behavioural and mental health problems in young people, e.g. depression, anxiety and post-traumatic stress disorder, like that of young asylum seekers or refugees. In some cases, young people experience abuse and may choose to leave home because of it.

A Mental Health Foundation report (Stephens, 2002) considers that insecure accommodation damages both mental and physical health. A lack of stable housing means that young people and/or families are likely to be moved regularly, often into housing that may not be entirely suitable. An example may be having only a single room for a family, having to share a bathroom and kitchen with others, having a lack of furniture and basic household items. There is often a stigma attached to living in these circumstances, and children may experience bullying at school. Moving to a new house may require changing schools and the consequent loss of friends and familiarity, that can feed into considerable anxiety about the future. Children may feel an obligation to care for parents who may themselves be experiencing mental health difficulties or struggling with addictions.

Young people who have been forced or chosen to leave 'home', this may be temporary accommodation or local authority care, are often vulnerable. Self-harming behaviours and substance misuse may be present as a means of coping with their current situation or a history of stress and/or abuse in the family home. These young people often lack the skills and opportunities to achieve socially and educationally, leading to unemployment and poor self-esteem. There are difficulties in transferring from child to adult services, particularly for those with diagnoses considered the property of children and young people, e.g. attention deficit hyperactivity disorder (ADHD).

Summary

For all homeless people, including asylum seekers, use of health services may be difficult. There are barriers to using mainstream services. These include not attending appointments due to the chaotic nature of their lifestyles, not receiving post, because of having no address or a shared address, illiteracy and mistrust of statutory services. For asylum seekers, there is the specific issue of speaking limited or no English. It is vital that health professionals obtain an independent interpreter and do not expect the young person to bring a friend or family member to interpret. It is important to recognise potential religious and cultural issues. In some cultures, there is no concept of depression and people present with physical manifestations, such as all-over body pain.

Case Study (1): Asad

Asad was born in Somalia and fled the violent conflict in his home country at the age of 16 and arrived in the UK seeking asylum. Upon arrival, he was placed in a Home Office-provided young asylum seekers home. In his early years in the UK, he was very quiet and mistrusting of others, especially those who represented the government, including the police and social workers.

Once he turned 18, Asad was granted indefinite leave to remain, i.e. refugee status. This change in status and his age meant that he was no longer able to remain in the young person's project and became street homeless.

Asad was very anxious about living on the streets, especially as his English was still quite limited. He was equally worried about moving into hostel accommodation, because of rumours he had heard about violence in those settings. Eventually Asad presented himself to the local street homelessness prevention team, who worked with him for some time to persuade him to move into a hostel. It was crucial not to pressurise Asad into hostel accommodation, but to build up a trusting relationship with him. He opened up about his interests and stated that he had a flair for art. His support worker was able to identify a smaller hostel where his artistic talent could be encouraged. They visited on several occasions to help Asad to feel more comfortable with the idea of being there.

Asad began to settle well, but, after a few weeks an argument between two other residents triggered traumatic flashbacks form the violence he had witnessed in Somalia. He left the hostel and was found by his street homelessness worker asleep in a local car park. With encouragement, he, his worker and the hostel manager met away from the hostel to discuss his fears and concerns. An action plan was formulated between the three of them, which involved him spending time with a member of the hostel staff if another confrontation occurred until he felt calmer. Asad was referred to his GP to discuss possible psychological reports with regard to the flashbacks he had experienced.

Case Study (2): James

James (16) lived in a family where high conflict had been present throughout his entire life. Until the age of ten he had witnessed his mother experiencing domestic violence at the hands of his father. On one occasion, his mother became extremely violent towards his father and after that the physical abuse ended. The verbal aggression continued.

As James grew older and developed physically, he had begun to respond to verbal aggression from his parents with similar responses and on a few occasions, with his father, it had become physical. The situation came to a head when James fell into a fight with his father and broke two of his father's fingers. James was immediately thrown out of the house by his father and told never to return.

James was able to stay on the sofas in friends' houses for a few weeks, but his friends' parents would eventually say that he needed to move on. Eventually, an adult friend took James to the local homeless unit. After the homeless unit tried and were unable to reach a resolution with James' parents, he was placed in emergency accommodation until a room in a young person's project could be found.

Once at the youth housing project, staff observed James displaying unusually high levels of verbal aggression towards other young people, often in response to the smallest of triggers. This had resulted in a fight with another male resident that put the tenancy at risk. James confided in a staff member, saying that he hated becoming angry so quickly, but felt unable to manage himself. James was referred by the project to the local community CAMHS team. He was assessed and allocated an individual therapist to begin exploring his experiences and their impact on his current behaviour.

After a course of sessions James was able to identify conflict situations and his patterns of response to them. With the therapist, he was then able to explore alternative responses in those situations. He tested those out and reported a positive outcome. With the support of his therapist he was able to contact his mother and father and meet up with them to begin rebuilding their relationship. James stated that he would not return home, but wished to find accommodation of his once he turned 18.

Once more settled, James was able to enrol on a course in plumbing at his local college.

Multiple-Choice Questions

See answers on page 669.

1. Which of the following should be considered when assessing an asylum-seeking child/young person?
   a. Whether they speak English
   b. Cultural issues and religious beliefs
   c. Whether or not they are entitled to NHS services
   d. Experience of traumatic events
   e. All the above
2. According to Vostanis (2002) what is the main cause of homelessness for mothers and children?
   a. Being made redundant
   b. Domestic violence
   c. Harassment from neighbours
   d. Relationship breakdown
   e. Rent arrears

3. Which of these is a young homeless person most likely to experience?
   a. Schizophrenia
   b. Self-harm
   c. Anxiety
   d. Bi-polar disorder
   e. Substance misuse

Key References

Hodes, M. (2008). Risk and Resilience for Psychological Distress Amongst Unaccompanied Asylum Seeking Adolescents. *Journal of Child Psychology and Psychiatry*, 49(7): 723–732.

Hodes, M. and Vostanis, P. (2018). Practitioner Review: Mental Health Problems of Refugee Children and Adolescents and Their Management. *Journal of Child Psychology and Psychiatry*, 60(7): 716–731.

Stephens, J. (2002). *The Mental Health Needs of Homeless Young People. Bright Futures: Working with Vulnerable Young People.* London: Mental Health Foundation.

Vostanis, P. (2002). Mental Health of Homeless Children and Their Families. *Advances in Psychiatric Treatment*, 8: 463–469.

31 Post-Traumatic Stress Disorder (PTSD)

Alex Christie

Introduction

Traumas are events that overwhelm an individual's ability to cope with the situation. When people experience a trauma, it can lead to the development of long-term psychological and physiological responses that can become debilitating, known as post-traumatic stress disorder (PTSD).

ICD-10 Classification

Table 31.1 outlines the current criteria for a diagnosis of PTSD to be given using the World Health Organization's ICD-10. The next revision (ICD-11) has been provisionally released and will come into effect from 1 January 2022. ICD-11 focusses on the symptoms most specific to PTSD, keeping the same three clusters of symptoms identified in ICD-10, i.e. re-experiencing, avoidance and hyper-arousal, but identifying only two core symptoms within each cluster: respectively, re-experiencing through nightmares and flashbacks, cognitive and physical avoidance of reminders, hypervigilance and exaggerated startle response, that make it distinct from a reactive depressive episode or from grief following a bereavement.

This may reduce the number of diagnoses of single-event PTSD (Barbano et al., 2019) but the addition of complex PTSD, not considered here, as another diagnosis is an acknowledgement of the significant impact of distressing life events on individuals where their multiple traumas have led to emotional dysregulation, interpersonal difficulties and negative self-concept (Knefel et al., 2019) and may be a very helpful diagnosis within the CAMHS setting.

Risk Factors and Aetiology

The dynamic nature of childhood development means that treatments can vary in efficacy depending on the age and cognitive ability of the child, increasing the difficulty in like-for-like comparisons across studies and treatments. Ethical considerations abound. Consent and capacity are key issues, and trauma work inherently includes the risk of re-traumatisation of the individual. There is the possibility that the child's social circumstances may make parental involvement in treatment impossible or unwise. This considered, the experimental evidence base for PTSD in children might reasonably be expected to be slim and much of the evidence is extrapolated from adult populations.

Prevalence

PTSD can vary enormously across studies, even those that examine post-trauma symptoms stemming from a single traumatic event, e.g. one meta-analysis examining PTSD following

Table 31.1 WHO (1992) Diagnostic Criteria for PTSD

A. There must have been exposure to a traumatic event	This could be experiencing or witnessing an event that either leads to death or serious injury, or in which death or serious injury appear likely It could be to the individual themselves, or to others in the immediate vicinity Events impacting on significant figures in the individual's life, parents, partner or close friends can be traumatic even if not directly observed
B. There must be reliving of the event through intense dreams, flashbacks, vivid memories or through acute distress on exposure to events resembling the initial trauma	Flashbacks are distinct from nightmares or bad dreams in that they can occur when awake as well as during sleep, and that they have the quality of feeling 'real', i.e. that the individual is actually back in the traumatic moment again
C. There must be active or attempted avoidance of situations that resemble or that are associated with the traumatic event	These avoidances can be either physical, e.g. not returning to the scene of an assault or avoiding using public transport after a road traffic collision, or psychological, e.g. never discussing the event or forcing oneself not to think about it The avoidance should not have been present prior to the traumatic event
D. There must be either: • **An inability to accurately recall some aspects of the event** • **Persistent psychological sensitivity and physiological arousal, from any two or more of:** **a. Difficulty getting to or staying asleep** **b. Increased irritability or anger** **c. Difficulty in concentrating** **d. Exaggerated startle response**	The impact on memory can be a significant factor in traumas resulting from criminal acts These increases in psychological and physiological arousal often present as hyper-vigilance, adopting a heightened level of alertness as a preventative measure, often disproportionate to the rate of likely reoccurrence of the initial trauma
E. For criteria B to D inclusive, the symptoms must have begun within six months of the stressor event	Some of the symptoms may be further delayed in onset beyond six months

road-traffic collision found prevalence rates varying in studies between 6% and 45% (Heron-Delaney et al., 2013).

Time Elapsed

It appears that the closer to the traumatic event an individual is assessed, the more likely they are to report symptoms suggestive of PTSD (Heron-Delaney et al., 2013).

Socioeconomic and Cultural Factors

Cultural and socioeconomic factors appear to be significant predictors of the prevalence of PTSD, given that areas with lower infant mortality rates tend to show lower rates of PTSD. Infant mortality is used here as an aggregate measure of a country's socioeconomic status, level of health care, technological development and other cultural factors relevant to psychological resilience.

Demographic

Women are consistently found to be at greater risk of developing PTSD in most prevalence studies (Keane et al., 2005) and show increased risk of developing PTSD even within studies focussed on a specific form of trauma, e.g. combat stress (Wolfe et al., 2003). In males, the elderly and young boys may be at greater risk of developing PTSD, with this effect appearing significantly lessened for women and girls (Kessler, 1995).

Nature of the Trauma

That certain types of traumatic event may increase the likelihood that the individual experiencing them will develop PTSD symptoms does have face validity. It is widely recognised that events such as the experience of sexual assault or combat stress are more likely to trigger PTSD than that of natural disasters. However, it is difficult to effectively categorise and define events across sample populations even within one study, let alone when undertaking meta-analysis across numerous studies (Keane et al., 2006), making it difficult to draw firm conclusions.

Previous Trauma

Several large analyses have examined the impact of repeated exposure to trauma and appear to suggest that past traumas and adverse life events have a predisposing effect for the development of PTSD in response to later traumatic events (Brewin et al., 2000; Ozer et al., 2003). The effect appears to vary as to whether the traumas are accidental or interpersonal violence, with lesser effect seen when the traumas are not personally directed at the individual experiencing them, e.g. natural disasters. It is possible that repeated exposure may, for individuals exposed to regular traumatic events, lead to a reduction in the physiological response to new traumas that may be protective against the development of PTSD (Bowman and Yehuda, 2004).

Pre-Existing Mental Health Difficulties

Having pre-existing difficulties with mental health appears to be linked to a higher prevalence of PTSD, with depression particularly appearing to be a significant risk factor (Ozer et al., 2003).

Treatment Interventions

Psychological

Guidance from the National Institute for Health and Care Excellent (NICE) for the treatment of PTSD (NICE Guidance 116; NG116) is clear that work should address the central trauma and in adults, recommends either trauma-focussed cognitive behavioural therapy (TF-CBT) or eye-movement desensitisation and reprocessing (EMDR). In children, EMDR is felt to be not as cost-effective as TF-CBT and less effective generally. It is recommended only if children have not responded to or cannot engage with TF-CBT.

In adults both TF-CBT and EMDR are well-evidenced, whilst non-trauma-focussed interventions can be effective to a lesser degree (Bisson, Roberts, Andrew, Cooper and Lewis, 2013; Sin, Spain, Furuta, Murrells and Norman, 2017). An evidence basis is emerging for EMDR in adolescents and children, suggesting it may prove as effective in under-18s. Recent meta-analysis of a small number of studies (8, n = 295) suggested that efficacy may match TF-CBT, but cautioned that larger samples and direct comparative trials are needed (Moreno-Alcazar et al., 2017).

Pharmacological

NG116 identifies limited evidence for treatment of PTSD in children and young people with PTSD and does not recommend drug treatment. Fluoxetine, sertraline and citalopram are recommended for treatment of depression in 12–18-year olds, alongside psychological treatment (NICE, 2019), and young people with PTSD presenting with a co-morbid depressive episode may find treatment of their low mood helpful in improving functioning and quality of life.

Practice-Based Evidence

Children and young people's mental health is a field with significant ethical constraints to be overcome when conducting research. As a result, specialist CAMHS services may offer treatments not specifically recommended by NICE in the treatment of trauma. Systemic family therapy may be helpful where parents are being highly critical of a child's behaviour, or where a desire to reduce their child's anxiety is leading to parental involvement in safety behaviours that maintain the heightened responses in the long term.

Case Study (1): Andrew

Andrew (eight) presents with low weight for his age and height, a very restricted diet and has recently stopped eating, unless he is with his mother. When he does eat, he is only able to manage 'soft' foods like soups, sauces and saturated breakfast cereals. When offered firmer or crunchy-textured foods he becomes increasingly distressed and at times, oppositional. His school nurse has referred him concerned that he may be developing an eating disorder.

Along with Andrew's parents, a developmental history is undertaken to rule out an underlying neurodevelopmental condition (e.g. autistic spectrum condition). His early years did not suggest it and there are no other difficulties related to sensory preferences or sensory processing. His parents are clear that he has not always been faddy with his eating, but that that he has changed from eating a varied diet to this severe level of restriction over the past eight to ten months.

Their accommodation of his new preferences has led to his range of foods becoming smaller and smaller. Andrew does not report any concern about his body shape and is frustrated and upset that he cannot eat foods that he used to enjoy. During the assessment it is revealed that Andrew had an episode of choking on a piece of apple whilst at an after-school club about a year ago, requiring back slaps from the club's facilitator and assessment at accident and emergency for physical check-up. He appears convinced that eating crunchy foods will make him gag or might even kill him and is having nightmares about being taken to hospital.

Andrew experienced a potentially life-threatening situation whilst he was away from his parents and that precipitated his first and only trip to a hospital. He is actively avoiding foods that are textually similar to the one he choked on. His heightened anxiety is leading to the fight-and-flight responses whereby he lashes out or runs from the room. His parents' accommodation of his avoidance has led to a worsening of his symptoms and is a maintaining factor in his current difficulties.

The care plan for Andrew is twofold. It involves monitoring his physical health and providing advice about menu planning to ensure that there is no further weight loss. Support from a paediatric dietician may be helpful, alongside periodic weighing either by a CAMHS nurse or his GP.

The psychological treatment is likely to involve several components:

- Parental education about the role of avoidance in maintaining his anxiety about choking.
- Practical teaching of anxiety-management and grounding strategies to help Andrew manage when he awakes from his nightmares and to allow him to manage the next intervention.
- TF-CBT or EMDR. Due to Andrew's age, he may find it difficult both to access and to challenge his thoughts, and EMDR may be a good alternative to TF-CBT.

The work with Andrew is focussed on his memory of the initial choking event rather than his current fear of specific foods since it is this that has led to the current pattern of avoidance. There may need to be some exposure-based work on the currently feared foods but, without addressing the root cause, simply helping Andrew to overcome his phobia of coarse foods may not resolve the other trauma-related symptoms.

Andrew's parents learn how to tolerate some of his discomfort and become skilled in coaching him to try foods that cause him to fear choking. They encourage him to score his worry about choking before and after each new food and over time, he can recognise that his anxiety reduces each time. In his therapy sessions, he is gradually encouraged to access the memory he has of the initial choking episode and can reprocess it, so that it no longer troubles him to think of it. He is helped to understand that the trip to hospital was just a precaution and not a sign that he was close to dying.

Case Study (2): Laxmi

Laxmi (17) was a passenger in a fatal road traffic collision. Since the accident, she has been largely unable to tolerate being in a vehicle as a passenger and has felt unable to start driving lessons herself. She experiences waking flashbacks, vivid nightmares and, when she is in a car, panic attacks. The impact on her sleep is significant, and as her sleep has become poorer, her mood has become very low. She is starting to withdraw and become more isolated as she is unable to use cars or public transport to meet with her friends. She is feels that her life is not worth living at present.

Laxmi's assessment focusses on trying to establish the nature, frequency and severity of her symptoms. It aims to assess the beliefs that she has about the accident. During the assessment, Laxmi describes that it is only a matter of time before she is in another collision as she 'got away' the first time when she was 'meant' to die.

She avoids being in cars not only for her own protection, but to protect other road users and the people she is travelling with. She can recognise that these thoughts are irrational, but when in a situation that triggers them, she has almost 100% conviction that they are true.

Laxmi has developed strong beliefs about the accident that are tied to both a real risk, traffic accidents being relatively common, and her past life experiences, but that have become catastrophic with a sense of inevitability not warranted in reality. Her depressive symptoms appear secondary to the trauma, triggered by the reduction in her opportunities to socialise, her significantly impaired sleep and the high level of anxiety she experiences day to day. The fact she was a passenger rather than the driver has potentially worsened the impact of the event for her because she has no sense of being in control of her life at the time of the accident.

Laxmi would be likely to benefit from TF-CBT as she is well able to access her thoughts about the trauma and can recognise that many of them are irrational. Prior to this work starting, Laxmi attends sessions on grounding techniques to help her remain present and focussed when her fight/flight response has been activated.

As her symptoms have a marked impact on her functioning and she appears to be significantly depressed, Laxmi is offered an antidepressant medication to help improve her mood and to reduce some of her anxiety. Close support and monitoring take place as she begins this medication, given her suicidal ideation.

In therapy, she is encouraged to challenge and restructure her beliefs about the accident and is helped to identify the ways in which she both physically and mentally avoids reminders of it. As she more frequently accesses the traumatic memory, she can address some of the beliefs she has developed about the accident, further challenging them.

By undertaking exposure tasks to 'test' some of her hypotheses, Laxmi can unlearn some of the heightened physiological responses and to remain calm while being in a vehicle. Laxmi's mood improves significantly once she can resume travel to college and socialise with friends, and she continues the antidepressant for around six months after she feels 'better'. Laxmi's anxiety about car travel remains higher than normal, but no longer prevents her living her life.

Multiple-Choice Questions

See answers on page 669.

1. Core, defining, symptoms for PTSD can be categorised into how many clusters?
   a. Two
   b. Five
   c. Seven
   d. Three
2. NICE guidelines for PTSD in young people and children recommend TF-CBT as the first-line psychological treatment, unless the patient is unable to engage with the treatment model. Which other therapy does NICE recommend in the absence of TF-CBT?
   a. Systemic family therapy
   b. Brief child and adolescent psychotherapy
   c. EMDR
   d. Acceptance and commitment therapy
3. In general, within what timescale after the traumatic event happening should symptoms have started to appear for a diagnosis of PTSD to be considered?
   a. Within six months after
   b. Between one and two years after
   c. Before a year afterwards
   d. In the six months before the event
4. The six core symptoms for PTSD identified in ICD-11 are? (Pick **three**.)
   a. Nightmares and flashbacks
   b. Irritation and aggression
   c. Cognitive and physical avoidance

   d. Depression and anxiety
   e. Hypervigilance and exaggerated startle response
5. A child with PTSD may present with strong fear responses to certain stimuli. Which of the following would help determine whether you were supporting a child with PTSD rather than one with a phobia? (Pick **two**.)
   a. They have experienced a life-threatening or highly disturbing past event.
   b. They are avoiding the thing that they are scared of.
   c. They are experiencing intrusive thoughts or memories of a moment from their past.
   d. They are having panic attacks.

Key References

de Thierry, B., (2016). *The Simple Guide to Child Trauma: What It Is and How to Help*. London: Jessica Kingsley Publishers.

National Institute for Health and Care Excellence, (2018). NICE Guidelines NG116: *Post-traumatic Stress Disorder*. London: NICE.

Smith, P., et al., (2009). *Post-Traumatic Stress Disorder (CBT with Children, Adolescents and Families)*. London: Routledge.

Part IV

The Assessment of Children and Young People's Mental Health

Cathy Laver-Bradbury

The importance of assessment in CAMHS can never be underestimated. The skill of the assessment is to understand from the parent and child's perspective what the difficulties are and how these have occurred and what they attribute these to. The referral letter is the start of the process, and how the referrer attributes the difficulties starts the process of assessment although should not direct it. There are many styles and models of assessments used in a CAMHS service; however we suggest that the initial assessment should understand the models used in CAMHS and be broad enough to result in a formulation that has considered these.

Assessment should not be something that is only done at the beginning of treatment but a continuous process that happens each time you meet with the family, child or young person. The assessment builds up over time as trust is built. As the assessment proceeds, it may be that the original presenting problem becomes less significant and other problems assume priority for treatment.

The skill of the assessor is paramount, exploration of the surrounding systems is essential and none should be seen in isolation. This is an enormous task, and the skills of working with families to bring about change are often under-recognised, either by the system in which the health and social care professions work or by the time restraints often in place.

In this section we start with the importance of formulation and the theories used to inform this; we then offer an outline of the approaches to assessment within CAMHS, using different therapeutic models.

Assessments are often a treatment their own right; raising awareness in the family about the issues they want help with and why these might have occurred can often in itself bring about a significant change. The importance of 'holding' the family through this process, remaining curious and being able to put aside one's own judgements, is paramount if the family is to feel safe in exploring their difficulties.

32 Making Sense of Behaviour

Carlos Hoyos

Diagnosis and Formulation

Healthcare practitioners, doctors and nurses regularly conduct assessments of patients. We gather information in order to rule out or to arrive at a diagnosis. Usually, a diagnosis does describe what the problem is, what has gone wrong and how to treat it. If we present to a doctor with abdominal pain and, after examining us, they diagnose appendicitis, we know that the pain is caused by an inflamed appendix and that, unless it is removed, we may die.

Other diagnoses describe a problem but do not give enough information as to its origin or treatment. If we present to a doctor with tiredness and pallor and we are diagnosed with anaemia, we have a description of what is wrong with us, beyond the symptoms we presented, but do not necessarily know if this is because of an internal bleed or because we are not eating enough iron. It indicates what the problem may be, but not an explanation. Finally, there are diagnoses that only offer a description of the symptoms but offer very little in terms of explanation or treatment, e.g. if we present with a swollen foot and we are diagnosed with idiopathic oedema, we have a name, but very little understanding of what is happening with our foot or what to do about it. The diagnosis describes the symptoms using another language.

Most medical diagnoses in mental health are like the diagnosis of anaemia or idiopathic oedema in that they do not have very much explanatory value. What patients are mostly interested in, the primary task of a mental health assessment, is the construction of an explanation for the behaviour that has proved to be problematic and beyond the understanding of the people who present it. If a family brings a five-year-old child that, for no apparent reason, has started to soil and spread the faeces on the walls of the house and is unable to explain why, a diagnosis of 'encopresis' or 'conduct disorder' offers little comfort. What the family seeks is an explanation of what drives this behaviour and a way of making sense of what this behaviour means so that something can be done about it. That explanation, the story that meaningfully explains this behaviour, is what we refer to as a formulation.

A diagnosis is often a word that summarises the problem. It is categorical and susceptible to classification. If we diagnose a stage three carcinoma of the liver, we have explained what is wrong, what the prognosis and the treatment is, and we are putting the problem into the 'cancer' category. Carcinoma of the liver can then be classified further as more information arises. Diagnoses are mostly a positive statement, i.e. you either have a cancer or you do not. It is not subject to interpretation.

Formulations tend to be opinions and come in the form of explanations. 'I think your child is spreading faeces on the wall of the house because he is upset at the attention you pay to your new-born twins' is not a categorical statement and is always an interpretation. Yet, it is a more meaningful explanation than 'he does it because he has a conduct disorder' or, if it existed, he has a 'faeces-spreading syndrome'.

Meaningful Explanations

It may be worth examining what we mean by constructing 'meaningful explanations'. 'Meaning' refers to significance. Something is meaningful when it merits our attention. It is important. 'Explanation' refers to justification, an account that makes something clear. A behaviour is explained when we have an account that attributes a reason or a cause.

There are three ideas that are central to understanding both meaning and explanation. First the idea of what is 'important', second is the concept of an 'account' (a story) and lastly, the attribution of 'causality'. A meaningful explanation is a story that makes a causal attribution that seems important to us.

What is important to us in a story will depend mostly on what we think is important before we tell or hear the story. If we think parental attention is important, we are more likely to find the story: 'he is doing this because he is not getting enough attention' meaningful. If we do not, we may be more inclined to find other stories like 'he is doing this because there is something wrong with his brain' more meaningful.

The values we hold before hearing a story will inform how meaningful that story is, what kind of information we look for and how likely we are to accept the causal attribution implied in the story.

Our values (what we think is important) will therefore inform what we find meaningful. There is something more complex than values at play when we make causal attributions, when we think something causes something else. Accepting which 'causes' have explanatory value, what we accept as the 'cause' of a behaviour, will depend on how we understand behaviour to 'work'. If we think that the main influence on children's level of excitement is whether they consume sugar, when we see an excited child we will immediately ask whether sugar has been consumed, and if it has, then we will attribute the excitement to the sugar they took. This is because consumption of sugar is important to us, we pay attention, and because our understanding of how excitement in children works implies that sugar 'causes' excitement. If we believe instead that children become excited when they anticipate a reward, rather than sugar levels, when we see an excited child we will ask what future event they are excited about. When we find that they are about to go on an exciting ride, we will attribute the excitement to that forthcoming event.

Models of Behaviour

We commonly refer to the ideas about how we understand things to work as 'models'. A model is technically a representation of reality. A model airplane is a small-scale representation of a large actual plane. Maps are models of reality, geography in particular. By looking at a map we can comprehend our surroundings. We can anticipate and predict what we will find beyond what we can see. Maps allow us to know what we find and help us plan journeys. Model planes and maps are physical models of reality, but we use the same word to refer to mental representations of reality. Once we know a geographical area we have a 'mental map' of that area. We do not need the physical map because we have a representation of the space in our minds. We know how different elements of geography are linked to each other. We have an internal model of the world.

How models affect the way we behave can be understood using physical maps as an example. If we are in London and need to go from St James Park station to Piccadilly Circus and all we have is a map of the Underground, we will go to Victoria, change towards Green Park, then switch train to Piccadilly. If we have an A to Z Map we will probably realise that we can drive through Parliament Square and arrive there sooner. If we have Google Maps, we may realise that, in the time it takes to flag a taxi, we can walk through St James Park and arrive there sooner still. Which map we use will inform our understanding of our surroundings and determine what route we take, but maps often have a greater influence in our understanding of reality. People who are used to moving around London using only a map of the Underground often perceive the city as a set of islands around popular stations that are only connected via underground trains. Maps not only help us find our way, they help us understand reality in a particular way. They influence how our internal representation of reality is constructed.

Just as we have mental maps of the geography around us, mental models of our surroundings, we all have models of why and how people behave. If our model of what causes excitement in children is based on the idea of hyperglycaemia activating muscles, we will understand why children become hyperactive after drinking a fizzy drink. When we see an excited child, we will ask, what has he drunk? If our model is based on the idea of anticipated reward, we will have a different understanding of the same phenomena. We will ask, what is he looking forward to? Two different models prompt two different questions. The models we have before encountering the behaviour will determine what questions we ask, what we assess and what explanations are meaningful to us (how we formulate).

We will examine five models for understanding behaviour used by professionals in mental health. These five models inform five different ways to understand how behaviour develops, five different ways to ask questions and five different ways to establish causal attributions. There are many more than five models in use, but we will focus on those most used and commonly accepted.

The Medical (Biological) Model

This model developed towards the end of the 18th century, when doctors took an interest in understanding the behaviour of the residents of lunatic asylums using the newly developed anatomopathological model. Medicine had made great advances in the previous decades through understanding the anatomy (how things were), and physiology (how things worked) of the body and then how it appeared (anatomopathology) and how it went wrong (pathophysiology). Armed with these new methods, doctors took over from alienists (the name given to the people who studied the residents of lunatic asylums, from the French, 'alieniste', meaning insane) in the running of 'lunatic' asylums and brought new understanding to the formulation of the behaviour of the asylum residents.

Up until the 18th century, the prevailing causal attributions around troubling behaviour had been religious, e.g. spirit possessions, say, or damnations, or astrological, i.e. lunatic literally means under the influence of the moon. Doctors brought the revolutionary idea that biological changes in the structure or function of the body, particularly the brain, were much better explanations for the deviant behaviour of lunatics. During the 19th and 20th centuries these new insights led to the development of phenomenology (the study of mental experiences), psychology (the study of mental processes and behaviour), psychopathology (the study of abnormal minds and abnormal behaviours) and psychiatry (the study of medical conditions affecting the mind) and with them the new understanding of abnormal behaviour in biological terms. Pure biological explanations, for example, syphilis, were able to explain, and eventually cure, the behaviour of the largest group of residents of lunatic asylums.

Understanding abnormal behaviour as a symptom of an underlying biological condition became a powerful and helpful tool and led to the creation of many syndromes, i.e. collections of symptoms, that eventually became the modern psychiatric disorders, e.g. bipolar, schizophrenia or depression.

If we did not fully understand the biological structures or mechanisms that explained those symptoms, we could at least find drugs that dramatically improved these behaviours, proving that even if we did not fully understand them, they did have a biological basis. In the process, we were able to relieve incalculable suffering and eventually close most of these gargantuan institutions.

The main feature of the biological model is that behaviour can be considered the product of a biological mechanism. This means that understanding that biological mechanism leads to the understanding of the behaviour. Abnormal behaviour can be explained by abnormality in the underlying biological structure (organic pathology), or the way that structure works (functional pathology). Often this is clearly useful. Loss of memory can be explained by deterioration of neuronal tissue in Alzheimer's disease; abnormal perceptions can be explained by the effect of hallucinogenic drugs.

This model is the basis of psychiatry, and doctors often hold responsibility for this model in multidisciplinary teams. It underpins common understanding of behaviour outside that discipline. Common popular understandings of behaviour often follow this model. The reason why teenagers are rebellious is 'hormones', clever people are referred to as 'big brains', hyperactive or excited children experience a 'sugar rush', addiction is referred as a 'dopamine hit' and low mood as a 'deficit in serotonin'.

Although often presented as the preeminent model in mental 'health' teams, the biological model has its limitations. It offers a mechanistic and simple way to understand behaviour without having to engage with psychological complexity. It allows us to translate complex psychological phenomena into the language of biology, creating an illusion of understanding. Low levels of serotonin are not just a biological phenomenon associated with the psychological phenomenon of low mood. In the biological model, they are thought of as the same phenomenon as low mood and eventually the cause of it. We could explain a complex phenomenon such as crying as an imbalance between the production of serum by the lacrimal glands and the capacity of the lacrimal duct to evacuate such serum, just as we could explain depression as an imbalance in serotonin in the brain. In both cases, we reduce a complex psychological phenomenon (crying, low mood) to one of its biological components, such as overflow of serum or imbalance of serotonin. We understand some of the mechanics, but we are none the wiser as to what it means or why it happens.

The Bio-Psycho-Social Model

Since it was first used by the alienists of the late 19th century the biological model has evolved. Once the low-hanging fruit of syndromes that translated directly to biological pathology, like syphilis or dementia, were identified, the biological underpinnings of other syndromes, e.g. schizophrenia, anxiety, bipolar disorder or depression, became much more difficult to explain as merely the product of distinctly pathological biological mechanisms. Despite huge efforts and great advances in the understanding of normal and abnormal psychobiology, we still do not have convincing comprehensive biological models of those disorders. We continue to refer to these disorders as biological entities whose mechanisms we do not 'yet' understand. Anergia, anhedonia and persistent low mood are the three core symptoms of a biological disorder called depression. We do not know how serotonin, noradrenaline and many other neurotransmitter imbalances 'cause' it, but assume we soon will. We know that chemicals that change those balances affect those three symptoms and assume the biological disorder must be the 'cause'.

Years of successfully treating depression with antidepressants and psychosis with antipsychotics have further convinced doctors, and most of the general public, that the behaviour of people who display anergia, anhedonia and low mood can be explained by the existence of a biological condition called depression or that hallucinations and delusions can be explained by the existence of a biological condition called schizophrenia. Our understanding of the underlying biology of those conditions has so far offered very few insights into causes or explanations of the behaviour.

At the same time, years of studying pathology, such as depression and schizophrenia, have shown us that social and psychological aspects in the lives of people suffering from such conditions do play a significant role in the behaviour and experiences of those who suffer them. True to the biological model of behaviour, we have concluded that those psychological and social factors must influence the biological structures and mechanisms underpinning the behaviour. The simple biological model has evolved to incorporate those psychological and social elements and become what we refer to as the bio-psycho-social model.

The bio-psycho-social model shares with the pure biological model the understanding that a biological condition is the main explanation for the behaviour. A person is low in mood, anergic and unable to enjoy things because they suffer from depression. The useful addition to the model is the understanding that the biological condition itself may be caused, at least partly, by other psychological processes or social circumstances that somehow affect the biology of the brain. We only have a vague understanding of how social factors such as poverty or psychological ones such as automatic negative thoughts affect the biology of the brain, but the model is able to incorporate those without this causal understanding being made explicit by referring to these psychological and social phenomena as 'factors' and proving their influence by statistical association rather than demonstrating a biological mechanism.

Factors refer to items of information that are ascribed to variables in multivariate analysis of variance, a very powerful statistical tool that allows us to establish links between separate phenomena, biological or not, as they are distributed in a population. In the 1970s, Chess and Thomas collected data on a population of women suffering from depression. They observed that those women who were mothers and had three children under five at home were showing symptoms of depression in higher numbers that those without. An analysis of the variance of the distribution of depression between those with and without three children under five showed that this was a 'factor' that explained a significant amount of the variance. They could not conclude that having three children under five was the cause of the symptoms or the presence of the disorder, even less how this may work at a biological level, but they demonstrated that it was associated with depression.

Over the years, associations between many such factors and psychiatric conditions have been demonstrated and replicated, adding to our understanding of such conditions. This is why when constructing a formulation using a bio-psycho-social model we include 'having three children under five' as a significant social factor predisposing to depression. We may stop short of attributing causality, but we imply it, and we use population data to make specific assumptions about an individual case.

A formulation constructed with the bio-psycho-social model treats causality with scepticism, focusing instead on aspects of the history or presentation that have been shown to be significantly associated with the underlying pathology in the wider population. It maintains biology as the main explanation for behaviour, but it allows some nuance and complexity to be involved in the formulation provided there is evidence that such factors have evidence of association in population studies.

The Psychological (Behavioural) Model

Around the same time as doctors were setting out to explain the behaviour of lunatics in biological terms, the science that studies behaviour itself was being created. Psychologists study behaviour and the psychological processes that underpin it. In the early part of the century, following groundbreaking insights into how animals learn through classical and operant conditioning, paradoxically acquired by biologists such as Pavlov, a new methodology was established.

Behavioural psychology understood behaviour as something to be studied on its own, not as a product of biology. It focused on observable behaviour, often in laboratory conditions, and it did not constrict itself to the behaviour of humans. It used laboratory-based experimental methods to isolate behaviours, usually in animals, in order to establish empirical relationships between stimuli and behavioural responses, often using mathematically defined correlations. They produced a substantial body of knowledge of how specific behaviours are acquired or extinguished, i.e. learned and stopped, through the complex interaction of rewards and punishments. They convincingly explained how simple behaviour in animals, e.g. feeding or grooming, can be manipulated by punishing or rewarding a particular behaviour or its alternatives.

These insights were then translated to human psychology and now form the basis of many educational, industrial and clinical psychological principles that are still valid today. Examples of these insights range from algorithms that govern the rewards rates in slot machines to programming schedules of advertisements in the media. A similar example in clinical practice is the learning theory explanation for phobias. Classified by doctors as a disorder of anxiety, phobias are a common presentation in children, defined as an unreasonable, focused and uncontrollable fear that leads to avoidance. Behaviouralists do not understand this phenomenon as an anxiety disorder, but as the unfortunate learning of a dysfunctional response, i.e. avoidance of a specific stimulus that is reinforced by a reward, i.e. the lowering of anxiety, every time the behaviour is displayed. The learning theory model of phobias is a causal explanation that leads to a direct, very successful treatment, i.e. progressive desensitisation, without offering any biological understanding.

The behavioural model understands behaviour as the product of stimuli that are associated with it (classical conditioning) or the rewards and punishments that follow it (operant conditioning). It can cite thousands of papers with experimental empirical evidence that back these statements and offers a way to explain behaviour as a product of a principal psychological mechanism, learning.

When a clinician who understands behaviour following a behavioural model is presented with a particular phenomenon, say, a child who smears faeces on the wall, he or she will ask: how has this behaviour been learned? How is it rewarded and how are alternatives being punished? This will allow for a causal explanation based on learning theory. The focus will be on observable behaviour, not on assumed biological mechanisms. In clinical teams, behavioural advisors or learning disability nurses are often more confident in understanding behaviour in these terms. Specific techniques, e.g. behavioural analysis, are mostly predicated on this model.

The limitations of this model, however, are similar to those of the biological model. Whilst it allows for some psychological complexity, narrowing the focus of explanation to observable behaviour and learning theory may allow for demonstrable causal attributions, but excludes many complexities of behaviour that go beyond what can be observed in laboratory conditions and ignores all mental processes except learning. A formulation such as, 'your child spreads faeces on the wall because he has learned that that is the only way he receives any attention' may have explanatory value, but it ignores many psychological factors that may be involved.

The Psychological (Cognitive-Behavioural) Model

Whilst behaviouralism succeeded in offering a plausible model for phobias, it struggled to produce a convincing model for other conditions, e.g. depression, sometimes called 'learned helplessness'. More complexity was needed in order to incorporate psychological phenomena beyond learning. During the 1960s and 1970s, behavioural psychologists began to treat speech as behaviour. This led to the incorporation of psychological processes, e.g. thought and emotion, into the understanding of behaviour. Psychologists no longer assumed the mind to be a black box whose study can only be undertaken by studying observable inputs (stimulus) and observable outputs (behaviour). They became interested in, and developed, the methodology that would allow the study of belief and emotional responses alongside behaviour itself.

The cognitive-behaviour model assumes that behaviour can be explained by the individual's beliefs and emotions and that any understanding of a particular behaviour necessitates the understanding of the thoughts and feelings linked to that particular behaviour. Thoughts and emotions respond to their own processes that cognitive psychologists can describe and influence. Thought processes, e.g. cognitive bias, that is common errors in thinking, offer plausible explanations of why most people will readily absorb information that confirms existing beliefs whilst ignoring the information that questions it. This in turn explains feelings and behaviours associated with those beliefs. Variations of these, mostly well-understood cognitive processes, can be used to inform our understanding of psychiatric conditions. One variation of confirmation bias explains how people who are feeling low will focus on negative thoughts and events and ignore positive ones, leading to further low mood and depression.

By understanding how mood (emotion), thought (cognition) and the lack of energy (behaviour) interact, cognitive psychologists developed a cognitive model of depression that allowed the development of cognitive-behavioural interventions to treat the disorder. They are as effective as antidepressants in the treatment of what psychiatrists think of as a biological condition, challenging the assumption that depression is primarily caused by a biological imbalance and suggesting that it may be a 'thought imbalance'.

When a clinician who understands behaviour, following a cognitive-behavioural model, is presented with a child who smears faeces on the wall, he or she will ask: what is he thinking? What is he feeling? What does he think he will achieve? The formulation that may ensue will not be 'He has a conduct disorder' (medical) or 'He has come to learn that this is how he gets attention' (behavioural), it will be a formulation focusing on beliefs and emotions, something like 'He believes he is a naughty boy and spreading faeces is what naughty boys do'.

The limitations of this model, particularly as it applies to children, are that, very often, we are unable to access the beliefs and emotions linked to a particular behaviour because we are often not aware of them. Thoughts and explanations are often only provided after the behaviour has taken place. A six-year-old child who has smeared faeces on the wall of the house and is asked why or what he was thinking, is very likely to respond 'I don't know' or to make up a post-hoc explanation on the spot to satisfy the questioner.

The Psychological (Psychodynamic) Model

The turn of the previous century saw doctors contributing to the development of a psychology of the mind. Alienists and neurologists such as Freud, whilst still assuming the biological nature of psychiatric pathology, developed a series of concepts and metaphors to describe and interpret the phenomena they observed in their patients. They postulated that most of the psychological processes underpinning behaviour are unconscious in nature, and they developed methods to observe and modify these processes.

The psychodynamic tradition has developed many useful concepts that have been influential in mental health, such as transference, countertransference, projection and conversion, many of which are used by non-professionals (defence mechanisms, denial or rationalisation). It contributed to the creation of some pathological categories such as conversion disorder, but its methodology relies on interpretivist approaches and subjectivity, making it quite incompatible with the positivistic and experimental culture adopted by the rest of psychology.

The psychodynamic model understands behaviour as the product of unconscious psychological processes that the individual is seldom aware of, but that exist before, and give rise to, thoughts and feelings. Psychodynamic psychologists conceptualised and described how these unconscious processes worked and proposed techniques, i.e. psychotherapy, to influence these processes in order to benefit the individual.

In order to construct a formulation, psychotherapists will closely observe behaviour, their own emotional responses and the responses by the patient to the therapist's interpretation and infer the unconscious drivers of the behaviour that needs formulating. Psychodynamic psychology comes in many formats. Some of the practitioners have extensive training and require very intensive, very long-term contact before they can have a formulation. Attributing unconscious motives to the behaviour of others is very common practice amongst professionals and lay people, particularly when we work with children. A child may ask for a glass of water at night-time, say and believe that he is thirsty, but the parents understand that the driver is really a wish for contact and the avoidance of separation from his parents.

A clinician using a psychodynamic model for formulation may meet the child who spreads faeces on the wall and who says he does it because he is a naughty boy. After observing him closely, seeing his drawings of his family, in which his new-born twin sisters are omitted, with an abundance of violent imagery, and coming to realise that his own response to the child is that of caution and worry, the clinician may offer the formulation that, although the child is not aware of it, he is furious with his parents for having twin siblings and spreading faeces on the wall is an expression of this anger. The explanation for the behaviour does not lie in the biology of his brain, the rewards or his thoughts, it lies in unconscious feelings of rejection and jealousy that are too painful for his conscious mind to accept.

Although the psychodynamic model offers formulations that often appear very helpful, the limitations of the psychodynamic model are significant. The understanding of the conceptual framework that this psychology requires is difficult and requires in-depth training, as does the skill required to closely observe behaviour and one's own emotional responses. However, the most significant issue is its methodological basis. Subjective interpretations may feel insightful and offer meaningful explanations, but they may be wrong and potentially unhelpful or even harmful. As they do not conform to the experimental positivistic and empirical prevailing model of psychology, they are impossible to falsify, and there is very little acceptable population-based evidence available that can justify its use in a health system that describes itself as 'evidence based'.

Many professionals in CAMHS train and use this model for their practice. Variations of the psychodynamic model inform the work of psychotherapists, counsellors and art and play therapists.

The Systemic Model

We have discussed a biological and three psychological models for the understanding of behaviour. The last existing model in mental health services is neither biological nor psychological. Its conceptual framework stems from engineering, cybernetics, the study of the relations between elements of complex connected systems, for example, control mechanisms for heating or the computers in a computer network.

The principles of cybernetics were adapted to the study of relations in families in the 1960s. The main premise is that the individual is the wrong unit of study when trying to understand behaviour. If we want to understand someone's behaviour we need to understand what that behaviour means to the people around them and how it affects the relationships of that individual. Behaviour is seen as a communication between at least two individuals and to be always reciprocal. This means that if we are trying to make a causal attribution for a behaviour, we need to understand circular or reciprocal causality. A teenager may say 'I don't listen to you mum, because you are always moaning', meaning: your behaviour (moaning) causes mine (ignoring). His mother may say: 'Son, I have to moan because you never listen', meaning: your behaviour (ignoring) causes mine (moaning).

A systemic approach to understanding this behaviour would not focus on the behaviour of individuals, their biology or their psychological processes, but on the nature of the relationship and the communication between mother and son. One behaviour does not cause the other, the causality is circular. We do not need a meaningful story that explains the behaviour, i.e. formulation, we need to understand what the behaviour means to mother and son within the context of their relationship. We need to understand the story the son tells and the story the mother tells and the wider context in which both of them interpret and draw meaning in their relationship.

When a clinician who understands behaviour following a systemic model is presented with a child who smears faeces on the wall, he or she will insist on seeing the whole family, then ask: what does this behaviour mean to each of you? Or less complex questions to that end. The formulation may be something along the lines of:

> It seems that since the twins were born, there has been a lot of stress in the family and everybody is struggling to find their new place and have their own needs met and this little boy is trying to help you hold him in mind while you come to terms with your new situation.

There are three important limitations of the systemic model. First, neither families nor clinicians are used to framing understanding of behaviour as a relationship. The 'problem' is usually thought of as belonging to a child or a parent. Clinicians are reluctant to invite the whole family in order to make sense of 'someone's problem'. Families often feel blamed when the whole family is invited to discuss the problems of a child that they see as having a problem. They often struggle to come to appointments as a family.

The second limitation is that in order to understand systems, we need to be aware of as many relationships as possible. The meaning of behaviour can be understood in the relationship between the members of the family, but often the context for a behaviour includes many more relationships within wider support networks and institutions, i.e. schools, care services and even CAMHS itself. Cultural, religious, ethnic and economic contexts are often very relevant to the understanding of the meaning of behaviour. This level of complexity will often make formulations difficult to understand and communicate efficiently.

The third limitation relates to the previous models and the influence they have on clinicians. All those models, especially the biological model, construct formulations that try to home in on 'the cause' of the behaviour. The systemic model does not focus on 'the cause' but on 'all the relationships'. This is a hard shift for most clinicians accustomed to following the lineal causality of biological models.

In multidisciplinary teams, it is family therapists who tend to use the systemic model to make sense of clinical presentations. Social workers and other clinicians used to seeing behaviour in context may use the model, often unaware of its provenance (See Table 32.1).

The Shapes of Formulations

We have seen how formulations are meaningful explanations for behaviours of clinical presentations. We have seen how what is meaningful and what is an explanation vary depending on

Table 32.1 Examples of Explanatory Models

Examples of Explanations and Questions in Different Explanatory Models	
Biological	Something has happened to his brain (encephalitis, epilepsy, autism…). We need to do a CT Scan, EEG, look for family history of brain problems.
Behavioural	He has learned to do this. How did this start? What is the family doing that is rewarding this behaviour?
Cognitive	He thinks this behaviour will achieve something. What does he believe he will achieve by doing this? What made him think that?
Psychodynamic	He is acting out emotions he does not understand. What are his real feelings? What are his fantasies about this behaviour?
Systemic	This behaviour serves a purpose for this family. What does it mean to this family that he does that? What problem does it solve?

the model that is used to make sense of the behaviour and that causality is a shifting concept depending on the model, sometimes mechanistic (biological or cognitive), sometimes only implied (bio-psycho-social) and sometimes avoided (systemic).

Multidisciplinary teams often work with parallel formulations for the same clinical presentation, based on different models in their construction. The flexibility of teams and individual clinicians to be able to incorporate insights from all models to inform management plans and the formulation that is fed back to the family is one of the strengths of well-functioning multidisciplinary teams. This is achieved by respect for different models and the use of certain conventions that facilitate communication between clinicians. One such convention is the presentation of formulations following a model initially postulated by cognitive psychologists often referred to as the '5 Ps'.

The '5 Ps' structure shapes the narrative that will meaningfully explain the presentation in three acts. First, it establishes what the problem, or the presentation to be explained, is. It assumes that this problem was precipitated by an exacerbation of issues that were there before the problem appeared and predisposed the individual to the problem. Second, it examines how the problem is maintained by examining what is likely to perpetuate the problem and what is protective to the point that it may improve the problem. The Ps in the 5 Ps stand for problem, predisposition, precipitation, perpetuating and protective.

The 5 Ps model offers a structure for a narrative that explains the nature of a problem. It is particularly suited to problems that follow the development of a disorder. Depression and schizophrenia are two disorders that often follow this structure. The structure does have its limitations. Problems where there is a neurodevelopmental problem, or even the so-called personality disorders, require some finessing to fit this structure. A child with autism or ADHD is not predisposed to having a disorder. It is not precipitated.

Each of the models described above, except for the systemic model, can produce a narrative, and generally these narratives are helpful. The 5 Ps structure is particularly suited to the bio-psycho-social model because each of the Ps offers a category in which to organise the 'factors' associated with the problem without having to make explicit direct causal attributions. This enables us to include explanatory elements in the story that are meaningful to a non-biological model, as if they were linked to an underlying biological condition. We may cite the birth of the twin siblings as a precipitating factor for a soiling disorder. The link to this behaviour is a causal attribution that implies unconscious jealousy in a psychodynamic model. Yet, in a bio-psycho-social model we can classify it as 'predisposing factor' to a conduct disorder, without

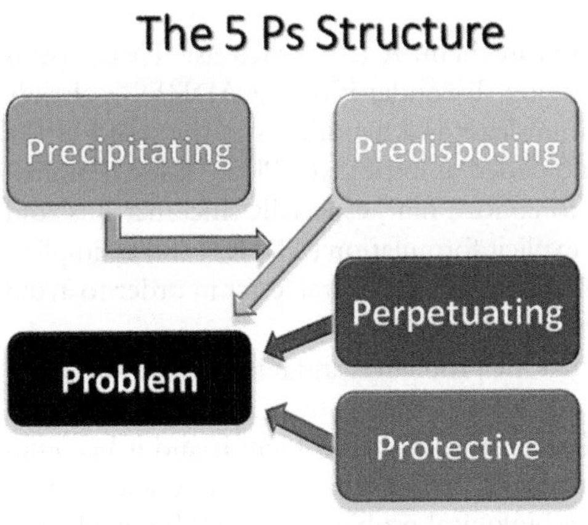

Figure 32.1 The 5 Ps structure for a formulation.

having to explain what exactly happens to the brain of a toddler when he is jealous, that triggers a psychiatric disorder (See Figure 32.1).

The bio-psycho-social model, where factors are organised along a 5 Ps structure and are subclassified into biological, social or psychological factors, has become the de-facto form for formulating presentations in psychiatry to the point where the grid is referred to as 'the formulation'. It is expected that, at the end of a presentation of a case, the clinician will offer a grid where each row will consist of one of the Ps and each column will consist of 'factors' divided into biological, social or psychological.

The advantages of the 5 Ps and the bio-psycho-social approach to formulation are that clinicians are encouraged to think beyond biological explanations even when the presentation is conceptualised as a biological problem. It is simple and understood by all, even by those who are not aware of the different models for conceptualising causal attribution of behaviour. The limitations are that it allows for factors to be included without a clear causal link or a sophisticated understanding of what the problem is. Living with three children under five is a social factor for depression in a depressed mother. It is right that this is thought about when constructing a formulation. The problem may not be so much depression in the mother as neglect from the father. Three children under five as a social factor may 'explain' depression beyond neurotransmitters, but miss what is essentially a social-relational problem.

Another limitation of that approach is that factors are rarely biological, social or psychological by themselves. It is the causal attribution that makes them so. If we think high IQ is a 'factor' in an eating disorder presentation, we may spend a considerable amount of energy deciding whether this is a psychological because IQ is a psychological construct, biological because it is largely determined by biology or social because IQ determines the quality of social interactions that underpin an eating disorder. We may be under the impression that we are using this energy to understand the presentation when we are only classifying a factor in a box.

Formulation in a Mental Health Assessment

Clinicians often understand formulation as the final product of the assessment process. We conduct an assessment and this allows us to understand what the problem is, what caused it and how to manage the case so that health is restored. Whilst this is true, it is important to understand that formulation is present at the start and is always fluid. There is a formulation before the referral is made, and the formulation at the end of the assessment may change once treatment is begun.

All referral letters contain at least a formulation in them. A letter such as: 'Please assess Tommy, he presents with hyperactivity and aggression. I wonder if he has ADHD' is already telling us what the problem is and what causes it, at least as a hypothesis in the mind of the referrer. Sometimes the formulation is implicit and coded as a subtext: 'Please assess Tommy. His mother says he is hyperactive, she struggles to control him, especially since her husband left the family. He may have ADHD'. There is an explicit formulation (ADHD) and an implicit one (mother not coping). It is important to identify these in the referral letter in order to avoid conducting an assessment that is organised by these formulations.

Often the family presents with a fixed idea of what the problem is and it is difficult to explore or assess aspects of the formulation that may point towards alternatives. Different members of the family may present with their own formulation of what the problem is and it becomes even more difficult to explore or conduct an assessment. The mother may be convinced that the child that she struggles to control must have a biological problem like ADHD, whilst the father may be convinced that his child's problems are caused by his mother's poor behaviour management skills. The child may attribute his difficulties to bullying at school and the school to parental discord. Constructing a formulation that incorporates all these narratives may be difficult and not satisfy anybody.

It is important to understand that the process of assessment is always guided by the formulations we have considered before the assessment even starts. Existing formulations and the clinician's own preferred models to explain behaviour will determine what the clinician and the family consider important and that therefore deserves curiosity. An example would be narrow, disorder-oriented assessments common in CAMHS, where the information gathered, the training of the professional conducting the assessment and the expected outcome are narrowed to a yes/no answer, e.g. 'ADHD assessments' or 'autism assessments' are set up in order to rule out or in one, and only one, explanation for the difficulties the child is experiencing. The outcome is not a formulation, but a narrow diagnosis.

Understanding that formulations exist before assessments, and that they change as information is gathered, allows clinicians the flexibility to think beyond what is presented at the start of the referral. Being able to understand the models underpinning the causal attributions that make the narrative in a formulation enables them to hypothesise and maintain curiosity about alternative explanations. This allows the clinician to stay curious about a wider range of important aspects of the presentation and to provide richer and more useful formulations that will eventually lead to better management plans. Formulations are essential to referrals, assessments, diagnosis and management plans. They are central to the activity of mental health professionals.

33 Child and Adolescent Mental Health Assessment

Margaret J.J. Thompson, Cathy Laver-Bradbury and Chris Gale

This chapter covers the principles behind a comprehensive assessment in CAMHS. It is then broken down into three sections to outline age-specific considerations:

- Assessment in the pre-school years
- Assessment in children aged 5–12
- Assessment in young people (12–18)

It should be read in conjunction with the chapter 'Making Sense of Behaviour', which focusses on the importance of formulation. This chapter focusses on how to conduct an assessment and the considerations needed in order to gain the information for a formulation to be made. There are many different ways to conduct an interview, but the primary skills involved are listening, curiosity and kindness – this is the start of a therapeutic encounter.

Principles of Assessment

A comprehensive assessment should lead to the CAMHS practitioner developing a working formulation about why the child/young person and family are experiencing difficulties, based on a careful history taking and drawing information from the widest possible range of sources, e.g. school/college or social services. This forms the basis of the intervention options available to the child/young person and their family, that may be offered by a specialist mental health service or other agency, if appropriate.

The initial assessment is considered to be an important opportunity to engage with the child/young person and family, if ongoing work is planned (Goodman and Scott, 1997). Assessments can vary in length, and it is not uncommon for them to take place over more than one session before a clear idea of the issues can be formulated. During the course of ongoing work new issues may emerge, making continuous reassessment a necessity.

For part of the assessment, consideration should be given to interviewing the child or young person without family members present, depending on age. Providing separate spaces for the young person and carers to discuss their perspectives on the referral issue can be a rich source of information and provide an insight into the family system. Any additional information gained from other sources, i.e. pre-school, school or college, should only be sought with the child/young person and/or carer's permission.

An example of a comprehensive assessment guide used at a local CAMHS level is given in the appendix. It provides a framework that practitioners can use with children/young people and their carers. The framework for a general assessment can differ from those employed at the start of intervention work, as the practitioner's approach will be governed by their professional background, clinical experience and the suggested modality as an outcome of the initial assessment. Treatment or issue-specific outcome measures can be employed to monitor the progress of work with a child/young person and their carers. It is important that all modalities are carefully considered in the initial assessment.

It is useful to have background information available about the child and if any interventions have already been tried with the family and how successful these have been. It is crucial to understand what the parent and young person understand about the difficulties and what they think will help, especially if these are in contrast to the clinicians' understanding. This will affect how the family view any treatment options offered. Knowing whether a treatment has already been tried and not seen as successful helps clinicians, the young person and their parents to make informed decisions about the difficulties and possible interventions.

Assessment of the Child/Young Person

The basis of any general assessment is to assess the mental state of the young person. A modified mental state examination is undertaken with children. This includes the following:

- Mood, affect and anxiety
- Behaviour and appearance/self-care
- Appetite
- Sleep
- Energy and motivation
- Speech
- Cognition
- Attention and concentration
- Perception and thought disturbances
- Self-harm or suicidal intent
- Obsessions, compulsions and rituals
- Insight orientation and judgement

The assessment needs to consider both the chronological age of the child/young person and the developmental age, as these may differ.

Observation of the Child/Young Person

- Are they physically well, appropriate height and weight?
- Subjectively, do they look happy or sad?
- What kind of temperament does the child/young person have? Active/passive? Emotionally labile or easy?
- What is the child/young person's concentration level? Attention? Speech and language? Comprehension? Use of gesture? Vocabulary? Pronunciation?
- Can the child/young person cope with frustration?
- Do they appear impulsive, can they inhibit their own behaviour?
- Can they distinguish reality from fantasy?
- Assess the child/young person's motor movement. Are they clumsy? Do they fall over or bump into objects?
- Do they have good fine motor control?

- Play skills for younger children: what is their ability to engage in symbolic, creative, constructional or physical play?
- Is play at the appropriate developmental level?
- Can the child persevere at play?
- How does the child/young person interact with parents, sibling/s, staff, peer group and other children/young people?
- What is their ability to follow rules?
- Can they wait, turn take, accept losing?
- How do they handle criticism and praise?
- Are they able to separate from their parent in a way appropriate for their age?
- Can they listen and follow instructions?
- Are they able to change activity?
- Is there eye contact between the parent and child? Is this spontaneous? Does the child look at the staff?
- Does the child/young person have the skills to negotiate with the parents, siblings, peers and other adults and does it work?

Individual Interview of Child/Young Person

Interviewing children and young people takes time and patience. Unlike adults, who usually understand that, when they go to see a health professional, they need to focus on a problem quickly, children and young people need time to feel reasonably relaxed before they discuss any worries they have. It is helpful if the focus initially is not on the referral problem, but on what makes them who they are, e.g. activities they enjoy, music they like, games they like playing, who plays with them, their favourite food, films. Once a child or young person is more relaxed the clinician can enter into questions about why they think they are seeing you, who is worried about them and why. It is important to use language relevant to the age of the child or young person, use aids, e.g. games, drawing material, question sheets.

Once the child seems more relaxed and reassured that you are here to help them, more direct questions can be asked:

- What is their view of the problem?
- How does this affect them on a day to day basis? Is it every day? Or are there days when it is okay?
- Does it affect their appetite?
- Does it affect their sleep?
- How are their peer relationships?

School

- Do they enjoy school? What is their favourite subject?
- How do they think they are doing in school? i.e. academic success
- How does he/she interact with teacher(s)?

Family Relationships (A Family Tree Might Be Helpful)

- Parents, carers, including both natural and stepparents
- Grandparents
- Siblings

The Child/Young Person's Mood and Motivation for Change

- Is this child/young person anxious?
- Is this child/young person depressed? What makes them happy or sad?
- Do they have ideas of what they can do to make them feel better?
- Have they anyone to talk to if they are sad?
- What is their capacity to reflect on their thoughts and actions?
- Do they take responsibility for change?
- Do they hope that things will be different?
- If they think things could be different, what will need to happen?
- What is the child/young person's motivation for involvement in any treatment plan?
- Does the child/young person think that their parent/s want things to be different?

Observation of Parent–Child Relationship

A useful schema for assessment of a parent–child relationship. Most interventions in the younger age group, and arguably in the older age group, involve the parents directly or indirectly, so it is important to consider the parent(s) attributions.

Aspects to Consider

- How long have the parent/s, biological, stepparent or adoptive parents, been with the child?
- How do they view the problem that the young person is presenting with?
- Their confidence in their own parenting skills.
- Their ability to set limits.
- Their consistency of approach and attitude.

The General Attitude of the Parent

- Are they warm to the child/young person or hostile?
- Does the parent 'cue' into the child/young person?
- Is the parent 'child-centred', i.e. aware of the child/young person?
- How does the parent gain co-operation? Are they coercive?
- Does the parent understand the developmental stage of the child/young person and interact or play appropriately?
- How would you describe the parent/s' affect and emotional health?

Resilience

In every assessment, consideration should be given to the resilience of the child/young person and their family. Many children, young people and families we work with have experienced considerable adversity and yet still manage to do well. It is worth noting the resilience of the child/young person and family when considering the care plan.

The following items were used in the International Resilience Project as a checklist for perceptions of resilience in children and young people:

- The child/young person has someone who loves them unconditionally.
- The child/young person has an older person outside the home with whom they can talk about problems and feelings.
- The child/young person is praised for doing things on their own.

- The child/young person can count on their family being there when needed.
- The child/young person knows someone they want to be like.
- The child/young person believes things will turn out all right.
- The child/young person does endearing things that make people like them.
- The child/young person believes in a power greater than seen.
- The child/young person is willing to try out new ideas.
- The child/young person likes to achieve in what they do.
- The child/young person feels that what they do makes a difference in how things turn out.
- The child/young person likes themselves.
- The child/young person can focus on a task and stay with it.
- The child/young person has a sense of humour.
- The child/young person makes plans.

Source: International Resilience Project

Strengths

The aim of an assessment is to gain an understanding of a difficulty and provide an explanation of why it is occurring. Assessment should highlight the strengths of the child/young person and their family. This is key to supporting them in managing their difficulties and in their family supporting them. Most behaviour change happens by encouraging the strengths of the individual and the family.

Care Plans

Each assessment should end with a formulation and a care plan that is agreed with the parent and child/young person. The care plan should include the following:

- Current aim of the care plan
- Intervention strategies documented
- Measurable goals
- When the progress towards goals is to be reviewed
- Patient and family views documented
- Copy sent to parent/young person
- Consent to treat obtained

Assessing the Child under Five

Additional considerations for this age group are:

Presenting Behaviour

- It always important to hear a description from the parents of their child's behaviour, in their own words, with a precise outline of this behaviour, i.e. type, triggers, outcome, consequences and severity.
- Ask about 'A day in the life of' their child. This is a useful way to gain insight about the problems faced on a daily basis and how the parent handles them. Are there routines and boundaries?
- As the parent describes the difficulties and the pleasures, you can obtain a sense of the parent's view of the child as outlined in the above discussion about the parental attitudes.

- There is a research tool called Expressed Emotion. The way the parent describes the child will give you a good idea of whether the parent views the child mainly positively, but is concerned, or is negative about the child and wants you to 'sort their child out'.
- This can lead to a discussion about the parent's attributions about the cause of the problems, i.e. is it their fault? the child's fault? the school's fault? and his/her schema about how the problem might have arisen.
- Include a discussion with the parents about why and when they think the behaviour happens. This is important as it will affect how receptive the parents are to treatment options. Different parents might have different ideas of the cause and the treatment needed. Further exploration may be necessary to see if they could agree a joint approach to support their child. It is important to find out how it affects their child and them and how they manage it.

A family tree can be useful but needs careful consideration as it can evoke painful memories. Permission from the parents is important when choosing how to illustrate findings, e.g. if a family member has died, ask parents how they would like this to be represented on the family tree. The tree can enable the assessor with the parent and child, if appropriate, to gain an understanding of the family and to ask about the health, both physical and mental, of siblings and other family members.

It can help to identify important relationships between family members and, with permission, is an opportunity to ask about relationships between parents and families of origin. The exploration of parental childhood memories provides an opportunity to explore how supportive the extended family is. It can be used to ask about different marital partners and any stepchildren and who has the care of the children during the week and weekends.

NB. If there is concern about a child with learning difficulties, ask about three generations of a family tree to establish any inherited conditions.

Case Study (1): Matthew

Mathew (four) is an only child. He is a very busy boy, up early in the morning and finding it difficult to settle to play, unless someone is with him. If either parent sits with him, he can play nicely for ten minutes, although he has to be encouraged to continue. He will run off, climb and put himself into dangerous situations, although he is rarely hurt. He can be stubborn about having his own way, e.g. if he is asked to stop what he is doing, he will have a temper tantrum and stamp his feet. If his mother becomes cross, he can cry for about ten minutes. If his mother remembers just to walk away, he will usually calm down.

At playgroup, Matthew rushes around, flitting from toy to toy. He hates sharing and will be cross if he does not have his own way or someone takes a toy he wants. His parents are puzzled as to why he behaves as he does, and his mother, in particular, is exhausted with him.

Ask parent(s)about:

- Pregnancy: health, illness and use of medication, history of alcohol, smoking and any other substance abuse.
- Birth history: gestation, was the labour natural or induced? Length, delivery type, Apgar scores, i.e. a measurement of the well-being of the baby at birth.
- Neonatal history: health of baby, neonatal unit or not, mother's feelings after the birth. Was he a cuddly baby or not?
- First year: health of baby and mother, including mother's mental state and how she feels she coped.
- Take a feeding and sleeping history.

Matthew was born after a normal pregnancy and delivery. He was well after the birth. His mother was delighted with her new baby. He was a poor settler and sleeper and fussy over feeding. He weaned with difficulty. As a result, the first year was difficult, but his mother was well-supported by her health visitor and by her own mother.

Child's development: include physical progress and speech development. Matthew's development was normal and he talked and walked at the right time. He is a cuddly child. He is beginning to say 'sorry' when he does something his parents do not like. He is beginning to 'read' his mother's mood, and he is sometimes able to stop what he is doing, when he is naughty.

Child's medical history: include history of fits, heart problems, hearing difficulties and accident history. Apart from the usual coughs and colds, Matthew has been a fit child with no illness. He has never had an accident.

Pre-school and school history: separation skills, behaviour and peer relationships, language and negotiating skills. At playgroup, Matthew rushes around. If a helper sits with him, she can keep him to task for about five minutes, then he wants to try something new. He hates sharing and will be cross if another child wants his toy. He cannot negotiate for what he wants.

Family history: include physical and mental health, important family life events past, present and future. Ask about the parents' own childhood and whether, in their opinion, it had been positive for them. This indicates the kind of parenting the parent himself/herself had. This would contribute to self-esteem and parenting skills. Ask about how the parents themselves fared at school.

Both parents work. Matthew's mother is a secretary and his father is an electrician. Both parents had good childhoods. Mother was the middle one of three children. Father was the eldest of four. Both sets of grandparents are helpful. Father was distractible at school and still finds it difficult to sit still. He 'channel-hops constantly with the TV buttons'. One of his nephews has since been diagnosed with ADHD. No other medical or psychiatry history of note.

Observation of the Child under Five

The child should be observed playing in the room and interacting with his parents. Observe the level of interaction. Does the child relate easily to the parents or is there some hesitation? Do the mother and father relate warmly to the child, appropriate for age and circumstance (novelty situation, strangers present, tiredness and hunger)? Do they use language appropriate to the child, and are their expectations of his behaviour within normal limits?

It is useful to have a schema for playing with the children that can used in the same sequence, so as to cover all the domains. If necessary, this can be varied if a child is very oppositional and compromise is called for. Language can be tested throughout, checking for, e.g. comprehension for vocabulary, level of sentence complexity and ability to follow commands.

For example, begin with bricks (colours, co-ordination); Lego with figures (fine motor control, imagination); cup saucer, spoon, plate and figures (imagination and can involve parents in tea party); drawing (fine motor control, shapes, draw a man, developmental level); floor jigsaw (fun, perseverance, shapes, colours, name objects).

Ask the parent to work on a jigsaw puzzle with the child. This should be appropriate to the child's ability, e.g. a big floor one for a younger child. This will enable you to assess the parent–child relationship:

- Does the parent encourage the child or take over?
- Is there good eye contact?
- Does she/he use specific praise?

- Does she/he use language to extend the play and make it fun?
- Does she/he have a method to do the jigsaw puzzle, so the child learns how to do it?
- Is she/he patient or does she become cross?
- Can she/he encourage to child to finish and not abandon it?

For older children, age-appropriate resources should be provided, e.g. drawing materials, jigsaws, action figures, Lego.

Observe the following and check that behaviour is appropriate to age and culture.

Behaviour

- Level of play. Include imaginative play, (both initiated by child and by observer).
- Language, use of language and comprehension.
- Interaction with observer and with parent.
- Eye contact.
- Concentration.
- Attention.
- Are they distractible, can they be brought back to task?
- Are they defiant?
- If they do not want to do something, can they be helped to do it or not?

Physical Development

- What is their hand co-ordination like? Are they right- or left-handed?
- Do they have good motor control? Can they hop, go up and down stairs, walk on tip toe?

Physical Examination

- Some clinics may want to make a physical examination. This would be particularly important before starting a child on medication for ADHD, i.e. to check blood pressure, pulse rate, height and weight.

Both parents related warmly to Mathew, giving reassurance and cuddles when appropriate. When Mathew was cross with the observer, who was playing with him, she was able to monitor the situation and managed to distract him back to task. Matthew was not good at listening and had poor eye contact, although he could be encouraged to look, when asked. He found it difficult to wait and was soon impatient. He could be kept to task, if encouraged, and his language skills were good. He could be encouraged to finish the jigsaw. He was imaginative in his play.

At the end of the assessment, the assessor will share her observations with the parents and a plan will be made as to the interventions, if any, that might be offered.

With the parents' permission, an additional assessment at nursery may take place, to obtain a view of Mathew in a different setting and to ask the nursery leaders their view of Mathew.

If the parents agree, it is useful that the parents are not told when the assessor is going in, so they do not warn Mathew, who may behave differently if he thinks someone he knows is going to be watching him.

Assessing the Child of 5–11 Years

Additional considerations for this age group are:

The most common conditions presenting in this age group are neurodevelopmental disorders, anxiety and developmental trauma or post-traumatic disorders. Any assessment undertaken in this age group should include screening tools (e.g. RCADs (2012), SNAP (1992), Conors (2016) or SDQ (2012) for the most recent versions) appropriate to the presenting difficulties and general information about how they are managing in school, in addition to a comprehensive early years history, as outlined above. Children presenting in this age group may struggle to articulate the difficulties they are having, and a considerable amount of information is acquired from the parents or guardian of the child. Screening measures can be useful to assess how the family is functioning.

With most neurodevelopmental disorders, seek the opinions of the child's wider network (e.g. teachers, after-school clubs, relatives), so that a variety of views are sought about what is contributing to the child's problems.

Engagement in this age group can vary depending on the developmental age of the child. Their understanding and reporting of problems can be variable, hence the need for information from a variety of sources. Given the opportunity, the child can indicate through play, drawings or in their behaviour what is worrying them or leading to a particular behaviour.

Children with both specific learning difficulties (e.g. dyslexia, dyscalculia, dysgraphia) and more general learning difficulties can present in this age group as they struggle to keep up with their peer group and become increasingly frustrated or disruptive in the classroom. Teachers may ask the parents to seek an assessment for the child, believing them to have underlying mental health difficulties. If a clinician is concerned about a discrepancy between the child's developmental and chronological abilities, then a cognitive assessment can be helpful.

Schools do assess children's progress as they go through school. The first request, if the clinician suspects such a discrepancy, should be to the school or the educational psychologist working with the school. If this is inconclusive, further assessment may be useful. Learning difficulties can be missed so this forms an important part of the assessment.

If the child has been exposed to violence or abuse, it may take them a while to trust the clinician and consistency in clinicians can be important, as they learn to trust adults to protect them. In this age group, it is possible that they may disclose abuse, in which case Child Protection policies must be followed.

Assessing the Young Person of 11–18 Years

Additional considerations for this age group are:

Consideration should be given to an interview separate from the parents/carers, especially in adolescence, where young people are encouraged to assume greater responsibility and autonomy in meeting their mental health needs. Separate interviews can be useful where there is a potentially high level of expressed emotion between the young person and other family members. Key areas that should be explored with a young person are outlined below, with the consideration of the individual's stage of adolescence:

- Has the young person been able to form appropriate attachment relationships with peers and, for older adolescents, boyfriend/girlfriends whilst becoming more independent from their parents/carers?
- How do they engage online and with social media? This can provide an insight into how often they engage with peers face-to-face, compared with online communication and in addition, to issues related to bullying.
- How does the young person identify in terms of gender and sexual orientation? In the UK, young people are growing up in a culture where the questioning of both is becoming

increasingly accepted, although LGBTQ+ young people can still experience significant harassment and discrimination. The contextual sensitivity of the clinician around this question is crucial, particularly in the initial assessment session or if family members are present.
- Is the young person sexually active? Again, the contextual judgement of the clinician as to the appropriateness of this question is important.
- Does the young person smoke, use alcohol or drugs? How does this impact on their life?
- What aspirations does the young person have for the future beyond school/college? This can be helpful in assessing hope/hopelessness in the young person and inform the level of risk they may present.
- Has the young person engaged in self-harming behaviours, had thoughts about ending their life and acted on these thoughts in any way?
- What is their motivation for things to change and for engagement in future work?

As with younger children, older children and young people are mainly referred to CAMHS in the light of concerns expressed by the adults in their life, e.g. parents, carers, school/college, social worker. They will need to assume responsibility for their own engagement in therapeutic work. A lack of motivation does not preclude an intervention being offered, particularly when the young person is presenting with significant mental health difficulties, e.g. an eating disorder or psychosis or engaging in self-harm and/or suicidal behaviours.

Key References

Goodman, R., Scott, S., (1997). *Child Psychiatry.* Oxford: Blackwell Science.
International Resilience Project. https://resilienceresearch.org/internationalresilienceproject/.

34 Genograms

Christine M. Hooper

Introduction

Genograms used during assessment can find out who is in the family and their relationships. They are a powerful tool for a clinician to use, and so care is needed when using them; if family members have died, asking how they would like this person indicated on the chart is respectful.

What Can We Learn from This Family Tree?

- Family trees should, whenever possible, illustrate at least three generations of the family. Children often enjoy helping out with drawing up the family tree and sometimes like to add in their friends and pets!
- We see here that Adrian and Jane were married and had two children, Paul (now 31) and Nina (now 28). Paul was married to Sue, but they are now divorced. They have three children, twin boys Joe and Jack (12) and a daughter, Paige (10).
- Nina is in a same-sex relationship with Kate, who at 42 is several years older than she is. They have a daughter, Thea (four).
- Adrian died young, aged only 51. Jane has since had a relationship with Kevin, a younger man, but he is no longer living with her.
- There is a pattern of early parenthood in this family.

Presenting Problem

Paul and Sue's three children have lived with their mother since their parents' divorce. Joe's behaviour has recently been out of control at school, and he has been aggressive at home towards his mother and his younger sister. The family GP has referred the family to CAMHS. Sue has come with the three children. Paul has told her he will come another time if he is asked to.

Possible Assessment Questions

- When did Joe's behaviour first begin to be so difficult to manage? What is their understanding of why the behaviour has occurred? What has been tried so far? Who has been helpful: family, friends, neighbours or professionals?
- How much did the children know about the potential for their parents to divorce? Was it a complete shock? What do they think went wrong? Have they taken 'sides'? How would they describe the relationship between their parents? Friendly, civil or hostile?

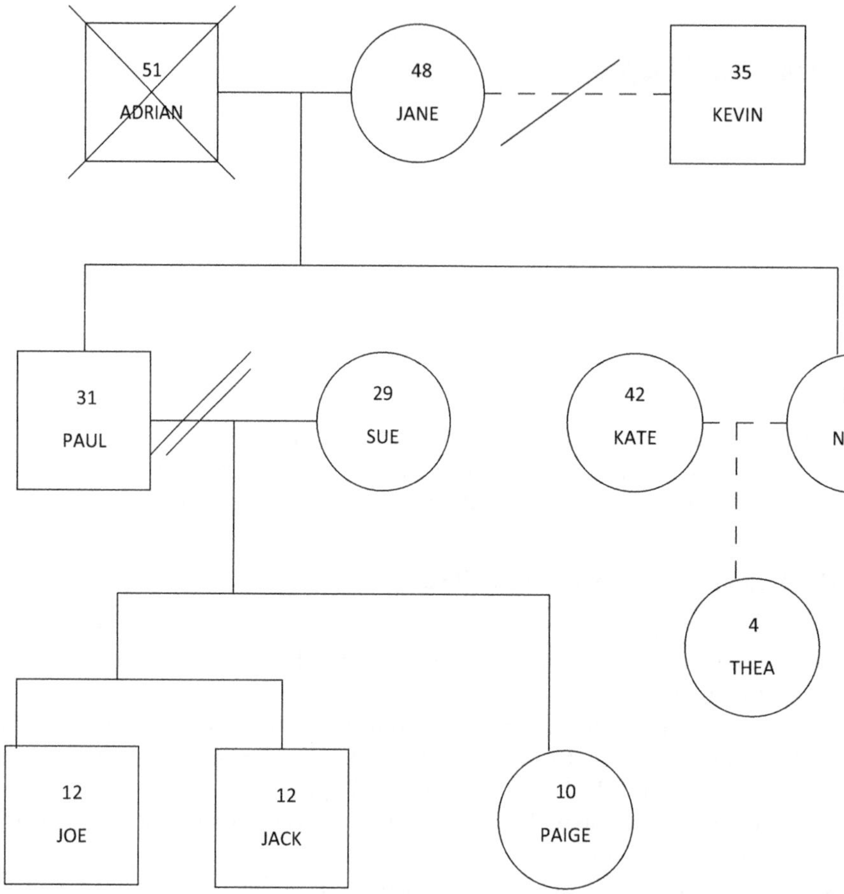

Figure 34.1 Illustration of a family tree (genogram).

- How often do Joe, Jack and Paige see their father since the divorce? How consistent is he about contact?
- How prepared were the children for the death of their grandfather? Was that a surprise? And sudden? Or had he been ill for some time? What would grandfather be saying to Joe if he were still alive?
- Had Adrian and Jane been involved in child care when Sue was at work? What part did Kevin play in their lives? How long was he around? How did Jane manage her life after Adrian died?
- How much contact is there with Nina, Kate and Thea? What was the family's reaction generally towards their same-sex relationship?
- What is Joe's attitude towards his behaviour? Regret? Remorse? Defiance?
- How much support has Sue's family been able to offer? (The maternal extended family can be added into the diagram.)

As questions are answered, further questions to clarify and understand what is being said will occur and the picture around the family will emerge.

Outcome

Looked at in this family context, it is obvious that Joe and his siblings have suffered several disruptions in their life, losing their grandfather, their father's day-to-day presence and, for Joe and Jack, their primary school. It seems that their grandmother was depressed after Adrian's death, which was very sudden, and withdrew her usual child care support. Sue still had to work, and the children were left under-supervised after school and in the holidays.

Joe felt lost and abandoned. Sue has two brothers who have offered to take more interest in Joe and Jack, to be male role models for them. Paul has agreed to come to the next appointment, an important message for Joe.

35 Family Assessment

Andrew O'Toole and Anne Brewster

Introduction

For family therapists, there is an overlap between assessment and intervention. 'The therapist's joining changes things in the family' (Minuchin and Fishman, 1981, p. 149). As part of the assessment session, the therapist introduces families to the service and talks about their hopes and expectations for attendance. It takes enormous courage to attend, and this might be the only time the family comes to an appointment. Blocks may include shame, the fear of being judged or of being seen as 'damaged' or 'ill', especially for people from minority groups.

Beginnings that stimulate interaction are desirable (Burnham, 1986). Burnham suggests looking at everyone and at no-one. Using an open, friendly approach, family therapists are curious about how people introduce themselves, who sits where, who takes charge, who does not speak. In 'warming the context', they might first engage the family in non-threatening areas of conversation within an atmosphere of purposeful interest. Haley (1973) describes this as the social stage.

KEY CONCEPTS

- How does this family work? Use a genogram to look at aspects of closeness and conflicts. Demographics over three generations looking at life cycle transitions, family strengths and vulnerabilities and patterns (e.g. dyadic and triadic). What are the family stories, myths, rituals, rules for living? How does the sibling subsystem relate to the parent subsystem?
- How does the problem or issue that has brought the family to therapy relate to the way the family is?
- How has the family affected the problem or issue? How has the problem or issue affected the family?
- What relationship changes are needed to improve the problem or issue?
- What resources does the family have to make these changes happen?

From Rivett and Street (2009, p. 132)

Developing a secure base and building an effective working alliance are essential ingredients for assessment. The family therapist aims to establish a collaborative partnership with shared, but different, expertise. The family members are experts on their history, and the family therapist is an expert on what has worked with other families and the up-to-date evidence base for difficulties.

What qualities do family therapists possess? Transparency, a respectful curiosity, sincerity and straightforwardness. Children and adolescents are the first to notice when there is a mismatch between what is said and the body language.

Each family member is invited to give their opinion on the presenting problem: its nature, frequency, intensity and successful or unsuccessful solutions. Family therapists track and follow the family's narratives and always act from an ethical standpoint.

In working with families, we need to pay attention to issues of power, authority and difference. A useful framework for working with difference is the Social GRRAACCEESS (Burnham). This acronym stands for gender, race, religion, age, ability, class, culture, ethnicity, education, sexuality and spirituality. These are frameworks within which we identify ourselves and are identified by others.

There are three standard assessment formats in family therapy. These are:

- The Circumplex model (Olsen, 2000) which assesses the dimensions of the family's adaptability and cohesion.
- The McMaster model (Ryan et al., 2005) which assesses communication.
- The Bentovim model which assesses problem-solving, behaviour control and affective responsiveness.

The aim is to focus intervention on whichever dimension will be most helpful. Byng-Hall (*Rewriting Family Scripts*, 1995) describes the framing of a family's history as a 'script' that may be acted out repeatedly, improvised or re-written. New situations need new scripts from the tried and tested responses of the past. Parents generally 'replicate the scripts' of their own childhood, if it was happy, and try a 'corrective' script, if it was miserable. Corrective scripts are less easy to devise. There is no blueprint to work from.

The quality of the parental relationship influences the security of the child's attachment. Children observe their parents' relationship as if they are the 'audience' and their parents the 'actors' on stage. This is how they learn the way to respond to their family environment. According to Byng-Hall, a secure family base is 'a family that provides a reliable network of attachment relationships which enables all family members ... to feel sufficiently secure to explore relationships with each other and with others outside the family'. He believed that the therapy situation could itself be a 'secure base' within which the family could explore new scripts.

A family assessment can carefully uncover the scripts that the family are working with, the better to understand their responses to the difficulties.

Case Study (1): Anna and Katie

Anna and Katie are a same-sex couple who have adopted a two-year old boy, Oliver. Both women come from conventional middle-class families where heterosexuality was the norm. Katie's father died when she was young, her mother re-married and has now moved abroad. Anna's parents live locally and, initially, expressed dismay at their daughter's sexuality and disapproval of the couple's decision to adopt. Anna's family script is of two parents of different genders and the belief that a child needs a mother and a father to thrive. Katie's script is of abandonment by her parents; her father 'left' her early in her life and, as soon as she could, her mother left Katie in England and made a new life for herself abroad.

Anna and Katie have had to adapt towards a different script for their family. They have decided that Anna will be 'Mummy' and Katie will be 'Katie', thereby improvising the script to 'fit' their circumstances. In other respects, their parenting style, of gentle correction and consistent rules, is similar to the one Anna observed as a child. Katie appreciates the certainties of Anna's approach to parenting. Her own experience of childhood was more chaotic. In a way, Anna is re-scripting Katie's experience.

Anna's parents have gradually been 'won over' to an acceptance of the situation, largely because Oliver is their first grandchild and is clearly contented. In addition, they and Anna's brother have attended two family therapy sessions to allow them (from that secure base) to explore their own pre-conceptions of what constitutes a normal family.

Case Study (2): Daniel and Chloe

Re-constituted families are less and less unusual in contemporary Britain. It is estimated that one in five young adult men are bringing up children to whom they are not a natural parent. Step-parenting does not have a recognised script. It does not have legal status unless the step-parent formally adopts the children of their new partner.

Daniel (ten) is Jane's only child. She is a single mother. Chloe (14) is Edward's daughter from his first marriage. Chloe has a brother, William (16). Both children chose to stay with their mother after the divorce, but Chloe has fallen out with her mother and come to live with her father. Daniel and Chloe are often at loggerheads, and the fledgling relationship between Jane and Edward feels threatened.

This family must invent a new script from those they have used before. Jane never lived with Daniel's father and is unused to compromising on parenting issues. She was an only child, and her parents often argued about how to manage her behaviour. She had found being a sole parent and in charge of discipline calmer than her experience of being a child herself. Daniel's father abandoned Jane once she was pregnant. It was several years before Jane felt able to abandon that 'script' and trust herself to live with a man again. Edward and his first wife had a conflicted relationship which upset their two children and means that Chloe is wary around Edward and Jane in case an argument breaks out and her own 'secure base' here is rendered unsafe.

Edward and Jane need to discuss thoroughly, out of earshot of Daniel and Chloe, which rules, rewards and punishments they can agree on. It is especially important that they do not quarrel in front of the children. Daniel has to learn to listen to Edward and not to seek to recruit his mother onto his side. Jane has to support Edward there. Chloe needs to experience a more harmonious parental relationship to restore her security. Jane and Edward must accommodate frequent weekend visits from William, who brings with him the different rules that operate at his mother's. Chloe would like to re-establish a relationship with her mother and to encourage that, Jane has to 'let go' of her feelings about Chloe's sudden arrival into the family and about Edward's first wife, whom she blames for the breakdown of his marriage.

An exploration of what everyone expects from family life would be the core of the family assessment here.

Multiple-Choice Questions

See answers on page 669.

1. How many generations should a genogram attempt to illustrate?
   a. Only the family of the individual with the presenting symptoms.
   b. Four generations, at least.
   c. A comprehensive historical family history covering the last century should be asked for.
   d. Three generations.
2. What is meant by 'joining with the family'?
   a. Sitting next to the oldest member of the family
   b. Making everyone a cup of tea

   c. Asking everyone the same question
   d. Making a home visit
3. What does the McMaster model assess?
   a. How well the family communicate together
   b. The severity of the problem
   c. The quality of parenting
   d. How well the children behave in the session
   e. What has already been tried
4. Who wrote about 'family scripts'?
   a. John Burnham
   b. Minuchin and Fishman
   c. Bentovim
   d. John Byng-Hall
   e. Rivett and Street

References

Burnham, J., (1986). *Family Therapy: First Steps towards a Systemic Approach.* London: Routledge.

Haley, J., (1973). *Uncommon Therapy: Psychiatric Techniques of Milton H Erickson, M. D.* New York: W.W. Norton.

Minuchin, S., Fishman, H.C., (1981). *Family Therapy Techniques.* Harvard, USA: Harvard University Press.

36 Parenting Styles and Family Scripts

Christine M. Hooper

Each family is unique in its unwritten rules, myths and anecdotes. Families are complex systems in the way that each part is dependent on, and influences, every other part. All family members are part of patterns that have derived from their experiences as an individual, their experiences of their own families and being parented, and by society in its expectations of parents. Some patterns can be helpful and others less so. Recognition of patterns is not always comfortable for parents and children.

Parents influence their children in many ways, by encouraging good nutrition, exercise and play and in guiding the child and helping them to socialise so that they can function in society. The beliefs that parents have about child-rearing provide the emotional context in which the child grows. This is known as a parenting style.

Parenting styles vary. This was first described in the 1960s by a psychologist Diane Baumrind, who described three types of parenting style, and later, researchers added a fourth style (Maccoby and Martin, 1983).

The four types of parenting styles:

- **Authoritarian parenting** – this style of parenting focusses on the child being obedient. The child is controlled through discipline and punishments, including the withdrawal of parental affection.
- **Permissive parenting** – this style of parenting offers emotional warmth, but with few boundaries or expectations. The child is generally free to do and act as they will.
- **Authoritative parenting** – this style is a balanced approach where there are some rules and behavioural boundaries, but the child is encouraged to explore and learn things by themselves in order to become independent.
- **Uninvolved parenting** – here the parents are not emotionally involved with their child. They provide the basics of food and shelter but are not interested in helping their child learn about society and how to function within it.

In the 1990s, Darling and Steinberg published a paper about parenting styles and their important effects on the development of children. Research has shown that generally this classification of parenting styles does hold up, albeit with some limitations. Baumrind's (1966) work was largely carried out in the USA with white middle class families. The categories were questioned, as they might not fit across all cultures. In addition, these are described as distinct categories, when most parents might fluctuate between them. It was also thought that the reciprocity of relationships between a parent and child (e.g. the child's effect on the parents and how they parent) was not considered.

Research into parenting styles is problematic and largely based on questionnaire reporting by parents and interpreted by researchers. Ambiguity in questions can lead to misinterpretation. Correlations between parenting and child outcomes can be studied controlling for other factors, i.e. economic status and using statistical methods that can give some indication of causality. Cohort studies of children presenting with problems followed up over time help to provide some of the evidence.

Given the difficulties of research in this topic based on the above types of research, authoritative parenting is thought to have the best outcomes for children. Uninvolved parenting appears to have the worst outcome with young people becoming involved with offending behaviour. Further studies examining the possible cultural differences have indicated differences both in the categorisation (not 'fitting' local parenting styles or that the description does not have an exact replica in a particular culture).

Pinquart and Kauser (2018) conducted a meta-analysis of 428 studies and found authoritative parenting to be associated with one positive outcome in every region of the world and that authoritarian parenting is linked with at least one *negative* child outcome.

Family Scripts

In *Rewriting Family Scripts*, John Byng-Hall (1995) discusses the idea of describing a family's narrative and history as a 'script', that can be acted out, improvised and re-written. He posits that family interactions are scripted over years and that new situations require new scripts. Children observe the adults in the family as if they are the audience, learning the roles as they are acted out from watching their parent-figures 'on stage'. Parents shape their children's behaviour by how they react to it, validating some behaviours and ignoring or punishing others. Families build up shared meanings through repeated rituals, each slightly different from each other (e.g. around mealtimes), 'until a generalized idea is built up'.

Byng-Hall (1995) speaks of 'replicative' scripts that take family experiences and re-enact them in the next generation. When their own experiences have been positive and happy, parents try to replicate them for their own children. When those earlier experiences have been intolerable or unhappy, they try to develop 'corrective' scripts, i.e. constructing a different way of family life and sometimes trying to 'make good' those previous experiences.

A family script belongs to the belief systems and practices that are shared with the extended family, the wider community and the culture. All children need to be sure that care is available at all times. The quality of the parents' relationship influences the security of the child's attachment. Opportunities for corrective scripts occur when adolescents leave home and review their parents' behaviour from a distance or when relationships extend beyond the family of origin and provide a new perspective to the individual's own past, e.g. new partners often ask one another about their childhoods, especially if they are thinking of starting a family.

A secure family base, says Byng-Hall (1995), is 'a family that provides a reliable network of attachment relationships which enables all family members, of whatever age, to feel sufficiently secure to explore relationships with each other and with others outside the family'. Sometimes, he says, the therapy situation can fulfil that need for a secure base from which the family, or individual family members, can feel free to explore new 'scripts' for themselves.

Key References

Baumrind, D., (1966). Effects of authoritative parental control on child behavior. *Child Development*, 37(4): 887–907.

Maccoby, E.E., Martin, J.A., (1983). Socialization in the context of the family: parent-child interaction. In P.H. Mussen (Ed.), *Handbook of Child Psychology* (Vol. 4, pp. 1–101). New York: Wiley.

37 Transition

Cathy Laver-Bradbury

This section has focussed on assessment, its principles and considerations through the age groups. It has stopped at 18 years because of the way CAMHS is currently structured to provide services. There has long been a call to extend the age of CAMHS to 25 years, and indeed some advocate a lifetime service.

Introduction

The definition of transition is both as a noun 'the process or a period of changing from one state or condition to another' and as a verb 'to undergo or cause to undergo a process or period of transition'. The health services structure between child and adult services causes young people to undergo a process of change between services. Whilst children and families face transition throughout childhood, it is the current configuration of health services that appears to cause distress to the young people we work with. The current child–adult split in mental health services has been described as appearing to create weakness in the care pathway where it should be at its most robust (McGorry et al., 2013) and is described as a major 'design flaw' in the current configuration (McGorry et al., 2014).

Reports from service users about the differences in care or commissioning of services between child and adult services has highlighted various difficulties. Young people have reported that they do not feel adequately prepared or supported during the transition period. They feel the loss of familiar service or personnel. They find understanding adult services difficult and do not feel they have a voice during the process of transition. Abrupt and unplanned transition has been likened to 'having to move house due to a flood' rather than as a planned process determined by choice, appropriate advice and informed decision-making (Wilson et al., 2015).

The Delphi study (Suris et al 2015) identified six essential elements of a successful transition programme:

- Assuring good co-ordination, e.g. timing of transfer, communication, follow-up, remaining available during transition between child and adult professionals
- Starting planning transition at an earlier stage, at least one year before the transfer boundary
- Discussion with patient and family about self-management
- Including the young person's views and preferences in transition planning
- If developmentally appropriate, seeing the adolescent alone at least for part of the consultation
- Identifying an adult provider willing to take on the young person before transfer

Studies from the UK and US show that mental health service use declines drastically when young people reach 16 years of age, i.e. by 24% and 45%, respectively, and even more so at the age of 18 years, over 60% in the UK (Potter et al., 2008, Singh et al., 2010).

Young people with severe mental disorders, such as psychosis, are more likely to transition to adult services, but a considerable number of young people with neurodevelopmental disorders or emotional difficulties due to trauma, and including children who have been looked after, have considerable transition difficulties (Singh et al., 2010)

In the UK about 15% of young people with attention deficit hyperactivity disorder (ADHD) make a transition (Ogundele M., Omenaka, 2012), but the figure for Ireland is 7% (Nicolas et al., 2015). In the US there is the additional problem of lack of, or inconsistent, health insurance coverage for ADHD (Montano and Young, 2012). Adult ADHD services are variable throughout the UK in both availability and capacity, and many professionals remain sceptical about the existence of ADHD in adulthood. Education for adult psychiatrists about the evidence for its continuation into adulthood is limited and often only accessed depending on their interest in the topic (Swift et al., 2014).

Looked after young people in the public care system are particularly vulnerable. They are less likely to have family support and often continue to have significant mental health and social problems, including a higher risk of self-harm and suicide. They are more likely to have poorer educational achievement and a greater risk of unemployment, homelessness and incarceration (Office of National Statistics, 2009). The complex mental health needs of care-leavers often remain unmet as the transition services or even support services end when they reach 18 years of age. They often disengage from services, and there is an increase in their use of crisis care, further impacting on any continuity of care.

In order to overcome this, commissioners are now considering extending CAMHS services to 25 years whilst some might argue that having a 0–25 service, as planned in Birmingham, UK (http://forwardthinkingbirmingham.org.uk), shifts the transition boundary to 25 years. The new proposal does provide continuity at the period of maximum risk both of discontinuity of care in early-onset disorders and of the peak incidence of emerging mental disorders. For young people with neurodevelopmental disorders, it continues to provide consistency as they transition from education into the workforce. There is likely to be a significant difference in the demand for adult services between those young people with neurodevelopmental disorders, due to the incidence of those with emerging psychosis.

Several similar models have sprung up in Australia, the UK, Ireland, Singapore and Denmark, with new ones proposed in Canada, the US and Israel, indicating that this is an issue of transition within countries worldwide (Singh et al., 2015). MILESTONE is a European Union (EU)-funded transition project (www.milestone-transitionstudy.eu) that explores the child–adult interface. It has looked at policies, service structure and organisation, and transition-related training in mental health care across Europe. It has identified a large cohort (N = 1000) and tracked the journey of transition-age youth in eight EU countries, reviewing their journey across the transition boundary. They are in the process of disseminating their findings.

Summary

Good transition should be a co-ordinated, purposeful, planned and person-centred process that ensures continuity of care, optimises health, minimises adverse events and ensures that the young person attains his/her maximum potential. It begins with preparing a service-user to leave a child-centred health care setting and ends when that person is received in, and properly engaged with, the adult provider. The service structure should be developed in support of these aims and around the needs of the individual.

Key References

McGorry, P., Bates, T., Birchwood, M., (2013). Designing youth mental health services for the 21st century: examples from Australia, Ireland and the UK. *British Journal of Psychiatry*, 202(Suppl. 54): s30–35.

McGorry, P.D., Goldstone, S.D., Parker, A.G., et al., (2014). Cultures for mental health care of young people: an Australian blueprint for reform. *Lancet Psychiatry*, 1: 559–568.

Wilson, A., Tuffrey, A., McKenzie, C. et al., (2015). After the flood: young people's perspectives on transition. *Lancet Psychiatry*, 2: 376–378.

associated with ... and affect growth. The same ... shown ... in support of these ... to the ... in the ... task.

Key References

[illegible], ..., Friedman, M. (2015). [illegible]

M. [illegible] ... (2016) [illegible]

[illegible]

Part V

Mental Health Issues Presenting in Children and Young People

Margaret J.J. Thompson and Christopher Gale

This section outlines the presentation of mental health difficulties that are referred into CAMHS. We have used either DSM or ICD categories for these chapters, as once the children, young people and parents have been assessed, a decision is made with them as how to progress further.

Using evidence practice where possible, we need to be clear as far as we can about the issues we are working with. Therefore, for these chapters we use a categorical decision-making process using criteria from the relevant coding system.

That is not to say we should not be aware of other factors that will contribute to the possible aetiology of the difficulties and what may maintain them (for example, family issues, temperament of the child, attachment issues). These must be addressed as well. Nor should we ignore the reticence of some CAMHS professionals to diagnose a mental 'disorder' to children and young people who are still developing (formulation is discussed elsewhere in this book).

Part V

Mental Health Issues Presenting in Children and Young People

[illegible]

[illegible]

38 Epidemiology

Summary of *Mental Health of Children and Young People in England* (2017)

Margaret J.J. Thompson

The Mental Health of Children and Young People (MHCYP) survey was previously conducted with 5- to 15-year olds in 1999, and with 5- to 16-year olds in 2004, all of whom were living in Britain and sampled from Child Benefit records. For the 2017 survey, a stratified multistage random probability sample of children was drawn from the NHS Patient Register in October 2016. Children and young people were eligible to take part if they were aged 2 to 19, lived in England and were registered with a GP.

Children, young people and their parents were interviewed face-to-face at home using computer-assisted personal interviewing (CAPI) and computer-assisted self-interviewing (CASI), between January and October 2017. A short paper or online questionnaire was completed by a nominated teacher for children aged 5 to 16 years old. The survey response rate was 52%. Prevalence estimates for 5- to 16-year olds were adjusted slightly upwards with a factor designed to take account of the fact that not everyone of this age group had data from teachers. The statistics for 5- to 19-year olds are official statistics, whilst the data for the 2- to 4-years olds are seen as experimental statistics, as this is a new survey in this age group to enable planning. It might need to be repeated. The survey was funded by NHS Digital and carried out by researchers from National Centre for Social Research: Office of National Statistics and Youth*in*Mind

Summary of Results

- One in eight (12.8%) 5- to 19-year olds had at least one mental health disorder when assessed in 2017.
- Specific mental health disorders were grouped into four broad categories, i.e. emotional, behavioural, hyperactivity and other less common disorders. Emotional disorders were the most prevalent type of disorder experienced by 5- to 19-year olds in 2017 (8.1%).
- Rates of mental health disorders increased with age: 5.5% of 2- to 4-year-old children experienced a mental health disorder, compared with 16.9% of 17- to 19-year olds.
- Caution is needed, however, when comparing rates between age groups due to differences in data collection, for instance, teacher reports were only available for 5- to 16-year olds. Please refer to the Survey Design and Methods Report for full details.
- Data from this survey series reveal a slight increase over time in the prevalence of mental health disorders in 5- to 15-year olds, i.e. the age group covered on all surveys in this series, rising from 9.7% in 1999 and 10.1% in 2004, to 11.2% in 2017.
- Emotional disorders have become more common in 5- to 15-year olds rising from 4.3% in 1999 and 3.9% in 2004 to 5.8% in 2017. All other types of disorder, such as behavioural,

hyperactivity and other less common disorders, have remained similar in prevalence for this age group since 1999.
- One in eight (12.8%) 5- to 19-year olds had at least one mental health disorder when assessed in 2017.
- One in 20 (5.0%) 5- to 19-year olds met the criteria for 2 or more individual mental health disorders at the time of the interview.

Mental health disorders were identified according to the International Classification of Diseases (ICD-10) standardised diagnostic criteria, using the Development and Well-Being Assessment (DAWBA). To count as a disorder, symptoms had to cause significant distress to the child or impair their functioning. All cases were reviewed by clinically trained raters.

Emotional Disorders

- Including anxiety disorders, characterised by fear and worry; depressive disorders, characterised by sadness, loss of interest and energy and low self-esteem; and mania and bipolar affective disorder.
- One in 12 (8.1%) 5- to 19-year olds had an emotional disorder, with rates higher in girls (10.0%) than boys (6.2%). Anxiety disorders (7.2%) were more common than depressive disorders (2.1%).

Behavioural/Conduct Disorders

- A group of disorders characterised by repetitive and persistent patterns of disruptive and violent behaviour in which the rights of others, and social norms or rules, are violated.
- About one in 20 (4.6%) 5- to 19-year olds had a behavioural disorder, with rates higher in boys (5.8%) than girls (3.4%).

Hyperactivity Disorders

- Include disorders characterised by inattention, impulsivity and hyperactivity. The number of children with a hyperactivity disorder, as defined by ICD-10, is likely to be lower than the number of children with ADHD, as defined by the Diagnostic and Statistical Manual of Mental Disorders (DSM-5), as hyperactivity disorders have a more restrictive set of criteria.
- About 1 in 60 (1.6%) 5- to 19-year olds had a hyperactivity disorder, with rates higher in boys (2.6%) than girls (0.6%).

Other Less Common Disorders

- Include autism spectrum disorders (ASD), eating disorders, tic disorders and a number of very low-prevalence conditions.
- About 1 in 50 (2.1%) 5- to 19-year olds were identified with one or more of these other types of disorder, 1.2% with ASD, 0.4% with an eating disorder and 0.8% with tics or another less common disorder.

Seventeen to Nineteen-Year Olds

- Young people aged 17 to 19 were 3 times more likely to have a disorder (16.9%) than pre-school children aged 2 to 4 (5.5%).
- About 1 in 6 (16.9%) 17- to 19-year olds experienced a mental health disorder in 2017. Girls were over twice as likely to have a mental health disorder than boys at this age (23.9% and 10.3% respectively). Emotional disorders were the most common type of disorder, experienced by 14.9% of 17- to 19-year olds. Nearly one in four (22.4%) girls experienced an emotional disorder.
- Around 1 in 16 (6.4%) of 17- to 19-year olds experienced more than one mental health disorder at the same time.

Pre-School Children

The early years are a critical time of rapid development. These experimental statistics are England's first estimates of disorder prevalence in two- to four-year olds, based on high-quality assessments with a national, random sample.

- One in 18 (5.5%) pre-school children were identified with at least one mental health disorder around the time of the interview, boys 6.8% and girls 4.2%.
- Behavioural disorders were evident in 2.5% of pre-school children, consisting mostly of oppositional defiant disorder (1.9%). Autism spectrum disorder (ASD) was identified in 1.4% of two- to four-year olds. Other disorders of specific relevance to this age group were assessed, of which sleeping (1.3%) and feeding (0.8%) disorders were the most common.

Key Reference

Sadler, K., Vizard, T., Ford, T., Marcheselli, F., Pearce, N., Mandalia, D., Davis, J., Brodie, E., Forbes, N., Goodman, A., Goodman, R., McManus, S., (2017). Responsible Statistician: Dan Collinson. *Mental Health of Children and Young People in England.* NHS Digital (accessed January 8th 2020 at https://digital.nhs.uk).

39 Autistic Spectrum Conditions

Jeremy Turk

Introduction

Autism spectrum conditions (ASC), or autistic spectrum disorders (ASD) as they are also known, are neurodevelopmentally determined states of mind described in the tenth revision of the World Health Organization International Classification of Diseases (ICD-10) and the fifth edition of the Diagnostic and Statistical Manual of the American Psychiatric Associations (DSM-5). DSM-5 uses one umbrella term, autism spectrum disorder, while ICD-10 lists several conditions:

- Childhood autism.
- Atypical autism with atypical age of onset, i.e. after three years of age.
- Atypical autism with atypical symptomatology, i.e. absence of autistic tendencies in one or more diagnostic domains, or insufficient symptom numbers, persistence or intensities.
- Asperger syndrome: see below.
- Childhood disintegrative disorder: a rare condition with deterioration in multiple developmental domains including social, language and intellectual, following initial seemingly normal development.
- Pervasive developmental disorder: atypical development in all key psychological domains, but not to the same degree as childhood autism or Asperger syndrome.

It is difficult to distinguish these subcategories, and ICD-11 will adopt a dimensional 'spectrum' approach similar to DSM-5.

Autism spectrum conditions comprise variants in a range of psychological processes:

- Social functioning, understanding and awareness challenges.
- Difficulties with language and communication, verbal and non-verbal, expressive and receptive (comprehension).
- More intellectually able individuals experience difficulties with higher language functions, its social use for mutually beneficial dialogue, its meaning (semantics) and its use and context (pragmatics).
- Repetitive and stereotypical, ritualistic and obsessional behaviours and interests.

  Less intellectually able individuals may present with repetitive behaviours, e.g. hand flapping, rocking, finger and whole body twisting and spinning and rhythmic vocal utterances. These are believed to serve self-stimulatory functions, often known colloquially as 'stimming'.

  More able individuals can present with encyclopaedic knowledge regarding often bizarre topics, for instance, bus numbers and routes, train timetables, mechanical

machinery, astronomy and history, perhaps preoccupied by these to the exclusion of other activities, including social ones. Insistence on routine and sameness of surroundings is common, often with catastrophic emotional and behavioural responses to these being altered.
- Sensory fascinations and aversions, covering the range of sensory modalities, sight, smell, sound, taste, touch and balance. There may be over-preoccupations with bright lights and shiny objects, finger gazing, strong odours, sounds including road drills, emergency vehicle sirens, water hissing in pipes, certain tastes and food textures, oversensitivity to skin sensations, e.g. intolerance of tight or textured clothes or touch or liking being spun round or jumping up and down.
- Imaginary and symbolic challenges, such as a lack of early imaginative and make-believe play, puzzlement over fancy dress and pretending to be another person or creature; may extend to more extreme behaviours, e.g. twirling wheels on a toy car or train rather than pushing it along making suitable sounds.

The above should be present from early life, though ascertainment may occur later.

Additional associations include:

- Anxiety states, frequent and often debilitating
- Phobias
- Sleep and eating disorders
- Tantrums and aggression
- Other psychiatric disorders, including depression, obsessive-compulsive features, tics and Tourette syndrome and, occasionally, catatonia

Individuals may show more 'mainstream' non-autistic social impairments including shyness and social anxiety, social faux pas, misreading social situations, social unease, preference for solitary pursuits and misinterpretations of others' motives and intentions. Gross and fine motor anomalies may occur, for instance, uneasy gait with lack of arm swinging and fine motor challenges up to and including dyspraxia.

Key Points

- ASCs/ASDs are biologically determined neurodevelopmental conditions, not the result of poor parenting, attachment disorder, adverse childhood experiences or unconscious psychological conflicts.
- They are life-long, although individuals can adapt and benefit from their strengths.
- There can be any level of intellectual ability.
- Individuals can present with a wide range of difficulties, each from mild to severe.
- The nature of clinical presentation is influenced by the level and profile of intellectual functioning.
- ASCs/ACDs are not mental illnesses, but individuals are more prone to psychiatric disorders for a range of biological, psychological, educational and social reasons.
- Assessment is complex, involving multi-disciplinary approaches.
- There is a range of treatment approaches.
- Management focusses on improving quality of life and maximising fulfilment of potential.
- There can be strengths, e.g. intensive focus on specific interests, activities or areas of academic study, and lack of distraction by social happenings.

Other developmental challenges are common, both general, for example, intellectual disability and ADHD, and specific, for example, dyslexia, dyscalculia and dyspraxia.

Background

Leo Kanner, a United States professor of psychiatry, published a clinical series of 11 children with 'inborn disorders of affective contact' in 1943. He argued that, just as some children are born with intellectual disabilities, others are born with difficulties socialising, understanding the nature of social interaction and experiencing language and communication challenges, in addition to other features described above, with a wide range of possible intellectual ability.

In 1944 Hans Asperger, working at the University Children's Hospital, Vienna, described the syndrome bearing his name. Individuals are usually of high intellectual ability, male, with normal early language development. They often speak with good, even impressive, vocabularies, and grammar and speech may seem advanced for their years. However, it can appear stilted and pedantic, with poor reciprocity in communication. There are often gross and fine motor co-ordination problems, social interaction difficulties and restricted, stereotyped and often unusual repertoires of interests and activities. The term Asperger syndrome is often used more broadly to describe intellectually gifted individuals on the autism spectrum. The label has fallen into disrepute recently because of a growing awareness of Asperger's associations with Nazism and the eugenics movement.

The concept of an autism spectrum was described in the 1970s by Lorna Wing, a psychiatrist in London, in what she called the 'Triad of Impairments': social understanding and awareness, language and communication challenges and ritualistic/obsessional tendencies.

Impairments in Social Interaction

Children and young people often make poor use of interpersonal social cues, e.g. facial expression, eye gaze, social smiling and gesture. They show lack of awareness of, or unusual responses to, other's feelings and their own. They have difficulty developing relationships and can appear disinterested in peers and adults, or only maintain interaction briefly. They can become more sociable with age, but behaviours often remain socially inappropriate, with little understanding of social cues and rules. They lack the ability to impute independent mental states to others which differ from their own, being unaware that others have their own likes, dislikes, wishes, feelings and emotions. This is known as lacking a theory of mind, or mentalising ability.

Wing identified five social interaction clinical categories:

- **Aloof** individuals neither initiate nor respond to social overtures. They are usually the most intellectually disabled, either passively withdrawn or severely challenging behaviourally, including chaotic and disorganised hyperactivity, aggression, tantrums and self-injury. They are the most difficult to help.
- **Passive** individuals do not initiate social interactions but do respond to social overtures from others. They can seem to engage normally with others, but further observation reveals their reliance on peer group behaviour to interact.
- **Active and odd** individuals both initiate and respond to social interactions and overtures garrulously, but often inappropriately, bombarding conversational partners with one-way conversations regarding their own interests with little understanding or awareness of other people's wishes, interests and needs. Despite often good intellectual capacity, they are often markedly socially naïve, immature, impressionable and hence vulnerable to being

manipulated and taken advantage of by others pretending to be friends, something they yearn for, so-called 'mate crime'.

- **Overpedantic and pseudo mature** 'little professors' may appear to have a maturity which belies their years for instance, saying 'I wish to thank you for the hospitality that you have extended to me today' rather than 'thanks for the cup of juice'. Their pseudo maturity can mask significant learning and social challenges.
- **Relates well but only to one or two individuals.** The person appears fine and average when with a close, trusted and loved adult, e.g. a parent, but things fall apart with others.

Impairments in Language and Communication

Speech and language development is often delayed and atypical. When severe, there may be no speech at all. Speech may be unusual with repetitiveness, use of stereotyped phrases, pronominal reversal, e.g. muddling up use of I/me with you, wrong word order, unusual intonation and vocal expression and one-sidedness in conversation, talking incessantly about one's own interests with little regard for the conversational partner's ones.

Commonly speech is not used in communicative and socially beneficial ways. It can be difficult to keep conversations going unless conversation topics are the child's interests. Non-verbal communication is impaired. Children with autism do not make good use of gesture to communicate, describe objects, influence others' behaviours and to express sympathy.

Children do not point at objects to share interests, though may point to ensure their needs are met. Even with marked speech delay, they can sometimes be taught simple signing or picture exchange communication systems. Eye contact is often limited or unusual, staring too long and hard at others, gazing unfocusedly through people into the distance or avoiding eye contact, looking sparingly out of the corners of the eyes. Play is less spontaneous and less imaginatively varied.

Restricted, Repetitive Patterns of Behaviour and Interests

Young people with autism spectrum conditions can become over-preoccupied with interests which absorb them, e.g. trains, numbers, buildings, car washes, machinery, even unusual objects like toilets, plugs or street signs. Many show repetitive use of objects, e.g. spinning wheels and lining up objects. They may develop rituals and fixed sequences of behaviour. They may have unusual sensory interests that occupy them incessantly, for instance, feeling textures, peering at things from unusual angles and smelling things. They can have problems with changes in routine, disliking taking different routes to places, changes in their clothing or insisting on eating a limited range of foods or only certain types or brands. They may dislike changes around them, e.g. how furniture is arranged. Some develop repetitive motor mannerisms, rocking, hand flapping, finger flicking, jumping up and down or spinning.

Epidemiology

Incidence and prevalence are difficult to determine because of differing diagnostic criteria, differing thresholds of feature severity for a diagnosis and increasing awareness of the conditions and hence, greater enthusiasm to make diagnoses. ASD may sometimes be used as the primary diagnosis instead of, for example, intellectual disability. Kanner speculated a rate of 4–5 per 10,000, though by 2001, rates were estimated as ten times that with figures of 1–2% being quoted now.

There is no evidence for autism spectrum conditions becoming more common but they are ascertained more often. There are no variances within social class or ethnic group. Males are identified more than females with an approximate ratio of 4:1 for childhood autism and 9:1 for Asperger syndrome. Gender ratio is more equal with other neurodevelopmental challenges, including intellectual disability, particularly if severe, cerebral palsy and epilepsy.

Females may be more difficult to diagnose, inflating the perceived uneven gender ratio. Speech articulation can appear more normal thereby masking underlying diagnosis. Girls may compensate for social challenges better, copying peers and assimilating socially.

Aetiology

Autism spectrum conditions are usually genetically determined in complex polygenic fashions. Evidence comes from identical versus non-identical twin studies, sibling risks, family prevalences, sub-diagnostic parental autistic features, i.e. psychological rigidities, anxiety, aloofness, hypersensitivity to criticism and adoption studies. Extended family trees often show evidence of the 'broader phenotype' with individuals displaying ASDs, in addition to sub-diagnostic social and language challenges, obsessionality, sensoriness, non-autistic social impairments and specific learning difficulties. Longitudinal twin studies suggest increasing concordance for autistic features, implying that the influence of genetics on social and communicatory functioning increases rather than decreases with age.

Some single-gene conditions predispose to ASDs, e.g. fragile X syndrome, tuberous sclerosis, untreated phenylketoneuria, neurofibromatosis, Williams syndrome, Angelman syndrome, Turner syndrome, XYY syndrome and, less expectedly, Duchenne muscular dystrophy.

Infectious causes include congenital rubella, herpes encephalopathy and cytomegalovirus. Far from causing autism, MMR immunisation minimises the risk of autism as a consequence of serious brain adversities. The best chances of children growing up without autism are for them to have received comprehensive immunisation programmes.

Toxic causes occur, most often fetal alcohol spectrum disorder with often severe, debilitating and long-term impairments covering a range of psychological abilities.

ASD rates are increased in other neurodevelopmental conditions including intellectual disability, cerebral palsy and epilepsy. The possible significance of perinatal adversities remains unclear. Neurotransmitter, EEG and brain imaging studies have produced equivocal inconsistent findings.

Exceptionally profound neglect and deprivation of sensory stimulation, love, care, affection and nurturing at early highly sensitive developmental phases may cause permanent abnormal central nervous system development, including ASDs.

Assessment

Assessment and diagnosis are complex. There are many diagnostic instruments including:

- Autism Diagnostic Interview (ADI), a detailed, lengthy, semi-structured interview administered to parents or carers by trained professionals, taking around three hours.
- Autism Diagnostic Observation Schedule (ADOS): often complements the above and is equally exhaustive.
- Diagnostic Interview for Social and Communication Disorders (DISCO), a semi-structured questionnaire completed collaboratively by parents/carers and professionals. It takes a clinically orientated dimensional approach, covers the entire intellectual ability range, provides coverage of commonly associated challenges and diagnoses and includes

algorithms allowing ascertainment of a range of diagnoses. It is completed in conjunction with behavioural observations and interactions with the child in both structured and unstructured settings. Supporting information from important sources, such as school, is necessary.
- The computerised 3Di interview is another valid and reliable diagnostic tool.

There are many screening instruments including:

- **Checklist for Autism in Toddlers** (CHAT), designed for GPs and health visitors, a quickly administered questionnaire to screen for autistic traits at very young ages during routine clinic visits.
- **Social Communication Questionnaire** (SCQ), a brief structured list of statements, rated true or false. A score is calculated estimating the likelihood of positive diagnosis.
- **Childhood Autism Screening Tool** (CAST), similar to the above.

Specialist clinics often have assessment protocols, with professionals including clinical and educational psychology, speech and language therapy, paediatrics, psychiatry and occupational therapy. Teacher observations are important as challenges often display at school. It is common for diagnosis to be delayed until junior or even secondary school, the nurturing, structured, supportive and caring infant school environment helping to shield autistic features until social demands increase.

Comprehensive and detailed guidelines for referral and diagnosis have been commissioned by the National Institute for Health and Clinical Excellence (NICE). They help in planning and commissioning evidence-based, cost-effective and clinically useful diagnostic, intervention and support services.

Psychological Challenges

Psychological challenges are common including:

- Generalised intellectual disability.
- Uneven cognitive profile with verbal/non-verbal skill discrepancies.
- Inability to read emotions ('alexithymia').
- Lack of theory of mind and poor mentalising abilities.
- Executive function deficits.
- Poor central coherence, diminished drive towards meaning with piecemeal information processing, being a 'proof-reader' rather than a 'big picture' person. The world can be perceived in fragmented and often incomprehensible and scary ways.

Case Examples

(1) A nine-year-old boy described as a 'loner' and teased by classmates spends break-time in the library looking up obscure details of astronomy. He hates sitting at tables with others, but if a subject interests him, he flaps his hands and rocks excitedly. He is rarely invited to birthday parties. He does not understand jokes. When the headmaster told him to 'pull your socks up' he looked down at his socks, seemed puzzled and then pulled up his socks.

(2) A four-year-old girl in playschool never speaks but screams if other children sit on the chair she regards as hers or approach her when she is playing incessantly with her favourite doll. She never makes eye contact, won't sit on the mat for 'snack time', but puts the teacher's

hand on the tap when she wants a drink. Her favourite playtime activity is spinning herself. She bites teachers if they try to make her wear a coat.

(3) A 14-year-old boy prefers to spend his leisure time at train stations, writing down train numbers in a notebook. He does this alone, rejecting efforts by others to join him. He has hundreds of notebooks, which he keeps in chronological order, and attacks anyone who disturbs them or suggests disposing of them. He knows train timetables off by heart and can recite 'Thomas the Tank Engine' stories from memory. It is impossible to stop him once he has started. He has an uncanny knack of being able to tell you which day of the week you were born on, simply by being told your date of birth.

Management

Aspects of management include

- Information-sharing, education and support for individual, family and others
- Contact with and membership of the National Autistic Society
- Fostering social development
- Enhancing learning and problem-solving
- Tackling information-processing difficulties and challenging behaviours
- Speech and language support, including social use of language, basic sign language (MAKATON) and picture exchange communication systems
- Occupational therapy for fine motor co-ordination, sensory sensitivities and adaptations and aids
- Social and welfare supports, e.g. Disability Living Allowance, autism-friendly supermarket and cinema sessions and support groups for individuals, parents, siblings, teachers and others

Education is often successful in mainstream schools. Social, interpersonal and communication experiences are essential parts of learning and can only be provided in communal education settings, meaning that school is usually better than home tutoring.

Specific educational programmes often use a high degree of structure, predictability and routine, for instance, Treatment and Education of Autistic and related Communication-Handicapped Children (TEACCH). Children can be educated in many different settings, depending on individual needs, ranging from special schools for autistic children and other special schools, to mainstream provision often with extra support and adapted teaching environments and curricula.

Psychotropic medications can in extremis be used in addition to the above to decrease severely challenging behaviours, such as extreme aggression, obsessive-compulsive symptoms, anxiety and ADHD.

Commonly prescribed drugs include:

- Selective serotonin reuptake inhibitors (SSRIs), e.g. fluoxetine, for depression, anxiety including social anxiety, and obsessive-compulsive phenomena
- Psychostimulants, usually methylphenidate or dexamphetamine in immediate- or modified-release preparations for ADHD
- Alpha 2 partial, e.g. clonidine and guanfacine for ADHD, sleep enhancement and as gentle calming agents
- Melatonin, for sleep induction difficulties

- Atypical antipsychotics, e.g. risperidone, quetiapine, olanzapine and aripiprazole for extreme challenging behaviours.

Choice of drug, dose and duration must be determined by specific behavioural goals and must be reviewed regularly by specialist clinicians.

Prognosis

Outcomes vary enormously. Some individuals make exceptional progress, adjusting to their challenges and celebrating their strengths, becoming comfortable with their 'neurodiversity' status differentiating them from 'neurotypicals'. Others, particularly those lacking in insight and often with complex, multiple and marked developmental challenges, may need considerable long-term support.

Positive prognostic indicators include:

- Degree and normality of language development
- Better intellectual functioning
- Minimal severity of challenging behaviours
- Presence of social awareness
- Well-developed concentration span, attentional abilities and mental organisation skills
- Warm, nurturing and structured family life
- Developmentally appropriate, suitably differentiated, focussed and structured schooling
- Progress to date

Children with non-verbal IQ abilities below 50 and with limited language are likely to require life-long high levels of adult support. Children with high IQs and satisfactory verbal skills can make good progress socially and linguistically. Children in between these two extremes may remain dependent on others as adults or may be capable of some degree of independent living. From adolescence onwards, there is increased susceptibility to psychiatric disorders, often depression and anxiety. Emotional limitations and unusual behaviours can result in relationship difficulties and workplace problems.

Being able to exploit a special interest or intellectual 'gift' can facilitate social integration and recognition, although this only applies to a few. The 2009 Autism Act lays out the legally required service provisions across age and ability ranges for individuals with autistic spectrum conditions.

Multiple-Choice Questions

See answers on page 669.

1. Which of the following suggest an autism spectrum condition in a young child?
    a. Lack of pointing to share interests
    b. Hearing voices
    c. Preference for routine/sameness
    d. Poor eye contact
    e. Overactivity, inattentiveness and impulsivity
2. Which of the following DO NOT play roles in causing autism?
    a. Genetics
    b. Fetal alcohol exposure
    c. Poor parenting
    d. Congenital infection
    e. MMR immunisation

3. Reasons ASC are diagnosed more commonly now include:
    a. Increased awareness in girls
    b. Increased prevalence in ethnic minorities
    c. Perinatal hypoxia
    d. Advantage in school to having ASC
    e. ASC diagnosis made in preference to other labels
4. Which of the following are recognised diagnostic tools?
    a. ADI and ADOS
    b. Strengths and Difficulties Questionnaire (SDQ)
    c. 3Di
    d. DISCO
    e. Conner's Questionnaires
5. Which of the following conditions occur commonly with ASD?
    a. Attention deficit hyperactivity disorder
    b. Personality disorder
    c. Hypomania
    d. Intellectual disability
    e. Anxiety

Key References

Attwood, T., (1998). *Asperger's Syndrome: A Guide for Parents and Professionals.* London: Jessica Kingsley Publishers.

Baron-Cohen, S., (2008). *Autism and Asperger Syndrome (The Facts).* Oxford: Oxford University Press.

Howlin, P., (2004). *Autism and Aperger Syndrome: Preparing for Adulthood.* Abingdon: Routledge.

Powell, S., Jordan, R., (2011). *Autism and Learning, A Guide to Good Practice.* London: Routledge.

Wing, L., (2003). *The Autistic Spectrum: a Guide for Parents and Professionals.* London: Robinson.

Sources of Further Information

National Autistic Society—Information, Publications, Conferences, Local Support Groups www.nas.org.uk.

40 Attention Deficit Hyperactivity Disorder

Margaret J.J. Thompson, Anan El Masry, Samuele Cortese and Wai Chen

KEY CONCEPTS

- Attention deficit hyperactivity disorder is a life-long condition.
- Even though it tends currently to be seen as a dimensional condition, there is a clear set of criteria to use for categorical diagnosis.
- It is the most researched condition in child and adolescent mental health.
- ADHD is present is pre-school children.
- ADHD usually presents with co-morbidity.
- Structural and functional changes can be seen in the brains of children with ADHD.
- Neuropsychological differences are present in some, but not all, children with ADHD and are heterogeneous.
- Medication helps at least 70% of the children to reduce the severity of ADHD core symptoms.
- Parenting and behaviour modification techniques should be introduced as treatment and support for the parents, especially for pre-school children.

Attention deficit hyperactivity disorder (ADHD) is a syndrome characterised by age-inappropriate impaired attention and/or hyperactivity and impulsivity to a degree that is maladaptive or inconsistent with the developmental level of the child (Posner et al., 2020). To meet the Diagnostic and Statistical Manual of Mental Disorders (DSM-5) criteria for diagnosis, symptoms should be pervasive across situations, persistent in time and start before the age of 12 years (American Psychiatric Association, 2013). DSM-5 includes three presentations: predominantly inattentive, predominantly hyperactive/impulsive and combined. The world-wide prevalence of ADHD has been estimated as 5.29%; the rates are stable across countries and in the past three decades when the same methods for the diagnosis are used (Polanczyk et al., 2014).

Some British clinics tend to use the stricter International Classification of Disease Version 10 (World Health Organisation, 2018) criteria for hyperkinetic disorder which demands that onset be before the age of seven years, with a set number of symptoms of inattention, overactivity and impulsivity. ICD-11 will include a diagnostic definition for ADHD similar to the one in the DSM-5, even though a prototypical approach (a general description of behaviour rather than an algorithm to define the disorder) has been proposed (Cortese and Rohde, 2019).

As such, it is not surprising that a recent national study (Digitalhealth.gov – Ford et al., 2019) found that the number of children with a hyperactivity disorder, as defined by ICD-10, is likely to be lower than the number of children with ADHD as defined by the DSM-5.

The survey found that about 1 in 60 (1.6%) 5- to 19-year olds had a hyperactivity disorder, with rates higher in boys (2.6%) than girls (0.6%). Girls with primarily an inattentive presentation tend not to be diagnosed until late primary school/adolescence. In pre-school children, behavioural disorders were evident in about 2.5% of the sample, consisting mostly of oppositional defiant disorder (1.9%). Autism spectrum disorder (ASD) was identified in 1.4% of two- to four-year olds. Other disorders of specific relevance to this age group were assessed, of which sleeping (1.3%) and feeding (0.8%) disorders were the most common developmental disorders.

Children with ADHD will have behavioural, emotional, social (resulting in a financial impact on services due to educational and society breakdown) and academic difficulties (Mannuza et al., 1993). The disorder often severely affects family life (Barkley, 2002). These children can be very aggressive. Forty percent of children with ADHD will continue to have problems into adulthood. Some may require referral to adult psychiatrists (Faraone, Biederman and Mick, 2006).

Children with ADHD have an increased likelihood of having other medical conditions. A narrative review found that there was an intriguing, but puzzling, association with adults with ADHD and obesity (Cortese, 2019). Cortese and colleagues carried out a systemic review and a large meta-analysis of Swedish samples and showed a definite association between asthma and ADHD (Cortese et al., 2018).

Aetiology: Current Thinking

Twin studies indicated that monozygous twins were more likely to have ADHD with a hereditary variance of around 60% (Greven et al., 2011).

- Categorical viewpoint with a molecular viewpoint of genetic causation, but although single genes have been implicated, the odds ratios are low.
- Dimensional viewpoint that suggests that the condition is caused by the quantitative extreme of the same genetic factors that are responsible for variation in the normal range, as well as the disorder range, known as quantitative trait loci (QTL) hypothesis (Plomin, Owen and McGuffin 1994; Chen and Taylor, 2006).
- The resulting trait is distributed quantitatively as a continuous dimension rather than qualitatively different as a discrete disorder.
- Gene–gene interaction (epitaxis is important).
- Gene–environment effect on the dimension of hyperactivity in all children, including children at the lower end of the expression.

NB. As only 75% of the variance can be accounted for by the genetic loading, the gene–environment interaction is important (Rutter, 2003).

Several genes may be implicated, but the dopamine and serotonin genes were the most researched (e.g. the DAT 1 – dopamine transporter genes, and the DRD 4 – dopamine receptor gene – Di Maio, 2003; Todd et al., 2005). The odds ratios for any one gene was very low. Gene–environment interaction is an important factor in causing the expression of the gene. To research causative genes, very large sample sizes are needed. Current research with the Genome-Wide Association Study (GWAS) suggests that ADHD will not be caused by a single gene but by a collection of high-risk genes working together (Stergiakouli and Thapar, A., 2010). A recent GWAS study found 12 genes clearly implicated in ADHD. Interestingly, they are not specific to ADHD, but, rather, they underpin the genetic vulnerability to other psychiatric and somatic disorders (Demontis et al., 2019).

The importance of gene–environment interaction is significant. ADHD is associated with low birth weight (Pettersson et al., 2015); toxins and infections in pregnancy, possibly mediated through the genetic profile of the baby (Mill and Petronis, 2008); alcohol in pregnancy (Sood et al., 2001); drug abuse (Wilens et al., 2005); smoking (Kotimaa et al., 2003; Thapar, 2003; Rodriguez and Bohlin, 2005); stress in pregnancy, probably mediated by cholesterol; and exposure to other toxins, e.g. lead after birth. A very useful paper by Thapar et al. (2013) suggests this aetiology might be casual, apart from the genetic input, with the only proven link with ADHD, i.e. changes in the brain, that has been found in young children who have suffered severe deprivation.

Follow-up studies of children from the Romanian orphanages (ERA) have found that children who were adopted from the orphanages after six months living there were more likely to have significant permanent symptoms, with functional magnetic resonance imaging evidence, of ADHD-type or autistic-type problems, than children who were adopted after less than six months in the orphanages (Sonnuga-Barke et al., 2017). Kay et al. (2016) have published similar findings with their study on children brought up in very deprived and neglectful situations in the UK.

The Brains of These Children Are Different

Multiple studies with structural magnetic resonance imaging (MRI) of groups of children with ADHD compared to control groups have documented anatomical differences (e.g. reductions of about 10% in the size of the caudate nucleus, right frontal and cerebellar vermis regions of the brain – Hoogman et al., 2017). A meta-analysis of 14 data sets indicated that the most replicable structural abnormalities are in the basal ganglia (Nakao et al., 2011). The authors suggest that ADHD medication may normalise the structural abnormalities in ADHD. When functional MRI scanning techniques are used, areas of the brain in children with ADHD function differently from the brains of children without ADHD (Hart et al., 2013).

Persistence in Symptoms Will Depend on

ADHD symptoms are more likely to persist if the disorder is severe (Sonuga-Barke et al., 1997 – community sample; Lahey, 2004 – clinical samples), if there is co-morbidity with behaviour problems, if there is neuro-developmental delay and/or neuro-cognitive delay, if the parenting style is hostile and coercive and if schools are unsympathetic.

- Children with ADHD are difficult to parent (Johnston and Mash, 2001).
- Conversely, hostile intrusive parenting with young infants can lead to a child presenting with hyperactivity (Jacobvitz and Sroufe, 1987; Morrell and Murray 2003; Forget-Dubois et al., 2009).
- Non-cooperation and negotiation by the parents will not help a child with ADHD to learn self-regulation (Frick et al., 1992; Reid and Patterson, 1989; Reuben et al., 2016) and may lead to long-term difficulties in a child already predisposed to ADHD (Campbell, 1995; 2006).

And on Co-Morbidity

Children with ADHD have many problems that may present in different ways. By the time they are referred to CAMHS, they may have very complex problems (Aebi et al., 2010). In the Multi-Modal Treatment Study of ADHD (MTA) study (Richters et al., 1995) 11% of the children had tics, 40% had oppositional disorder, 14% had conduct disorder and 34% had anxiety disorder. Children with ADHD may have language disorder and a reading disorder.

Nutrition

Evidence of whether nutrition is associated with ADHD is still equivocal. A trial reported in *The Lancet* suggested that preservatives can cause irritability in all young children (McCann et al., 2007). There may be gene–environment interaction, possibly the histamine gene (Stevenson et al., 2010). One or two rigorous trials do suggest that nutrition may encourage hyperactive symptoms, but this hypothesis is not supported by other studies and meta-analytic evidence (Stevenson et al., 2014).

Neuropsychological Findings

Different pathways are proposed to explain the way children with ADHD might present. Sonuga-Barke (2002) suggested a dual pathway:

- A dorso-lateral-striatal pathway that is associated with executive function difficulties, i.e. problems with planning, set-shifting and organisation (Barkley, DuPaul, McMurray and Murphy, 1990).
- A frontal-ventral striatal pathway that is involved with delay aversion and motivation, i.e. difficulty in waiting (Sonuga-Barke, 2002).
- Sonuga-Barke et al. (2010) propose the addition of a third neuropsychological pathway hypothesised to represent temporal processing deficits (TPD) in ADHD. Indeed, there is some evidence that ADHD children show TPD across a range of timing tasks (Rubia et al., 2003).
- Giedd and colleagues (Giedd et al., 2001) have proposed a cerebellar-prefrontal-striatal network, the cerebellar vermis, to fit with the findings of a smaller cerebellum. The cerebellum is associated with timing, cognition, affect and motor movement.
- The neuropsychology findings in pre-school children (Dalen et al., 2004) are the same as in older children with a similar dual neural pathway model proposed (Solanto et al., 2001).

Is ADHD a Categorical or a Dimensional Condition?

Current literature discusses whether the condition is categorical, i.e. if a child presents with a number of symptoms, will he definitely have the disorder or is it dimensional, i.e. that all children have some attention problems, but it becomes a functional difficulty with a high impact for the child when he has problems in all the domains of ADHD and in all settings. Most professionals would recognise the problems as being dimensional (Coghill and Sonuga-Barke, 2012).

Pre-School Children with ADHD

Parents may contact their GP with concerns about very young children who seem to be overactive, especially if they are non-compliant. By the time the child is referred to CAMHS services, the referred behaviour is usually non-compliant and aggressive, in addition to overactive. The problems are generally present in both school and home.

Symptoms

These will vary depending on any underlying neuropsychological difficulties and possible other co-morbid conditions. It is important that the initial assessment takes place within a developmental framework and observes the child in different settings (Daley et al., 2014).

- Constantly 'on the go'.
- Dashing into obstacles, not watching where they are going. This differs from clumsiness, which can be a sign of dyspraxia, a potential co-morbid finding.
- Attention and concentration problems. This might be less obvious in young children, except perhaps at story time.
- Poor at sharing.
- Difficulty with waiting and turn-taking, wanting to do everything immediately.
- Difficulties with:
    - Negotiation skills
    - Sleep pattern
    - Early language
    - Fine and/or gross motor skills

Current Thinking about Pre-School ADHD

- Prevalence in younger children is the same as that in older children, using an interview Schedule, the Pre-school Age Psychiatric Assessment (PAPA), i.e. between 3 and 6% (Egger and Arnold, 2006).
- Hyperactivity is more common in younger children.
- Inattention is more apparent as the child becomes older (Lahey et al., 2004).
- 50% of these children will still have symptoms at school entry (Campbell and Ewing, 1990; Lavigne et al., 1998).
- Pre-school hyperactivity will not necessarily go away (Barkley et al., 2002; Lahey et al., 2008; Mannuzza et al., 1990).
- This behaviour is different from disruptive behaviour (Sonuga-Barke et al., 1997).

Presentation of Hyperactivity in Young Children Is Important

Children who were originally seen at three years old in 1990 as part of a study of a birth cohort of children in the New Forest, England (The New Forest Development Project; Thompson et al.,, 1996) and at three years in 1994 and 1997, as part of a screening for parenting trials, were followed up with their parents between 14 years and 22 years. The researchers found that pre-school hyperactivity in the three-year olds, specifically, elevated long-term mental health risks more strongly in males than females (Smith et al., 2017). Additionally, pre-school hyperactivity was associated with long-term economic burden (Chorozoglou et al., 2015).

Resulting Problems for Children with Pre-School ADHD

- ADHD is associated with lower pre-academic skills and language problems (Sonuga-Barke et al., 1994).
- Social problems and exclusion from day care (Campbell, 1995).
- Speech and language problems may co-exist, as may problems with reading, writing and arithmetic.

- Many children will have fine and gross motor problems (Lahey et al., 2004).
- Associated behaviour problems are present, commonly oppositional defiant disorder and conduct disorder (Gadow and Nolan, 2002).
- Co-morbid depression and anxiety may be present (Egger et al., 2006).

It may be that it is this co-morbidity that causes most of the parenting difficulties and possibly the persistence of problems (Campbell and Ewing, 1995; Caspi et al., 1990; Woodward et al., 1997). A thorough assessment is necessary, paying special attention to the development of the child, and speech and learning development.

The use of questionnaires can be helpful for assessment and outcome measures. General questionnaires would be Strength and Difficulties, four to six years (Goodman, 1997) or the Conners questionnaire (Conners,1998). Questionnaires that can be used for young children's behaviour are: for hyperactivity, the Routh modification of the Werry–Weiss–Peters rating scale (a score of over 20) (Routh, 1974), and the Emotionality Activity Shyness temperament scale (a score of over 4.5 on the activity subset) (Buss and Plomin, 1986); see Thompson (2001) and the SNAP Questionnaire for hyperactivity and oppositional disorder (Swanson et al., 2012).

In the New Forest Development Project (Thompson et al., 1996; Thompson, 2001), a community project screening a birth cohort of three-year-old children, 11.5% of children were found to be overactive (a score of 20 or more on the Werry–Weiss–Peters (WPP) Scale Routh, 1978) and a score of 4.5 or more on the Emotionality Activity Scale (Buss and Plomin, 1984). About half of the three-year olds were found to have marked problems on further testing. Using only the WWP activity scale, 18% will have a score of 20 or over. This is a useful community screening scale.

Treatment: For Pre-School Children

Parenting advice should be the treatment of first choice (NICE, 2018; Sonuga-Barke et al., 2001; Thompson et al., 2009). For this to succeed, the work should be delivered in an organised manner and the parents must be motivated and able to change, with few other problems in their life at the time. Parents who have ADHD themselves may cope less well (Sonuga-Barke et al., 2003).

Medication is effective (PATS) (Greenhill et al., 2006) but with increased side-effects in young children of which the most common were decreased appetite, emotional outbursts, difficulty falling asleep and weight loss (Wigal et al., 2006). Medication should be titrated slowly, and smaller doses used than those for older children.

Case Study (1): James

James (four) has been referred to the young child clinic by his health visitor. James seldom sits still to play, despite his mother's best efforts to encourage him. Pre-school staff have noticed the same behaviour at nursery and say that James has difficulty in sharing toys, becoming aggressive towards other boys at times. Management advice from both the health visitor and the nursery nurse has so far made no difference.

Following a careful assessment, the staff in the clinic thought that James was exhibiting signs and symptoms of pre-school ADHD.

James's mother was offered the New Forest Parenting Programme (Weeks, Laver-Bradbury and Thompson, 1997; Sonuga-Barke et al., 2001; Thompson et al., 2009), and she thought that the programme made a difference to James's behaviour. He settled well into his reception class.

ADHD in School-Age Children and Adolescents

ADHD is a common childhood disorder that has been estimated to affect 3 to 5% of school-age children (Busch, 2002).

In School

The primary school child with ADHD is frequently seen as being different. A sensitive teacher may be able to adapt the classroom to allow an able child with ADHD to succeed, but more often the child experiences academic failure, rejection by peers and low self-esteem (Landgraf et al., 1999). A negative relationship between ADHD and educational achievement has been observed in both clinical and population samples (Polderman et al., 2010). Children who displayed more ADHD symptoms, as rated by their mother at the same time or five years earlier, scored lower on an educational achievement test. Comparing the different components of ADHD, inattentiveness and hyperactivity suggests variation in the magnitude of the association with educational achievement. Inattentiveness is to a much greater extent related to educational under-achievement than hyperactivity (Eveline de Zeeuw et al., 2017).

One explanation might be that a relatively stable pattern of inattentive symptoms is often seen in children with ADHD compared with a decline of hyperactivity symptoms with increasing age (Biederman et al., 2000). Another explanation is that the time children spent doing their schoolwork is related to their educational achievement and having poor attention skills makes it more difficult for them to focus on classroom activities (Duncan et al., 2007). In addition, inattentive symptoms might hamper students in developing basic skills in the early grades that are often needed to learn higher level skills (Breslau et al., 2009).

Parents should inform the school if their child has been diagnosed with, and is receiving treatment for, ADHD. If a child enters school and is experiencing difficulties that lead parents or the school to suspect he or she may be suffering with ADHD, then parents should ask the school to evaluate their child. A child may qualify for special education services once he has been diagnosed with ADHD. The school should assess the child's strengths and weaknesses and design an Individualised Educational Programme (IEP) or their school equivalent. Ideally, this should be re-evaluated at each new school and stage of learning.

Within the Family

ADHD within a family has profound effects. Parents have little time for themselves and family relationships may become extremely strained and, in some cases, break down, bringing additional social and financial difficulties. This may make the child feel sad or, even, show oppositional behaviour (Harpin, 2005). The siblings of children with ADHD report being victimised by aggressive acts of physical violence, verbal aggression, manipulation and control. Siblings reported that parents expected them to care for their ADHD sibling because of the social and emotional immaturity associated with ADHD (Kendall, 1999).

Conversely, family-level factors may contribute to more positive outcomes in ADHD. There is evidence for the promotive effects of positive parenting for young people diagnosed with ADHD and for family cohesion and support for promoting positive outcomes for adolescents with ADHD. Specific positive parenting mechanisms are critical during the early years and family cohesion/support may be especially relevant during adolescence. It seems likely that positive parenting and family cohesion foster a sense of attachment and commitment to parental values that help young people avoid risky situations and behaviour, e.g. substance use and delinquency.

For adolescents with ADHD or ADHD symptoms, positive parenting can be an important source of social support and social modelling, leading to reduced problems in their interactions with peers and teachers. This assertion is consistent with the studies in their review that found that parental support and authoritative parenting promote higher levels of social competence for young people with ADHD (Dvorsky et al., 2016).

Emotional Understanding, Reactivity and Regulation in Children and Adolescents with ADHD

Emotional competence predicts later socioemotional functioning (Blandon et al., 2010; Denham et al., 2012), and emotional competence deficits place children at risk for psychopathology (Steinberg and Drabick, 2015). Emotional problems in ADHD consist of a broad array of deficits in emotional functioning, including poor emotion regulation, excessive emotional expression, low frustration tolerance, reduced arousal to emotional stimuli and anomalous allocation of attention to emotional stimuli (Bunford, 2015; Serrano et al., 2018). Such emotional symptoms are common in children with ADHD. In the United States, approximately 30% of children with ADHD were reported to have co-occurring emotional and behavioural difficulties and impairments in daily functioning (Strine et al., 2006). In Europe, studies have shown that children and adolescents with ADHD symptoms exhibit increased emotional problems, i.e., excessive worry, depressed mood, heightened nervousness in new situations, increased fears and/or somatic symptoms, compared with children without ADHD (Becker et al., 2006; Coghill et al., 2006). Previous reports have highlighted the association between increased emotional lability, i.e. rapid, exaggerated changes in mood, and ADHD symptom severity, particularly in children and adolescents with more hyperactivity/impulsivity symptoms and co-morbid psychopathology (Sobanski et al., 2010).

Specific Issues for ADHD in Adolescence

ADHD is the most common emotional, cognitive and behavioural disorder treated in teenagers. Though previously thought to remit in adolescence, a growing literature supports the persistence of the disorder and/or associated impairments into adulthood in a majority of cases (Kesler at al., 2005).

ADHD is a major public health problem because of its associated morbidity and disability in children, adolescents and adults. Children with the disorder are at greater risk for longer-term negative outcomes, e.g. lower educational and employment attainment.

As children with ADHD grow older, the way the disorder impacts upon them and their families changes. The core difficulties in executive function seen in ADHD result in a different picture in later life, depending on the demands put on them by their environment, including school and family. This is affected by the insight and cognitive abilities of the child or young person (Harpin, 2005).

Adolescence may bring about a reduction in overactivity, but inattention and inner restlessness remain major problems (Spencer et al., 2007). Young people with ADHD are at an increased risk of academic failure, dropping out of school or college, teenage pregnancy and criminal behaviour (Harpin, 2005). When children enter high school, they have less adult supervision, multiple teachers, an increased volume of homework and more complex assignments. Early academic problems may be amplified by the increased demands that are placed on children in high school (Barbaresi, 2007).

Driving poses an additional risk. Individuals with ADHD are easily distracted when driving slowly, but when driving fast they may be dangerous (Barkley et al., 1996; Woodward et al., 2008).

What to Remember about ADHD in Adolescence

- In adolescents there is a decline in hyperactivity/impulsivity.
- Inattentive symptoms persist into adulthood.
- Associated with school failure, emotional difficulties, poor peer relationships and trouble with the law.

Associated Disorders

Autism Spectrum Disorder (ASD)

ASD regularly co-occurs with other psychiatric and neurodevelopmental disorders; upwards of 70% of individuals with ASD meet diagnostic criteria for an additional psychiatric or neurodevelopmental disorder (de Bruin et al., 2007; Simonoff et al., 2008). ADHD is particularly common; 28–60% of individuals meeting criteria for ASD meet the diagnostic criteria for ADHD (Yoshida and Uchiyama, 2004; Simonoff et al., 2008), and subclinical traits associated with these conditions show considerable covariation in the general population (Ronald et al., 2008).

Oppositional Defiant Disorder (ODD) and Conduct Disorder (CD)

ADHD and ODD/CD have been found to co-occur in 30–50% of cases in both epidemiologic and clinical cases.

Mood Disorder

Lifetime rates of co-morbid depression in children with ADHD increased from 29% at age 15 to 45% at a 4-year follow-up. A baseline diagnosis of major depression predicted lower psychosocial functioning, higher rates of hospitalisation and impairments in interpersonal and family functioning (Beiderman et al., 1992).

Recently it has been found that, although childhood ADHD increases the risk for adolescent depression, stimulant treatment for ADHD neither heightens nor protects against such risk (Moncrieff and Timimi, 2013).

It is often difficult to differentiate adolescent onset mania from ADHD, CD, depression and psychotic disorders, because of overlapping developmental features. However, the symptoms of ADHD may precede the first manic episode by many years. The prevalence of mania in children with ADHD was found to increase from 11% to 23% in a four-year follow-up in an American study. Children with ADHD with co-morbid mania had other correlates associated with mania, including additional psychopathology, psychiatric hospitalisation, severely impaired psychosocial functioning and a greater family history of mood disorders (Spencer et al., 2007). In the UK, many of these children might be diagnosed as having dysregulation, rather than mania. Dysregulation often coexists with ADHD (Ryckaert et al., 2018).

Anxiety Disorder

Childhood anxiety disorders are often not suspected in an overactive child, even though some of the behavioural features of anxiety include agitation, tantrums and attention-seeking behaviour. Children with ADHD and co-morbid anxiety disorder need more psychiatric treatment. They tend to have more impaired social functioning and a greater family history of anxiety disorder (Mennin et al., 2000).

Substance Use Disorder (SUD)

Young people with ADHD are at increased risk of cigarette smoking and substance abuse during adolescence. Individuals with ADHD tend to maintain their dependence longer compared with their non-ADHD peers. Treatment for ADHD with stimulant medication decreases the risk of substance use disorders by 50% (Willens et al., 2003). Children diagnosed with ADHD mid-adolescence who were not treated with stimulants had the greatest occurrence of SUD. Studies have shown that 25–33% of adolescents diagnosed with SUD meet the diagnostic criteria for ADHD (Wilens et al., 2004).

Sleep Disorder

Sleep disorder is a major issue for children and adolescents with ADHD. Cortese and colleagues, in a meta-analysis of 16 studies looking at the sleep patterns of children with ADHD against controls, found that children with ADHD were more resistant to going to bed, had more sleep onset difficulties, were more likely to wake during the night and had sleep disordered breathing. They were slow to rouse in the morning and often had daytime sleepiness (Cortese et al., 2013).

Treatment and Assessment Which May Be Helpful with Children with ADHD

- Occupational assessment
- Cognitive assessment for cognitive ability, word processing, working memory assessment, assessment for dyslexia
- Social skills training
- Parenting groups or individual work with parents
- Family work, especially for adolescents where there may be relevant family stress issues and/or hostility towards the child
- Individual work, having first assessed for motivation, and counselling and/or psychoeducation
- Attention training, to help the child cope with delay
- Work with the school/college, e.g. work with reading, mathematics, writing, work study skills

Medication

The MTA study (Richters et al., 1995), the largest randomised control trial ever undertaken for children with ADHD, found that for most children with the disorder, medication alone was successful. However, the authors added important caveats that the medication should be carefully monitored and adjusted, to control symptoms appropriately. The best results came from university clinics, where staff presumably had the special expertise and staffing resources to monitor their families frequently. Behaviour and family work alone, or as an added therapy, did not affect the efficacy but did influence the amount of medication that was necessary. It must be remembered that the behaviour work was beyond what any clinic in the USA or the UK could provide.

Some children with ADHD and co-morbid symptoms of anxiety and depression fared as well with behaviour work alone and possibly better in the long run (Jenson et al., 2007). Interestingly, medicated children in community clinics improved in line with children offered behaviour and family work only, but less well than the children who attended the university clinics (Jensen et al., 2001). Long-term follow-up, when intensive monitoring stopped, caused all the groups to end up on the same trajectory. Those children who did worse were those with the more severe symptoms and co-morbidity. Those who did best were those who were still taking medication and being monitored regularly. In the long-term follow-up, behaviour work was clearly helpful for those young people who had major behaviour problems and/or anxiety and depression (Molina et al., 2009).

During trials lasting between three and seven months, Schachar and Tannock (1993) found that stimulants were more effective at treating the core behavioural symptoms of ADHD than placebos, non-pharmacological treatments or no treatment. In addition, stimulants may improve cognitive performance and help to reduce conduct problems and peer relationship difficulties (Woolraich et al., 1990). ADHD symptoms were less well controlled as medication was adhered to less well without the benefit of the careful monitoring in university clinics.

In the UK, the prescription of stimulant medication is governed by law, and clinical guidelines have been set down by the National Institute for Clinical Excellence (NICE, 2018). These guidelines recommend that medication is helpful for children with ADHD, but stressed the importance of careful assessment, behaviour modification and regular monitoring to achieve optimum results. The message seems to be clear that appropriate children should be treated with the correct medication and that other work should be tailored to the needs of the children and the family. This is important, as assessing and treating children who are on the ADHD spectrum is becoming an increasing burden on CAMHS.

More in-depth assessment of parents, children and families might aid the decision about treatment pathways, i.e. assessing the child and his/her parents' understanding of the condition and the parents' empathy towards their child and the treatment process, and to ascertain parent and child preferences and attributions towards medication. This will include an important discussion of the medication that could be used and the possible side-effects. This will assist both parents and children to 'own' the treatment decisions and encourage compliance. Not all parents wish to use medication and would prefer behavioural work (Tarver et al., 2015). A thorough assessment should take place before medication is started with baseline measurements of height, weight, pulse rate and blood pressure, at a minimum. It is important to take a history of baseline symptoms of stomach aches, headache, bruising and frequent nosebleeds, tics, sleep and eating patterns, as these symptoms may be present as side-effects of medication. A careful history should rule out a child and/or family history of heart disease, fits, tics and glaucoma (see European guidelines: Taylor et al., 2004; Banaschewski et al., 2006). Titration of the medicine dosage is important with regular monitoring of effect and of blood pressure, pulse rate, height, weight and a list of possible side-effects to determine whether to continue the medication, increase the dosage or change to a different preparation, either a long-acting brand or a different brand.

Stimulant Medication

Stimulant medications currently used in the United Kingdom are:

- Methylphenidate (Ritalin): not licensed for use for children under six years of age
- Extended-release SR Ritalin, Concerta, Equasym XL, Medikinet (not licensed for use for children under six years of age)
- Dexamphetamine (Dexedrine): licensed for use for children from three years of age
- Lisdexamfetamine

Non-Stimulant Medication

- Atomoxetine is a selective norepinephrine reuptake inhibitor.

- Guanfacine is an adrenergic alpha receptor agonist originally developed for treating high blood pressure. It works by influencing the receptors in the brain that strengthen working memory and by reducing distractibility and improving attention and impulse control.

Sometimes other medications might be helpful alongside medications for ADHD, e.g.

- Clonidine hydrochloride (Catapres, Dixarit), especially with concomitant tics.
- Risperdal: could be used if the adolescent is exhibiting very aggressive behaviour.
- Fluoxetine (Prozac): if the adolescent is depressed.
- Carbamazepine (Tegretol); sodium valproate for associated mood disorders.

A recent large meta-analysis of trials of medication for ADHD in children, adolescents and adults suggests that for children methylphenidate is the first choice of medication with the best efficacy, tolerability and safety (Cortese et al., 2018).

Other Issues Specific to ADHD in Adolescence

There are several key themes relevant to ADHD transition in adolescence. First, overt hyperactivity and impulsivity may desist to be replaced by a subjective sense of restlessness. It is not uncommon for the presentation of the 'combined' subtype of ADHD to evolve into that of the 'predominantly inattentive' subtype. Second, some patients may present *de novo* in adolescence, because previously their high IQ and/or supportive family structure have protected them from developing significant impairments, despite displaying symptoms in childhood or primary school, whereas the increasing demands in secondary school and adolescence unmask their impairments.

Thirdly, ADHD-related emotional dysregulation may become more prominent, shading into 'adolescence turmoil' or an emerging adolescent affective disorder, when the prevalence of a mood disorder rises sharply. Fourth, the influence of delinquent peers becomes more prominent when parental supervision and control recede, while on-going educational failure or negative schooling experience accelerates the risk of conduct problems. This risk further superimposes upon the transient rise of delinquency in adolescence observed amongst even non-ADHD individuals. Fifth, medication control may become out of control, mirroring the well-documented adolescent brittle diabetes, when rebellion and resentment intensify any non-adherence to medication. Sixth, adolescence is a period of rapid maturity of executive function in non-ADHD adolescents. The development of executive function is delayed amongst ADHD subjects, lagging about three to four years behind their normative peers. The executive function deficit and lag further widen the gulf between ADHD and non-ADHD individuals, accentuating any behavioural and functional deviance.

Finally, the increasing autonomy associated with adolescence entails intensified conflicts with parental and adult authority, in addition to leading to a greater exposure to drugs, alcohol, reckless driving, sexuality and association with delinquent peers. Impulsivity and sensation-seeking traits amplify these risks, resulting in driving offences, crimes, substance misuse and increased rates of teenage pregnancies and contracting sexually transmitted disease and HIV. For some ADHD subjects, adolescence is a time associated with significant hazards presenting major challenges to both parents and clinicians. Specialist care is often indicated.

Case Study (2): Peter

Peter (15) was referred by his GP, as he was experiencing marked difficulties in keeping to task at school. Peter has always found school challenging, especially in keeping to task and concentrating.

When Peter was younger, he found it difficult to sit still in class and required regular prompting from the teachers and teaching assistants. His mother has been able to manage him at home with the help of Peter's father, who is very supportive and firm. Sadly, Peter's father had been recently diagnosed with cancer and he is less able to contribute. Peter's behaviour had undergone major changes, with him becoming increasingly angry, with violent outbursts and defiant behaviour.

Assessment

Peter is an only child with older parents. The pregnancy was normal, and the baby was healthy. He was breast fed for six months, and then his mother began weaning him. He was an easy baby but found it difficult to settle at night. As a toddler, Peter started at nursery, where he enjoyed playing with other children, but he was always the one running around, dancing or knocking things over. Despite this, his nursery teachers felt he was a bright child who learnt to speak clearly and well early on.

At school, although clearly a bright child, Peter would often be restless in class, with constant fidgeting. He answered questions prematurely, interrupting other students. Nevertheless, he received very good support from school, with more intense input from the teaching assistants. Despite his difficulties, he clearly had a good grasp of the subjects taught and performed exceptionally well in mathematics, art and music.

In senior school, Peter's fidgetiness seemed to lessen, although his ability to concentrate for long periods of time in class continued to be a problem. Although his grades had gone down, he was still doing well in his preferred subjects.

Since his father's illness, Peter's concentration in class seemed to have worsened and he appeared less vivacious and lively in the classroom. At home, he would spend hours in his room, playing computer games and not attempting to achieve in his studies, despite regular prompting from his parents. Indeed, their attempts to engage him led to angry and verbally violent outbursts that are out of character for him.

Observation in Clinic

Both parents attended with Peter. They seemed warm and genuinely concerned about him. Peter was sitting quietly most of the time, but he appeared to be fidgeting constantly with his jumper sleeves. He replied clearly and coherently to the questions.

Peter described feeling empty and unable to feel much for the last three months. His sleep, usually poor, continued to be a problem although lately he has started to have an interrupted sleep pattern. Peter described having lost his appetite, which was good before. Peter told us that he felt useless and hopeless about the future and saw no point in trying hard at school, as 'we were all going to die anyway'.

Peter described always having a sense of restlessness, although he feels this has improved with time. He said that he has always found it difficult to concentrate, but as the subjects were generally not too difficult, he could 'get away with' little work. Lately, he has been unable even to do that.

Following consent to contact the school, school staff were able to confirm many of the symptoms that Peter presented with in clinic. A Connor's teacher and parent questionnaire confirmed high scores on inattention and poor concentration.

Initial Formulation

It seemed very possible from the history given that Peter had ADHD, when younger. The hyperactivity symptoms seemed to have waned, but the concentration problems were still an issue. Peter appeared to have managed well at school through the concentrated efforts of supportive schoolteachers, who saw his potential, and through the loving and firm efforts of his parents. Lately, however, there has been a marked shift in Peter's presentation, with symptoms suggestive of a major depressive illness, probably precipitated by his father's diagnosis. It was vital not to interpret all the difficulties facing Peter and indeed, any young person with ADHD, as being due to ADHD and not to consider any other precipitating factors, social, personal or educational, for additional mental health issues.

Management Plan

In this instance, treatment of the depressive illness was the initial step in the management of the symptoms. Anti-depressant medication was prescribed and Peter was referred for counselling to help him deal with the issues arising from his father's illness. Following the improvement of his depressive symptoms, the option of medication for ADHD was discussed with Peter and the family, who declined the offer, as they felt Peter was able to manage better at school now that his mood had improved.

Case Study (3): Tania

Tania (13) attends a local school. She was referred to CAMHS due to her disruptive and defiant behaviour at school and at home. Tania has always had problems listening to instructions and keeping to task.

Assessment

Tania lives with her mother, stepfather and younger brother, aged two.

Her parents separated when Tania was only three years old. She sees her father occasionally at weekends. Tania was born when her mother was only 18 years old. Her mother smoked for at least the first trimester. The pregnancy was uneventful, but the delivery was prolonged and intervention via a ventouse extraction was necessary. Tania required no special care.

Tania was a difficult baby to put to down to sleep and often cried. As a toddler, she continued to have difficulties with her sleep, was constantly having accidents and was very difficult to manage. Tania went to nursery at age three and exhibited an obvious inability to sit still or engage gently with other children. This continued to be a problem when she went to primary school, with the teachers finding her very disruptive in class and very difficult to keep to tasks. At home, she exhibited defiant behaviour.

This pattern of problem behaviour continues. The defiant behaviour has escalated to aggression, both at school and at home. Tania's mother described how she was very similar to Tania as a child, but that, despite this, she found Tania very difficult to manage. She said that she often 'gave up' trying to promote discipline and would often give in to Tania's demands, which upset her husband who was trying to re-enforce the rules

Observation in Clinic

Tania attended with her mother. She interrupted her mother constantly during the interview and would leave her seat regularly to fiddle with different toys and objects in the room. Tania was not keen to be seen on her own, and her mother gave permission for us to contact the school.

The school report showed repeated incidents of disruptive behaviour and difficulty keeping to task. Conner's Parent and Teacher questionnaire revealed high scores on inattention, hyperactivity and oppositional behaviour.

Initial Formulation

The history and presenting symptoms suggest an early onset of behavioural manifestations suggestive of ADHD. There appears to be a family history of ADHD in mother, in addition to the increased risk of developing ADHD, due to maternal smoking.

The social circumstances, relating to parental separation, and the different parenting styles adopted by Tania's mother and stepfather, may have assisted in the emergence of the ODD in recent years.

Management Plan

Tania was started on an extended methylphenidate preparation, to help with her ADHD symptoms. This was regularly monitored, and Tania's height, weight and blood pressure were measured regularly. Appointments with parents to introduce them to parenting strategies were arranged, and they eventually joined a parent ADHD group. Later, the family began family therapy sessions to help improve family systems and dynamics. There was regular contact with the school to promote the understanding of Tania's problems and to assist the teachers in the development of management strategies in the classroom. Tania's mother sought a statement of Special Educational Needs for Tania.

Persistence of ADHD into Adulthood

Before the 1990s, ADHD was considered to be a disorder confined to childhood, undergoing spontaneous remission during the transition to adolescence and adulthood. The seminal longitudinal research studies derived from six major cohorts published in the 1990s showed that ADHD is a lifelong disorder in the majority of patients, persisting into adulthood with social, occupational and psychological impairments. These cohorts, and their representative authors, include those from New York (Gittlelman, Mannuzza), Montreal (Weiss, Hechtman, Milroy), Wisconsin (Barkley, Fletcher), California (Lambert) and East London (Taylor). Their fuller findings were reviewed by Chen and Taylor (2005). In brief, these studies suggested that about 30% of childhood cases underwent spontaneous remission, 30% persisted into adulthood with mild to moderate impairments, whilst the remaining 30% developed severe impairments with additional co-morbidities including substance misuse, depression, anti-social personality disorder and law infraction. Overall, conduct problems, impulsivity, low IQs, external locus of control, i.e. always blaming someone else for one's problems, and more negative self-esteem predicted poorer outcomes.

In contrast to the earlier research, more recent work has focussed on the impact of the definition of adult ADHD on the persistence rates of childhood ADHD. In other words, the thinking has moved away from applying the childhood criteria of ADHD to study the persistence of adult ADHD. Biederman, Mick and Faraone (2000) found persistence rates to vary: at 40%, if defined by childhood syndrome criteria; at 80%, if defined by sub-syndromal presence of ADHD symptoms; and approaching 90%, if defined by functional impairments. A meta-analysis (Faraone, Biederman and Mick 2006) of 32 follow-up studies showed a pooled persistent rate at around 15%, if defined by the full syndromal criteria, but around 65% by the adult ADHD 'partial remission' criteria. Overall, ADHD is now regarded as a non-benign and life-long disorder, rather than a self-limiting one confined to childhood.

Issues Specific to Adult ADHD

Patients may present to an adult ADHD service as a childhood ADHD 'graduate' or as a *de novo* adult referral seeking assessment and treatment for the first time, having come through childhood undiagnosed. Alternatively, some parents of ADHD children self-diagnose as having ADHD and come forward to seek treatment. Amongst these, some have marked disorganisation and poor time-management, leading to poor childcare and child protection concerns. The extreme cases could be involved in court proceedings where the Social Services Department seek to remove their children from their care. A court assessment may present another route of referral.

Recent surveys in prisons show that a significant proportion of male adult inmates have undetected and untreated adult ADHD (Chitsabesan et al., 2006; Young et al., 2011). They may be referred for ADHD treatment via a forensic psychiatry service. Alcohol and substance misuse are common, because of their use as self-medication for primary ADHD symptoms and/or for secondary depression and anxiety arising from chronic ADHD impairments. Some adult patients are misdiagnosed as having a personality disorder or an affective disorder, including a bipolar disorder, because of the symptoms of impulsivity, emotional dysregulation and poor self-control. They may be referred as a long-standing psychiatric patient non-responsive to a series of treatments offered, because of misclassification.

In general, the impairments of adult ADHD are much more pervasive, affecting the functions in self-control, learning, occupation, organisation, time-management, financial management, social and occupational relationships. Adult ADHD is a real, valid and debilitating condition and warrants a well-resourced service that provides both good-quality assessments and comprehensive treatment of all the accompanying disorders.

As in adolescents, behavioural work is helpful either in a group or individually (Ferek et al., 2009). Life coaching is very helpful, in particular, for students.

Medication Use in Adults

Medication is equally useful for adults with ADHD. As in younger people, a careful history has to be taken to exclude other psychiatric syndromes that might account for the symptoms or might make it more complicated to treat, e.g. bipolar disorder and substance abuse should be screened for.

Physical contraindications to medication should be established. Adults should receive ongoing care from their GP as well as from an interested adult psychiatrist.

A recent large meta-analysis of trials of medication for ADHD in children, adolescents and adults suggests that for adults, amphetamines are the first choice of medication with the best efficacy, tolerability and safety (Cortese et al., 2018).

Multiple-Choice Questions

See answers on page 670.

Which is correct?

1. The prevalence of ADHD in the population is:
   a. 5% of the population
   b. 20%

   c. 30%
   d. 15%
   e. 25%
2. Which is correct?
   a. Inattention is the usual finding.
   b. Medication is the treatment of choice for pre-school ADHD.
   c. Pre-school hyperactivity is difficult to diagnose.
   d. Co-morbidity is not common.
   e. The neuropsychology findings are different in pre-schoolers.
3. Which is correct?
   a. A single gene has been identified in children with ADHD.
   b. Tics are rarely found in young children with ADHD.
   c. Behaviour modification should be started as first treatment, even when the symptoms are very severe.
   d. High IQ will make no difference to outcome for children with ADHD.
   e. In young children, the normal co-morbidity with ADHD is oppositional defiant disorder.
4. Which is *not* correct?
   a. ADHD may appear *de novo* in adolescence.
   b. Medication is not effective with adults with ADHD.
   c. Adults with ADHD are very likely to be smokers.
   d. Driving offences occur more often in the population with ADHD.
   e. Adults with ADHD may first present with problems at work.

Key References

Banaschewski, T., et al., (2006). Long-acting medications for the hyperkinetic disorders. A systematic review and European treatment guideline. *European Child & Adolescent Psychiatry*, 15: 476–495.

Belsky, J.A.Y., Hsieh, K.H., Crnic, K., (1998). Mothering, fathering, and infant negativity as antecedents of boys' externalizing problems and inhibition at age 3 years: differential susceptibility to rearing experience? *Development and Psychopathology*, 10(2): 301–319.

Biederman, J., Mick, E., Faraone, S.V., (2000). Age-dependent decline of symptoms of attention deficit hyperactivity disorder: impact of remission definition and symptom type. *American Journal of Psychiatry*, 157(5): 816–818.

Bunford, N., Evans, S.W., Wymbs, F., (2015). AD/HD and emotion dysregulation among children and adolescents. *Clinical Child and Family Psychology Review*, 18: 185–217.

Campbell, S.B., (1995). Behaviour problems in preschool children: a review of recent research. *Journal of Child Psychology and Psychiatry*, 36: 113–149.

Coghill, D., Sonuga-Barke, E.J., (2012). Annual research review: categories versus dimensions in the classification and conceptualisation of child and adolescent mental disorders—implications of recent empirical study. *Journal of Child Psychology and Psychiatry*, 53(5): 469–489.

Daley, D., Jones, K., Hutchings, J., Thompson, M., (2009). Attention deficit hyperactivity disorder in pre-school children: current findings, recommended interventions and future directions. *Child: Care, Health and Development*, 35(6): 754–766.

Daley, D., Van Der Oord, S., Ferrin, M., Cortese, S., Danckaerts, M., Doepfner, M., ... Banaschewski, T., (2018). Practitioner review: current best practice in the use of parent training and other behavioural interventions in the treatment of children and adolescents with attention deficit hyperactivity disorder. *Journal of Child Psychology and Psychiatry*, 59(9): 932–947.

Faraone, S.V., Biederman, J., Mick, E., (2006). The age-dependent decline of attention deficit hyperactivity disorder: a meta-analysis of follow-up studies. *Psychological Medicine*, 36: 159–165.

NICE 2018 guidelines for AD/HD. Available at https://www.nice.org.uk/guidance/NG87 (New Forest Parent Programme cited on page 107 and 123).

Sonuga-Barke, E.J., Brandeis, D., Cortese, S., Daley, D., Ferrin, M., Holtmann, M., ... Dittmann, R.W., (2013). Nonpharmacological interventions for AD/HD: systematic review and meta-analyses of randomized controlled trials of dietary and psychological treatments. *American Journal of Psychiatry*, 170(3): 275–289.

Tarver, J., Daley, D., Thapar, A., Cooper, M., Eyre, O., Langley, K., (2013). Practitioner review: what have we learnt about the causes of AD/HD? *Journal of Child Psychology and Psychiatry*, 54(1): 3–16.

Taylor, E., Dopfner, M., Sergeant, J., Asherson, P., Banaschewski, T., Buitelaar, J., Coghill, D., Danackaerts, M., Rothenberger, A., Sonuga-Barke, E., Steinhausen, H.-S., Zuddas, A., (2004). European guidelines for hyperkinetic disorder-first upgrade European *Child & Adolescent Psychiatry*, 13 Supplement 1: 7–30.

41 Juvenile Disruptive Behaviour Disorders

Oppositional Defiant Disorder (ODD) and Conduct Disorder (CD)

Graeme Fairchild (updated by Lucy Wilford)

Introduction

Oppositional defiant disorder (ODD) and conduct disorder (CD) are together considered as the disruptive behaviour disorders. Children with ODD and CD struggle to respect authority and behave in ways that go against societal rules in ways that disrespect or harm others. These behaviours significantly disrupt family life, schooling and friendships and place these children and young people at high risk of developing later mental health and substance abuse diagnoses.

These disorders often lead children and families to present to multiple professional groups and require long-term interventions. Due to the complexity of the aetiology and presentation of ODD and CD, these diagnoses should be part of a comprehensive assessment and formulation.

This chapter aims to describe the classification and diagnosis of ODD and CD. The prevalence and aetiology of the disorders are presented together with issues of assessment and diagnosis. A brief description of treatment and intervention options is provided.

KEY CONCEPTS

- The behaviours associated with ODD and CD are severe and cause significant distress to children and families, with an increased risk of educational, social and criminal outcomes for young people.
- The aetiology of the disorder is multi-factorial with genetics, temperament, parenting, social stressors and early adverse experiences all contributing.
- Intervention should take into account the complex causes of ODD and CD, with long-term family-based interventions having the best outcomes.

Classification and Diagnosis of Juvenile Disruptive Behaviour Disorders

ODD involves a recurrent pattern of defiant and disobedient behaviour towards parents and other authority figures leading to the impairment of day-to-day activities and is typically viewed as a milder condition than CD.

CD commonly involves behaviours that are pervasive across settings and against the law, e.g. physical assaults, serious theft and violations of societal norms, perhaps pathological lying or serious truancy. Although there is considerable overlap between these conditions, with many children with CD meeting the full criteria for ODD and a proportion of those with ODD fulfilling sub-threshold criteria for CD, evidence from factor analytic studies suggests that these clusters of behaviour are, at least partly, separable.

Developmentally, ODD-type behaviours are more characteristic of younger children, whereas CD occurs more commonly in older children and adolescents (Loeber et al., 2000). Longitudinal studies that have followed children from a young age into adolescence and young adulthood have revealed that many children who fulfil criteria for ODD in childhood do not develop CD at a later stage, whereas almost all of those who meet the criteria for CD previously fulfilled criteria for ODD.

There is considerable overlap between CD, ODD and ADHD, with approximately 50% of those with CD or ODD meeting the diagnostic criteria for ADHD and vice-versa (Kutcher et al., 2004). The ICD-10 includes a specific diagnostic sub-group for this group of children referred to as 'hyperkinetic conduct disorder'. The diagnosis of the disorder should always be part of a wider formulation of the child's difficulties, considering potential diagnostic overlap, particularly of ADHD. The clinician should consider the family situation and parenting styles and should liaise with other agencies, where involved. It is important to receive feedback from the child's school and to consider educational psychology involvement to assess whether there is a concurrent learning disability or specific learning needs.

CD/ODD Diagnostic Criteria According to the WHO ICD-10

There are two classification systems for these disorders, the DSM-5 (American Psychiatric Association, 2013) and the ICD-10 (World Health Organization, 1996). Both of these systems are relatively similar in terms of emphasising the persistent duration of the behaviours with a categorical approach to describing the presence of these disorders. They differ in that DSM-5 considers ODD and CD as separate conditions, whereas the ICD-10 symptom criteria are similar to the combined criteria for both the DSM-5 CD and ODD disorders. The revised DSM-5 criteria differ from DSM-4 in placing a greater emphasis on mood, impulse control and irritability and classifies the disorders under 'Disruptive, impulse control and conduct disorders'. According to the WHO ICD-10, to be classified as having either CD or ODD, the following criteria need to be met:

- A repetitive and persistent pattern of behaviour, in which either the basic rights of others or age-appropriate societal norms or rules are violated.
- This pattern of behaviour must be present for at least six months, during which some of the following symptoms are present (individual sub-categories for rules or numbers of symptoms; WHO ICD-10 1993).
- Symptoms 11, 13, 15, 16, 20, 21 and 23 need only to have occurred once for the criterion to be fulfilled (See Table 41.1).

Specification of Possible Sub-Divisions

Conduct disorder can be further categorised into the following subgroups: CD confined to the family context, unsocialised CD and socialised CD.

For **conduct disorder** confined to the **family context** the following criteria must be met:

- The diagnostic criteria for conduct disorder must be met.
- Three or more of the symptoms listed for conduct disorder must be present, with a least three from items 9–23.

Table 41.1 Table of Individual Symptoms

No.	*Symptom Description*
1	Has unusually frequent or severe temper tantrums for his or her developmental level
2	Often argues with adults
3	Often actively refuses adults' requests or defies rules
4	Often, apparently deliberately, does things that annoy other people
5	Often blames others for his or her own mistakes or misbehaviour
6	Is often 'touchy' or easily annoyed by others
7	Is often angry or resentful
8	Is often spiteful or vindictive
9	Often lies or breaks promises to obtain goods or favours or to avoid obligations
10	Frequently initiates physical fights. This does not include fights with siblings
11	Has used a weapon that can cause serious physical harm to others, e.g. bat, brick, broken bottle, knife, gun
12	Often stays out after dark despite parental prohibition, beginning before 13 years of age
13	Exhibits physical cruelty to other people, e.g. ties up, cuts or burns a victim
14	Exhibits physical cruelty to animals
15	Deliberately destroys the property of others, other than by fire-setting
16	Deliberately sets fires with a risk or intention of causing serious damage
17	Steals objects of non-trivial value without confronting the victim, either within the home or outside, e.g. shoplifting, burglary, forgery
18	Frequently truants from school, beginning before 13 years of age
19	Has run away from parental or parental surrogate home at least twice or has run away once for more than a single night **NB This does not include leaving home to avoid physical or sexual abuse**
20	Commits a crime involving confrontation with the victim, including purse snatching, extortion, mugging
21	Forces another person into sexual activity
22	Frequently bullies others, e.g. deliberate infliction of pain or hurt, including persistent intimidation, tormenting or molestation
23	Breaks into someone else's house, building or car

- At least one of the symptoms from items 9–23 must have been present for at least six months.
- Conduct disturbance must be limited to the family context.

For **unsocialised conduct disorder** the following criteria must be met:

- The diagnostic criteria for conduct disorder must be met.
- Three or more of the symptoms listed for criteria must be present, with at least three from items 9–23.
- At least one of the symptoms from items 9–23 must have been present for at least six months.
- There must be poor relationships with the individual's peer group, as shown by isolation, rejection or unpopularity and by a lack of lasting close reciprocal friendships.

For **socialised conduct disorder** the following criteria must be met:

- The diagnostic criteria for conduct disorder must be met.

- Three or more of the symptoms listed for conduct disorder must be present, with at least three from items 9–23.
- At least one of the symptoms from items 9–23 must have been present for at least six months.
- Conduct disturbance must include settings outside the home or family context. Peer relationships are within normal limits.

It is recommended that the age of onset be specified:

- **Childhood-onset type**: at least one conduct problem before the age of ten years.
- **Adolescent-onset type**: no conduct problems before the age of ten years.

For determining a prognosis, the WHO guidelines suggest that 'severity', indexed by number of symptoms, is a better guide than the precise type of symptomatology.

It is recommended that cases be described in terms of their scores on three dimensions of disturbance, these include

- Hyperactivity, i.e. inattentive, restless behaviour
- Emotional disturbance (anxiety, depression, obsessionality, hypochondriasis)
- Severity of conduct disorder:
    - Mild: few, conduct problems only enough to make the diagnosis and the conduct problems cause only minor harm to others.
    - Moderate: the number of conduct problems and the effects on others are intermediate between 'mild' and 'severe'.
    - Severe: many conduct problems present more than those required to make the diagnosis, or the conduct problems cause considerable harm to others, e.g. severe physical injury, vandalism or theft.

Oppositional Defiant Disorder

- The general criteria for CD must be met.
- Four or more of the symptoms listed for conduct disorder must be present, but with no more than two symptoms from items 9–23.
- The symptoms must be maladaptive and inconsistent with the developmental level.
- At least four of the symptoms must have been present for at least six months.

Prevalence

Epidemiological studies suggest that around 6.5% of school-aged children meet criteria for ODD and 2.2% for CD (Merikangas et al., 2010). The prevalence of these disorders is difficult to quantify in the community, as many children will present with extremes of behaviour, but there are a number of factors that distinguish a child with ODD or CD. These include an extreme number of symptoms, the frequency of symptoms, chronicity and the degree of impairment for the child and/or their family.

A weak association between lower socioeconomic status and prevalence of ODD and CD has been shown, but varies between studies (Piotrowskia, 2015). Sex differences have been reported with a sex ratio of approximately 2.5 males for each female, with males furthermore exceeding females in terms of frequency and severity of symptoms (Moffitt and Scott, 2008).

The causes of these disorders are generally the same for both sexes, however males experience more CD as they experience more of the risk factors, e.g. hyperactivity and cognitive deficits.

Associated Conditions

Symptoms of ODD and CD are the leading cause of referral to children's mental health services with at least half of these young people meeting the criteria for another psychiatric condition, most commonly ADHD, but often internalising disorders, such as depression and anxiety (Nock et al., 2007; Burke et al., 2005). Co-occurring behaviours include psychopathy (Lynam and Gudonis, 2005), autistic traits (Gilmour, et al., 2004), bullying (Olweus, 1997) and adolescent partner violence (Ehrensaft et al., 2004).

Many children with ODD have an emotionally labile temperament, with irritability being an important feature of the disorder. Their parents often find such children difficult to care for. Children with ODD find it difficult to regulate their emotions and cope with challenging situations by being aggressive and oppositional.

Aetiology

Genetics

There is increasing evidence from behavioural genetic studies for a role of genetic influences in the aetiology of CD/ODD, with 40–50% of variance in these conditions explained by heritable factors and a relatively large contribution of shared environmental factors relative to other psychiatric disorders (Rhee and Waldman, 2002). Heritability is even higher (60–70%) for aggressive forms of CD and for CD with high levels of callous-unemotional or psychopathic traits (Viding et al., 2005). In terms of specific genes, a functional polymorphism in the monoamine oxidase A (MAOA) gene that codes for an enzyme responsible for breaking down the neurotransmitters serotonin, noradrenaline and dopamine in the brain has been implicated in the aetiology of CD. It appears to have only weak effects on the risk for developing CD when it occurs in isolation, but in combination with exposure to childhood maltreatment, the low activity form of the MAOA gene appears to confer increased susceptibility to developing CD (Abrahamson et al., 2002).

This gene is X chromosome-linked and its effects on vulnerability to negative rearing environments appear greatest in, or possibly confined to, males. It is likely that, as with other psychiatric disorders, many genes are involved in the aetiology of CD and complex interactions between susceptibility genes and environmental factors will be the rule, rather than the exception.

Neuropsychology

Neuropsychological and neuroimaging studies have provided important insights into the aetiology of CD/ODD. Children with conduct problems have been found to have increased rates of verbal and language-based deficits and poor executive functioning (Peterson et al., 2016). It is likely that such children have difficulties organising their thoughts and expressing themselves. Such children may attempt to gain control over such situations by using aggression.

Children with these conditions have been found to be more sensitive to positive or rewarding stimuli, and less sensitive to negative or punishing stimuli, when making decisions or learning, than typically developing children (Fairchild et al., 2009a). They have been shown to have weaker psychophysiological responses to punishing or painful stimuli (Luman et al., 2010).

A number of brain-imaging studies have revealed reductions in amygdala and anterior insula grey matter volume in the brains of children with CD compared to healthy controls (Sterzer et al., 2007; Huebner et al., 2008; Fairchild et al., 2013), that potentially helps to explain why they show deficits in empathy and facial expression recognition (Fairchild et al., 2009b). Functional brain-imaging studies have shown reduced amygdala responses to emotional facial expressions in adolescents with CD (Passamonti et al., 2010) or conduct problems and callous-unemotional traits (Jones et al., 2009; Marsh et al., 2008). It is likely that these changes in brain structure and function in children with CD contribute to their difficulties with social cognition, although longitudinal studies are needed to investigate whether these neural differences cause or contribute to the symptoms of CD or are merely a secondary consequence of other causes of CD (Breeden et al., 2015). Attempts to link antisocial behaviours with neurotransmitters have been successful in adults (Nelson and Trainor, 2007), but findings with children have not been consistent (Hill, 2002).

Perinatal Insults

Prenatal alcohol exposure is a risk factor for externalising behaviours, executive functioning difficulties and learning disability (Ware et al., 2013), and a large proportion of children with fetal alcohol syndrome have ODD or CD (Koren, 2015). There is evidence that maternal smoking during pregnancy is associated with increased risk of CD in offspring (Brennan, Grekin and Mednick, 2003). Complications surrounding the time of birth, e.g. low birthweight (Brennan, Grekin and Mednick, 2003), are thought to be associated with some of the neuropsychological difficulties associated with CD and ODD.

Temperament

The innate temperament of a child will make a difference to how they view the world and conversely how the world will view and interact with them. Hyperactive children are difficult to parent and often exhibit behaviours that can escalate into chains of conflicts, that can in turn often result in coercive parenting (Patterson, 1982). This refers to a pattern of interactions whereby a parent may unknowingly reinforce coercive behaviours in their children by nagging, scolding and yelling when the child misbehaves. These behaviours initiate the coercive interaction. If the child continues to misbehave or escalates the conflict despite the parent's aversive behaviours, the parent eventually reaches an exhaustion point. At this point, the child's misbehaviour is negatively reinforced when the parent fails to follow through with their promised consequences or ceases punishing them. Then the parent backs down and fails to discipline the child adequately and the child quickly learns that they can manipulate the parent into meeting their needs by using coercive strategies.

Rule-breaking and apparent disobedience in children with poor listening skills and poor ability to predict the consequences of their behaviour can lead to punishment and negative reinforcement. A highly emotionally fragile child will be inappropriately sensitive to criticism and cry easily, setting him/herself up to be teased and often used as a scapegoat. These are often children who tend to say 'no' rather than 'yes', creating situations for the development of ODD.

Parenting and Early Trauma

Parenting practices and attitudes will affect children with CD and ODD. Positive parenting practices foster good self-esteem, confidence and problem-solving techniques in children, whilst inconsistent, negative or 'coercive' parenting fosters the opposite. Children need predictability from parents, together with consistent, clear and understandable limits. Inconsistent parenting is often present in families with a conduct disordered child, e.g. extremes of lax to harsh and unpredictable discipline, with the child not knowing from one day to the next what is expected from him or what punishment will follow, should he transgress that day's rules. Any factors that add to stress and unpredictability in parenting will make clear and consistent parenting more difficult to implement. Parental mental illness has been shown to correlate with conduct disorder in children (Kazdin, 1997).

Children in any family will pick up on the ways in which the adults around them speak and interact with each other and with authority figures. There is a strong correlation between conduct disorder in children and criminal behaviour in parents (Farrington, 1995). Many children experience or witness neglect or physical, emotional or sexual abuse, and these adverse childhood experiences are strongly linked with later psychopathology (Bielas et al., 2016).

Early adverse experiences or trauma are strongly correlated with emotional instability, irritability and externalising behaviours and are a risk factor for ODD, CD and juvenile offending (McLaughlin, 2016). This is likely to be linked to the effect that trauma has on the core regulatory systems with up-regulation of autonomic response to threat, and to the child's early experience of authority figures as being unreliable and dangerous.

Attachment theory offers a means of understanding a child's response to threat by looking at their early experience with caregivers. It has been postulated that insecure and disorganised attachment could be correlated with the development of ODD/CD, with a mechanism of interfamilial stressors and unpredictable parental response leading to insecure attachment that in turn leads to difficulty with emotional regulation and empathic responses in the child (Marron, 1998). A recent meta-analysis showed that insecure and disorganised attachment is more likely to be found where a child has been diagnosed with ODD and CD, but that it was not possible to show a direct causal link (Theule, 2016).

Maintaining Factors

Children with CD or ODD are often from families with financial difficulties, lacking access to transport and living in overcrowded households and unsafe neighbourhoods. These stressors can add to lack of control and feelings of uncertainty for the family, making strong consistent boundaries difficult to implement, and the potential for a feeling of chaos being replicated within the family relationships.

When a family is experiencing practical hardships and difficult dynamics, they may come into increased contact with professionals from social and health care agencies that have the potential to be adversarial. Similarly, the child may have difficult relationships with teachers at school, where these factors may exacerbate bad behaviour and bring more attention on the child.

A complex cycle may arise where the child becomes the focus for perceived difficulties in the school or the family, when that might not always be true. Children will target and scapegoat a child who annoys them, compounding the difficulties for the child. In some cases, teachers might do the same.

These children have poorer peer relationships than non-disordered children. There is evidence to support that (a) children's antisocial behaviours lead them to have peer problems, (b) their deviant peer relationships lead to antisocial behaviours or (c) some common factor leads to both these factors (Moffitt and Scott, 2008). It is important to keep in mind the reciprocal manner in which conduct problems can influence who a child's friends are and in turn, how such friends might promote the child's conduct problems.

Prognosis

In childhood, ODD and CD carry a risk of low attendance and attainment at school, criminality and alcohol and drug use. This is a risk that continues into adulthood, with greater rates of unemployment and criminality in adulthood, in addition to higher than average rates of antisocial personality disorder, anxiety, mood and somatoform disorders (Scott et al., 2001). It carries an increased risk of attempted suicide in young adulthood (Ogden and Hagen, 2018).

However, even in early-onset forms of conduct disorder these risks are not certainties, as only 25–40% of individuals go on to show serious forms of criminality and/or antisocial personality disorder in adulthood (Zoccolillo et al., 1992). Later onset of the disorder, at about age 15, characterised by less of a gender split, but by delinquent, i.e. theft or vandalism, rather than aggressive behaviour, has a better prognosis.

Treatment

Treatment methods have been developed for this group of children, but as the root causes of the disorder are complex and involve the child's temperament, family factors, the environment, the school and the child's peers, change is difficult and needs a multi-factorial approach. Treatment techniques need to address more than one domain for lasting, effective change to happen (Bakker et al., 2017).

The NICE guidelines highlight the need for individualised care with early identification and treatment and an emphasis placed on engagement due to the likelihood that young people will have had negative experiences of authority figures (National Institute of Clinical Excellence, 2013).

The guidelines suggest:

- Early identification of 'at risk' young people, with classroom-based emotional learning and problem-solving skills where there are a high number of 'at risk' pupils.
- Comprehensive assessment, taking into account the young person's background and identifying any co-morbidities, especially ADHD and autism.
- Parent or foster care/guardian training programmes, that can be group based or 1:1 when focussed on children with complex needs.
- Group social and cognitive problem-solving training for children where parent training alone is insufficient.
- Multi-systemic therapy should be a considered as a means of tailoring treatment needs to the individual child.
- Medications should not be considered as routine management and should only be considered where the benefits clearly outweigh the risks.

Parent Management Training

Parenting will influence children's behaviour. However, the relationship between the parent and child is a two-way process. Parents who have difficulty understanding why their child does not listen may find themselves in a very negative cycle with their child, i.e. children who are receiving little attention might behave badly to gain any attention, but, of course, this can produce an unpredictable result, reinforcing the negative cycle.

Parenting packages promote positive parenting, encouraging parents to recognise behaviours for what they are, i.e. reframing the problem. This enables the parents to anticipate the cycle of difficulties in order to learn to intervene with positive parenting strategies. Coercive and negative parenting strategies are discouraged. The family as a whole is encouraged to use positive rewards and plenty of praise with their children together with clear, well thought-out sanctions, when necessary.

Parent training emphasises the importance of clear, consistent, predictable parenting. It is often helpful for families with young children to bring them along to the session so that the therapist can demonstrate helpful techniques, e.g. setting limits and developing listening skills. Such parent training for parents of children with CD/ODD has been well researched (Scott et al., 2001) with positive results at ten-year follow-up (Long et al., 1994). Earlier interventions lead to better results than interventions in adolescence (Kochanska and Kim, 2013).

Functional Family Therapy

This therapeutic approach addresses how the family communicates. Its theoretical viewpoint draws together an understanding of family systems, underlying cognitive processes and behavioural functioning. The aim of this approach is to help families understand an individual family member's behaviour. This approach focusses on how each family member's communication pattern affects the rest of the family. The therapist's task is to aid the learning process and reinforce positive approaches with praise and interpretation, both verbally and non-verbally.

Outcome studies indicate that this treatment method can be very successful, especially with delinquent children. Family processing does show change and 'successful' families show positive change in communication style.

Multi-Systemic Therapy

It is often helpful to take a multi-systemic approach with children and their families as these children often cause distress to themselves, their families and their environment. The multi-systemic approach makes a positive decision to address the wider context and all the systems surrounding the individual. Such an approach will address the child individually, the family, including the marital system, the peer group and the school. Although it uses many of the techniques already referred to, it is not simply an amalgamation of packages, but a positive attempt to offer a package to help resolve the difficulties. Outcome studies suggest that for children with extreme problems, e.g. those involved with the youth justice system, this approach works well (Huey et al., 2000).

Medication

Medication has a place for children with hyperactivity. Although stimulant medication might help the symptoms of extreme temper and aggression, it may not alter the conduct disorder behaviour, e.g. defiance, lying or stealing. Other types of medication have been used to try to target a variety of problems, but no clear benefits have been obtained. Clinicians often find that cases of extreme aggression are very difficult to control.

Mood stabilisers, e.g., carbamazepine or sodium valproate, have been found to be effective in such individuals. Risperidone has been used in trials with conduct disordered children, most commonly in those with co-morbid intellectual disabilities, and has been shown to have a moderate effect on violence and aggression across IQ groups (Pringsheim et al., 2015). It appears effective in reducing aggressive symptoms in this group but should be used with caution, as it is associated with side-effects such as extrapyramidal symptoms, somnolence, weight gain and dyspepsia in a significant minority of cases. The long-term side-effects of this medication are still to be determined, thus base-line measures of blood sugar, cholesterol, liver function tests and possibly lipids should be taken and repeated, if concerned, or at least every six months.

Kazdin lays out a useful framework for considering whether a particular treatment is the correct one for a condition, bearing in mind that we should not be using treatments that have not been shown to produce change in well-conducted trials. This conceptualisation of treatment is particularly helpful when we consider how best to change the behaviour of children with conduct disorder. Kazdin and colleagues discuss why some treatment approaches might not work (Kazdin, 1997; Kazdin and Wassall, 1999; Kazdin, 2001a; Kazdin, 2001b; Nock and Kazdin 2001).

Framework for Considering Valid Treatment Approaches

- The disorder and the mechanisms underlying the disorder need to be conceptualised correctly in order to target treatment appropriately.
- Is there research to back up the above conceptualisation? e.g. is there clear research evidence that family factors correlate with the development of conduct disorder? Do particular family communication patterns correlate with the development of difficult behaviour in the children?
- Have there been sound controlled trials or well-evaluated treatment studies indicating that a particular treatment method works?
- Have there been studies looking at treatment targeted at the processes underlying the development of the disorder, e.g. the family communication pattern or the distorted cognitive processing mechanisms in children, and that have shown clinically effective change in proportion to positive change in the processes?

The above criteria are very strict, and no treatment can show change in all domains. The aim of treatment outcome for this group of children should be to improve the child's functioning in both the short and long term.

What Affects Outcome?

Unfortunately, families with conduct disordered children often encounter a wide range of additional problems. Such problems can often prove to be significant barriers to treatment. Therapists need to find ways of engaging family members as well as 'holding' them in therapy. Helping with transport issues, telephoning before appointments and engaging all family members separately, for instance, are important factors to consider and represent good practice.

Group work with children, all with similar delinquent problems, is not recommended, as the children tend to model each other's behaviour. If the group is mixed, i.e. including pro-social children, results seem to be better, as the children have pro-social norms from the non-conduct disordered child to follow (Bailey, 1996).

Research has found that the factors that mitigate against positive and lasting gains include:

- An early onset of the conduct disorder
- Aggressive behaviour
- Poor executive functioning in the child
- Being male and having an increased number of symptoms

The best way to work with these children and families seems to be to assess carefully the domains in which the child has difficulties and whether there are any co-morbid problems present. Following this, treatment can be targeted appropriately.

ODD Case Study (1): Charlie

Charlie (six) was referred to CAMHS with concerns around his disruptive and verbally aggressive behaviour at home and at school. He had been fostered at the age of three due to neglect and had witnessed domestic violence in the home. There was a strong suspicion that he had been physically abused. He was placed in a foster family with committed foster parents, who were struggling to cope with his insulting language, frequent tantrums and 'devil may care' attitude to rules, including smashing property and running away.

At school he struggled with friendships and was frequently in fights. His teachers said he was likeable but deliberately antagonistic towards other pupils and teachers, and had a very quick temper.

Charlie was assessed jointly by a therapeutic social worker and psychiatrist, with input from his school and social work team. He was diagnosed with ODD and ADHD and was referred for an educational psychology assessment. This identified difficulties in working memory and executive functioning. The role of his early trauma and attachment difficulties was explored and a comprehensive formulation of his difficulties fed back to his foster parents and the network.

Charlie was transferred to a specialist school where the assessments informed a comprehensive package including 1:1 support and a nurture group with an emphasis on social stories, aimed at promoting positive interactions with others and reducing fights. Treatment for ADHD with methylphenidate gave some improvement and he was able to concentrate more in class, fidget and run around less and begin to enjoy his lessons. As a result, he received positive feedback from teachers and his attitude to school gradually changed. Charlie's foster parents were offered a 12-week parenting programme with parents of similar children and worked hard at establishing clear rules at home. They found the support of other parents invaluable in developing an understanding of Charlie's particular needs. Social care arranged regular, consistent respite placements for Charlie. Charlie did well in the new school and is likely to move to mainstream secondary school. That transition will need careful planning as he continues to respond to stress and change with anxiety and often anger.

CD Case Study (2): Tom

Tom (15) and his family had been open to social services for ten years, initially due to concerns about maternal drug use. The family had engaged well with social services and the children remained with their birth parents, but family life was chaotic. The area they lived in was known for high levels of drug-related crime.

Tom was diagnosed with ADHD in primary school but was no longer taking medication. His attendance at school was 60%, and he was often rude to teachers and disruptive in lessons, a pattern throughout his schooling. He had been re-referred to CAMHS after being excluded for setting light to a bin in school and threatening a teacher with a knife.

His family were concerned that Tom had become involved with a local gang and might be running drugs, as he was frequently missing from home and appeared to have a lot of money. He was referred to the local youth offending service after being arrested for theft and after a rocky start, began working with a mentor and the police, to stop his criminal activities.

He and his mother began to attend family therapy sessions. Initially, Tom appeared unconcerned about the impact of his behaviour, but after several sessions with a family therapist Tom revealed that he was very anxious about the risks he taking and the risks posed to his family by his involvement in gangs. His mother was shocked as she had thought he was unable to see anyone else's point of view, and together they explored how their communication had reinforced her opinion and made Tom resentful.

The diagnosis of CD was helpful for Tom and his parents in understanding how his behaviours may have started and been reinforced and was helpful in moving the focus away from Tom's 'naughtiness' and onto the wider difficulties that the family were facing. Tom continues to receive support from the Youth Offending Team. He is attending college and studying mechanics.

Multiple-Choice Questions

See answers on page 670.

1. The division between conduct disorder: childhood onset, and conduct disorder: adolescent onset, occurs at what age?
   a. 14 years
   b. 12 years
   c. 10 years
   d. 11 years
   e. 13 years
2. What is the estimated prevalence of ODD and CD in school-aged children?
   a. >5%
   b. 5%
   c. 30%
   d. 10–20%
   e. 30–35%
3. Which of the following is *not* a recommended treatment option for CD and/or ODD?
   a. Multi-systemic therapy
   b. Selective serotonin reuptake inhibitors (SSRIs)
   c. Parent management training
   d. Functional family therapy
4. What is the current reported heritability for CD and ODD?
   a. <10%
   b. 70–80%
   c. 20–30%
   d. >80%
   e. 40–50%
5. Which candidate gene has been particularly implicated in the aetiology of CD?
   a. BRCA1
   b. DAT1
   c. MAOA
   d. BDNF
   e. APOA5

Key References

Bakker, M.J., et al., (2017). Practitioner review: psychological treatments for children and adolescents with conduct disorder problems—a systematic review and meta-analysis. *Journal of Child Psychology and Psychiatry*, 1: 4–18.

Farrington, D.P., (1995). The twelfth Jack Tizard memorial lecture: the development of offending and anti-social behaviour from childhood: key findings from the Cambridge study in delinquent development. *Journal of Child Psychology and Psychiatry*, 360(6): 929–964.

Kazdin, A.E., (2001). Treatment of conduct disorders. In Jonathan Hill and Barbara Maughan (Eds.), *Conduct Disorders in Childhood and Adolescents* (pp. 408–448). Cambridge University Press.

Theule, J., (2016). Conduct disorder/oppositional defiant disorder and attachment: a meta-analysis. *Journal of Development and Life Course Criminology*, 2: 232–255.

42 Tic Disorders and Tourette Syndrome

Valerie Brandt and Samuele Cortese

KEY CONCEPTS

- Tic disorders are not necessarily associated with distress, and a lot of children who display tics in childhood appear to be tic-free in adulthood, irrespective of whether the tics were treated or not. The most important aspect of treating tics is therefore psychoeducation.
- Tics are highly heritable and commonly associated with ADHD, OCD and other disorders, which can cause distress. Patients with tics should therefore undergo a broad assessment.
- Tics are associated with changes in the basal ganglia, a structure that is responsible for appropriate action selection processes.

Diagnosis and Characteristics

Tic disorders are common, childhood-onset neuropsychiatric disorders and are characterised by motor tics (e.g. eye blinks) and/or phonic (e.g. coughing) tics. Tics can be simple (e.g. an eye blink or a nose wrinkle) or complex (e.g. jumping, touching things in a specific order, repeating words). The most salient tic is coprolalia, i.e. involuntary swearing, but only approximately 10–33% of patients with a tic disorder have coprolalia (Eddy and Cavanna, 2013). There are several different diagnostic categories for tic disorders (American Psychiatric Association, 2013):

a) Transient tic disorders are defined by one or more tics that last under a year and occur for the first time before the age of 18.
b) Chronic motor or vocal tic disorder is defined by one or more motor or phonic tics that last longer than a year and occur for the first time before the age of 18.
c) Tourette syndrome (TS) is defined as one or more phonic tics and two or more motor tics that last longer than a year and occur for the first time before the age of 18.

There are two other categories for rarely occurring tic disorders, such as tics with an onset in adulthood. Tics have to occur on most days, they typically wax and wane in frequency and intensity and were not caused by another source, such as drugs or a head injury. Distress is not necessary to diagnose tic disorders, and not all individuals with tics experience stress or even necessarily notice their tics. However, tics can be perceived by others as disruptive or odd and are often associated with psychosocial difficulties and discrimination against the patient (Conelea et al., 2013), which can lead to depressive symptoms (Lin et al., 2007).

The entirety of current tics that can be identified in a patient is called the 'tic repertoire'. The tic repertoire changes over time, that is, new tics can develop, some tics may disappear. The tic repertoire is more stable in adults than in children.

The estimated population prevalence of TS is 0.3–0.9% (Scharf et al., 2015); the prevalence of other tic disorders is higher but estimates vary widely between 1 and 25%, depending on the sample and the assessment tool used (Black, Black, Greene and Schlaggar, 2016; Robertson, 2008; Scharf et al., 2015). Tic disorders are three to four times more common in male than in female children (Hirschtritt et al., 2015; Robertson, 2008) but interestingly, there is some evidence that they are only 2:1 more common in male to female adults (J. Yang et al., 2016). Tics typically start around the age of four to eight, reach their peak in early adolescence and then decrease in frequency and intensity (Hirschtritt et al., 2015; Schlander, Schwarz, Rothenberger and Roessner, 2011). It is currently thought that the majority of patients who experience tics as children grow up to be tic-free adults (Hassan and Cavanna, 2012; Pappert, Goetz, Louis, Blasucci and Leurgans, 2003). However, this assumption is based on little data and needs to be re-evaluated. A recent study showed that all 39 children who were diagnosed with a transient tic disorder and seen a year later still had tics, albeit most of them had improved (Kim et al., 2019). This indicates that transient tic disorders are not as transient as their name suggests. Furthermore, very little is known about the predictors of tic severity in adulthood, although this is typically one of the main concerns of families who have a child with a tic disorder. Currently identified predictors include a smaller caudate volume, more severe childhood tics and untreated co-morbidities (Hassan and Cavanna, 2012; Pappert et al., 2003), but these are again based on small studies. In patients where the tics persist, they can become more severe over the course of life and have a detrimental effect on the patients' social life and work opportunities (Pappert et al., 2003). It is therefore important to assess patients with tic disorders longitudinally. Approximately 90% of patients who seek medical help have co-morbidities, most commonly ADHD (54%) and OCD (50%) (Hirschtritt et al., 2015), and these co-morbidities can cause more distress than the tics.

Premonitory Urges

In 1980, approximately 100 years after TS was formally described for the first time by Georges Gilles de la Tourette (Gilles de la Tourette, 1885), Joseph Bliss described for the first time that tics might not be entirely involuntary, movements but might be driven by an urge to tic (Bliss, 1980). Research has since found that more than 90% of adult patients with TS experience the urge to tic (Kwak, Dat Vuong and Jankovic, 2003; Leckman, Walker and Cohen, 1993). In the majority of patients, the urge appears to increase until the tic is executed and then decreases (Brandt et al., 2016). The urge becomes particularly strong when patients suppress their tics consciously. The current behavioural model assumes that there is a vicious circle that maintains tic behaviour: the urge increases, the tic is then executed; the urge decreases as a result and thereby negatively reinforces the tic behaviour. The next time the urge increases, the patient is more likely to exhibit a tic again in order to avoid the uncomfortable urge (Evers and van de Wetering, 1994).

However, evidence for this model is scarce, and there is some conflicting evidence. Urges occur on average three years after tic onset (Leckman et al., 1993), suggesting that the urge may be a consequence of suppressing tics rather than a cause of tics (Draper, Jackson, Morgan and Jackson, 2015). But this finding could also be due to difficulties of four- to five-year olds to describe a concept such as urges. Furthermore, the pattern between tic suppression and urge ratings is not consistent across patients, particularly youths (Brabson et al., 2016), indicating that there may be no commonly applicable urge-tic mechanism across patients. In summary, the negative reinforcement model is currently useful for therapeutic interventions (see cognitive behavioural therapy) but still needs to be confirmed or refuted. A further open key question is how tics and urges develop in the first place.

Neuropathology

Tic disorders are associated with changes in the cortico-striato-thalamo-cortical (CSTC) loop (Kalanithi et al., 2005; Kataoka et al., 2010; Worbe et al., 2012). The loop includes motor cortical areas, then leads to the striatum, encompassing the basal ganglia, to the thalamus and then back to the cortex. The basal ganglia are a structure that is important for action selection processes. Whenever a person enters into a situation, they have several possibilities to act (e.g. seeing a picture in a museum). The basal ganglia are responsible for selecting a context-appropriate action (e.g. looking at the picture) and to suppress context-inappropriate actions (e.g. touching the picture). Some evidence points to an imbalance in the inhibitory and excitatory pathways in the CSTC loop in patients with tics (Kalanithi et al., 2005; Kataoka et al., 2010; Worbe et al., 2012), possibly leading to a constant over-output of context-inappropriate actions.

It has also been suggested that tics may be associated with alterations in the dopaminergic system, mainly because anti-dopaminergic medication can be used to successfully attenuate tic severity, but experimental evidence is not yet strong enough to show that this is indeed the case or how the dopaminergic system might be affected (Buse, Schoenefeld, Munchau and Roessner, 2012; Hienert, Gryglewski, Stamenkovic, Kasper and Lanzenberger, 2018).

Heritability and Environmental Factors

There is strong evidence for a genetic contribution to tic disorders. The risk for a first-degree relative of someone with a diagnosed tic disorder to also have a tic disorder is 19 times higher compared to an unaffected individual (Mataix-Cols et al., 2015), and the risk decreases substantially for second- and third-degree relatives. Twin studies show very high concordance rates in monozygotic twins, 53–94%, and lower rates in dizygotic twins, 8–23% (Hyde, Aaronson, Randolph, Rickler and Weinberger, 1992; Price, Kidd, Cohen, Pauls and Leckman, 1985). Correlations for any tic disorder are 0.63 in monozygotic twins and 0.34 in dizygotic twins (Polderman et al., 2015).

Despite strong evidence for the heritability of tics, genetic studies have had difficulties pinning down the genes that are involved in tics disorders. It appears that the genetic component of tic disorders is complex, including rare (high-impact) and common (low-impact) genetic variants; it probably involves a number of genes (polygenetic) and environmental factors (Yu et al., 2019), as well as epigenetic factors (Muller-Vahl, Loeber, Kotsiari, Muller-Engling and Frieling, 2017). A meta-analysis showed that genes that have been associated with risk for tic disorders in genome-wide association studies (GWAS) are commonly expressed in the dorsolateral prefrontal cortex and that TS and the other tic disorders are likely on the same spectrum, sharing polygenetic risk (Yu et al., 2019). However, it has to be noted that results of candidate gene studies could not be replicated (Abdulkadir et al., 2018) and that GWAS have had difficulties providing genome-wide significant findings, possibly due to relatively small sample sizes (Fernandez, State and Pittenger, 2018). It is expected that genetic studies will render significant findings in the coming years.

Several environmental factors in tic disorders have been proposed, but studies have shown only very small associations, if any, between environmental factors and the likelihood to develop tics (low birth-weight, maternal smoking (Chao, Hu and Pringsheim, 2014) and maternal pre-natal anxiety (Ben-Shlomo, Scharf, Miller and Mathews, 2016)) and these factors are not specific predictors of tic disorders. The long-held assumption that streptococcal infections may cause the onset or exacerbation of tic disorders has recently been refuted by a large, longitudinal, European multicentre study (EMTICS). Patient reports that stress or emotional excitement exacerbates tics has also not been confirmed experimentally (Buse, Enghardt, Kirschbaum, Ehrlich and Roessner, 2016; Silva, Munoz, Barickman and Friedhoff, 1995).

Treatment

Psychoeducation

Several treatment options exist but it should be stressed that tics do not necessarily need to be treated. For all treatments, psychoeducation is very important. It is often a relief for patients and their parents to learn that in many children, tics will disappear in early adulthood, with or without intervention. Furthermore, it is often helpful for children to learn that their tics are possibly inherited and to think about other family members that may have tics or had tics when they were children. It is also helpful to point out that tics are associated with changes in the brain. It is important for children and parents and sometimes teachers to understand that tics are not executed on purpose or to disrupt the classroom and that the child cannot help their tics. Some children find it helpful to tell their classmates about their tics to increase openness and understanding about their behaviour. The (potentially severe) side-effects of medical interventions need to be well explained.

It is also important to take a careful history of the patient's symptoms. Tics are often salient but not necessarily the most debilitating symptoms that a patient experiences. ADHD and OCD often have more detrimental effects on a child's school performance or well-being than the tics. In that case, the disorder that is most debilitating should be treated first. Improvement in other symptoms can often lead to an improvement in tics. For instance, recent research shows that treating children suffering from ADHD and tics with stimulants leads to improvements in both ADHD and tics in most children (Osland, Steeves and Pringsheim, 2018).

Cognitive Behavioural Therapy

Cognitive behavioural therapy is recommended as the first-line treatment (Verdellen, van de Griendt, Hartmann, Murphy and Group, 2011) for tic disorders in children and adults. However, it can be difficult to get access to a trained clinician that is nearby. The current gold standard behavioural treatments are habit reversal training (HRT) and exposure with response prevention (ERP) (van de Griendt, Verdellen, van Dijk and Verbraak, 2013; Verdellen, Keijsers, Cath and Hoogduin, 2004). Both treatments target the negative reinforcement cycle of tics and urges. During ERP, patients are asked to suppress their tics for as increasing amounts of time and to tolerate the urge to tic. It is assumed that urge to tic habituates (decreases) after a while, similar to anxiety during exposure. However, whether urges do indeed habituate is currently unclear (Capriotti, Brandt, Turkel, Lee and Woods, 2014; Specht et al., 2013; Verdellen et al., 2008). HRT involves establishing a hierarchy of tics that bother the patient. The most bothersome tic is then selected and the patient practices a competing movement that makes it impossible to execute the urge. For this, patients need to be aware of their tics and of their urge to tic, to interrupt the tic movement before it starts. Awareness training can enhance tic awareness. A meta-analysis of randomised controlled trials (RCT) has confirmed that both behavioural interventions successfully reduce tics with a medium to large effect (McGuire et al., 2014).

Medication

The pharmacological treatment is one of the components of the multimodal treatment of tics. To date, the most comprehensive evidence synthesis on the pharmacological treatment is provided by the network meta-analysis (NMA, an advanced meta-analytic approach allowing the comparison of two or more treatments even when they have not been compared head-to-head in individual trials) conducted by Yang et al. (2019). The authors included 60 RCTs, for a total of 4,077 participants (aged 2–65 years) with a clinical diagnosis of tic disorders as per the Diagnostic and Statistical Manual of Mental Disorders-3 (DSM-3), DSM-4, or DSM-4-Text Revision, the International Classification of Diseases-10 (ICD-10) or the Chinese Classification and Diagnostic Criteria of Mental Disorders (CCMD). Haloperidol (standardised mean difference, SMD = –3.20, 95% CI [–6.52, –0.14]), olanzapine (SMD = –6.11, –11.86, 0.55), ziprasidone (SMD = –5.57, –11.15, –0.048), risperidone (SMD = –3.47, –6.87, –0.37), aripiprazole (SMD = –4.74, –8.67, –1.06) and quetiapine (SMD = –12.32, –19.09, –5.63) were significantly more efficacious than placebo in improving tic severity. Quetiapine was significantly more efficacious than haloperidol, pimozide, risperidone, tiapride, aripiprazole and penfluridol. Aripiprazole was significantly more efficacious than tiapride. Unfortunately, this NMA did not report comparative tolerability of drugs and did not conduct subgroups analyses in children/adolescents only. Therefore, the reader should interpret with caution the overall findings of this meta-analysis and refer to guidelines based on evidence and expert consensus as well.

Guidelines

The most recent expert guidelines highlight that tics should be treated when they cause 'subjective discomfort (e.g. pain or injury)', 'sustained social problems for the patient (e.g. social isolation or bullying)', 'social and emotional problems for the patient (e.g. reactive depressive symptoms)' or 'functional interference (e.g. impairment of academic achievements)', and the pharmacological treatment should be considered if non-pharmacological treatments are ineffective or unavailable (Roessner et al., 2011). As for the choice of the agent, the guidelines highlight the paucity of comparative evidence. When taking into account expert opinion and experience, the guidelines recommend risperidone as a first-choice agent, but they also highlight that aripiprazole has a more favourable profile in terms of risk of weight gain. As for the other drugs, the guidelines recommend pimozide over haloperidol, due to its more favourable tolerability profile, and clonidine, especially when there is co-morbid ADHD. Finally, the guidelines suggest risperidone as first line when there is a co-morbid OCD.

Table 42.1 reports the doses of the most commonly used medications for tics as recommended in the practice parameters of the American Academy of Child and Adolescent Psychiatry (Murphy et al., 2013).

Case Study (1): Joe

Joe, an eight-year-old boy, presented with motor tics (blinking, shoulder shrugs, arm movements and grimacing) and vocal tics (frog noises, throat clearing and barking sounds). The parents reported that the tics had first occurred around the age of four and that symptoms waxed and waned, a common sign of a tic disorder. The tics exacerbated when Joe watched TV or

Table 42.1 Doses of the Most Commonly Used Medications for Tics

Drug	*Starting Dose (mg)*	*Usual Dose Range (mg/day)*
Aripiprazole	1.0–2.5	2.5–15
Clonidine	0.025–0.05	0.1–0.4
Guanfacine ER	1.0	1.0–4.0
Risperidone	0.125–0.5	0.75–3.0

came home from school, while tics were barely noticeable in school. Joe reported that his tics were preceded by a rising, uncomfortable urge to tic that increased when he tried to suppress his tics. It could be clinically observed that the tics were suggestible, i.e. Joe executed tics when they were mentioned. Some impulsive behaviour could also be observed, such as interrupting others. However, Joe's parents reported that these behaviours did not to extend to school and that Joe had no trouble concentrating or sitting still.

Joe reported liking school and not being too bothered by his tics socially. He was chatty and showed no symptoms of anxiety. He reported finding his tics exhausting when they occurred with a high frequency but not suffering from them. He also reported that his tics distracted him when reading and writing in school. Joe's parents reported his school performance was in the normal range and no problems had been flagged by the school.

The symptoms described and observed were consistent with Tourette syndrome. Criteria for an ADHD or anxiety disorder diagnosis were not fulfilled.

Regarding the family history, Joe's parents reported that Joe's dad may have had tics as a child but that they were never diagnosed and had disappeared during adulthood. Joe did not have any siblings. Joe's mum reported not having been diagnosed with tics, ADHD or OCD.

It was decided with Joe and his parents that Joe did not need treatment at this point. He did not suffer from his tics and did not wish to pursue treatment. He also had no debilitating co-morbidities at the time of assessment and his school performance was not affected. However, he did decide to give a presentation at school to explain his disorder to his class, and his school agreed to accommodate his symptoms by granting him extra time when writing.

Joe is a typical example of a child with an uncomplicated tic disorder and a possible family history of tics disorders. Unfortunately, no predictions can be made about the course of his symptoms because research in this domain is still lacking.

Multiple-Choice Questions

See answers on page 670.

1. Patient A presents with the following symptoms: eye blinking, nose wrinkling and couching tics with an onset at age five; the symptoms have been present for more than two weeks and less than a year. The correct diagnosis would be:
   a. Transient tic disorder
   b. Chronic motor tic disorder
   c. Tourette syndrome
2. The following statement is correct:
   a. Tic disorders are more common in adulthood than in childhood.
   b. Tic disorders are equally common in children and adults.
   c. Tic disorders are more common in childhood than in adulthood.

3. What are the two most common co-morbidities of Tourette syndrome?
   a. Anxiety disorder and attention deficit hyperactivity disorder
   b. Attention deficit hyperactivity disorder and obsessive-compulsive disorder
   c. Obsessive-compulsive disorder and learning disorder
4. Which one of the following statements is not a sign of heritability of tics?
   a. Concordance rates for tic disorders are higher in monozygotic twins than in dizygotic twins.
   b. Low birth weight is a predictor of tic disorders.
   c. First-degree relatives of patients with a tic disorder have an increased risk of also having a tic disorder.
5. Which one of the following is a common treatment in patients with tics?
   a. Habit practice
   b. Cognitive restructuring
   c. Exposure with response prevention

Key References

van de Griendt, J.M.T.M., Verdellen, C.W.J., van Dijk, M.K., Verbraak, M.J.P.M., (2013). Behavioural treatment of tics: habit reversal and exposure with response prevention. *Neuroscience & Biobehavioral Reviews*, 37(6): 1172–1177.

Hirschtritt, M.E., Lee, P.C., Pauls, D.L., Dion, Y., Grados, M.A., Illmann, C., et al., (2015). Lifetime prevalence, age of risk, and genetic relationships of comorbid psychiatric disorders in Tourette syndrome. *JAMA Psychiatry*, 72(4): 325–333.

Roessner, V., Plessen, K.J., Rothenberger, A., Ludolph, A.G., Rizzo, R., Skov, L., et al., (2011). European clinical guidelines for Tourette syndrome and other tic disorders. Part II: pharmacological treatment. *European Child and Adolescent Psychiatry*, 20(4): 173–196.

43 Depression in Children and Young People

Anna Gibson

KEY CONCEPTS

- Depression is a common mental disorder that can affect children of all ages, although it becomes more common with age, particularly in adolescence (Poznanske and Zrull, 1970).
- Diagnosis can be affected by cognitive developmental level and in younger children may be made by observations of behaviour across settings.
- First-line treatments in mild depression would include supportive treatments, reserving medication for moderate to severe depression. Medication is recommended in conjunction with therapeutic approaches. Offering combination treatment can be more effective than medication or therapy alone.

Classification

ICD-10 classification of depressive episodes describes symptoms that should be present on most days, represent a change from normal for that person and that include core symptoms of low mood, anergia and anhedonia. Other symptoms include reduced concentration, sleep and appetite disturbance, poor self-esteem, feelings of guilt and of worthlessness. In addition, 'somatic' symptoms can include early morning wakening, diurnal variation in mood, i.e. mood lowest in the morning, psychomotor retardation or agitation, loss of appetite, weight loss and loss of libido.

Depression is classified as mild, moderate or severe. Mild depression would be experienced as two or three distressing symptoms, but the individual is able to function. Moderate depression would include four or more symptoms present to a degree where it is very difficult to continue functioning. Severe depression would include several significant and distressing symptoms, usually including some 'somatic' symptoms. Suicidal thoughts and acts are common.

The DSM-5 (APA, 2013) classifies major depressive disorder as including at least five of nine symptoms, at least one of which is depressed mood, although in children and adolescents this may present as irritable rather than sad, or anhedonia. The other seven symptoms are:

- Changes in appetite/weight
- Sleep disturbance
- Change in psychomotor activity
- Decreased energy

- Feelings of worthlessness or guilt
- Difficulty concentrating/thinking
- Recurrent thoughts of death/suicidal ideation

There must be significant impact on functioning for a diagnosis, and it must not be due to substances or another medical condition.

In both ICD-10 and DSM-5, depression can be classified with or without psychotic symptoms and can be classified as recurrent if there has been a previous episode. In both classifications, it is important to ensure there has been no previous manic or hypomanic episode that would lead to a diagnosis of bipolar disorder.

In children under the age of 12 years, a history should be taken both from the child and the parents in addition to seeking information from the child's school. In adolescents 12–18 years, a history should be taken from the young person, and a collaborative history from the parents and school context can be extremely helpful.

Symptoms should be present across contexts. Although not in the classification systems, in children and adolescents, social withdrawal may be present and in younger children, there may be several somatic complaints, e.g. headaches or stomach aches. In younger children, who are less able to articulate complex feelings such as worthlessness and guilt, it is important to ask parents/carers about observable behaviours, such as social withdrawal, loss of interest in activities and tearfulness.

Semi-structured interviews such as the Kiddie Schedule for Affective Disorders and Schizophrenia (K-SADS), which is aimed at children aged 6–18 years, or the Child and Adolescent Psychiatric Assessment (CAPA), aimed at children aged 9–17 years, are recommended as potentially useful in aiding diagnosis, although they may need modification to be useful in the clinical setting of a busy CAMHS community team.

Epidemiology

A recent UK survey of the mental health of children aged 2–19 found the prevalence of depressive disorders to be 0.3% in the age group 5–10 years, 2.7% in 11–16-year olds and 4.8% in 17–19-year olds. This shows a clear trend for an increase in the prevalence of depression as children grow older. Depressive episodes, including mild, moderate and severe depression and other depressive disorders, were present in 1.5% and 0.6% respectively of children aged 5–19. Major depressive episodes were twice as common in females than in males (2% vs 1%), although other depressive disorders showed no significant gender difference. Other studies have shown no gender difference in children until adolescence, when depression becomes twice as common in females as in males. Depressive disorders did not vary in prevalence by ethnic group. Children with special educational needs (SEN) are more than twice as likely to suffer depression that those without (3.6% vs 1.5%) (NHS Digital Health, 2017).

The general health of the child relates to rates of depressive disorder. Worse general health is correlated to a higher risk of depression. Parental mental health was measured with the General Health Questionnaire (GHQ), and higher scores, denoting poorer mental health, were associated with increased rates of depression in children and young people. Families with less healthy functioning were associated with a higher prevalence of depressive disorders in their children. Households with the lowest incomes were associated with higher rates of depressive disorders. Higher rates of depressive disorders in children and adolescents were associated with parental receipt of disability benefits, but not of income benefits.

In children aged two to four the diagnosis of depressive disorder was not separated from anxiety disorders, but included in a group of 'emotional disorders', and the prevalence of this was around 1% with no gender difference. A community pre-school study in Spain found a prevalence of major depressive disorder of 1.12% with no gender difference (Domènech-Llaberia et al., 2009) although a community study in the USA found lower prevalence rates for major depressive disorder of 0.3% (Lavigne et al., 2009).

Recommended Outcome Measures

NICE guidelines (2005, updated (CG28), 2017) recommend general outcome measures, e.g. the Strengths and Difficulties Questionnaire or the Health of the Nation Outcome Scale for Children and Adolescents to monitor progress. NICE recommends an outcome measure specific to depression, the Mood and Feelings Questionnaire (MFQ). The MFQ has a short and long version (33 and 13 items long respectively), each item being rated 'not true', 'somewhat true' or 'true'. There are both child and parent versions of the questionnaire, which gives helpful collateral history. It is suitable for administration for children aged 6–17 years.

Another useful questionnaire to monitor depressive symptoms and response to treatment is the Revised Children's Anxiety and Depression Scale (RCADS), which has the benefit of screening for anxiety disorders, which are commonly co-morbid with depression. There are parent and child versions, and it is suitable for children aged 8–18 years.

The questionnaire consists of 47 items rated 'never', 'sometimes', 'often' or 'always'. When entered into an appropriate scoring programme, this gives scores for depression and total anxiety in addition to the following subtypes of anxiety: separation anxiety, social phobia, generalised anxiety, panic and obsessive-compulsive disorder. Once a young person has been diagnosed with specific difficulties, subsets of questions can be used in ongoing monitoring, rather than completing the whole questionnaire each time.

Relevant Treatments

NICE guidelines for depression in children aged 5–18 years recommend that treatment of depression begins with careful assessment and diagnosis, to include any co-morbidities, e.g. anxiety, ADHD or conduct problems. Part of this assessment should include screening for reversible causes of depression including anaemia, thyroid deficiency and micronutrient deficiencies, i.e. vitamin B12, iron, folate and vitamin D.

Once diagnosed, the first-line treatments would be psychoeducation offered to patients and their families, including information about the nature, course and treatment of depression. This needs to be age-appropriate information. For younger children, this may take the form of information the parents can share with their children or relevant storybooks.

Self-help websites (e.g. moodgym.com.au) and support groups and organisations, including Young Minds, are useful resources that patients and families should be encouraged to access for support.

Mild Depression

Basic supportive treatment is recommended, alongside lifestyle advice and watchful waiting. Lifestyle advice would include a structured programme of exercise for 45–60 minutes three times a week for 10–12 weeks, advice about sleep hygiene and anxiety management, plus advice about nutrition and a balanced diet. Young people with mild depression should be monitored for progress, and if there is no improvement with lifestyle advice and time, psychological therapies should be offered. For 5–11-year olds there is limited evidence, but guidelines suggest that appropriate therapeutic options for 5–18-year olds would include digital cognitive behavioural therapy (CBT), or group therapy which might be CBT, non-directive supportive therapy (NDST) or interpersonal therapy (IPT). Other options would include attachment-based family therapy or individual CBT, adapted for age. These therapies can be offered in community settings other than CAMHS, for instance, in schools or by primary mental health workers.

Moderate to Severe Depression

NICE recommends that young people with moderate to severe depression should be referred into CAMHS for review and offered lifestyle advice and psychological therapy. For 5–11-year olds, psychological therapies to be considered would include family-based IPT, family therapy, psychodynamic psychotherapy or individual CBT. For young people aged 12–18 years, individual CBT, for at least 3 months, should be offered. However, if this would not meet an individual's needs then other options can be considered, including IPT for adolescents, family therapy, either attachment-based or systemic, brief psychosocial intervention or psychodynamic psychotherapy.

If a young person is not responding after four to six sessions of psychological therapy then a multi-disciplinary review is recommended to consider other factors that might need to be addressed to aid treatment, perhaps if a parent is depressed, encouraging them to seek psychological support for themselves.

Medication (see below) can be considered for moderate to severe depression, either if psychological treatment is not showing improvement after four to six sessions or, sometimes, in combination with psychological treatment from the beginning.

Psychosis and High-Risk Depression

If a young person presents with psychotic symptoms in depression, their medication can be augmented by a second-generation antipsychotic medication, although there is little evidence for which doses are helpful in this age group or for how long treatment should continue (Poznanske and Zrull, 1970).

In high-risk depression, inpatient treatment may be considered, although usually a trial of intensive community treatment, where available, would be preferable. A careful assessment of risk and severity of the depression and the benefits of inpatient treatment need to be balanced against the risks, e.g. escalation of self-harming behaviour, loss of family and community support.

In rare cases of severe and life-threatening depression, or severe depression unresponsive to all other treatments offered, ECT may be considered in 12–18-year olds (but not in under 12-year olds). This would only be after careful assessment by a practitioner experienced in the use of ECT in this age group and in a specialist environment.

Medication

The first-line medication in treatment of depression in under 18-year olds is Fluoxetine. The evidence of its effectiveness in children aged 5–11 years is not established, and it should be used with caution, clear information and consent and only after depression has been unresponsive to four to six sessions of psychotherapy. In young people aged 12–18 years, Fluoxetine is only recommended after multi-disciplinary review and as an adjunct to psychological treatment. It should only be prescribed by a child and adolescent psychiatrist and young people should be monitored weekly in the early stages of treatment, by their therapist or prescribing doctor, looking for side-effects including increased suicidal behaviour, self-harm or hostility.

Second-line drug treatments would be Sertraline or Citalopram, and the depression would need to be sufficiently severe to justify a trial of a second anti-depressant.

Paroxetine, Venlafaxine, tricyclic anti-depressants and St John's wort should not be used to treat depression in children and young people.

Children under Five Years

There is very little evidence for treatment of depression in the under fives, although supportive treatment and lifestyle advice would remain important. There are pilots of interventions in this age-group, e.g. parent–child interaction therapy, emotional development module (PICT-ED). This is a psychotherapeutic approach being trialled, working with parent–child dyads, using behavioural and play therapy techniques (Luby et al., 2012; Lenze et al., 2011).

Maintenance of Remission

NICE recommends that children in remission from depression should remain under regular follow-up in CAMHS for a year after a single episode of depression or two years after recurrent depression, before a clear discharge to primary care with appropriate information-sharing. Should they later need a referral back into CAMHS services, they must be prioritised.

Case Study: Meg

A 14-year-old girl, Meg, was brought to see the GP by her mother, who was concerned that she was becoming withdrawn, going out less, frequently tearful and became angry over small things. On questioning Meg, the GP found that she was feeling sad all the time and felt she was a rubbish person. On direct questioning Meg admitted to having thoughts of not wanting to be alive anymore and of using self-harm, cutting her arms, as a way of coping when she felt distressed. These symptoms had been present for the last six months and were worsening. Meg had tried some counselling at school, but this did not help, and the GP referred to the local CAMHS service for further assessment and treatment.

At CAMHS Meg was assessed by a clinician who diagnosed several symptoms of depression, including feeling persistently low in mood and anhedonia. Meg used to enjoy dancing but had lost interest in this and stopped attending her dancing class. In addition, she no longer enjoyed her favourite TV show and was feeling constantly tired. Meg had little motivation, and although she used to be particular about her hairstyle and make-up, she no longer had the energy to care. Meg was struggling with her concentration, often drifting off in class at school, and as a result, had started to achieve lower grades in her work. She was missing occasional days off school, feeling too tired to leave her bed.

There were concerns at school and at home about irritability, with Meg finding herself in arguments with friends and family over small things that would not have bothered her a year ago. Meg was suffering initial insomnia of two to three hours, lying awake feeling useless and thinking about suicide. Her mother was a strong protective factor and so Meg believed she would never act on these thoughts. Nevertheless, they were extremely distressing for her.

Meg was treated with CBT, but when after six sessions there was little improvement, she saw a psychiatrist and it was felt appropriate to add an antidepressant. Fluoxetine was started. In the coming weeks, Meg's symptoms and functioning began to improve. She went back to her dancing class and attended school more regularly. She completed her CBT and stayed on antidepressant medication for a further year, before reducing and eventually stopping it after completion of her GCSE exams.

Multiple-Choice Questions

See answers on page 670.

1. According to the DSM-5, which of the following is not a core symptom of depression?
   a. Changes in appetite/weight
   b. Change in psychomotor activity
   c. Self-harm
   d. Feelings of worthlessness or guilt
   e. Decreased energy
2. Major depressive episodes are:
   a. The same in prevalence between boys and girls
   b. Twice as prevalent in girls
   c. Twice as prevalent in boys
3. The usually recommended therapeutic intervention with young people (12–18) experiencing depression is:
   a. Cognitive behavioural therapy
   b. Dialectical behaviour therapy
   c. Cognitive analytical therapy
   d. Person-centred counselling

Key References

Domènech-Llaberia, E., Vinas, F., Pla, E., Claustre Jané, M., Mitjavila, M., Corbella, T., Canals, J., (2009). Prevalence of major depression in preschool children. *European Child & Adolescent Psychiatry*, 18(10): 597–604.

Lavigne, J., LeBailly, S., Hopkins, J., Couze, K., Binns, H., (2009). The prevalence of ADHD, ODD, depression, and anxiety in a community sample of 4-year-olds. *Journal of Clinical Child & Adolescent Psychology*, 38(3): 315–328.

Lenze, S.N., Pautsch, J., Luby, J., (2011). Parent–child interaction therapy emotion development: a novel treatment for depression in preschool children. *Depression and Anxiety*, 28(2): 153–159.

Luby, J., Lenze, S., Tillman, R., (2012). A novel early intervention for preschool depression: findings from a pilot randomized controlled trial. *Journal of Child Psychology and Psychiatry*, *53*(3), 313–322.

NICE, (2017). *Depression in children and young people: identification and management (CG28), 2005, updated 2017.* London: NICE.

Poznanske, E.O., Zrull, J.P., (1970). Childhood depression: clinical characteristics of overtly depressed children. *Archives of General Psychiatry*, 23(1):8–15.

44 Bipolar Disorder in Children and Young People

Cara Sturgess

Introduction

Although there has been a rise in reporting of children and adolescents with bipolar disorder over recent years, it remains a controversial diagnosis and has been heavily debated. There are a number of reasons suggested for this increase, including a genuine rise in prevalence, over-diagnosis or an improvement in accurate diagnosis in practice (Meter et al., 2016, Findling et al., 2018). It is important to note that in the 2013 update of the DSM-5 the criteria for bipolar disorder have been modified from previous versions. Consequently, those who may otherwise have been sub-threshold, as a result of not meeting the full criteria, can now be diagnosed.

Diagnostic Criteria

There are two clinically distinct mood states in bipolar disorder: depression and (hypo)mania. Depression in bipolar disorder is assessed against the same criteria as unipolar depression. For a diagnosis of bipolar disorder to be made, both the ICD-11 and DSM-5 state that at least three of the following symptoms indicating a manic episode must be present:

- Increased activity or physical restlessness
- Increased talkativeness, 'pressure of speech'
- Flight of ideas or the subjective experience of thoughts racing
- Loss of normal social inhibitions, resulting in behaviour that is inappropriate to the circumstances
- Decreased need for sleep
- Inflated self-esteem or grandiosity
- Distractibility or constant changes in activity or plans
- Behaviour that is foolhardy or reckless and whose risks the individual does not recognise, e.g. spending sprees, foolish enterprises, reckless driving
- Marked sexual energy or sexual indiscretions

A hypomanic episode occurs when the symptoms of mania are less severe and there are no psychotic experiences present. Mixed states may be observed in which symptoms of both extremes occur simultaneously. Evidence suggests that children and adolescents with a diagnosis of bipolar disorder may suffer with co-morbid conditions, e.g. anxiety (54%), attention deficit hyperactivity disorder (ADHD) (48%) and substance use disorders (31%) (Frias et al., 2015).

It is imperative that an accurate diagnosis is made as soon as possible as latency between onset of symptoms and commencement of treatment has been shown to have a significant impact on the trajectory of the illness (Malhi, 2017). Early diagnosis and subsequent intervention may decrease the risk of co-morbid diagnoses, suicide, wider social difficulties and employment barriers associated with the illness (Baune and Malhi, 2015). Evidence suggests that it currently takes an average of 12.5 years to receive an accurate diagnosis, by which point many of the benefits of early intervention will have been lost (Joyce et al., 2016).

Case Study: Lucy

Lucy (17) has been seeing child and adolescent mental health services for three months. She was referred by her GP following an episode of low mood in which she had started to experience a marked increase in sleep and reduced appetite. She described feeling sad and 'numb' all the time. She explained that she was gaining no pleasure from her usual interests, was frequently tearful and was having recurrent thoughts of ending her life by taking an overdose or jumping from the top of a car park.

However, recently she has experienced a notable improvement in her mood. In fact, Lucy described feeling the happiest she had ever been. She was socialising more, staying out late and was sleeping for around two to three hours a night. She described her thoughts as 'racing' and she had several new ideas that she wanted to execute. She talked non-stop, annoying her friends and siblings, and she fell out with her friends because of making inappropriate comments towards them.

Her parents described her as being 'out of control' and 'like a different person'. She was in trouble with her lecturers due to disruptive behaviour towards other students, and she had lost interest in her college work, instead favouring her own ideas for new projects. Up until this point Lucy had been a quiet, hardworking and conscientious student. This behaviour was markedly out of character for her. This episode lasted for two weeks.

Assessment

Early intervention can be the key to bringing symptoms of bipolar disorder under control. There are several assessment tools that can be used when assessing for bipolar disorder in children and adolescents. These include the University Kiddie Schedule for Affective Disorders and Schizophrenia (WASH-U-KSADS), the Childhood Behaviour Checklist and the Child Mania Rating Scale – Parents (CMRS-P). Each of these have been shown to be effective tools in helping to identify symptoms indicating bipolar disorder (Gellar et al., 2001; Fitzgerald et al., 2018).

Although diagnostic tools are a fundamental component of the assessment process, they should not routinely be used in isolation. Whilst adolescents can meet the diagnostic criteria for bipolar disorder, they are less likely to identify changes in their own mood and evidence suggests that they have less insight into identifying fluctuations, compared with their adult counterparts (Angst 2013; Findling et al., 2018).

As a result, input from families or other professionals working with the young person is essential to making an accurate and informed diagnosis. Narratives from parents and wider family members, teachers and other health care professionals can add vital information to the overall assessment process, consequently leading to a more accurate diagnosis. It is recommended during this process that parents/carers and the child are met with both separately and together in order to gain the views of each party independently, followed by the opportunity to discuss any inconsistencies as a group (Baroni et al., 2009).

Irritability and poor judgement are likely to present in children and adolescents with bipolar disorder but they can be observed in other conditions such as ADHD, post-traumatic stress disorder (PSTD) and conduct disorder. These symptoms alone may not therefore be indicative of bipolar disorder.

Alternative diagnoses and organic causes need to be ruled out. A reduced need for sleep and elevated mood in addition to the symptoms associated with other diagnoses are strong indicators that a bipolar disorder diagnosis may be accurate (Youngstrom et al., 2008).

In addition to ruling out other diagnoses with overlapping symptoms, it is important to explore whether Lucy has used any substances that may be responsible for the symptoms she is presenting with. If it is found that substances may have contributed to her current presentation, this does not mean that a diagnosis should be ruled out as substance use is frequently observed in the early stages of bipolar disorder (Duffy et al., 2012).

Formulation and Intervention

As Lucy had presented during a depressive episode with no reported symptoms of mania, this is what she was initially monitored for. However, she has now described symptoms that are clearly indicative of a manic episode, including elated mood, reduced sleep, disinhibited behaviour and pressured speech. Therefore, she has had the minimum of three symptoms and the two mood episodes required to receive a diagnosis of bipolar disorder.

Pharmacological treatment for depressive disorders in children and adolescents is likely to include an antidepressant for a 6–12-month period, during which time symptoms will be regularly reviewed (National Institute for Health and Care Excellence [NICE], 2017). However, antidepressants can induce episodes of mania. Therefore, Lucy would not be routinely prescribed an antidepressant as she has reported symptoms that may suggest a diagnosis of bipolar disorder.

The recommended intervention for bipolar disorder is to prescribe medication with mood-stabilising properties, e.g. atypical antipsychotics, anticonvulsants or lithium. This is the recommended treatment for both adults and adolescents. Doses must be adjusted according to the British National Formulary for Children and should be reviewed after 12 weeks (NICE, 2018).

In contrast to treatment for unipolar depression, pharmacological treatment for bipolar disorder may be considered a longer-term intervention as evidence to date suggests that it is a lifelong condition. Mood-stabilising medication is used as both a prophylactic treatment and in response to episodes of mania or depression (Severus and Bauer, 2013). It must be noted that female patients of child-bearing potential should not be prescribed valproate as a mood stabiliser, as it is teratogenic.

NICE guidelines (2018) suggest that a psychological therapy such as cognitive behavioural therapy (CBT) or interpersonal therapy should run concurrently with pharmacological interventions. The child's development, cognitive ability and emotional functioning must be taken into account when deciding the best course of treatment, along with their views and capacity to consent. Evidence suggests that, when treating children and adolescents with bipolar disorder, family involvement in therapy can be beneficial to treatment (Salinger et al., 2018). In addition to psychological therapies, psychoeducation is a key factor in helping people to control and manage their illness. As young people can find it difficult to objectively notice changes in their own mood, strategies, e.g. a mood diary, can be important tools to help the young person self-identify changes in their presentation.

It has been shown that both pharmacological and psychological treatments are more effective when begun in the early stages of the illness (Joyce et al., 2016). It is vital that interventions are offered as soon as a diagnosis is established.

Prognosis

It is currently thought, based on available evidence, that bipolar disorder is a chronic and, at times, disabling condition with poor rates of remission (Ferrari et al., 2016). However, with the right combination of treatment, it is possible for people to experience periods of stability, and studies have shown that approximately one-third of people diagnosed can experience euthymic mood up to 80% of the time (Birmaher, 2017).

Higher rates of suicide have been noted in bipolar disorder compared with any other psychiatric diagnosis. Current evidence suggests that an earlier age of onset further increases this risk (Joslyn et al., 2015). This, in addition to long-term physical health implications, social difficulties and overall functioning, all indicate that if untreated bipolar disorder can be a destructive illness in which the individual's quality of life can be severely affected.

For these reasons, and those mentioned throughout this chapter, early diagnosis, prompt, evidence-based interventions and person-centred care are key factors in helping the young person to manage their illness successfully across their lifespan.

Multiple-Choice Questions

See answers on page 670.

1. How many symptoms of mania need to be present for a diagnosis of bipolar disorder to be made?
   a. 2
   b. 3
   c. 4
   d. 5
2. Which medications are not recommended when treating bipolar disorder?
   a. Antidepressants
   b. Anticonvulsants
   c. Antipsychotics
3. Which of the following are symptoms of mania?
   a. Pressured speech
   b. Flight of ideas
   c. Extreme mood changes throughout the day
   d. Decreased need for sleep
4. Which of the following psychological therapies are recommended by NICE to treat bipolar disorder?
   a. Cognitive behavioural therapy
   b. Dialectical behavioural therapy
   c. Acceptance and commitment therapy
   d. Interpersonal therapy
5. Which factors may have contributed to the rise in young people being diagnosed with bipolar disorder?
   a. A rise in prevalence
   b. A change in diagnostic criteria
   c. Over-diagnosis

Key References

Baron, A., Lunsford, J., Luckenbaugh, D., Towbin, K., Leibenluft, E., (2009). Practitioner review: the assessment of bipolar disorder in children and adolescents. *Journal of Child Psychology and Psychiatry*, 50(3): 203–215.

Findling, R., Stepanova, E., Youngstrom, E., Young, A., (2018). Progress in diagnosis and treatment of bipolar disorder among children and adolescents: an international perspective. *Evidence-Based Mental Health*, 21(4): 177–181.

National Institute for Health and Care Excellence [NICE], (2018). *Bipolar disorder: assessment and management (CG185)*. Available from: https://www.nice.org.uk/guidance/cg185.

45 Fear and Anxiety

Julie Hadwin and Roxanne Magdalena

KEY CONCEPTS

- Anxiety disorders reflect increased fear and anxious affect.
- Fear reflects an adaptive and instinctive response that prepares individuals to 'run or escape' from threat and danger (Cannon, 1932, p. 227).
- Anxiety signifies a chronic emotional state often associated with uncertainty and increased vigilance for potential threat (Steimer, 2002).
- Fear and anxiety are linked to physiological arousal and avoidance of situations perceived to be threatening (American Psychiatric Association (APA), 2013, p. 189), and when an individual is unable to manage symptoms, feelings of stress increase (Putwain, 2007).

Core Symptoms

While the focus of concern between anxiety disorders is different, core physical, cognitive/emotional and behavioural symptoms are common and can occur in anticipation of or when faced with feared objects or events.

Physical

Heart racing/pounding, sweating, shaking, dizziness, 'butterflies', nausea, vomiting, dry mouth, headaches, hyperventilation. In younger children, symptoms may present as somatic complaints, e.g. stomach ache.

Cognitive/Emotional

Worry, fear, crying, feeling 'on edge' or under threat, irritability/tantrums, uncertainty, reduced attentional focus/control.

Behavioural

Feared situations are avoided or 'endured with intense fear or anxiety' (APA, 2013).

A recent review reported that the mean age of onset of anxiety is 11 years, and symptoms reach a peak in middle age and decline thereafter (Bandelow and Michaelas, 2015). Across anxiety disorders the authors reported a lifetime prevalence rate of around 30%, with a female to male ratio of approximately 1.5:1.

Anxiety Disorders in Children and Adolescents

Feelings of anxiety and fear emerge and dissipate across typical development (Muris et al., 2000). Anxiety disorders reflect developmentally atypical anxious affect and associated distress, that is enduring and impacts on daily functioning (Mohr and Schneider, 2013). Anxiety disorders occur in around 6% of children and adolescents and have a significant negative impact on development, including reduced achievement in school and poor physical health (Battaglia et al., 2017), in addition to increased unemployment and challenges with social adaptation (Copeland et al., 2014; de Lijster et al., 2018).

Several anxiety disorders emerge in childhood and adolescence, including selective mutism, separation anxiety disorder, specific phobia, social anxiety disorder, panic disorder and agoraphobia and generalised anxiety disorder (APA, 2013). Anxiety disorders are often co-morbid with each other, and with neurodevelopmental disorders (Franz et al., 2013) and depression (Cummings et al., 2014). Around one-quarter of children diagnosed with attention deficit hyperactivity disorder (Jarrett and Ollendick, 2008) and half of those diagnosed with an autism spectrum disorder (van Steensel et al., 2011) meet the diagnostic criteria for an anxiety disorder.

There is often disagreement in the reporting of anxiety symptoms between different informants (parents and teachers versus children or adolescents themselves), and a multi-informant approach in its assessment is recommended (Spence, 2018). Key epidemiological features and core symptoms of anxiety disorders are outlined in diagnostic manuals (APA, 2013; World Health Organization, 2004), including:

Separation anxiety – linked to significant distress associated with actual or anticipated separation from an attachment figure. Lifetime prevalence is around 4%, and recent data suggest a bimodal age of onset in childhood and early adulthood, with respective prevalence rates of around 4% and 6% respectively (Silove et al., 2015).

Selective mutism – occurs in fewer than 1% of children. It is typically identified when a child starts school. Its core symptom reflects a lack of speech in situations where there is an expectation to speak, i.e. in the school environment and when this absence is not evident in different contexts, i.e. when the child is at home (Muris and Ollendick, 2015).

Specific phobia – occurs in around 6% of children and adolescents (Ollendick et al., 2017) and is characterised by an acute and immediate fearful reaction linked to a specific object or event, that is out of proportion to the reality of the situation. Diagnostically, fears are separated into animal, natural environment, blood-injection-injury, situational (e.g. enclosed spaces or fear of choking types – APA, 2013).

Social anxiety disorder – symptoms include worries and fears associated with being scrutinised by others. These symptoms can relate to different social situations or can be restricted to those that include a performance element, e.g. giving a presentation. It typically emerges in late childhood or early adolescence, and its development is uncommon after the age of 25 years (Spence and Rapee, 2016).

Generalised anxiety disorder – worry is the core cognitive component of generalised anxiety disorder, and individuals experience fear and worry on most days and across different topics and events. The typical age of onset is 15 years, with prevalence rates of around 5% (Newman, Llera, Erickson, Przeworski and Castonguay, 2013). It is often co-morbid with other anxiety disorders and with depression (Moffitt et al., 2007). Generalised anxiety disorder and depression are referred to as chronic 'anxious-misery states' (Kendler, Prescott, Myers and Neale, 2003, p. 929).

Panic disorder, with or without agoraphobia – children diagnosed with separation anxiety disorder are at increased risk of developing panic disorder (Kossowsky, 2013). The typical age of onset is 15–19 years, and the prevalence rate is around 1–2%. Panic disorder is associated with repeated panic attacks, described as an 'abrupt surge of intense fear or intense discomfort that reaches a peak within minutes' (APA, 2013, p. 214). Worry about panic attacks leads to an avoidance of situations where escape would be difficult or embarrassing. This behaviour is associated with a diagnosis of agoraphobia. Agoraphobia typically emerges in adolescence or adulthood and has a prevalence of around 5% (Magee, Eaton, Wittchen, McGonagle and Kessler, 1996).

Key Features of Anxiety in Development

Anxiety is atypical if it is out of proportion to the situation at hand, persisting or interferes with daily functioning and quality of life. Around 8% of children and adolescents meet the diagnostic criteria for at least one or more anxiety disorder. They are more common in females and are often co-morbid with neurodevelopmental disorders and depression. Anxiety disorders in children include selective mutism, separation anxiety and specific problems and in adolescence, social anxiety disorder, panic disorder and agoraphobia and generalised anxiety disorder. Evidence suggests that CBT is effective for most anxiety disorders and can be used in conjunction with adjunct psychological and pharmacological therapies.

Risk Factors for Anxiety

Research has explored narrow risks associated with specific anxiety disorders, e.g. disgust sensitivity is most linked to specific phobia (Oar, Farrell and Ollendick, 2015). It has highlighted risks that are common, i.e. transdiagnostic, across different anxiety disorders, e.g. temperament, poor attentional control, cognitive biases for threat, intolerance of uncertainty (Norton and Paulus, 2017) or between internalising and externalising disorders, e.g. low socioeconomic status, experience of early adversity and trauma, disorganised or insecure attachment relationships with significant others (McLaughlin et al., 2012; Ein-Dor et al., 2016).

Genetic influence – has been highlighted via family studies, showing that anxiety disorders are evident across generations within the same family (Sydsjö et al., 2018). Twin studies consistently report heritability rates of around 30–40% for anxiety disorders and related traits, e.g. parental overcontrol (Eley et al., 2010). There is an emerging literature on genome-wide association studies (GWAS) that have reported some, though limited, evidence on genetic variation associated with different anxiety disorders, and there is a need for further studies in this area of research (review by Otowa et al., 2016).

Temperament – temperamental differences in development are assumed to have a biological basis and often sit at the core of theoretical frameworks in anxiety (e.g. Oar et al., 2015; Spence and Rapee, 2016). Research studies consistently show that children who display behavioural inhibition, i.e. a temperamental style characterised by increased negative affect and avoidance in novel/unfamiliar situations and associated personality traits, i.e. neuroticism, are at increased risk for the development of anxiety (Lonigan et al., 2011). Research suggests that temperament is likely to interact with genetic, cognitive and environmental factors to increase risk (e.g. White et al., 2017).

Environmental influence – several studies have highlighted that specific aspects of the environment place children and adolescents at increased risk of anxiety. Within families, maternal overprotection and an absence of paternal behaviour that challenges offspring to move beyond their comfort zone have been associated with anxiety (review by Möller et al., 2016). Parent modelling of fearful behaviour and the sharing of negative verbal information that conveys threat about some aspect of the environment have been associated with the development of anxiety (Percy et al., 2016). Further studies indicate that negative experiences can act as conditioning events to place children at risk of specific phobias (review by Shechner et al., 2014). Adverse peer experiences (e.g. low support and acceptance) have been associated with the development of anxiety in adolescence and with specific elements placing girls at most risk (e.g. relational victimisation) (Pickering et al., 2019).

Interventions for Anxiety

Following National Institute for Health and Care Excellence (NICE, 2014) guidelines, children and adolescents diagnosed with anxiety disorder are typically offered evidence-based psychological interventions (cognitive behavioural therapy – CBT) via child and adolescent mental health services (CAMHS). Across anxiety disorders, CBT, irrespective of the nature of its delivery, whether in groups, individually, with or without parent involvement, via the internet or in person, is typically effective for around 60% of children and adolescents (James et al., 2013).

Recent reviews suggest that CBT may be less effective for children and adolescents diagnosed with social anxiety disorder (Leigh and Clark, 2018). In some cases, and where symptoms are severe, young people are prescribed selective serotonin reuptake inhibitors (SSRIs) to augment or replace psychological interventions (Patel, 2018). The recognition of common risk and core symptoms and co-morbidity between anxiety disorders with depression, for instance, has led to an increase in the use of transdiagnostic CBT interventions (Ehrenreich-May et al., 2017).

Recent interventions have been developed to target symptoms that characterise specific anxiety disorders, e.g. one-session treatment for specific phobia (Farrell et al., 2018) and meta-cognitive therapy for the treatment of generalised anxiety disorder (Esbjørn et al., 2018). Though the evidence base is less extensive, further studies have explored the effect of novel or adjunct therapies on anxiety symptom reduction, including bibliotherapy (review by Yuan et al., 2017), attention-based interventions (review by or mindfulness-based psychotherapies (review by Zenner et al., 2014).

Case Study (1): Joe

During his early years Joe was removed from his parents' care for a year-long period due to significant domestic violence from his father towards his mother, that he witnessed first-hand. He had then returned to live with his mother. Aged seven, Joe presented with tiredness, stomach ache and nausea in the mornings, resulting in reduced school attendance. He was unable to fall asleep until the early hours of the morning because of 'seeing shadowy figures' in his room.

The response to anxiety symptoms, e.g. avoidance of school when feeling unwell, maintained and reinforced Joe's anxiety. This avoidance may have served the unconscious function of ensuring his mother's physical safety and that his father did not return. Joe's poor sleep and night-time experiences reflected a state of hyperarousal that resulted from his traumatic early experiences and led to hypervigilance for threat and misinterpretation of typical stimuli as threatening.

A history of Joe's early experiences and milestones was taken, during separate interviews with Joe and his mother. Younger children may report physical symptoms of anxiety rather than describing anxiety cognitions. An assessment of Joe's physical health was explored to exclude a physical illness.

A broader approach was taken to treatment, given the presence of anxiety and trauma. Family therapy sessions were arranged with Joe's mother to discuss their traumatic experiences and to consider how needs were being communicated within the family. The family was reassured that the shadowy figures were not an indicator of psychosis. A CBT approach to anxiety management was taken. Due to Joe's age and his difficulties with identifying and verbalising his anxious thoughts, this approach focussed more on behaviour than cognitions. Joe's mother was included in CBT sessions to enable the two of them to develop techniques to use at home and to find a better understanding of how Joe's anxious thoughts and feelings were reflected in his behaviour.

Case Study (2): Lauren

Lauren (16) reported feelings of anxiety when speaking to others, both in social situations and performance (speaking in front of others). Lauren described fears of being humiliated in public and being preoccupied with thoughts that others were staring at her and judging her. Following a worsening of anxiety and developing panic attacks, she had recently started to drink excessive amounts of alcohol at weekends on a regular basis, to manage her difficulties around others.

Lauren met criteria for social anxiety disorder, reflecting an avoidance of social relationships, particularly with unfamiliar people, and the intense fear of public scrutiny and humiliation. The assessment considered whether other anxiety disorders were present and asked about substance use.

A CBT-based intervention allowed Lauren's thoughts to be challenged and her beliefs about others tested. Due to the impact on her functioning, Sertraline was started, alongside regular CBT, with good effect. Lauren was given specific advice on managing her alcohol use.

Case Study (3): Nico

Nico (11) was diagnosed with an ASD. Nico experienced social communication difficulties, but had been managing well in primary school. He recently began at mainstream secondary school and described feeling worried at break times. Symptoms included heart racing and a shortness of breath.

Peer social relationships had become more complex, and Nico was struggling to understand the subtler nature of interpersonal communication. Moving from a smaller nurturing environment in primary school where his difficulties had been well managed, to a larger secondary school where he was expected to be more independent, had left him feeling more vulnerable.

This process involved considering which aspects of anxiety were related to Nico's ASD and whether he had a separate anxiety disorder, distinct from his ASD.

Treatment included meeting with Nico's teachers to explain how his ASD affected him and to consider how he could be supported during unstructured activity time. CBT was started, using an adapted approach taking Nico's autism into consideration. Adaptations included using familiar and factual scenarios, rather than using metaphors or abstract exercises. A clinician met with the family to discuss how anxiety can arise from ASD and to consider ways his environment could be adapted, e.g. preparing him visually for transitions between activities.

Useful Online Resources

- Self-help and therapy resource: https://www.get.gg/
- A self-help guide for phobias: http://www.moodjuice.scot.nhs.uk/phobias.asp
- The Child Anxiety Network: http://childanxiety.net/
- Anxiety and phobias in teenagers: http://kidshealth.org/teen/your_mind/mental_health/phobias.html

Multiple-Choice Questions

See answers on page 670.

1. Separation anxiety can develop:
   a. In childhood
   b. In adolescence
   c. In early adulthood
   d. In early childhood or early adulthood
2. Transdiagnostic risk factors are important for understanding:
   a. The diagnosis of two or more anxiety disorders
   b. The diagnosis of co-morbid anxiety and depression
   c. The diagnosis of co-morbid anxiety and neurodevelopmental disorders
   d. All of the above
3. A child is asked to report on her symptoms of anxiety. One of her parents and her teacher are also asked to provide an anxiety report. Considering the child's anxiety symptoms:
   a. The child is most likely to agree with the parent.
   b. The child is most likely to agree with the teacher.
   c. The teacher and parent are most likely to agree with each other.
   d. It is unlikely that the child, parent or teacher will agree.
4. Studies have suggested that cognitive behavioural therapy (CBT) is likely to be least effective for a child or adolescent who has been given a diagnosis of:
   a. Separation anxiety disorder
   b. Social anxiety disorder
   c. Generalised anxiety disorder
   d. Panic disorder
5. 'Anxious-misery states' is a term used to refer to:
   a. Generalised anxiety disorder and depression
   b. Selective mutism and social anxiety disorder
   c. Any two co-morbid anxiety disorders
   d. Panic disorder and agoraphobia

Key References

American Psychiatric Association, (2013). *Diagnostic and statistical manual of mental disorders* (5th ed.). Washington, DC: American Psychiatric Association.

Copeland, W.E., Angold, A., Shanahan, L., Costello, E.J., (2014). Longitudinal patterns of anxiety from childhood to adulthood: The Great Smoky Mountains study. *Journal of the American Academy of Child and Adolescent Psychiatry*, 53: 21–33. doi: 10.1016/j.jaac.2013.09.017.

Spence, S.H., (2018). Assessing anxiety disorders in children and adolescents. *Child and Adolescent Mental Health*, 23: 266–282. doi: 10.111/camh.12251.

46 OCD and Related Disorders

Phill Nagle, Christopher Gale and Jo Barker

Introduction

The DSM-5 and most recent ICD-11 diagnostic manuals have re-classified obsessive compulsive disorder (OCD) from an anxiety disorder and collected it with disorders indicating similar presenting symptoms and causal factors. This group includes OCD, body dysmorphic disorder (BDD), hoarding disorder, trichotillomania, i.e. hair-pulling, and excoriation, i.e. skin-picking, disorder.

These disorders share cognitive phenomena, e.g. preoccupations, obsessions and intrusive thoughts, with accompanying compulsive behaviours. Hoarding's central cognition is a compulsion to keep things. There is less of a cognitive aspect for habitual action-driven repetitive behaviour disorders, such as skin or hair pulling. Each disorder's symptoms result in significant distress or functional impairment. The focus of this chapter is OCD and BDD, the most common presentations within children and young people.

KEY CONCEPTS

- Obsessive thoughts lead to anxiety; compulsive behaviours temporarily reduce the anxiety, but this reinforces the obsessive thought.
- OCD can be very debilitating, can be misdiagnosed and requires willingness for treatment in order for symptoms to improve.
- BDD is a somatoform disorder, where the individual is excessively preoccupied with a perceived or minor bodily defect. It can have a chronic course and prognosis, if untreated.
- The prevalence of BDD in under 18s is difficult to ascertain, because of normal angst around body image experienced by many developing young people.
- The evidence base for the assessment and management of BDD is limited, especially so in children and young people, and relies on wider research into OCD and adult-based studies and theory.
- The first line intervention for both OCD and BDD with children and young people is CBT with ERP, with an SSRI medication as an adjunct, if deemed clinically appropriate.
- Related disorder trichotillomania's interventions differ, as adapted CBT, e.g. habit reversal therapy, is recommended and antidepressants are not.

Obsessive-Compulsive Disorder

Obsessive-compulsive disorder (OCD) is characterised by recurrent obsessions and/or compulsions, most commonly both, that cause significant distress and/or impairment of functioning. Obsessive compulsive disorder can be chronic, continuous or episodic.

Key Features

An obsession is defined as a frequent and repetitive intrusive thought, image or urge that causes an increase in distress or anxiety. Typical obsessions in children and adolescents include a fear of contamination, fear of offending God, unwanted sexual thoughts often around family members or children, thoughts of harming others and transformation worries. OCD thoughts are no different from other thoughts. It is the significant meaning attached to the thought that causes distress, as it might clash with the personal values of the young person or create a fear of responsibility for something 'bad' happening.

Compulsions are repetitive physical behaviours, mental acts or avoidance behaviours that the person feels driven to perform, are difficult to resist and carried out in an attempt to reduce the anxiety or distress caused by the obsession. A compulsion can either be an external action, such as checking that the door is locked, or internal action, e.g. repeating a certain phrase in one's mind. They are not enjoyable and do not result in the completion of any useful task. Children may often involve their family in their compulsive acts, e.g. in checking, counting or cleaning, or may persistently demand reassurance. Compulsions help maintain OCD as they provide temporary relief from distress and prevent disconfirmation of belief.

The symptoms of OCD are time-consuming, can cause significant distress and disrupt social and academic functioning.

Epidemiology

- OCD has been estimated to affect 0.25–2% of children and adolescents.
- It is the fourth most common mental health disorder in young people.
- It is thought that OCD can start at any time from pre-school to adulthood, but there are two peaks of presentation, i.e. between the ages of 10 and 12 and between late teenage and early adulthood.
- The World Health Organization (WHO) ranked OCD in the top ten most disabling illnesses of any kind.
- There is no single proven cause, although theories suggest that causes include genetics, life stresses, neurobiology and psychological factors or cognitive biases.
- Evidence shows that early diagnosis and assertive treatment are likely to improve the outcome. OCD is unlikely to improve without treatment. One in three children with OCD will make a complete recovery; 50% of cases persist into adulthood and 10% follow a chronic deteriorating course.

Assessment

The NICE guidelines (2005) recommend that when OCD is suspected direct screening questions should be asked such as:

- Do you wash or clean a lot?
- Do you check things a lot?

- Is there any thought that keeps bothering you that you would like to get rid of but can't?
- Do your daily activities take a long time to finish?
- Are you concerned about orderliness or symmetry?
- Do these problems trouble you?

Detailed assessment should include:

- An accurate description of presenting symptoms, i.e. content of thoughts, types of compulsions, onset, severity and frequency. The Children's Yale-Brown Obsessive Compulsive Scale (C/YBOCS) is a validated assessment measure that is widely used in specialist centres to rate symptom severity and functional impairment (Goodman et al., 1991).
- A consideration of the **predisposing**, e.g. genetic factors, **precipitating**, e.g. traumatic events, **perpetuating** factors, e.g. parental reinforcement, and **protective** factors, e.g. high self-esteem.
- Exclusion of other diagnoses and assessment of possible co-morbidity. The POTS (2004) study suggests 80% co-morbidity and of family disturbance.
- It is vital to assess any risk of self-harm and suicide, particularly if depression has been diagnosed.
- Evaluation of family dynamics and the degree of family involvement in OCD.
- Assessment of parental anxiety and other mental illness.
- Consideration of developmental issues. Some superstitious behaviour and routines may be developmentally normal.

Challenges in Assessment

- Shame or embarrassment associated with thoughts or behaviours may reduce engagement.
- Lack of insight/masking extent of difficulties.
- Impaired concentration.
- Hesitance of verbalising thoughts, due to thought–action fusion.
- Apparent risk, i.e. thoughts about harming others.
- The bizarre nature of symptoms may appear like other disorders.

Differential Diagnoses

- Normal developmental variation. Children commonly have non-intense routines/rituals that are normal up to the age of four.
- Primary depressive disorder with secondary obsessive/compulsive symptoms.
- Tic disorders, e.g. more likely to be touching, counting and blinking.
- Pervasive developmental disorder. Stereotypes can appear similar to rituals.
- Neurological, e.g. brain injury, post-encephalitis, tumours
- Paediatric autoimmune neuro-psychiatric disorders (PANDAS) associated with streptococcal infection
- Body dysmorphic disorder (BDD)
- Eating disorders
- Psychosis

Possible Co-Morbid Conditions

- Depression (35%)
- Anxiety disorders (40%)

- Tic disorder/Tourette syndrome (50–60% of TS patients have OCD)
- Substance misuse
- ADHD (30%)
- Oppositional defiant disorder (43%)
- Developmental disorders including autism
- Hoarding
- Eating disorder

Intervention

The NICE guideline on the treatment of OCD (2005) recommends a stepped care approach with increasing intensity according to clinical severity and complexity.

Mild Functional Impairment

Guided self-help may be effective in early or mild OCD (see links below for resources). Psychoeducation about the diagnosis should be given, and the young person and family should be helped not to feel blame or shame. If self-help is refused or ineffective, the young person should be offered CBT.

Moderate or Severe Impairment

Cognitive behavioural therapy (CBT), and especially exposure plus response prevention (ERP), is an effective treatment for OCD and should be offered first. If CBT is ineffective or refused, a selective serotonin reuptake inhibitor (SSRI) should be considered after multi-disciplinary review.

If the CBT+SSRI combination is ineffective, then switching to a different SSRI or augmentation with Clomipramine or anti-psychotic medication may be considered in a specialist setting.

Inpatient treatment may be required in severe cases.

CBT with Exposure and Response Prevention (ERP)

CBT should include thorough assessment and collaborative formulation, psychoeducation, ERP and relapse prevention. Research suggests that the active element of CBT for OCD is ERP and the cognitive element of CBT treatment is not needed, unless in difficult-to-treat OCD (Tolin et al., 2008). In ERP, the young person makes a list of feared situations and begins with the least feared. They then repeatedly practise facing the fear (EXPOSURE) without carrying out a ritual (RESPONSE PREVENTION). The aim is for the young person to experience their anxiety reducing over time, whilst remaining in the feared situation. The young person learns that their anxiety will reduce with repeated exposure. 'Overlearning' and relapse prevention are important parts of the treatment for long-term efficacy.

The family/carers should be involved. This may lead to greater success due to the reinforcing accommodations family develop and the link to parental anxiety in the perpetuation of the disorder. Family involvement is essential for children under 11. Manual-based treatments can be usefully drawn upon (March and Mulle, 1998).

Treatment with Medication

OCD is thought to be associated with altered brain functioning in the basal ganglia and orbitofrontal cortex. OCD responds specifically to drugs that inhibit the synaptic reuptake of serotonin. The only SSRIs licensed for use with children and young people experiencing OCD are Sertraline and Fluvoxamine. Where there is significant co-morbid depression, Fluoxetine can be prescribed. Response may take up to 12 weeks, maximal doses may be required and improvements can continue for up to one year. Medication should be continued for at least six months after remission to reduce the risk of relapse, although maintenance therapy may be at a lower dose. Withdrawal from SSRIs should be very gradual to minimise adverse side-effects.

Case Study (1): Liam

Liam (13) presented to child and adolescent mental health services (CAMHS) following a referral from his mother. She reported that Liam experienced sexual thoughts about people in authority, such as his teachers and his parents. Liam felt guilty every time he had these thoughts and felt compelled to inform his mother of every thought he had, seeking reassurance that his thoughts did not mean he was 'dirty-minded' or a 'pervert' and checked if these thoughts were 'okay'. Liam's concentration at school suffered as a result and he would send messages to his mother throughout the day explicitly stating each thought.

Liam found this so difficult that he began to avoid looking at his teachers and his attendance at school dropped. He avoided his parents at home and stayed in his room to reduce contact.

Liam was seen by a CBT therapist at CAMHS, who worked with Liam and his mother. He was seen for 12 sessions of CBT with the focus on tolerating the distress caused by the thoughts and reducing the maintenance factors of reassurance seeking. Liam and his family disengaged from the sessions once they believed that the OCD was at a 'manageable level' that was not significantly interfering with Liam's life. This was against clinic advice as the treatment was incomplete.

Case Study (2): Helga

Helga (16) presented to CAMHS following a referral from her GP. After a number of close family bereavements and her sister developing a chronic illness, Helga began experiencing high levels of anxiety regarding becoming ill and around cleanliness. Her handwashing increased to over 30 times daily, and her hands became red and chapped. She reduced her dietary intake due to fears of food being contaminated and needed to prepare all her own food. She took anti-bacterial wipes with her in order to wipe down any surfaces that she touched. She was unable to use public transport, and her attendance at college reduced. She developed panic attacks and due to these problems persisting over 18 months, her mood deteriorated and she began having suicidal thoughts. Helga felt responsible for her sister's health and reduced her socialising and performed actions in threes to prevent harm coming to her.

Helga was seen for an initial assessment at CAMHS and was placed on a waiting list for CBT. Whilst waiting for this intervention, Helga was prescribed Sertraline by her GP. Once allocated to a CBT therapist, Helga was seen weekly for 18 sessions and had 2 follow-up sessions, spaced at 2-month intervals.

Following psychoeducation, Helga and her therapist worked up Helga's 'fear ladder' through exposure response prevention (ERP) tasks. Helga's cognitive process during the tasks became:

> 'acknowledge the OCD thought. This is only the amygdala sending a danger signal to the brain when it is not needed. Therefore, I do not have to do anything and can just get on with my day'.

Helga was able to complete tasks including catching the bus and touching railings without cleaning first, touching bin handles without handwashing, performing actions in twos, then once, then not at all, eating food without handwashing first and as 'overlearning' tasks, eating biscuits from places generally thought of as 'unclean' (e.g. the floor), without performing any compulsive ritual before or after. Helga's Y-BOCS scores fell to virtually zero, her attendance at college increased, she was no longer handwashing excessively and was able to socialise without feeling a responsibility for others. Helga was discharged with a relapse plan, having reclaimed her life from OCD.

Body Dysmorphic Disorder

Young people with body dysmorphic disorder (BDD) will experience an obsessive preoccupation with an imagined flaw in their physical appearance, when other people cannot see it or the physical anomaly is slight. These worries develop into compulsive behaviours or routines to deal with the emotional distress caused by the worries. These behaviours can be very time-consuming, e.g. several hours in any one 'routine', significantly impacting on a young person's attendance at school or work and on their ability to socialise with peers. He or she may wake exceptionally early in the day to perform the routines of checking or camouflaging, thus disturbing their sleep patterns and energy levels.

Key Features

- **Intrusive thoughts** about one or more areas of the body such as being out of proportion, too big or too small, disfigured, lacking symmetry or a belief about a defect that makes one ugly or deformed.
- **Compulsive behaviours**, e.g. constantly checking in the mirror, camouflaging with make-up, touching the body part, measuring the defect, excessive grooming, skin picking, reassurance-seeking, surgery or medical consultations, excessive exercise often directed to one particular area, avoiding social situations, comparing appearance to other people and changing posture.
- The young person's concern is markedly **excessive**. Excessive physical appearance concerns causing emotional distress. Significant impact on functioning and on day-to-day life.

Many young people do not seek help because they are worried that they will be perceived as self-obsessed or vain. Others may not do so due to embarrassment, if concerned with the appearance/size of their genitals, for instance. As adults, many will seek intervention from cosmetic surgeons as an alternative (Ashraf, 2000). This may explain the gap between age of onset of BDD, commonly held to be during adolescence, and its diagnosis and treatment, often during an individual's 20s or 30s.

Epidemiology

- NICE suggest that 0.5–0.7% of the population have BDD.
- The prevalence of BDD ranges from 1–2% (Arthur and Monnell, 2005) to 13% (Biby, 1998) of the general population and 13% of the psychiatric adult inpatient population (Reynolds, et al 2001). This range may be accounted for by the inclusion or exclusion of body image issues associated with eating disorders, in addition to the feelings of shame that prevent many BDD sufferers from seeking professional help from mental health services (Reynolds, et al 2001; Veale, 2002).

- Another explanation for the lack of identification in adolescence is the perceived crucial role of body image and issues of identity development, peer relationships, dating and sexuality (Levine and Smolak, 2002). This lack of identification would suggest that any prevalence rates in this age group are potentially underestimated (2.2% – Mayville et al., 1999). The presentation of symptoms/behaviours in adolescence does not appear to differ from that of adulthood (Phillips et al., 2006). There is often a chronic nature and course to the illness, with an average of 16 years' duration.

Possible Causal Factors

Fully establishing the causal factors relating to BDD is difficult, as research in this area remains sparse and conducted mainly with adult clinical populations, due to the feelings of shame that can delay presentation to mental health services. Mental health services do not routinely include body image screening questions during initial assessments. Despite these challenges, genetic, neurobiological and psychological (e.g. bullying, low self-esteem and perfectionism) have all been proposed as causal factors.

Assessment

Because of the increased risk of suicidal behaviour in individuals with BDD, NICE (2005) recommend that a thorough risk assessment and risk management plan is conducted at the earliest possible opportunity. As part of a CAMHS assessment, the following five questions should be included, if BDD is suspected in a young person:

- Do you worry a lot about the way you look and wish you could think about it less?
- What specific concerns do you have about your appearance?
- On a typical day, how many hours a day is your appearance on your mind? More than one hour a day is considered excessive.
- What effect does it have on your life?
- Does it make it hard to do your work or be with friends?

Much of the literature about BDD emphasises the importance of using diagnostic screening tools, e.g. the Body Dysmorphic Disorder Questionnaire (BDDQ), the Yale Brown Obsessive Compulsive Scale for BDD (BDD-YBOCS) and the Body Dysmorphic Diagnostic Module (BDDM).

Veale (2001) outlines the CBT model for assessing BDD, looking at a trigger, i.e. reflection in the mirror, causing the processing of self as an aesthetic object, that leads to a negative appraisal of one's body image, e.g. depression or disgust, and the avoidance and safety behaviours, i.e. mirror checking or camouflaging.

In addition, it is important to consider the impact of the BDD symptoms on other members of the family: how does each family member respond when the young person is 'stuck' in their checking/grooming routine?

BDD and Other Mental Disorders

As stated earlier, BDD has been classified within the OCD umbrella in the DSM-5 and ICD-11. NICE has grouped OCD and BDD together in its guideline for assessment and treatment (NICE, 2005).

There are distinct differences, however, highlighted alongside the commonalities in Table 46.1.

Table 46.1 Similarities and Differences between BDD and OCD

Similarities between BDD and OCD	*Differences between BDD and OCD*
• Persistent and intrusive thoughts, e.g. is my nose to big? Am I ugly? • Compulsive behaviours, e.g. grooming, mirror checking • Treatment approaches, i.e. SSRI anti-depressant medication and cognitive behaviour therapy	• BDD suffers generally have poorer insight (Phillips et al., 1995) • Checking behaviours increase rather than decrease anxiety (Phillips et al., 1995) • BDD has a greater co-morbidity with depression and social phobia (Frare et al., 2004) • BDD sufferers are less likely to form long-term relationships or hold down employment (Goldsmith et al., 1998)

BDD is often misdiagnosed as an eating disorder, as the symptoms may appear similar, i.e. preoccupation with body image, worry about appearance and compensatory behaviours. Eating disorder cognitive preoccupations are more likely to be about weight and shape, rather than the specific features that feature in BDD.

Other co-morbid presentations include:

- Borderline personality disorder Gunderson, J. G. (2011)
- Depression (Labuschagne et al., 2010)
- Anxiety (Labuschagne et al., 2010)
- Suicidal thoughts or suicide attempts: 22–29% in BDD sufferers (Arthur and Monnell, 2005)

Intervention

A clear feature of the NICE (2005) recommended interventions with BDD is its links to OCD. As with OCD, the two key interventions in the management of moderate to severe BDD are the use of cognitive behaviour therapy (CBT), with the inclusion of exposure and response prevention strategies. Emphasis is placed on the importance of family/carers being involved in the therapeutic process and supporting experimental activities away from the therapeutic setting. As an adjunct, the introduction of an SSRI or Clomipramine is suggested, especially if the young person is experiencing low mood. The stepped care model of intervention outlines the appropriate treatment at each level of severity of the disorder.

The use of SSRI antidepressant medication with young people under the age of 18 is contentious, because of the perceived potential for an increased risk of suicidal ideation. The British National Formulary for Children (2010) recommends that when prescribing Fluoxetine, the SSRI considered best tolerated in young people, a maximum dose of 20 mg daily is considered. For adults, the maximum dose is 80 mg for cases of severe depression or OCD. One of the few studies about the adolescent presentation of BDD (Phillips et al., 1995) saw a significant reduction of BDD symptoms after ten weeks, with a dose of only 60 mg a day. Veale (2004) suggests that these doses should be prescribed for at least 12–16 weeks before considering whether the medication has proved effective.

Although NICE (2005) do not specifically recommend the introduction of family therapy with those children and young people experiencing BDD, as with many other mental disorders in under 18s, an exploration of its impact on the family and any possible maintaining influences within the family system should be explored.

Case Study: Tilly

Tilly (15) has expressed concerns about her physical appearance since the age of five, asking her parents if she looked 'okay'. Her concerns have increased in the past three years since some boys in her class at school told her she looked like a horse. This led her to carry out lengthy washing, make-up and grooming routines, for up to three hours at a time in the morning, and made a difference to her day-to-day life. She was frequently late for school and social events. Her routines have left her physically and mentally exhausted and caused conflict with her parents and younger brother at home.

Multiple-Choice Questions

See answers on page 671.

1. In obsessive compulsive disorder (OCD), which of the following would be the true definition of compulsions?
   a. Repetitive or ritualised behaviour patterns that the individual feels driven to perform in order to prevent some negative outcome happening.
   b. Repetitive thoughts about harming or distressing others.
   c. Overwhelming desires to behave in an inappropriate fashion.
   d. Ritualised worrying about negative outcome of events.
2. Which statements are true about the content of the thoughts young people with OCD experience?
   a. Young people with OCD are responsible for everything.
   b. Their thoughts contain delusions of grandeur.
   c. The belief that one has power that is pivotal to bring about or prevent subjectively crucial negative outcomes.
   d. The thought content is the same as those without OCD.
3. Which of the following is NOT a key feature of BDD?
   a. Constantly checking oneself in the mirror
   b. Camouflaging with make-up
   c. Pulling out of hair
   d. Touching the body part
   e. Measuring the defect
4. Which two treatments are considered most effective in treating moderate to severe cases of OCD/BDD?
   a. A selective serotonin reuptake inhibitor (SSRI) medication
   b. Guided self-help/relaxation
   c. Cognitive behaviour therapy
   d. Cognitive behaviour therapy with exposure and response prevention
   e. A-typical antipsychotic medication
5. What are some of the challenges in the assessment or treatment of OCD and BDD (choose three)?
   a. Embarrassment or shame regarding thoughts or behaviours reduces engagement with services.
   b. There are no effective pharmacological treatments.
   c. Unintentional parental maintenance of symptoms.
   d. Co-morbidities increase complexity.
   e. You can't create a fear hierarchy in OCD/BDD.
   f. Having thoughts to hurt others means they are more likely to act on them.

Useful Resources for Children, Young People and Families

Derisley, J., Heyman, I., Robinson, S., Turner, C., (2008). *Breaking Free from OCD: A CBT Guide for Young People and Their Families.* London: Jessica Kingsley Publishers.

March, J., Benton, C.M., (2007). *Talking Back to OCD.* New York: Guilford Press. (A self-help guide for young sufferers and their families).

Huebner, D., Matthews, B., (2007). *What To Do When Your Brain Gets Stuck: A Kids Guide to Overcoming OCD.* Magination Press. (An interactive self-help book for children and their parents).

National and Specialist OCD, BDD and Related Disorders Service, Maudsley Hospital, (2019). *Appearance Anxiety: A Guide to Understanding Body Dysmorphic Disorder for Young People, Families and Professionals.* London: Jessica Kingsley Publishers.

Helpful Websites

www.ocdisnotme.com
www.ocduk.org
www.bddfoundation.org

Key References

Franklin, M.E., Freeman, J.B., March, J.S., (2018). *Treating OCD in Children and Adolescents: A Cognitive-Behavioral Approach.* New York: Guilford Press.

Heyman, I., Mataix-Cols, D., Fineberg, N.A., (2006). Obsessive-compulsive disorder. *British Medical Journal,* 333: 424–429.

Pediatric OCD Treatment Study (POTS) Team, (2004). Cognitive-behavior therapy, sertraline, and their combination for children and adolescents with obsessive-compulsive disorder: the Pediatric OCD Treatment Study (POTS) randomized controlled trial. *Journal of the American Medical Association (JAMA),* 292(16): 1969–1976.

Phillips, K.A., Didie, E.R., Menard, W., Pagano, M.E., Fay, C., Weisberg, R.B., (2006). Clinical features of body dysmorphic disorder in adolescents and adults. *Psychiatry Research,* 141: 305–314.

Veale, D., (2002). Shame in body dysmorphic disorder. In Gilbert, P., Miles, J. (Eds.), *Body Shame: Conceptualisation, Research and Treatment* (pp. 267–228). Hove & New York: Brunner-Routledge.

47 Psychosis in Children and Young People

Tony James and Lakshmeesh Muttur Somashekhar

Introduction

Psychotic symptoms and experiences are not uncommon in childhood and adolescence. In children these experiences may not be of pathological significance. However, in adolescence, psychotic symptoms are more likely to occur in a range of emotional and other disorders, in addition to major psychotic disorders. Paranoid experiences occur along a continuum in the adolescent population (Taylor et al.,2016), can be transient and many respond to psychological approaches. By contrast, schizophrenia, a serious psychiatric disorder, that involves multi-system disturbances of perception, thinking, volition and cognition, is extremely rare before the age of ten (Eggers and Bunk, 2009). However, the incidence rises steadily through adolescence to reach a peak in early adult life to become one of the major causes of morbidity and mortality worldwide. Childhood- and adolescent-onset schizophrenia shares many characteristics with the later onset forms, but are more severe with early neurodevelopment abnormalities and a poorer response to treatment.

Aetiology

The aetiologies of psychosis and schizophrenia are complex, multifactorial and to a large degree unknown. Early-onset schizophrenia can be regarded as a neurodevelopmental disorder (an early, often prenatal deficit, that manifests later, typically in late adolescence or early adulthood). It is not entirely clear why changes occur later in life, although one hypothesis is that synaptic pruning of pyramidal level III dendritic neurones (Sellgren et al., 2019) affects connectivity. Neuroimaging studies confirm large-scale system connectivity problems and small world or local deficits (Alexander-Bloch et al., 2013) in childhood-onset schizophrenia.

Schizophrenia is a genetic disorder with heritability of 80% (Gejman et al., 2011), although the majority of new cases are sporadic and not familial (Yang et al., 2010). A polygenetic transmission, with many genes of small effect, is most likely. A *Nature* report (Schizophrenia Working Group of the Psychiatric Genomics, 2014) of 123 genes at 108 loci, although hailed as a breakthrough, raised many questions. The single nucleotide polymorphisms (SNPs) were mostly non-coding, and the most prominent gene involved, perhaps surprisingly, was the histocompatibility complex (MHC) on chromosome 6.

A variety of environmental factors play a vital role in the onset and maintenance of psychosis and schizophrenia (Table 47.1). Gene environment interactions (GxE) and gene environment correlations (G-E) are involved.

Table 47.1 Aetiological Factors for Psychosis and Schizophrenia

Genetic	Multiple genes of small effect. Rarer genes of large effect, copy number variations (CNVs) 22q11 (velocardial facial syndrome).
Environmental early	Pregnancy infections; toxoplasmosis gondii; obstetric complications; advanced paternal age; famine (Holland, WWII; China, Great Leap Forward).
Environmental childhood and later	Childhood maltreatment; urban deprivation and isolation, migration. Receptive language disorders.
Environmental later	Illegal drug use, e.g. cannabis, especially heavy use from age 13 or before.
Associated medical conditions	Steroids and other prescribed drugs (psychosis); autoimmune encephalitis, including Hashimoto's encephalitis, adrenoleukodystrophy and other white matter diseases.

Clinical Presentations

The clinical presentations for psychosis are very varied (Table 47.2). At one extreme is the acute disturbance of perceptions, most often auditory hallucinations, second or third person, speaking in a derogatory manner and commenting on the subject. Visual hallucinations are frequent, especially following drug use. In the acute state, paranoid ideation of delusions can drive the patient to become extremely agitated, frightened and to act in a defensive or aggressive manner.

Further, passivity symptoms and thought disorder, loosening of associations, derailed thinking and even a gross thought disorder, a word salad, are seen. The latter are termed 'positive symptoms'. Patients with these symptoms can present acutely to mental health services, or following public disturbances involving teachers, police, judicial system or social services. Alternative presentations are seen with 'negative symptoms' of apathy, gradual withdrawal and isolation, with poverty of thought and action. Patients with these symptoms often show a gradual, but relentless, decline in social functioning, and do not come to attention for some while. These patients do not cause a disturbance in school and can be overlooked until the

Table 47.2 Clinical Symptoms

Hallucinations are sensory perceptions in the absence of external stimuli, most often auditory hallucinations, which can be second person or third person. Visual hallucinations are also common in this age group.

Delusions are false beliefs, incompatible with the patient's social, religious or educational background, which are not amenable to reason.

Paranoid delusions; delusions of reference and delusions of control.

Passivity phenomena: thought broadcast, thought insertion and thought withdrawal and control of body functions.

Disordered thought and speech: incoherent speech (loosening of associations), neologisms or a paucity of content and ideas, i.e. poverty of speech.

Reduced or inappropriate emotional reactivity and lack of volition: negative symptoms.

Motor abnormalities: mannerisms, catatonia (rare) and stereotypies.

situation is troublesome for the patient's family or until the patient begins to display positive symptoms as well.

A proportion of young cannabis-users come to attention, or may seek help, when paranoid symptoms or hallucinations become too intense. Paranoid ideation occurs fairly frequently with non-prescribed or recreational drug use, but is mostly transient and self-limiting, that is unless the person has a particular genetic sensitivity and/or a history of maltreatment (Vinkers, 2013) or there is prolonged heavy use of the more potent types (i.e. Skunk), especially if used from an early age of, e.g. 13 years. Interestingly in the authors' experience, patients often stop using cannabis two to three months before the onset of a frank psychotic episode. Research, both population studies and neuroimaging studies, has shown the association of cannabis with the onset of psychosis and schizophrenia. Despite common belief, it does not appear to be the case that patients use cannabis as a means to alleviate developing symptoms of psychosis; rather cannabis use can precipitate or bring forward a psychotic episode.

Patients presenting with acute neurological disturbance, i.e. fits, neurological signs and symptoms suggesting encephalitis with clouding of consciousness, may display psychotic symptoms. Brain antibodies, voltage gated potassium channels (anti-VGKC-complex-antibodies) and N-methyl-D-aspartate-receptor (anti-NMDAR-antibodies) detected in blood and CSF would suggest an auto-immune encephalitis (Al-Diwani, 2017). This is an important diagnosis to make as the treatment for the associated psychosis is markedly different from traditional treatments with antipsychotic medication and includes high-dose steroids and plasmapheresis.

Case Study (1): Alice

Alice was a 14-year-old girl who developed an acute catatonic state made more concerning because she was not eating or drinking. She looked frightened and appeared at times to be responding to auditory hallucinations. She was initially admitted to a paediatric ward where she underwent physical investigations, including blood tests, EEG and an MRI scan, all of which were normal. She was considered too ill to undergo a lumbar puncture. However, blood tests for brain antibodies were negative.

Alice had been a bright girl, and she had attended a high-achieving secondary school. However, at school she had been bullied. There were no neurodevelopmental problems and no family history of psychosis. She had not used cannabis or other illegal drugs.

Alice was later admitted to a psychiatric unit where she was treated with antipsychotic medication, two types on a gradual increasing titration regime without great improvement in her auditory hallucinations, although the catatonia and negative symptoms resolved. Psychometry indicated a drop in IQ, particularly performance speed. Later Alice was started on clozapine and made a good recovery.

Case Study (2): Peter

Peter was a 17-year-old boy who was admitted to an adolescent psychiatric unit after an acute psychotic breakdown with paranoid delusions, delusions of reference and clear second-person auditory hallucinations and tactile hallucinations. Peter had been using cannabis quite heavily for several years. However, he had stopped using illegal drugs three months beforehand, because of increasing paranoid ideation when smoking cannabis. There was no family history of mental illness. However, Peter had become increasingly anxious and depressed prior to the onset of the psychotic episode.

On admission, physical investigations, including drug screening, were negative. Because he was agitated, initially he was treated with low-dose benzodiazepines, which helped him settle.

He remained acutely distressed and paranoid, and a low-dose antipsychotic medication was given. He responded well within a week or two. There was no evidence of cognitive decline, and all his psychotic symptoms resolved fairly rapidly. Further enquiry did not indicate any previous psychotic symptoms, except paranoia when smoking cannabis. He was given counselling about the use of illegal drugs and was discharged home and back in college within one to two weeks.

Follow-up enquiries revealed that Peter had not resumed smoking cannabis, as far as one can ascertain. However, he had further psychotic episodes, and a formal diagnosis of a paranoid delusional disorder was made.

Investigations

Patients require a full physical examination, blood tests (routine, plus thyroid function tests, brain antibodies, caeruloplasmin levels), psychometry and, for some individuals, EEG and an MRI scan.

Differential Diagnosis

Severe mood disturbance, with depression or mania, the latter as part of a bipolar disorder, can present with acute polymorphic psychotic symptoms. The key diagnostic issue is the history of mood disturbance, often preceding the onset of psychosis. The psychotic symptoms may be mood congruent, but not always, in which case further observation, including response to treatment, is necessary to avoid a misdiagnosis of schizophrenia.

Psychotic symptoms are seen with autistic spectrum disorder (ASD), especially in adolescence, and can be difficult to differentiate from a psychotic illness or schizophrenia, which do co-occur. Psychotic symptoms are seen in medical disorders, Wilson's disease, Hashimoto's encephalitis and with white matter diseases, such as adrenoleukodystrophy, amongst others. Psychotic symptoms can be precipitated by the use of prescribed drugs, high-dose steroids and so on, and most commonly recreational drugs, e.g. cannabis, synthetic cannabinoids, methamphetamine, LSD or ketamine.

Treatment and Outcome

In line with modern medical practice, there is an emphasis on earlier identification of at-risk mental states (ARMS) and brief, limited intermittent psychotic symptoms (BLIPS). However, the transition rate of these acute psychotic states to a frank disorder appears to be low in adolescence. Negative symptoms and anxiety states are more often seen to be precursors of psychotic disorders. Patients presenting with brief psychotic symptoms are best kept under review. The NICE guideline for psychosis and schizophrenia in children and young people (NICE guideline CG 155, 2013) does not endorse antipsychotic treatment in this group, but CBT may be helpful for associated anxiety and depressive symptoms. Counselling against the use of cannabis or other drug use is important.

Early intervention psychosis services (EIS) have been set up nationwide with an emphasis on a community basis for quick non-stigmatising referrals with the delivery of CBT, medication, psychoeducation and school and vocational support, outside of traditional hospital settings. Preliminary evidence points to the effectiveness of this pattern of service delivery in terms of acceptability, effectiveness and cost-effectiveness. It should complement other services in CAMHS and hospitals.

Paranoid symptoms are distributed on a continuum across the population (Taylor et al., 2016) and, therefore, the assumption underlying the categorical diagnostic systems (DSM and ICD) that there is a disjunction, or break, between those who are ill with paranoid symptoms and the remaining population, may not be the case in practice. This is an important point in psychoeducation, as one tries to normalise unsettling and often disturbing experiences as a start to treatment with cognitive behaviour therapy for psychosis (CBT-P). Recent work has targeted worry and sleep disturbances as precursors or precipitants for psychosis (Reeve et al., 2018).

It is important to recognise that patients presenting with at-risk mental states (ARMS) most commonly do not transition to psychosis, but nonetheless suffer anxiety or depression, which need treatment, often CBT, in their own right.

The NICE guideline for psychosis and schizophrenia in this age group (NICE guideline CG 155, 2013) highlights the need for antipsychotic medication, initially at low dose and gradually increasing, and psychological approaches including family therapy (mostly behavioural) and cognitive behavioural therapy (CBT-P) alongside psychoeducation for the patient and carers. Antipsychotic medication essentially involves dopamine D2 blockade, although research work with positron emission tomography (PET) indicates the primary problem in schizophrenia is hyperactive presynaptic striatal synthesis (Howes et al., 2011) which these drugs do not directly tackle. Atypical antipsychotics (e.g. olanzapine, risperidone) are used, rather than older traditional antipsychotics (e.g. trifluoperazine, haloperidol) due to a lower risk of extrapyramidal side-effects, especially tardive dyskinesia, but they have worrying side-effects of severe and rapid weight gain and dyslipidaemias. Aripiprazole, amisulpride and lurasidone seem to produce less weight gain.

Although recent trials in adults indicate that amisulpride may be more effective than other antipsychotics, there is little to choose between these medications, and the patient's choice may be guided by the side-effect profile. Convention dictates that a failed trial of up to six weeks, since research suggests early benefit should be seen by three weeks, of two antipsychotics should be followed by a trial of clozapine, recognised as the most effective antipsychotic. A recent study in adults suggests that a single trial of amisulpride may be all that is necessary and that a second trial of another antipsychotic confers little, or no, advantage (Kahn et al., 2018). Clozapine is not used first line (except in China), because of the risks of agranulocytosis and cardiac effects which require regular blood and ECG monitoring. Unfortunately, around 30% of patients remain refractory to treatment, possibly higher in children and adolescents with schizophrenia, who have a higher rate of treatment resistance and corresponding poorer prognosis. Indeed, the outlook for childhood-onset schizophrenia is very poor, with 50% remaining ill at long-term follow-up (Eggers and Bunk, 2009). There is very little evidence for the use of a combination of antipsychotics, or higher than recommended doses. An important practice point for the treatment in hospital of disturbances often involving violence is that benzodiazepines are preferred for sedation, rather than high-dose antipsychotics.

In light of the poor treatment response seen with early-onset schizophrenia, we need a conceptual leap forward in order to make progress. An addition to standard CBT-P, AVATAR therapy (virtual reality with the therapist imitating the hallucinatory voices – Freeman et al., 2019) has been shown to be effective against auditory hallucinations in adults, but there is no reason to believe it should not work with adolescents. To date, drugs have centred on the dopamine system. However, the glutamatergic system is involved (Howes et al., 2015). Unfortunately, we do not yet have drugs to effectively alter the glutamatergic neurotransmitter system for the treatment of psychosis. Novel therapies including cannabidiol in addition to antipsychotics are being researched in adults.

Key References

Eggers, C., Bunk, D., (2009). Early development of childhood-onset schizophrenia. *Fortschr Neurol Psychiatr*, 77(10): 558–567.

NICE, (2018). Psychosis and schizophrenia in children and young people: recognition and management. NICE guideline CG155 2013, www.nice.org.uk/CG155.

Reeve, S., et al., (2018). Insomnia, negative affect, and psychotic experiences: modelling pathways over time in a clinical observational study. *Psychiatry Research*, 269: 673–680.

48 Eating Disorders

Jo Barker and Lynne Oldman

Introduction

Eating disorders usually develop in adolescence and early adulthood. Eating disorders are more common in females, but numbers are increasing in pre-pubertal children, older women and males. Cases that present in childhood or adolescence have a better prognosis that those that present or persist into adulthood.

Eating disorders are split into broad categories according to the Diagnostic and Statistical Manual of Mental Disorders 5th Edition (DSM-5) and the International Classification of Diseases 11th Revision (ICD-11), including anorexia nervosa, bulimia nervosa, binge-eating disorder and avoidant and restrictive food intake disorder (ARFID). Pica and rumination disorder are included but will not be discussed here as they tend to be conditions in younger children or those with a learning difficulty.

KEY CONCEPTS

- Anorexia nervosa is characterised by a morbid fear of gaining weight and concerted efforts to reduce weight through restricting food intake and in some case, purging/vomiting and excessively exercising.
- Bulimia nervosa is characterised by episodes of bingeing on food, followed by concerted efforts to rid the body of food, through vomiting or use of purgatives.
- Binge eating disorder is characterised by episodes of bingeing on large quantities of food, followed by feelings of extreme guilt and self-loathing.
- Avoidant restrictive food intake disorder is a new classification within eating disorders in both ICD-11 and DSM-5 classification systems.
- There is no one treatment of choice for eating disorders in children and young people. Typically, a combination of interventions is required to bring about a positive outcome. The involvement of the family in treatment is paramount to its success.
- Research evidence suggests that treatment in the community rather than in inpatient adolescent units is most effective.

In 2013, the Diagnostic and Statistical Manual of Mental Disorders, Fourth Edition (DSM-4) was replaced by its successor, the DSM-5, yielding a number of adjustments in diagnostic criteria across psychiatric diagnoses. A main intention of the DSM-5 adjustments was to decrease the number of cases falling into the former diagnostic category ‘eating disorder not otherwise specified' (EDNOS), a poorly defined and heterogeneous residual category representing the majority of DSM-4 eating disorder cases (Keel et al., 2011).

This was done by removing binge-eating disorder (BED) from the DSM-4 EDNOS category and reintroducing it as an independent and specified DSM-5 diagnosis and by expanding the boundaries of anorexia nervosa (AN) and bulimia nervosa (BN). The DSM-5 retained practically all core anorexia nervosa features but clarified the weight criteria by changing the wording from 'a body weight less than 85% of that expected' to 'significantly low weight'. The amenorrhoea criterion was removed.

For bulimia nervosa, the minimum frequency of binge-eating episodes and inappropriate compensatory behaviour was reduced from twice a week to once a week. In addition to these changes, three disorders previously reserved for children and classified as 'Feeding and Eating Disorders of Infancy or Early Childhood' were revised and introduced in the DSM-5 as independent diagnostic categories, i.e. pica, avoidant/restrictive food intake disorder (ARFID) and rumination disorder.

Eating disorders are often not recognised or only diagnosed when the patient's condition becomes critical. Nicholls and Becker have said that one of the challenges to recognising the condition earlier lies in correcting the inaccurate and unfortunate framing of eating disorders as niche disorders affecting a limited demographic. They stress that eating disorders must be understood as the common and serious mental health problems they are, and that every clinician should be familiar with recognising and managing them. Evidence suggests that by 20 years of age, up to 13% of people have met the diagnostic criteria for an eating disorder, with UK adolescent girls being the group most at risk (Nicholls and Becker, 2020). Bould and colleagues in a study of UK girls' school health records found that 40.7% had some form of disordered eating behaviour, e.g. fasting, purging or binge eating, of which 11.3% were at a level compatible with an eating disorder diagnosis (Bould et al., 2018). Nicholls and Becker point out that eating disorders are not only a risk for adolescent girls. The incidence among young males is rising, as is recognition of the disorder among older women and men (Nicholls and Becker, 2020).

Low body weight is maintained by a persistent pattern of behaviours to prevent restoration of normal weight by reducing energy intake and increasing energy expenditure. The quantity of food eaten is increasingly restricted and is frequently accompanied by calorie counting, checking food labels and weighing food. Initially, certain food groups, i.e. sugars, carbohydrates and fats, are reduced and cut out of the diet. Low-calorie options are frequently chosen. Exercise to significantly increase energy expenditure is typical and can become obsessive. Purging, e.g. self-induced vomiting and/or misuse of laxatives or diuretics are strategies used.

Anorexia Nervosa

The term 'anorexia nervosa' was coined by the English physician, William Gull, in 1968. He emphasised the psychological causes of the condition, the need to restore weight and the role of the family. Anorexia nervosa is characterised by a significantly low body weight for the individual's height, age and developmental stage that is not due to another health condition or to the unavailability of food.

A review of almost 50 years of research confirms that anorexia nervosa has the highest mortality rate of any mental disorder (Arcelus et al., 2013; Demmler et al., 2020). Intense fear of weight gain is typical and persists as an intrusive, overvalued idea. Low body weight or shape is central to the person's self-evaluation. Sufferers develop a distorted sense of their own body size, often inaccurately perceiving themselves to be a normal weight or even excessively overweight when they may be dangerously underweight.

A review of the literature found the incidence of anorexia nervosa to be 8 cases per 100,000 population per year, and the incidence of bulimia nervosa was 12 cases per 100,000 population per year. The prevalence rates for bulimia nervosa were 1% and 0.1% for young women and young men, respectively. The estimated prevalence of binge eating disorder is at least 1%. The authors found that only a minority of people who met the stringent diagnostic criteria for eating disorders had been seen in mental health care. The prevalence of anorexia nervosa varies from 0.5% to 1.0% of the adolescent population. The peak incidence for anorexia nervosa is in the 15 to 19 years age group.

NB. Due to changes in diagnostic criteria outlined above for eating disorders including anorexia nervosa, the numbers of which prior to 2013 would have been defined under 'eating disorder not otherwise specified' (EDNOS), the incidence and prevalence rates are likely to show an increase (Hoek and Van Hoeken, 2003). A later paper looks at the world-wide rates and shows similar figures (Smink et al., 2012).

Diagnosis

Anorexia nervosa is diagnosed in the UK by using the ICD-10 (WHO, 1992).

For a definite diagnosis, all of the following are required (Al-Adawi et al., 2013).

- Body weight is maintained at least 15% below expected weight, either lost or never achieved or the body mass index (BMI) is 17.5 or less. Pre-pubertal individuals may show a failure to make the expected weight gain during the growth period.
- Weight loss is self-induced by avoidance of 'fattening foods'. One or more of the following may be present: self-induced vomiting, self-induced purging, excessive exercise, use of appetite suppressants and/or diuretics.
- There is body image distortion whereby a dread of 'fatness' persists as an intrusive, overvalued idea and the patient imposes a low weight threshold on him- or herself.

  A widespread endocrine disorder involving the hypothalamic–pituitary–gonadal axis manifests in women as amenorrhoea and in men as a loss of sexual interest and potency. An exception is the persistence of vaginal bleeds in anorexic women on hormone replacement therapy, e.g. contraceptive pills. There may be elevated levels of growth hormone, cortisol, changes in the metabolism of thyroid hormones and abnormalities of insulin secretion. Amenorrhoea has been dropped as a criterion as its cause may be not due to anorexia nervosa.
- If onset is pre-pubertal, the sequence of pubertal events is delayed or even arrested, i.e. growth ceases, in girls, breasts do not develop and there is primary amenorrhoea; in boys, the genitals remain juvenile. With recovery, puberty is often completed normally, but menarche is late.

BMI is calculated as: BMI = weight (in kg)/height (in metres). Normal BMI falls within the range of 20–25. This can be a crude measure. It is an adult measure and does not allow for the varying rate at which children and young people physically develop, including body frame size. A more useful measure in children and young people would be weight- for-height charts, or percentage median BMI.

The DSM-5-TR (Eddy et al., 2008) further classifies anorexia into:

- **Restricting type** in people who restrict their dietary intake
- **Binge eating/purging type** in people who engage in bingeing and purging behaviours

DSM-5 removed the need of fear of weight loss to be verbalised if it was clear that eating was being curtailed. Amenorrhea was no longer required, and it changed the criteria for weight loss to a BMI-based severity rating.

Aetiology

Anorexia nervosa has a multi-factorial aetiology (Herle, 2020). Eating behaviours in childhood are considered as risk factors for eating disorder behaviours and diagnoses in adolescence. Researchers investigated associations between childhood eating behaviours during the first ten years of life and eating disorder behaviours, i.e. binge eating, purging, fasting and excessive exercise, and diagnoses, i.e. anorexia nervosa, binge-eating disorder, purging disorder and bulimia nervosa, at 16 years of age. Data from 4,760 participants from the Avon Longitudinal Study of Parents and Children were included. They recorded parent and self-recorded questionnaires over eight time points. Objectively measured anthropometric data were obtained at 16 years.

Childhood overeating was found to be associated with increased risk of adolescent binge eating and binge-eating disorder.

Persistent undereating was associated with higher anorexia nervosa risk in adolescent girls only. Persistent fussy eating was associated with greater anorexia nervosa risk. The authors suggest these eating patterns in early childhood should be considered seriously (Herle et al., 2020).

Biological Factors

The incidence of anorexia is 6–10% in the female siblings of patients, more so in identical twins than in non-identical twins. Apart from the genetic contribution, shared familial environment may be significant. Family genetic studies have shown that there is an association between eating disorders and mood disorders (Clarke et al., 2012).

Psychological Factors

These young people are often struggling for control, a sense of identity and effectiveness, with the relentless pursuit to achieve thinness as a result. They can be perfectionists, high achieving, conscientious, popular, successful, overly compliant and have low self-esteem. They often struggle with expressing negative emotions, such as anger, sadness or anxiety, especially if these are not tolerated within the family system.

The bodily changes that return it to a pre-pubertal state, or to maintaining one in younger children, can be interpreted as a regression to childhood, escaping the emotional problems of older childhood and adolescence. This may include the process of developing an identity as a sexual being, particularly if there have been unwanted sexual experiences.

Familial Factors

There may be disturbed relations in the family. Patterns of relationships could include enmeshment, over-protectiveness, rigidity and lack of conflict resolution whereby strong negative emotions are not well tolerated. It is sometimes unclear whether these patterns of dysfunction predate the onset of the illness or are a response to it. The young person's illness and the need for closer supervision and care may be holding the family together, if it is perceived to be at risk of breaking down.

Social Factors

The cultural pressure on women to be thin and on men to be muscle-toned may be an important predisposing factor in the development of eating disorders. The disorder is predominantly seen in western cultures. There are, however, reports of increased incidence of anorexia in rapidly developing economies, e.g. India and China, where western cultural influences are becoming more widespread.

Most adolescents and young women will diet at one time or the other, but people with anorexia nervosa usually come from a family or social background where weight, shape and eating concerns are promoted, e.g. family members' dieting or consciousness about weight and shape. Those young people who aspire to enter certain sports or industries, e.g. dance, gymnastics or modelling, where a certain body shape is required, are at particular risk of developing the disorder.

Physical/Psychological Signs/Problems in Anorexia Nervosa

- Sensitivity to cold and possible hypothermia.
- Constipation and slow gastric emptying.
- Low blood pressure and low heart rate.
- Vomiting and laxative abuse may lead to signs of electrolyte imbalances including severe hypokalaemia, i.e. low potassium levels in the blood, that may cause seizures and death by cardiac arrhythmia.
- Hair becomes brittle, and there can be the appearance of fine hairs on the face, arms and legs, known as lanugo, as the body attempts to maintain a safe core temperature.
- Poor concentration and cognitive processing ability that may increase the distress if the young person has historically been a high academic achiever.
- Changes to mood and anxiety levels. Sufferers can become highly anxious and irritable/ angry, especially in situations involving food.
- Increased social isolation in an attempt to avoid situations involving food.

Prognosis and the Need for Prompt Treatment

In adolescence there is a critical growth period during which the young person completes vital physical development. This period is considered to be essential for optimum physical and mental growth as an adult. Any disruption at this stage may have serious long-term health implications, e.g. stunted growth and infertility and osteoporosis in women. In the shorter term, anorexia is perhaps the most fatal of psychiatric disorders with a mortality rate of up to 22%.

In a systematic review of studies into anorexia nervosa, Steinhausen et al (2005) found the following rates of recovery among adolescents (n = 784): with full recovery in 57.1%; improvement after treatment 25.9%; chronicity 16.9%.

This does not account for those young people who do not access services to manage their illness. Some may cease the restricting behaviour but go on to develop bulimia nervosa. A large study of two cohorts of Swedish children, screened when they were 15 years old, identified 51 children with eating disorders who were matched with 51 children with no disorders from the same class and followed up for 30 years. Ninety-six percent participants were available at 30 years, and 19% still had an eating disorder, i.e. 6% anorexia nervosa, 2% binge-eating disorder, 11% other specified feeding or eating disorder; 64% were now symptom free for at least six months. Participants had had an eating disorder for at least ten years on average. Interestingly, 23% received no psychiatric treatment. Thirty-eight percent had other psychiatric disorders. Sixty-four percent had full eating disorder symptom recovery, i.e. free of all eating disorder criteria for six consecutive months. One in five had a chronic eating disorder. The authors said that a good recovery was predicted by later onset in the adolescents of anorexia and pre-morbid perfectionism (Dobrescu et al., 2020).

Bulimia Nervosa

Bulimia nervosa refers to episodes of uncontrolled excessive eating called 'binges', followed by vomiting or the use of purgatives. The onset of bulimia nervosa is usually in late adolescence, often after a period of concern about weight and shape and following a period of food restrictions. Twenty-five percent of patients have a past history of anorexia. The number of episodes of bingeing increases over time, returning the weight to near normal (MacDonald et al., 2014).

Diagnosis

ICD-10 (WHO, 1992) criteria for bulimia nervosa: NB. The ICD-11 will propose slightly different criteria (Al-Adawi et al., 2013).

- A persistent preoccupation with eating and an irresistible craving for food. The patient succumbs to episodes of overeating in which large amounts of food are consumed in short periods of time.
- The patient attempts to counteract the 'fattening' effects of food by one or more of the following: self-induced vomiting, purgative abuse, alternating periods of starvation, use of drugs, e.g. appetite suppressants, thyroid preparations or diuretics. When bulimia nervosa occurs in diabetic patients, they may choose to neglect their insulin treatment.
- The psychopathology consists of a morbid dread of fatness. The patient sets herself/himself a sharply defined weight threshold, well below the premorbid weight that constitutes the optimum or healthy weight in the opinion of the physician. There is often, but not always, a history of an earlier episode of anorexia nervosa (in 25%), the interval between the two disorders ranging from a few months to several years. The earlier episode may have been fully expressed or may have assumed a minor cryptic form with moderate loss of weight and/or a transient phase of amenorrhoea.

The DSM-5 further classifies bulimia nervosa into:

- **Purging type** in people who have regularly employed self-induced vomiting/misuse of laxatives, diuretics or enemas.
- **Non-purging type** in people who have used other compensatory mechanisms, e.g. starvation, excessive exercise.

Other Features

The young person may exhibit a profound loss of control. Episodes of bingeing can be brought about by stress or by the breaking of self-imposed dietary control. Binges usually occur when alone, with initial relief of stress followed by feelings of guilt and disgust. The young person may then induce vomiting or take laxatives. Co-morbid depression can occur that may improve with the improvement of the eating disorder.

Aetiology

The aetiology for bulimia nervosa is in many ways similar to that of anorexia nervosa, a possible exception being the dynamics within the family system. In contrast to the anorexic family, where strong negative emotions are not easily tolerated, bulimic families can often be high in conflict and distress (Wonderlich et al. 1996).

Physical and Psychological Signs/Symptoms

- Repeated vomiting can cause severe hypokalaemia, i.e. very low levels of potassium in the blood, resulting in weakness, kidney damage and potentially fatal cardiac arrhythmias, i.e. abnormal electrical activity in the heart leading to cardiac arrest. The mortality rate across all age ranges is approximately 0.4% (NICE, 2004).
- Decreased motility of the colon and constipation.
- Teeth may become pitted with gastric acid erosion due to repeated vomiting.
- It has been suggested that long-term vomiting can increase the risk of permanent damage to the oesophagus.

Avoidant-Restrictive Food Intake Disorder

Avoidant-restrictive food intake disorder (ARFID) often presents in the younger age group and is characterised by abnormal eating or feeding behaviours that result in the intake of an insufficient quantity or variety of food to meet adequate energy or nutritional requirements. Restricted eating and avoidance of eating certain foods can cause significant weight loss, failure to gain weight as expected in childhood or pregnancy and clinically significant nutritional deficiencies. Dependence on oral nutritional supplements or on tube feeding is typically needed to maintain adequate nutrition and health.

There is a marked impact on psychosocial functioning, e.g. the young person may be too anxious to go to school or on school trips. The pattern of eating does not reflect concerns about body weight or shape. Restricted food intake is not better accounted for by lack of food availability or another health condition. There is often a co-morbid diagnosis of autism spectrum condition. Other co-morbid conditions including anxiety disorders may appear in up to 58%. Often individuals would prefer to have a higher body weight, but their anxiety stops them from eating adequately.

Presentations of Eating Disorders and Making a Referral

It is important that young people are referred early for assessment where there are any concerns about a possible eating disorder. Early intervention offers the best outcomes. Referrals can be made by the GP, school, family, carers or self-referral by the young person.

It is commonly parents rather than young people who seek help initially, often following a long period of the problem unfolding. Parents may notice a change in the young person's eating behaviour, including social withdrawal from situations that involve food. The young person may appear lethargic. Parents may not initially notice any weight loss particularly if the young person is wearing layers of loose-fitting clothes. Parents may notice the young person has excessive concerns about their weight and shape. They may have concerns that a young person is dieting or restricting their eating, even if they are already underweight.

Young people are typically reluctant to visit the surgery in these cases. By the time help is sought, the young person can be very unwell, and a single consultation about weight and eating concern is a strong indicator of a possible eating disorder (Lask et al., 2005). Often the young person will not discuss weight loss without direct questioning and even then, may refuse to do so and become angry and upset when asked about weight and eating problems. The young person is typically resistant to being weighed and examined physically. Compensatory behaviours, e.g. laxative or diuretic misuse or vomiting, need to be asked about specifically, as this information is unlikely to be volunteered by the young person.

Children and young people with an eating disorder may present with faltering growth or delayed puberty. Presentations to health workers, such as the GP, may include menstrual disturbances, although this will be masked if they are on hormonal treatments, such as the contraceptive pill. Unexplained gastrointestinal symptoms are common. Dentists may see dental erosion in bulimia nervosa.

Red flags for urgent referral to paediatricians and consideration for admission to a paediatric ward are physical signs of malnutrition, including poor circulation, palpitations or low pulse rate, fainting and low blood pressure, and where there are problems managing a chronic illness that affects diet, e.g. diabetes or cystic fibrosis.

What Makes a Good GP Referral?

Information in the referral should include a detailed history of the presentation including any diagnostic features (refusal to maintain body weight or failure to gain weight during a period of growth, intense fear of gaining weight, disturbed body perception, undue influence of body weight or shape on self-esteem, denial of seriousness of current low body weight).

Initial assessment should include general physical examination, including current weight and height. Information on previous weights and heights should be included to assess the severity and how longstanding the problem is. Observations including lying and standing blood pressure, lying and standing pulse and temperature should be done. An ECG should be done particularly if there has been rapid weight loss, continuing weight loss or low weight on first presentation. Baseline blood tests should be taken, including electrolytes, calcium, phosphate and magnesium, liver function, thyroid function, renal function and a full blood count.

Differential diagnosis includes diabetes mellitus, hyperthyroidism, glucocorticoid insufficiency, carcinoma, lymphoma, leukaemia, intra-cerebral tumour or chronic infection, e.g. tuberculosis, HIV, viral. Cases where there is a physical problem with no evidence of an eating disorder should be referred to paediatricians.

Information on current mental state including mood and self-harm is important as there are often co-morbid mental health disorders coexisting with eating disorders.

Referral to Specialist Services

In line with the National Institute of Clinical Excellence, all young people under 18 years with a suspected eating disorder should be seen by a specialist eating disorder team within 4 weeks of first contact (National Institute for Clinical Excellence NICE Guidance, September 2018). In recent years, waiting times have improved for children and young people, with more than 80% now starting treatment within four weeks of referral. This is an increase from less than 65% before 2016.

If weight is below 80% of percentage median BMI for age and gender, the referral should be considered urgent and seen within a week or sooner. A percentage median BMI of 70% indicates that a referral should be made direct to paediatric services for initial assessment. Other factors, in addition to weight, need to be considered, including cardiovascular state and degree of malnutrition. Referral may be to a specialist eating disorder service or to a specialist eating disorder team within community CAMHS. Community treatment is the most effective, and standard treatments are outlined later in this chapter.

Risk Indicators

Body Mass Index (BMI)

BMI is calculated as: weight (in kg)/height (in metres). BMI centile charts can be used to report BMI centiles in young people. Charts can be obtained on www.healthforallchildren.com. There are separate charts for boys and girls aged 6 months to 20 years. BMI is a crude measure in children and does not allow for the varying rate at which children and young people physically develop, including body frame size. For young people with a BMI below the 0.4th centile, as is the case in all young people with severe anorexia nervosa, there is a need to quantify the degree of underweight.

Much of the literature on adolescent eating disorders uses some form of percentage weight for height. The use of a single method of calculating percentage weight for height (WFH), based on the percentage median BMI, in line with the World Health Organization is recommended. Median BMI for age can be read from BMI centile charts or there are Excel programmes that will calculate percentage BMI using the UK BMI reference data, e.g. the Weight for Height programme developed at Great Ormond Street Hospital, London. The reference data are not ethnically sensitive, so some ethnicities, e.g. Asian young people, will be overrepresented in underweight groups. For a fuller discussion on methods of defining underweight, see Cole et al. (2007).

$$\frac{\text{Percentage BMI} = \text{Actual BMI}}{\text{Median BMI } (50^{\text{th}} \text{ percentile}) \text{ for age and gender}} \times 100$$

Change in weight is a marker of illness trajectory. Rate of weight loss increases cardiovascular risk and electrolyte instability, especially if there is associated purging. Rapid weight gain increases the risk of re-feeding syndrome. Generally, weight loss of 0.5 kg to 1 kg per week is cause for concern, but should not be considered in isolation but alongside blood pressure and any postural drop and pulse rate to assess cardiovascular risk. Similarly, rapid weight loss from overweight to the normal range can result in medical instability. On the other hand, slow, chronic weight loss can manifest as growth retardation, and previous growth charts should be examined where possible. If weight is below 80% of median BMI for age and gender, the referral should be considered urgent, and if 70%, a referral should be made direct to paediatric services for initial assessment and possible admission to a paediatric ward.

Assessing and Defining Severe Malnutrition

In adolescents, a United Nations Administrative Committee Report on Nutrition defined severe malnutrition in adolescents requiring therapeutic intervention as less than 70% weight for height, plus either bilateral pitting oedema (nutritional), inability to stand or apparent dehydration (Woodruff and Duffield, 2000). The risk of death in 'acute' malnutrition is closely related to its severity. Several studies have shown that low mid-upper arm circumference (MUAC) less than 115 mm and/or weight for height <70% predicts a high risk of mortality (Alam et al., 1989; Dramaix et al., 1996; Lapidus et al., 2009). The presence of bilateral (nutritional) oedema improves predictability. Independently, low serum albumin (<16 g/l) is a major risk factor for mortality.

Cardiovascular Risk (Smythe et al., 2020)

Bradycardia is a very common, well-documented condition in young people with anorexia nervosa. A heart rate of 50 beats per minute (bpm) should raise concern, and a consistent heart rate of 40 bpm or below is grounds for assessment by a paediatrician and consideration of admission for monitoring, including blood testing. This absolute value is only a guide. A more worrying indicator is when the pulse rate is normal or high despite low weight or with low blood pressure. There may or may not be variability with the tests undertaken with the young person standing or when under stress. Some drugs, e.g. antipsychotics, can lengthen the QTc interval on an ECG and hence enhance the cardiac ill-effects of malnutrition.

Management of Really Sick Patients with Anorexia Nervosa (MARSIPAN)

Junior MARSIPAN was developed for under 18-year olds with anorexia nervosa to provide guidance on a number of areas, including initial risk assessment, physical examination, including weight indicators for diagnosis, monitoring and treatment and assessment of medical complications, including re-feeding syndrome.

MARSIPAN Guidance outlines criteria for admission, location of care, who should be involved and transition between services. It gives guidance on compulsory treatment, paediatric admission and local protocols, management of re-feeding, management in paediatric inpatient and specialist inpatient child and adolescent settings and advises on management in primary care and paediatric out-patient settings.

Re-Feeding Syndrome

Re-feeding syndrome is a life-threatening risk to be considered when starting treatment for anorexia nervosa. Severe weight loss over time reduces the amount of insulin released and electrolytes become depleted. When re-feeding starts, insulin levels increase and electrolytes are taken into cells, reducing the level of these chemicals in the blood. Of high concern is a reduction in phosphate that can affect heart and brain function. Weight loss results in low blood pressure and reduction in the size of the heart muscle. This combined with a low phosphate level can cause heart failure. There may be swelling, shortness of breath, rapid or irregular heart rate, low blood pressure and confusion. The initial phase of re-feeding requires close monitoring of blood electrolytes and the cardiovascular system.

Re-feeding syndrome is most likely to occur in the first few days of re-feeding but may occur up to two weeks after. It is extremely rare, but is more likely to occur in a young person with rapid weight loss and a BMI of 0.4th centile or less, who has eaten little or nothing in the past week or who has abnormal biochemical parameters. In these circumstances, the young person should be admitted to a paediatric ward. Support from a dietician with expertise in managing eating disorders should be sought. Patients and parents should be advised not to increase nutritional intake rapidly, even if motivated to do so. If the risk for re-feeding syndrome is high, regular, e.g. up to daily or twice daily, blood tests are needed during the initial phase of re-feeding, particularly from day three, and should include electrolytes, calcium, phosphate and magnesium. Monitoring should continue for a fortnight or until electrolyte parameters are stable.

Re-Feeding

Starting intake should not be lower than intake before admission. For most young people, starting at 20 kcal/kg/day or higher, such as 1000 kcal per day, or quarter/half portions appears to be safe. Electrolytes and clinical state need careful monitoring, and transfer to a paediatric unit may be required if, for example, phosphate falls to <0.4 mmol/l. In the individuals who are at highest risk, and usually in paediatric rather than psychiatric settings, it may be necessary to use lower starting intakes, e.g. 5–10 kcal/kg/day, especially in the presence of severity indicators, e.g. ECG abnormalities or evidence of cardiac failure, electrolyte abnormalities before re-feeding starts, active co-morbidities, e.g. diabetes or infections, or very low initial weight. If low initial calorie levels are used (5–10 kcal/kg/day), clinical and biochemical review should be carried out twice daily at first, with calories increasing in steps and continuing to increase until weight gain is achieved.

Treatment in the Community

Treatment in community eating disorder teams, as opposed to inpatient adolescent units, has been shown to be most effective. Community teams with expertise in managing eating disorders may be distinct teams or specialist teams within CAMHS. Early referral of any young person with possible signs of disordered eating is essential, as early intervention offers the best outcomes.

When a young person is under the care of the community eating disorder services, a GP or paediatrician may continue to be involved to monitor their physical health, including weight and cardiovascular state. Regular communication between the professionals involved is essential.

Psychological Treatment for Anorexia Nervosa in Children and Young People

Anorexia-Nervosa-Focussed Family Therapy (Ft-An)

FT-AN can be delivered as single-family therapy or a combination of single- and multi-family therapy. Young people should have the option to have some single-family sessions separately from their family members or carers, in addition to together with their family members or carers. FT-AN for children and young people with anorexia nervosa should typically consist of 18 to 20 sessions over 1 year with regular review to establish how regular sessions should be and how long treatment should last. This can last over a year.

It is important to emphasise the role of the family in helping the person to recover and not to blame the person or their family members or carers. Early in treatment, it is essential to support the parents or carers to take a central role in helping the person manage their eating and to emphasise that this is a temporary role. It is important to establish a good therapeutic alliance with the person, their parents or carers and other family members. Psychoeducation about nutrition and the effects of malnutrition should be included.

As treatment progresses, it is important to support the young person, with help from their parents or carers, to establish a level of independence appropriate for their level of development. In the final phase, the focus is on plans for when treatment ends, including any concerns the person and their family have, and on relapse prevention

Individual Cognitive Behaviour Therapy (CBT-ED)

CBT-ED for children and young people with anorexia nervosa should typically consist of up to 40 sessions over 40 weeks, with twice-weekly sessions in the first 2 or 3 weeks and 8 to 12 additional brief family sessions with the individual and their parents or carers, as appropriate. Psychoeducation about nutrition and the effects of malnutrition should be covered both in individual sessions and with the family. In family sessions, identify anything in the person's home life that could make it difficult for them to change their behaviour and find ways to address this.

Sessions on cognitive restructuring, mood regulation, social skills, body image and self-esteem, create a personalised treatment plan based on the processes that appear to be maintaining the eating problem, including self-monitoring of dietary intake and associated thoughts and feelings. Include homework, to help the person practice in their daily life what they have learned.

Adolescent-Focussed Psychotherapy for Anorexia Nervosa (AFP-AN)

AFP-AN for children and young people should typically consist of 32 to 40 individual sessions over 12 to 18 months, with more regular sessions early on, to help the patient build a relationship with the practitioner. Additional family sessions with the young person and their parents or carers, as appropriate, may be needed. In family sessions and in individual sessions, psychoeducation about nutrition, the effects of malnutrition and worries about weight gain are discussed. Individual sessions focus on the person's self-image, emotions and interpersonal processes and how these affect the eating disorder. A formulation is developed with the young person about the anorexic behaviour, and in later stages of treatment, issues of identity and building independence can be discussed.

Psychological Treatment for Binge-Eating Disorder

For children and young people with binge-eating disorder, the principles of treatment are the same as for adults with binge-eating disorder, but tailored to the young person's developmental needs. Binge-eating-disorder-focussed guided self-help programmes include cognitive behavioural self-help materials and supportive sessions, e.g. 4 to 9 sessions lasting 20 minutes each over 16 weeks, running weekly at first.

If guided self-help is unacceptable or ineffective after four weeks, group eating-disorder-focussed cognitive behavioural therapy (CBT-ED) can be offered, if this is available.

Individual CBT-ED should typically consist of 16 to 20 sessions to develop a formulation of the person's psychological issues, to determine how dietary and emotional factors contribute to their binge eating, and should be based on the formulation advice on regular meals and snacks to avoid feeling hungry. The treatment will tackle the emotional triggers for their binge eating, using cognitive restructuring, behavioural experiments and exposure . Include weekly monitoring of binge-eating behaviours, dietary intake and weight, and address body-image issues.

Psychological Treatment for Bulimia Nervosa

Bulimia-nervosa-focussed family therapy (FT-BN) for children and young people with bulimia nervosa should typically consist of 18 to 20 sessions over 6 months, using a collaborative approach between the parents and the young person, to establish regular eating patterns and minimise compensatory behaviours. Information about regulating body weight, dieting and the adverse effects of attempting to control weight with self-induced vomiting, laxatives or other compensatory behaviours is important, including self-monitoring of bulimic behaviours and discussions with family members or carers.

CBT-ED for children and young people with bulimia nervosa should typically consist of 18 sessions over 6 months, with more frequent sessions early in treatment, including additional sessions with parents or carers. The focus in sessions with parents and carers is psych-education about eating disorders and discussion of family factors that may reinforce behaviours, and how the family can support the person's recovery.

In individual sessions, the role bulimia nervosa plays in the young person's life and in building motivation to change is significant. Psychoeducation about eating disorders and how symptoms are maintained is important, whilst encouraging the person to gradually establish regular eating habits. The young person is taught to monitor their thoughts, feelings and behaviours and to set goals and is encouraged to address problematic thoughts, beliefs and behaviours with problem-solving.

Cognitive Remediation Therapy (CRT)

CRT was originally developed for psychosis and is available online as a Resource Pack for Children and Adolescents with Feeding and Eating Disorders. It is based on challenging thinking styles and processes rather than the content of the thoughts. It has been used in situations where people are unmotivated to change or contemplate CBT and is often used in inpatient units (Tchanturia et al., 2013).

Medication

Medication is not indicated for the treatment of eating disorders except where there is a co-morbid mental disorder. There is an increase in other mental disorders associated with eating disorders, including autism spectrum conditions, depression and obsessive-compulsive disorder (OCD). Medication including selective serotonin reuptake inhibitors (SSRIs), e.g. fluoxetine or sertraline, would be appropriate to use to treat a co-morbid disorder, such as anxiety or depression. Antidepressants are likely to be less effective when the brain is malnourished.

Case Study (1): Natalie

Natalie (16) was referred to her local CAMHS team for persistent weight loss. She had a history of dietary restriction for one year and had not menstruated for the past six months. Natalie lived with her mother and younger brother and had little contact with her father, whom her mother divorced when Natalie was ten. Natalie's father had moved to Australia soon after the divorce and was recently re-married.

Natalie reported feeling anxious and stressed about her exams and described withdrawing from her friends in order to spend her time revising. She talked about becoming more aware of her weight following a family holiday to Greece where she had been told she looked 'chunky' in a bikini. She described being preoccupied with thoughts of being fat and ugly.

Natalie's mother became concerned about Natalie's weight loss and encouraged her to eat, but without success. At mealtimes, Natalie's mother would put a plate of food in front of Natalie and they would argue about whether or not she should eat it. Natalie's mother describing 'giving in' because she thought the arguments were upsetting Natalie's younger brother, who sat with them at the meal table.

Natalie's mother encouraged Natalie's father to approach the issue of weight loss with her, but he insisted it was just a 'phase' that she would grow out of.

Natalie reported intensive physical activity, amounting to hundreds of star- jumps and sit-ups each day.

Natalie was mildly dehydrated with cold extremities and a weight for height ratio of 78%. Her blood pressure was within normal limits, but with a postural drop.

Natalie and her mother were informed of her diagnosis of anorexia nervosa and met with the dietician to agree a weight restoration meal plan of three meals and three snacks a day to gain weight to her target healthy weight range, 95–105% weight for height. Natalie was advised to stay at home until she was able to reverse her weight loss, and the school liaised with her mother to provide homework and study, prior to Natalie's exams later that year.

Natalie was referred for individual psychotherapy, but initially refused to attend the sessions. Both Natalie and her mother attended family sessions, and this helped to reduce the conflict at mealtimes. Natalie began to eat more. Eventually, Natalie asked to see her individual psychotherapist and explored themes of rejection and feeling 'left out' both in her family and in her peer group relationships. Natalie's father joined family sessions once a month via Skype, and Natalie reported feeling closer to her father, along with her mother finding his support and understanding, as a result of the sessions, helpful.

Natalie began to show significant cognitive changes and regained weight to the point where she began menstruating. She was motivated to continue her recovery. Natalie returned to school to take her exams and remained in contact with her therapist for a year following her initial assessment, to work through some of the interpersonal issues linked with her eating disorder.

Case Example (2): Noah

Noah (15) lives at home with his father, mother and younger sister. His older sister, and closest family member, is 19 and has recently left for university. Noah is an average-good achiever at school, whereas his older sister was very much a high-flyer. Noah and his younger sister have a reasonably good relationship, but she is the baby of the family and in Noah's mind, receives more attention from their parents than he does. Since Ruth left for university, Noah has been spending more time with a group of friends of whom his mother and father disapprove. He has returned home drunk on a few occasions, which has led to heated arguments, especially with his father. His parents have said that he should not be spending time with these friends.

For the past six months, Noah has been bingeing on food whilst everyone else is out, then making himself sick, three or four times a week. More recently, he has been going to the bathroom after meals and bringing up his dinner almost on a daily basis.

Noah has been seeing the school counsellor to whom he has told everything. This includes thoughts that he may be gay and concern about how his parents would respond if they knew. The counsellor refers Noah onto the local community CAMHS team after speaking with Noah and his mother.

At the assessment, Noah talks about 'not fitting in' within his family because he is neither the highest achiever nor the good student like the youngest sibling. This feeling of alienation is heightened by the thoughts/feelings that he may be homosexual, as this would go against his father's idea of what a man should be. Noah reported feeling out of control, bingeing and then vomiting to regain a sense of control over himself. Unfortunately, this leaves him with feelings of guilt, shame and disgust and impacts on his mood. This cycle of behaviour is becoming a daily occurrence.

Noah's mother and father had recently noticed some odd behaviour, such as Noah disappearing to the bathroom soon after each meal and realised that food had been rapidly disappearing from the kitchen cupboards. Their primary focus with Noah had been his association with 'undesirable' friends and the arguments this had caused. Noah has stated that he does not use laxatives or any other purgatives.

Noah's potassium level is low, but not at a dangerous level. There is some acid erosion to the enamel on his teeth, and his fingers are sore from putting them down his throat to induce vomiting.

Although Noah experiences low moods, it was not felt that an SSRI medication was appropriate initially. He and his parents were advised that this could be a future option should any therapeutic work be unsuccessful in moving Noah forward. Noah agreed to a course of cognitive behaviour therapy during which he and the therapist explored the core beliefs underpinning his distorted cognitions and behavioural experiments. He was asked to try to abstain from vomiting after meals. In the early stages of treatment, Noah was encouraged to spend at least 45 minutes in the company of another family member after each meal. At no time was he given the message that he had to stop vomiting completely, only to reduce it incrementally through the behavioural experiments.

Noah was advised to visit his dentist on a regular basis for check-ups and the best cleaning products available for weakened teeth.

Noah and his family, including his older sister when she was home from university, were invited to family therapy sessions where all family members were given the opportunity to explore the dynamics within their family system and how this may have brought about or maintained the bulimia nervosa.

It was during these sessions that Noah's father was able to have his concerns around Noah's friends heard and for Noah to offer reassurance that he was able to discern the potential influences they may have and respond in a mature manner. Noah was able, with the encouragement offered in his individual sessions, to talk about his feelings related to his sexuality. Although initially shocked, his parents were able to accept Noah's current feelings around his sexuality and promised to support him in any way they could.

Within six months of initial engagement with CAMHS, Noah's bingeing and vomiting has virtually ceased, although he reports feeling an urge to resume those behaviours when something particularly stressful happens. As a family, they feel able to communicate in a better way, certainly when potential conflict arises, listening to one another's views and working towards a mutual resolution.

Multiple-Choice Questions

See answers on page 671.

1. Repeated vomiting in bulimia nervosa can cause hypokalaemia, i.e. low potassium levels in the blood. This can increase the risk of what?
   a. Brain haemorrhage
   b. Respiratory failure
   c. Muscle weakness
   d. Kidney damage
   e. Cardiac arrhythmias
2. Which of the following is NOT a key feature of binge-eating disorder?
   a. Recurring episodes of binge eating, where a larger than normal amount of food is consumed in a relatively condensed period of time, although eating may be continuous over several hours.
   b. The individual has no control over the amount and type of foods they are eating.
   c. The episodes may be hidden from others due to shame and embarrassment.
   d. An episode is followed by feelings of guilt and disgust, which highlights possible underlying depression or anxiety and may be the cause or the result of the disordered eating.
   e. Eventually the young person will undertake compensatory behaviours, such as excessive exercise or vomiting and purging.
3. Selective serotonin reuptake inhibitors (SSRIs) can be useful in treating distorted cognitions in which eating disorder(s)?
   a. Anorexia nervosa only
   b. Bulimia nervosa only
   c. Binge eating disorder and anorexia nervosa
   d. Binge eating disorder and bulimia nervosa
   e. All three disorders

4. In relation to eating disorders, it is correct that:
   a. ED have decreased their prevalence over the last decades.
   b. AN has the highest mortality across all mental disorders.
   c. BED occurs exclusively in obese subjects.
   d. Individuals with BN are predominantly impulsive and have co-morbid borderline personality disorder.
5. Which of the following is not considered a diagnostic feature of anorexia nervosa?
   a. Depressive symptoms
   b. Significant weight loss
   c. Body image distortion
   d. Fear of becoming fat

Key References

Arcelus, Mitchel, Wales, Nelson, (2011). Mortality rates in patients with Anorexia Nervosa and other eating disorders. *Archives of General Psychiatry*, 68(7): 724–731.

Currin, L., Schmidt, U., Treasure, J., et al., (2005). Time trends in eating disorder incidence. *British Journal of Psychiatry*, 186: 132–135.

Dahlgren, C.L. et al., (2017). Feeding and eating disorders in the DSM-5 era: a systematic review of prevalence rates in non-clinical male and female samples. *Journal of Eating Disorders*, 5: 56.

Hoek, H.W., (2006). Incidence, prevalence and mortality of anorexia nervosa and other eating disorders. *Current Opinion in Psychiatry*, 19(4): 389–394.

National Institute for Health and Care Excellence, (2017). *Overview of Eating Disorders: Recognition and Management.* London: NICE.

Nicholls, D.E., Lynn, R., Viner, R.M., (2011). Childhood eating disorders: British national surveillance study. *British Journal of Psychiatry*, May 2011.

RCP, (2012). *Junior Marsipan Guidance CR168 Management of Really Sick Patients Under 18 with Anorexia Nervosa.* London: Royal College of Psychiatrists.

49 Somatoform and Related Disorders in Children and Young People

Sally Wicks

KEY CONCEPTS

- There is a strong interplay between psychological and physical symptoms in many disorders.
- Repeated presentation of physical symptoms not explained by a medical condition is known as a somatoform disorder.
- Assessment using predisposing, precipitating, presenting, perpetuating and protective factors can be helpful.
- Management of somatoform and related disorders often involves a multi-disciplinary team.

Key Terms and Definitions

- **Somatisation**: the process by which psychological distress is experienced and communicated through physical (somatic) symptoms which are attributed by the affected individual to physical illness.
- **Somatoform disorder**: a disorder in which the main feature is 'repeated presentation of physical symptoms, together with persistent requests for medical investigations, in spite of repeated negative findings and reassurances by doctors that the symptoms have no physical basis' (ICD-10, WHO, 1992).
- **Dissociative disorders (/conversion)**: share the main features of the somatoform disorders but have as their main presentation a partial or complete loss of the normal integration between memories of the past, awareness of identity and immediate sensations and control of bodily movements (ICD-10).

In the International Classification of Diseases 10 (WHO, 1992), somatoform disorders include:

- **Somatisation disorder**, in which the main feature is the presentation of multiple symptoms to health professionals over at least two years for which there is insufficient or no underlying medical cause. Few children meet criteria for this diagnosis due to the criteria of chronicity and multiple symptoms.
- **Hypochondriacal disorder**, in which the essential feature is a persistent preoccupation with the possibility of having a serious physical disorder (very rare in children).
- **Somatoform autonomic dysfunction**, in which symptoms are presented by the patient as if they were due to a physical disorder of a system or organ that is largely or completely

under autonomic innervation and control, i.e. the cardiovascular, gastrointestinal, respiratory and urogenital systems.

- **Persistent somatoform pain disorder**, in which the predominant complaint is of persistent, severe and distressing pain, which cannot be explained fully by a physiological process or a physical disorder, and which occurs in association with emotional conflict or psychosocial problems that are sufficient to allow the conclusion that they are the main causative influences.

Dissociative disorders in ICD-10 which present with physical symptoms include:

- **Dissociative motor disorders** – usually present with loss of ability to move the whole or a part of a limb or limbs.
- **Dissociative convulsions** – these mimic epileptic seizures but tongue-biting, bruising due to falling and incontinence of urine are rare, and some level of consciousness is usually retained.
- **Dissociative anaesthesia and sensory loss** – may be loss of skin sensation, possibly accompanied by paraesthesiae, or may be loss of sight or hearing.

In DSM-5 (APA, 2013) the class of somatoform disorders has been replaced by 'somatic symptom and related disorders' whilst in ICD-11 the term 'bodily distress disorder' is expected to largely replace the term somatoform disorder.

Functional Somatic Symptoms in Children

Somatic symptoms are common in children and adolescents and most are not related to a medical disorder but are physiological or 'functional' in origin. Common symptoms include:

- Abdominal pain
- Headaches
- Limb pains
- Nausea and vomiting
- Fatigue

It is helpful to think in terms of there being a continuum, from mild self-limiting symptoms common throughout the normal population at one end to persistent symptoms causing high levels of distress and/or disability at the severe end where criteria for diagnoses of somatoform or dissociative disorders are met. In between these two are recurrent symptoms which cause enough concern to the child and their parents that they are presented to health care professionals in primary care and outpatient settings.

Different symptoms seem to occur at different developmental stages, with pre-pubertal children presenting more often with abdominal pain (mostly in 5–12-year olds, peaks around age 9 years), and older children with headaches (peaking at age 12 years). Adolescents are more likely to present with limb pain, fatigue or neurological symptoms.

Recurrent Abdominal Pain

- Occurs in 7–25% of children and accounts for more than 50% of paediatric gastroenterology consultations. Only 5% of these have an organic cause, with additional symptoms and signs such as blood in stools, weight loss, localised tenderness, etc., indicating increased likelihood of an organic cause.

- Non-organic cause is more likely if the pain is vaguely localised or diffuse and if there are associations with specific times, e.g. Sunday evenings or school day mornings. Children are likely to report excess daily stressors and associations may be apparent between stressful events and pain symptoms.
- Recurrent abdominal pain in childhood is associated with anxiety and/or depression in adulthood as well as increased medical consultations.

Headache

- Approximately 60% of children report at least occasional headaches, with recurrent or severe headaches occurring in 17% of 4–18-year olds in one study (Lateef et al., 2009). Careful history and examination will indicate whether further investigation is required to look for an organic cause. It is important to note that non-organic headaches and migraine are uncommon in children under the age of five and therefore, an organic cause should be carefully looked for in this age group.
- Migraine, which is believed to be a neurovascular disorder, may occur in about 5% of all children at some time, usually at age eight years or older. A family history of migraine, plus typical symptoms of throbbing headache, photophobia, visual disturbance and nausea, point to this diagnosis.
- Non-organic headaches typically fit the description of 'tension headache' with a tight feeling around the head and possibly associations with emotive situations (similarly to recurrent abdominal pain), e.g. school days. This is the most common form of headache diagnosed.

Adolescents

- Physical symptoms are common, especially in girls (Eminson et al., 1996). In Eminson's epidemiological study, common symptoms were the feeling of a lump in the throat, dizziness, heart pounding, limb pains, headaches and chest pains.
- 8.3% of the adolescents reported experiencing 13 or more symptoms and again, this was more common in girls than in boys.
- The more symptoms the adolescents reported, the more likely they were to have serious concerns about illnesses (hypochondriacal beliefs) and a preoccupation with health. In some adolescents, the symptoms had a significant effect on lifestyle, e.g. preventing the adolescent from going to school or enjoying themselves. Thus, in some adolescents, somatisation is associated with significant disability in terms of general functioning, and an important aim in treatment must be to prevent this from becoming chronic.

Dissociative Disorders

The term 'dissociative' came from the presumption that the psychological mechanisms occurring in these disorders were the dissociation of one part of the individual from the rest, and 'conversion' from the conversion of emotional conflict into physical symptoms. These disorders are/include:

- Characterised by loss of function in any modality.
- Seen from middle childhood onwards, more commonly in adolescence and in girls.
- Low in incidence at 1.3–4.2 per 100,000.

- Complaints may be limb weakness, inability to see, talk or hear, unusual movements and epileptiform fits ('pseudoseizures', now more usually referred to as non-epileptic attacks). Some patients with epileptic seizures may also have non-epileptic attacks.
- Examination and observations may show that the symptoms and signs do not correspond to known disorders; rather the symptoms correspond to the patient's idea of physical disorder, which may not coincide with physiological or anatomical principles, e.g. an area of loss of feeling on a limb may display 'glove' or 'stocking' distribution of anaesthesia, rather than corresponding to the anatomy of the nervous system.
- There may be inconsistencies in the symptoms and signs, e.g. the child cannot weight bear when asked, but is observed to when not watched directly.

Management

Assessment

- Professionals involved must work collaboratively.
- Joint assessments can be beneficial, so that physical, developmental, psychological and social aspects can be considered in parallel, rather than the family being 'shunted around' professionals.
- It is essential to acknowledge the validity of the child's symptoms and not to dismiss them out of hand or suggest that the child is deliberately 'making them up'.
- It is usually unproductive to challenge the patient's subjective reality of the complaint.
- It is important to acknowledge the family's concerns, and to engage the family. With the family engaged, the history taking is carefully continued.

Predisposing, Precipitating, Perpetuating and Protective Factors

- **Predisposing Factors:**

  These include biological vulnerability, e.g. bronchial hyper-reactivity in asthma, early life experience including previous exposure to illness, parental over-concern with bodily functions or minor illnesses, parental mood disorder, temperamental traits of perfectionism, obsessionality or anxiety and socio-cultural influences. In some cultures, physical ill health may be more 'acceptable' than psychological ill health.
- **Precipitating Factors:**

  These include events, e.g. falling out with friends, being bullied, parental ill health (physical or psychological), a physical illness, e.g. a chest infection or viral illness, disruption of an attachment relationship (loss and bereavement) and traumatic experiences, e.g. accidents, assault or homelessness.
- **Perpetuating Factors:**

  What precipitates distress may also perpetuate it, e.g. continued bullying or family discord. There may also be a gain for the child in expressing the symptom and the symptom may be thereby perpetuated.

  Gain can be considered as being primary or secondary (Lask and Fosson, 1989). Primary gain is the relief of anxiety or distress by symptom production. Secondary gain is the benefit obtained from the symptoms, often the avoidance of undesirable situations. Consider an 11-year-old child who is anxious about attending school. The onset of abdominal pain draws attention from the anxiety (primary gain) and if the child misses school, then this can be seen as secondary gain. Symptoms may be perpetuated by reinforcement, e.g. if the parents give more positive attention to the child when they appear unwell, the child is more likely to continue expressing the symptom.

- **Protective Factors:**
  Some factors may protect children exposed to stress, e.g. adaptability, good self-esteem, good peer relationships and good family relationships with open communication.

It may be necessary to undertake physical investigations on the basis of the detailed history taken. If negative, they can be reassuring to the child and to the family. Repeated and prolonged investigation is unhelpful and can perpetuate the problem unnecessarily.

Having gathered the necessary information, the next step is to formulate an explanation for the family to explain what may be going on. It is sometimes helpful to use analogies, e.g. the idea of a tension headache being brought on by stress, a concept that most people would understand and accept.

- Treatment methods vary according to the assessment in each case.
- It is important to form a good therapeutic relationship with the family, whatever the treatment approach.
- Family therapy, individual therapy, including cognitive behaviour therapy (CBT), behaviour therapy, group therapy and relaxation could all be helpful.
- Medication, e.g. antidepressants, may be tried. It has been suggested that they are of benefit in adults with somatoform pain disorders. However, there is a lack of evidence to suggest that they are effective in children, and of course, they are themselves occasionally associated with side-effects, e.g. nausea, anxiety and headache.
- Physical treatments, e.g. physiotherapy and dietician advice, may be helpful.
- Several treatment methods can be used at any one time, but only if this approach is planned, with good communication between the professionals.
- It is important to consider the social circumstances of the child, e.g. there may be a need for liaison with the child's school, especially if there has been a prolonged absence, and a planned reintroduction is essential.

Case Study: Christina

Christina, aged eight, was taken to her GP by her mother, because of concerns about her recurrent abdominal pain. This had increased in frequency, causing serious worry in the family and leading to poor school attendance.

Christina is a quiet, sensitive and shy child, who lives at home with her parents and two-month-old baby sister. Christina's mother suffers from migraine, and her father, who works as a travelling engineer, is often away from home.

The GP could not find a physical cause for the pain, but acknowledged Christina's very real distress and the fact that she was not 'putting it on'. The GP suggested that the local child and adolescent mental health service was ideally well placed to provide a comprehensive assessment and an effective treatment programme.

The assessment then considered that Christina's temperament might have predisposed her to this presentation. Precipitating factors included the increasing lack of her mother's attention as she attended to the new baby and the worry of her father succumbing to a terrorist attack. The condition was thought to be perpetuated by the 'reward' of avoiding school and therefore receiving more care from her mother. It had also meant that Christina's father had cancelled a couple of his long-distance trips in order to help out at home.

The reassurance and explanation of what might be going on for Christina was enough to enable the parents to acknowledge her stress, and to pay more attention to her in a positive way. It also prompted them to consider communication patterns in the family. Christina was kept more clearly informed as to her father's movements. Liaison with her school helped to provide a smooth return, and the school was reassured that Christina's previous symptom of abdominal pain was not considered life threatening.

Multiple-Choice Questions

See answers on page 671.

1. What are some of the common symptoms seen in children presenting with somatising disorders?
   a. Abdominal pain
   b. Headaches
   c. Limb pains and fatigue
   d. Nausea and vomiting
   e. All of the above
2. What percentage of children presenting with recurrent abdominal pain in childhood have an organic disorder causing their symptoms?
   a. 10%
   b. 1%
   c. 5%
   d. 20%
   e. None
3. What factors may be helpful in assessing children with psychosomatic disorders?
   a. Predisposing factors
   b. Precipitating factors
   c. Protective factors
   d. Perpetuating factors
   e. All of the above

Key References

Eminson, D.M., (2007). Medically unexplained symptoms in children and adolescents. *Clinical Psychology Review*, 27: 855–871.

Garralda, M.E., (2011). Unexplained physical complaints. *Pediatric Clinics of North America*, 58: 803–813.

Lask, B., Fosson, B., (1989). *Childhood Illness: The Psychosomatic Approach: Children Talking With Their Bodies.* Chichester: John Wiley & Sons.

50 Chronic Fatigue Syndrome/ Myalgic Encephalomyelitis in Children and Young People

Sally Wicks (updated by Margaret J.J. Thompson)

KEY CONCEPTS

- Children and young people have better outcomes than adults.
- Poorer outcomes are associated with:
  - Lower socio-economic skills
  - Chronic maternal health problems
  - Lack of well-defined acute physical triggers
- Fifty to 75% make a full recovery or a marked improvement.
- Symptoms can persist.
- Many young people show a dramatic improvement.

Introduction

Chronic fatigue syndrome (CFS) is the name for a condition with the principle symptoms of fatigue and easy fatiguability. The other recognised name is myalgic encephalomyelitis or encephalopathy (ME). CFS is recognised in children and adolescents, where it can have a profound effect on physical, emotional, social and academic functioning (Garralda and Rangel, 2002).

Demography

Population surveys for CFS/ME suggest the prevalence in teenagers is between 0.4% and 2.4% depending on whether the definition used is of six or three months of fatigue, respectively. The reported prevalence of CFS/ME is much lower (0.06–0.1%) in studies that collect data from GPs or paediatricians (Chalder et al., 2003; Crawley, 2014).

Mean age of onset in clinic samples is 11 to 15 years, perhaps lower in community samples. Some studies report a higher proportion of girls.

Social Class

In clinic samples there are more cases in higher socio-economic classes, although current research suggests that is not necessarily the distribution in the community (Crawley, 2014). Approximately 60% of episodes of CFS may be triggered by viral-type illnesses.

Diagnostic Criteria and Symptomatology

Below are the symptoms listed in the NICE clinical guideline for chronic fatigue syndrome/ myalgic encephalomyelitis (NICE, 2007). This guideline applies to the diagnosis and management of the illness in both adults and children. Diagnosis should not be made on the basis of symptoms alone. Investigations to exclude other conditions should be performed first. The guideline recommends the diagnosis not being made until the illness is of four months' duration in adults, but advises earlier diagnosis, at three months, in children and adolescents (Garralda and Rangel, 2002).

Chronic Fatigue Syndrome

Fatigue with all of the following features

- New, or had a specific onset, i.e. not life-long
- Persistent and/or recurrent
- Unexplained by other conditions
- Has resulted in a substantial reduction in activity level, characterised by post-exertional malaise and/or fatigue, typically delayed by at least 24 hours, with slow recovery over several days

AND one or more of the following:

- Difficulty with sleeping, such as insomnia, hypersomnia, unrefreshing sleep, a disturbed sleep-wake cycle
- Muscle and/or joint pain that is multi-site and without evidence of inflammation
- Headaches
- Painful lymph nodes without pathological enlargement
- Sore throat
- Cognitive dysfunction, such as difficulty thinking, inability to concentrate, impairment of short-term memory and difficulties with word-finding, planning/organising thoughts and information processing
- Physical or mental exertion makes symptoms worse
- General malaise or 'flu-like' symptoms
- Dizziness and/or nausea
- Palpitations in the absence of identified cardiac pathology

Further points about diagnosis of CFS/ME in children and adolescents:

- Depressive and/or anxiety symptoms may be present and do not exclude the diagnosis of CFS, especially if they appear after the onset of fatigue.
- School phobia/refusal can be common in CFS, but could be a differential diagnosis.

Assessment

It is essential when taking the history to validate the child's complaints. Children with CFS and their families are extremely sensitive to a dismissive attitude on the part of professionals. A trusting relationship between the family and professional is important in subsequent management,

Table 50.1 History from Child and Parent

Presenting complaint	Principal symptoms, length of illness, school attendance, withdrawal from activities, typical day, (weekday and weekend), current level of functioning and independence
Past medical history	Previous illnesses and course of recovery; allergic history
Family history	Illness in other family members, including CFS and psychiatric, family adaptation to current illness, description of family relationships and communication style, current family stresses
Social history	Usual activities, peer relationships, degree of independence, school performance, enjoyment of school, previous school attendance
Illness history	Previous treatment and treatment experiences, child and family belief about the illness and effect of activity, dietary habits and beliefs
Psychological history	Mental health problems, especially anxiety, depression and school refusal, temperament

and the professional's acknowledgement of and concern about the symptomatology at the outset help to foster such a relationship. Children and families may have experienced a lack of knowledge and understanding of the disorder from professionals, repeated investigations, delay in referral and diagnosis or ineffective treatments. They may have fears about undiagnosed serious organic conditions. They may need explanation and support in understanding why a mental health team is involved. Joint paediatric and psychiatric assessments have been shown to be useful (See Table 50.1).

Physical Examination

Physical examination is important to exclude other pathology and to reassure the child and family. Marked physical abnormalities are rare in CFS and should be investigated.

Investigations

There is no specific diagnostic test. Investigations should be done to exclude other diagnoses suggested by the history or clinical examination but should be kept to a minimum. Investigations can be reassuring to children and parents, but once completed, further investigations should be avoided as this continues to raise parents' anxiety about possible misdiagnoses.

Blood tests indicated are full blood count, erythrocyte sedimentation rate, C-reactive protein, urea, creatinine and electrolytes, serum calcium, liver function tests, creatine kinase, thyroid function tests, random blood glucose, serum ferritin, screening blood tests for gluten sensitivity, serological testing if there is a history indicative of infection, e.g. for glandular fever, toxoplasmosis, etc. Occasional other tests as clinically required, to exclude specific diagnoses, e.g. inflammatory bowel disease. Vitamin D should be added for housebound patients.

School Report

A report from the child's school should be obtained with details of the child's academic achievements, social functioning, attendance record and any concerns the school may have.

Other Useful Assessments: these may only be possible in specialised treatment centres:

- **Cognitive Assessment**
  Formal testing of the child's cognitive/intellectual abilities, plus the level of function, e.g. in reading and spelling. Children with chronic fatigue syndrome may, in the past, have pushed themselves to do well. A comprehensive assessment of their abilities can ensure help is targeted and expectations are realistic.
- **Physiotherapy and Occupational Therapy Assessment**
  An initial assessment of the child's muscle tone, muscle power, exercise tolerance, balance and co-ordination help provide the baseline for the child's graded exercise programme. An occupational therapy assessment may be helpful in picking up subtle problems, e.g. poor fine motor control.
- **Detailed Psychological Assessment**
  Children who show very significant impairment in functioning, a long duration of illness or clear depressive/anxious symptomatology should have a further assessment from a professional in the mental health field.

Aetiological Factors

The aetiology of CFS in children, adolescents and adults remains controversial. The 1996 report from the Royal Colleges stressed a multi-factorial (biological, psychological and social) approach in defining the predisposing, precipitating and perpetuating factors in each patient. It is not helpful to view CFS as either purely physical or purely psychological, and it is often unhelpful to enter into long debates with the family and young person about this issue (Wessely, 1996). Examples of aetiological factors in children and adolescents are given below. For a detailed discussion of the role of infection as a precipitating and/or maintaining factor, see the report from the Royal Colleges.

Physical Factors

Viral illness may precipitate CFS. In particular, fatigue may follow infection with the Epstein–Barr virus (EBV), with rates of CFS of 13%, 7% and 4% at 6, 12 and 24 months, respectively, after EBV infection.

It is important for the young person and their family to understand that fatigue and weakness are exacerbated by excessive rest and inactivity. The effects of inactivity are:

- Significant effects occur within one to four weeks of bed rest.
- Reduced muscle volume and strength.
- Reduced muscle protein and increased connective tissue.
- Reduced bone mineral density.
- Joint stiffness.
- Reduced BMR.
- Altered white cell function.
- Changes in immune response.
- Effect on mood and circadian rhythm.

Psychological Factors

Once out of normal activities, children can quickly lose confidence in their physical and social activities and become anxious or miserable about the loss of time in school and reduced contact with their peers. Many of these young people are compliant and perhaps perfectionist by nature and find failure hard to tolerate. Returning to school after a prolonged absence is difficult. A professed desire to return to school does not mean there are no problems with it. Some young people with CFS may become depressed and the depression may be a perpetuating factor of CFS. Symptoms of depression in adolescents include irritability and anger, in addition to the more commonly recognised depressive symptoms. Psychological difficulties (e.g. the effects of bullying and/or poor peer relationships) may be predisposing, precipitating or perpetuating factors. Abuse or major life events are not often found to be aetiological factors.

Family Factors

The family's response to the illness, and beliefs about the cause of the illness, are important. Families who are keen to pursue an entirely physical cause, with an insistence on a large number of physical investigations, may be contributing to the perpetuation of the symptoms.

Family dynamics are often relevant (e.g. overprotection of the child), possibly as a result of the illness rather than present before the onset, identification with another sick member of the family and a change in family roles, e.g. a parent who has altered their work pattern to look after the child.

Treatment

A combined approach addressing the physical and psychological issues together is best (e.g. in primary care or combined paediatric/psychiatric clinics). It is essential to believe the child and family's description of the symptoms and to establish a trusting relationship between the child, family and professionals. The child should be central to any decisions made about management. A positive approach to treatment and outcome is vital with an emphasis on good prognosis, although full recovery may take some time.

The concept of gradual rehabilitation should be introduced, i.e. a steady and controlled increase in physical activity, social activities and schoolwork.

A Rehabilitation Programme

- Complete a daily timetable to structure the day.
- Activity should be set at a level that, at baseline, can be achieved without causing an increase in fatigue the next day.
- Periods of activity should be spread evenly through the day and balanced by rest periods.
- Discourage sleeping during rest periods.
- Levels of activity and rest each day should be as similar as possible across different days of the week.
- Start the timetable at the child's current level of functioning with small increases, e.g. 5–10% weekly.
- Stress the need to go at a pace agreed between the clinician and the child and family, not too fast or too slow.
- As the child's tolerance improves, the increases in activity can increase.

Graded Exercise Programme

- Exercise should not be short bursts of very strenuous activity, but more gradual exercises, carried out daily. In very severe cases, this may start with simple sitting up and gentle stretches.

- Mental activity, e.g. schoolwork, reading, social activity.
- Review goals regularly.

Individual Support for the Young Person

Some young people may require more intensive psychological treatment than general counselling or supportive therapy. Cognitive behaviour therapy (CBT) has been shown to be effective in the treatment of adults with CFS, and there is evidence of benefit in children, with further trials underway. Treatment of co-morbid psychiatric conditions should be addressed.

Family Support

Regular liaison and involvement of the family in the rehabilitation programme is essential, as the rehabilitation process is a slow and taxing one. Work with the family to address identified issues of family dynamics may be important. Gaining the family's confidence by working with and acknowledging their concerns is a priority. Family therapy can be helpful in exploring factors maintaining the illness or more serious underlying family dysfunction. As family life, and life outside the home for the parents, may have ceased because of the worry about the young person, encourage the parents to pick up life again, perhaps encouraging the mother (or father) to return to work where possible.

Friends

Young people who are off school for any length of time often lose friendships. Encourage the young person and the family to keep contact with friends by phone and visits, so that he/she can keep in touch with the gossip and friendship groups. The loss of friendships often makes it more difficult to return to school.

School

Discourage home tuition for any length of time, if possible, as this can perpetuate the illness. Encourage a very gradual return to school, if necessary, with a tutor who accompanies the child into a school or small school unit. Good liaison between the school, parents and other professionals is essential. Any discrepancies found on cognitive testing and any specific school-related problems, e.g. bullying, need to be addressed. Young people are often very anxious about time in school, and careful attention to managing details of the school day, e.g. carrying heavy bags, helps progress.

Drug Treatment

There is no systematic evidence for any drugs benefiting the core disorder. Pain relief (e.g. paracetamol), and non-steroidal anti-inflammatory drugs, may occasionally be necessary for headaches and muscle pain. Anti-depressant therapy may be indicated, if there are clear depressive symptoms, e.g. low mood with irritability and lack of pleasure in activities. There is, as yet, no clear evidence for alternative therapies offering substantial long-term benefits. It is important to anticipate setbacks and difficult transitions and to maintain encouragement and optimism.

Treatment Setting

Most young people can be managed as outpatients, with combined input from primary care, education, paediatric and child mental health services. Good liaison between all professionals involved is essential with regular (e.g. weekly) goal setting and monitoring. Referral to specialist services is recommended in the NICE guidelines within six months for mild CFS/ME, within three to four months for moderate CFS/ME and immediately in severe illness.

Inpatient treatment is necessary in some cases, especially if there is a lack of progress, a long duration of illness or if the child is particularly affected, e.g. not attending school at all or housebound. A specialist unit with experience in the treatment of CFS in young people and with access to a number of professionals, e.g. paediatricians, child psychiatrists and psychologists, physiotherapists, occupational therapists and nurses, is desirable, so that there is a multidisciplinary approach to assessment and management.

Case Study (1): Caitlin

Caitlin (12) was referred to the paediatric liaison team with a four-month history of fatigue and headaches and a fluctuating school attendance. She was trying to continue to attend school on a regular basis, but frequently had to return home early or would have days when she felt too ill and tired to manage to go in at all. She was unable to participate in the sports she normally enjoyed. The weekend before she was seen, a friend had come over for a sleepover that Caitlin very much enjoyed, but which kept her up later than usual. This left her with worsened symptoms of fatigue and headache for several days afterwards.

Caitlin and her mother were asked to keep a diary for two weeks, showing all her activity in half-hour chunks and grading it as low-energy activity, high-energy activity or rest. There was some discussion about how to categorise different activities and the need for rest to be 'true' rest and not watching television or texting friends.

This exercise showed something of a 'boom and bust' cycle, with Caitlin being much more active for two or three days at a time, then showing much reduced activity for the next few days, due to redoubled symptoms. This information was used to find a baseline for activity levels, and a structured plan, including short periods of high- and low-energy activities and rest, was constructed.

Caitlin's school were happy to agree to her attending school each day for a much shorter length of time with an expectation that this would be manageable and could be increased. A short walk was included daily. Caitlin initially found it difficult to have periods of absolute rest during the day, but soon found that these did help her to feel better. She found it frustrating not to be allowed to do more with friends on days that she felt better, but did understand the rationale.

Once it was clear that Caitlin was able to cope with her baseline plan, small changes were introduced every one to two weeks to increase activity and reduce some of her rests, with careful attention paid to how Caitlin coped with each change. She was gradually able to increase her time in school, but a brief relapse on returning to full-time schooling showed that the pace of change had become too fast and she reverted to attending for a little less than a full school day for an extended period of time before successfully resuming full-time attendance. Caitlin continued to have a short rest on return from school each day. She was able to participate in sports again, but on a less competitive level than before.

Case Study (2): Bryony

Bryony's (15) illness started with a period of a few months when she had a series of sore throats, at times with fever. She managed to attend school through much of this time, but on returning to school one day after time off, still fatigued, she had to return home the same day due to feeling exhausted. Her parents were alarmed at how pale she looked. A number of investigations failed to reveal any abnormality, and as the fatigue, headaches and intermittent sore throats continued in spite of rest, a diagnosis of chronic fatigue syndrome was made.

Bryony had increasing difficulty with mobility, only leaving the house in a wheelchair, and although home tuition was arranged, was only able to participate minimally in it. Her mother was taking extended periods of leave from work, and that was a source of stress for the family. Bryony was not improving with an outpatient approach and was admitted for a period of rehabilitation.

A daily timetable was drawn up that matched her levels of activity at the time, with careful structuring to spread activity and rest across the day. Daily physiotherapy was included, involving stretches and some gentle muscle-strengthening exercises. Time with a psychologist was included, initially for only 15 minutes at a time. Bryony managed to cope with this baseline programme, and subsequently small increases in activity and decreases in rest were made each week. She began attending the unit's school and gradually started to walk short distances both outside and inside the unit.

Bryony's rehabilitation continued for several months before a plan was made for school reintegration. A discharge date was agreed, after which physiotherapy input was maintained on an outpatient basis for some time.

Multiple-Choice Questions

See answers on page 671.

1. Chronic fatigue syndrome is often precipitated by a viral illness.
   True or False
2. Children with chronic fatigue syndrome have a higher recovery rate in comparison with adults.
   True or False
3. Graded exercise is often recommended in the treatment of chronic fatigue syndrome.
   True or False

Key References

Crawley, E., (2018). Pediatric chronic fatigue syndrome: current perspectives. *Pediatric Health, Medicine and Therapeutics*, 9: 27–33.

Chalder, T., Goodman, R., Wessely, S., et al., (2003). Epidemiology of chronic fatigue syndrome and self-reported myalgic encephalomyelitis in 5–15-year olds: cross sectional study. *BMJ*, 327: 654–655.

Garralda, M.E., Rangel, L., (2002). Annotation chronic fatigue syndrome in children and adolescents. *Journal of Child Psychology and Psychiatry*, 43(2), 169–176.

Kennedy, G., Underwood, C., Belch, J.J.F., (2010). Physical and functional impact of chronic fatigue syndrome/myalgic encephalomyelitis in childhood. *Pediatrics*, 125(6): e1324–e1330.

National Institute for Health and Clinical Excellence, (2007). *Chronic fatigue syndrome/myalgic encephalomyelitis (or encephalopathy); diagnosis and management. CG53.* London: National Institute for Health and Clinical Excellence (NICE).

Rangel, L., Garralda, M.E., Levin, M., Roberts, H., (2000). The course of severe chronic fatigue syndrome in childhood. *Journal of the Royal Society of Medicine*, 93(3): 129–134.

Wessely, S., (1996). Chronic fatigue syndrome: summary of a report of a joint committee of the Royal Colleges of Physicians, Psychiatrists and General Practitioners. *Journal of the Royal College of Physicians of London*, *30*(6), 497.

51 School Attendance Problems

Helen Carlow

Introduction

Persistent absence from school is defined by the Department for Education as missing 10% of possible school sessions in a given period of time (DfE, 2019) and is recognised as a worldwide issue. There are many reasons why a child may present with persistent absence, or school attendance problems (SAPs), including

- Long-term ill-health
- Reasons imposed by family or wider circumstances, e.g. being a young carer
- Parents' capability
- School-based reasons, e.g. part-time timetables
- Child-motivated reasons, e.g. truancy or anxiety around school

Once significant schooling is missed, the consequences of such absence have been well-documented and include increased risks of poor academic attainment, conflict with family and social isolation in the short term, and in the longer term, substance abuse, mental health and financial difficulties, unemployment and imprisonment (Heyne, 2019). This means that once established, unless they are successfully managed, school attendance problems can lead to a spiral of social isolation and poor outcomes across life.

Recent statistics suggest that, despite such far-reaching consequences, prevalence is increasing in England, with one in nine pupils persistently absent in the academic year 2017/18 (DfE, 2019). Males and females are equally likely to exhibit school attendance problems, with prevalence sharply rising in adolescence. Statistics reported by the DfE indicate that across England some vulnerable groups have higher percentages of persistent absenteeism, including those receiving free school meals, those with statements of SEN or an Education, Health and Care Plan (EHCP) and those for whom English is not their first language (DfE, 2019).

KEY POINTS

- School attendance problems (SAPs) refer to any degree of repeated non-attendance or attempted non-attendance, regardless of the factors that motivate its onset and continuation.
- While historically schools have dealt with non-attendance by implementing a series of 'blanket' interventions, research advocates taking account of both form and function of the behaviour and devising a tailored intervention based on this information.

Forms of Behaviour Include

- School withdrawal (parent motivated)
- School exclusion (school motivated)
- School refusal (child motivated)
- Truancy (child motivated)

Functions of Behaviour Include

- Avoidance of stimuli that provoke negative feelings
- Avoidance of aversive social or evaluative situations
- Attention seeking
- Pursuit of tangible reinforcement outside school

Best practice is to consider all cases individually and to devise a targeted and tailored management plan with the support of the pupil, family and school staff.

Beyond this, there is still limited evidence for any one intervention in the effective management of SAPs, though CBT, DBT and working with schools to support those influential school factors have the most promising findings. Open lines of communication, and involvement where appropriate, with local authority agencies (e.g. family support workers, educational psychologists and CAMHS) should be ensured.

What Do We Mean by School Attendance Problems?

One of the most challenging issues in the area is the inconsistency with which it is defined and described. The DfE classify persistent absence as missing 10% of school time in any given period, while authors researching the area cite a range of criteria, the most widely accepted being 25% of school time missed. Additionally, Tobias (2019) outlines a range of behaviours that can all be described as school refusal, some of which may be missed in the threshold criteria above:

- Persistent lateness
- Pattern of low or patchy attendance
- Morning behaviours that prevent leaving home
- Difficulty remaining at school for a whole day
- Refusal to attend classes/non-compliance
- Attendance under duress (e.g. crying at school gate)
- Authorised absence for serial illness

Complete absence for a significant block of time

In addition to threshold criteria there is inconsistency of terminology. Terms such as school refusal, school phobia and truancy are used interchangeably, but may refer to an umbrella term for all SAPs or to a specific pattern of behaviour.

Current Perspectives on Classification

There are two main perspectives around how SAPs are most helpfully distinguished, classification either by form or by function. In considering a child's difficulties with attendance, it is recommended that both form and function are considered.

Form of SAPs

Heyne (2019) outlined four categories of SAP:

- **School withdrawal**. This refers to the motivation of a parent to keep the child at home, for example, a child being a young carer.
- **School exclusion**. This refers to absences imposed by school, for example, fixed-term exclusions or part-time timetables.
- **School refusal**. The definition of this has varied over time, but Berg's 1996 definition is the most widely used and accepted (Heyne, 2019). This outlines four criteria including:
  - (i) Parental awareness that the child is not attending.
  - (ii) Diagnosis or existence of antisocial behaviour is not present.
  - (iii) Parents make efforts to get their child to school.
  - (iv) The child is emotionally upset at having to attend school.
- **Truancy**. This refers to absence when the child is making attempts to hide their non-attendance and parents are usually unaware of absence. A lack of observed anxiety around attendance is a feature.

Of these four categories, the latter two are child-motivated (CM-SAPs), as opposed to the first groups where parents or school are the primary motivation. Research in the field of SAPs generally refers to and focusses on SAPs that could be classified as school refusal or truancy.

Function of School Attendance Problems

The second perspective is not to classify SAP by type, but the function behind the behaviour. This perspective looks only at CM-SAPs. Kearney (2002) devised a measure to ascertain this, the School Refusal Assessment Scale (SRAS-R), which is widely used in the field. This suggested four main functions that serve to maintain attendance problems:

- **Avoidance of school related triggers**, which may include avoidance of a particular place, such as a school bus, a specific teacher or lesson.
- **Escape from social or evaluative situations at school**, which may include difficulties with peer relationships, including exams.
- **Receiving attention from significant people** – this does not relate to aversive factors inside school and more to the draw of remaining with a parent or significant person outside of school.
- **Tangible reinforcement outside of school** – this does not relate to aversive factors inside school, but to the draw of activities or reinforcements that can be gained outside of school, for example, socialising with peers.

Assessment

It is important to consider all cases and their unique characteristics and variables on an in-depth, individual basis. To guide initial thinking and gather information, tools exploring the form and function of behaviour have been developed. The most commonly used tool is the Revised School Refusal Assessment Scale (Kearney, 2002). Other scales include the Inventory of School Attendance Problems (ISAP; Knollmann, Reissner and Hebebrand, 2018) and the School Non-Attendance Checklist (SNACK; Heyne, 2019).

To form hypotheses regarding the nature of a pupil's SAPs, it is necessary to consider information from a variety of sources, including the pupil, the pupil's family and members of teaching staff, and through a variety of media (e.g. observation, interview and discussion, analysis of attendance records, etc.).

Areas that warrant exploration may include:

- Whether there is evidence of a key 'event' or incident which triggered, or preceded the period of school refusal.
- Whether there are any patterns to the school refusal (i.e. is attendance linked to particular times of day, teachers, curriculum areas).
- What the pupil is doing when they are not in school.
- The quality and nature of the pupil's relationships with their peers.
- The quality and nature of the pupil's relationships with their family members.
- Whether there is any history of school refusal behaviour (SRB) with other members of the family.
- Whether there are any other areas of concern within the child's life; for example, is school the only area in which the behaviour manifests, or do they show difficulties in other areas (e.g. work, social situations)?
- The level of attendance and the length of time that the SRB has persisted for.

Management and Intervention

Interventions for CM-SAPs are wide ranging, including pharmacology, family therapy, social work, legal interventions, parent training and individual child-centred therapies (Tobias, 2019). A systematic review of psychosocial intervention effectiveness was carried out by Maynard et al. (2015), drawing together findings from studies published between 1980 and 2013.

The review found few rigorous studies in the area, with cognitive behaviour therapy (CBT) being the focus in the majority. The review concluded that there is some tentative evidence that CBT may be effective for improving attendance, but there is little evidence for the longevity of any effects. Moreover, wide variation in the type of CBT across studies means it cannot be concluded which aspects were helpful for even short-term effects.

Recent research into DBT with web-based coaching has yielded some promising results (Chu et al., 2015). This is in part due to the flexibility provided through web-based support when the problem is most prevalent, e.g. in the child's home and outside of typical working hours, particularly early mornings. More research needs to be carried out to explore this further.

Due to the lack of clear research findings, many educational psychologists have reported uncertainty in knowing which intervention is best to recommend. Schools have historically responded to cases by putting in place a series of 'blanket' interventions, including offering rewards to the pupil for attendance, or spending time with a key member of pastoral staff. Qualitative studies exploring interventions for CM-SAPs from the perspectives of both children and adults have suggested that children do not feel listened to when being supported through an SAP (Baker and Bishop, 2015; Tobias, 2019) and did not feel as though their individuality was recognised.

As is widely accepted amongst psychology and behaviour professionals, it is necessary to consider the function of behaviour in order to implement an effective intervention. The nature of the research has indicated that this is particularly important for pupils exhibiting SAPs and pursuing similar routes for all cases is not helpful and may exacerbate the situation.

Having developed the SRAS-R, Kearney (2002) developed some tentative guidelines suggesting interventions that might warrant consideration for each different type of SRB. These were as follows:

- **Type 1 (avoidance)** may be best targeted by a child-based approach; exposure to school through systematic desensitisation or relaxation techniques to alleviate feelings of anxiety when presented with an anxiety 'trigger'.
- **Type 2 (escape)** may be best targeted by exposure to school in addition to cognitive restructuring or social skills training to support the child in situations that produce anxiety.
- **Type 3 (attention seeking)** may be best targeted by focussing on implementing routines and providing training in parenting skills, to equip parents with the skills to deal with attention-seeking behaviour.
- **Type 4 (tangible reinforcement)** may be best targeted by family-based therapies or contingency contracts to provide positive reinforcement for desired behaviours. Forced school attendance may be effective here.

Prescriptive interventions that make use of these guidelines have shown encouraging results (e.g. Kearney and Silverman, 1999), but there remains very little research from which to draw conclusions.

More recently, the influence of school factors in both the onset and treatment of SAPs has been increasingly prominent (Brouwer-Borghuis et al., 2019; McKay-Brown et al., 2019). Across the literature, where successful reintegration has taken place, such factors have played a key role, including the identification of a key adult, understanding staff, smaller class sizes and safe spaces identified within school. For this reason, it is important that the issue is not seen as purely a 'within-child' issue to manage.

To helpfully intervene for a child, there need to be clear systems in place on a local and school level. This will allow prevention and early intervention work to take place, prior to working at a more individual level with a child and their family. Kearney and Graczyk (2014) suggest a tiered model of intervention that outlines such an approach.

Tier One

Tier one takes place on a whole-school level for every student. This includes staff awareness of attendance policies and systems to regularly review attendance data to highlight any pupils who may be at risk. To encourage attendance, schools should foster climates that communicate safety and consistency by educating pupils in key areas linked to their social and emotional needs, including anger management, peer mediation and coping with difficult life events, e.g. divorce. Kearney and Graczyk flag the importance of secondary transition for identifying those pupils who may experience difficulties.

Tier Two

At tier two, 'at risk' pupils for CM-SAPs should benefit from additional support. This would include closer communication with parents and assessment around the function of CM-SAPs in individual cases, with early attempts to address these as appropriate, e.g. CBT approaches. Weekly monitoring of individual attendance is advised at this tier.

Tier Three

Kearney and Graczyk suggested that pupils who reach the legal limit for truancy, which they cite as ten absences per semester, or those who miss 20% of class time over a period of six weeks would require support at tier three. They suggest that such support would be extensions of the individual interventions put in place at tier two in addition to more work alongside parents.

School Attendance Problems across Age Groups

SAPs are rarely reported as a problem in the 0–5 age group, as there is no requirement for mandatory school attendance. Issues around attendance at this age generally relate to anxiety, particularly separation from parents, much of which may be age appropriate or managed between pre-school and parental strategies.

While present during the primary and junior school years (5–11), there is an increase in prevalence in secondary school (11–18). In addition to developmental, academic and social pressures that occur during these years, the secondary school environment is vastly different to primary, larger, with movement between peers, teachers and classrooms, all of which might contribute to the increase.

Despite the rise in prevalence in the adolescent age group, research suggests that treatment of this group is generally less successful than for primary-aged children. This may be a reflection of the complex factors mentioned above that interplay at this age, particularly in light of the transition to secondary school and the influence of school factors on SAPs. There is tentative evidence that developmentally sensitive CBT may be helpful for this age group, e.g. Heyne et al. (2014), though more research is needed.

Case Study (1): Niall

Niall was five and in his third term of reception. Niall's attendance at pre-school was very good, and his transition to school had gone smoothly. His absence began increasing shortly before the end of his first term at school. School staff and Niall's mother reported that he was never reluctant to attend school in the mornings, separated well from her on arrival and generally seemed happy on returning home. However, he was absent due to stomach aches on the days he did not attend.

Once flagged by senior management as 'at risk' of SAPs, closer examination of patterns demonstrated that absences tended to occur on Tuesdays and Thursdays, when there were whole-school assemblies. Staff reported that during lunch times, Niall tended to stay close to an adult rather than playing with his peers, though he happily interacted with them during class time.

It was hypothesised that Niall was finding whole-school environments overwhelming. Niall began working on relaxation techniques with an ELSA during assembly time. The ELSA then moved towards attending the assemblies alongside him. Over time, she began to leave the assemblies at an earlier point. Niall's attendance difficulties resolved after this point.

Case Study (2): Jasvinder, Age Nine

Jasvinder's attendance and attainment at school had not been of concern until Year 4. Just before the first half term, she had a period of absence lasting a school week and following this, her attendance records showed that she averaged one or two days off per week. During the next term, her absences increased, and she was often away for the whole week, perhaps attending for just one morning or afternoon. She often arrived at school with her mother, but refused to go in, becoming very distressed and anxious, hitting out when her mother attempted to leave. Jasvinder developed an excellent relationship with the Deputy Head Teacher, who assumed the responsibility of supporting her to separate from her mother at the start of the school day

As her attendance deteriorated, she was reluctant to leave the Deputy Head and spent what little time she was in school in her office. Similar to with her mother, any attempts to support Jasvinder to join her class were met with panic attacks, hyperventilation or upset and anger.

Jasvinder had a particularly close relationship with her mother. Her parents had separated and divorced in the previous academic year, and it was hypothesised that this may have triggered the onset of separation anxiety with her mother and related attention-seeking behaviour. Without the attention of her mother at home, she sought the individual attention of the Deputy Head, which appeared to worsen the situation, as she no longer attended class. Although Jasvinder's mother had been threatened with legal action, this only appeared to add to Jasvinder's level of anxiety.

Due to the severe nature of her anxiety, Jasvinder was referred to the child and adolescent mental health service, through which she and her mother accessed some cognitive behavioural-based family therapy. This focussed on working through issues around the separation of her parents and looked at the new routines in the home. Although the process was a lengthy one, coupled with secondary transition, Lauren's attendance rose over time and she was attending well by Year 9.

Case Study (3): Matty, Age 15

Matty attended primary school well but received a number of fixed-term exclusions for aggression and was permanently excluded from two secondary schools by the time he reached Year 10. He was placed on roll at the local education centre, but his attendance was only around 25%. During the time he was not in school, Matty was often picked up by the police, who were carrying out 'sweeps' of the local area, looking for 'truanting' pupils. Although he would leave the house in the mornings promising to attend school, he would reply honestly when challenged about his whereabouts in the evenings. He tended to spend his time with a group of older children who had left school the previous year, and they would play video games or walk around the local shopping centre.

Although reluctant to engage with school staff, Matty developed a positive relationship with an assistant psychologist, who was working in the centre with pupils on a programme designed to support pupils at risk of exclusion, and with the centre's family support worker. He appeared to enjoy the discussion and activity-based group sessions, designed to challenge thinking and encourage independence and attended these. This proved the trigger for him to engage in decision-making around his future at the centre, and he showed interest in a mechanics apprenticeship. Although his attendance improved, he continued to need support to motivate himself, and the centre effectively used a contingency contract, in which he earned 'vouchers' for every session he attended, which could be exchanged for rewards or activities. By the end of Year 11, Matty's attendance had risen to 85%, and he earned a place at the sixth form college.

Multiple-Choice Questions

See answers on page 671.

1. Which statement is correct about management of school attendance problems?
   a. School attendance problems should be treated at an individual level, from a within-child perspective. School systems and staff can have little influence.
   b. It is important to ensure that all pupils who exhibit school refusal behaviour in school are treated the same way.
   c. It is important to consider the form and function of a child's school refusal behaviour and plan an intervention tailored around this.

   d. Given that it is the responsibility of the parent to ensure that a child attends school, all cases of school refusal should result in parents being threatened with prosecution.
   e. Cognitive behaviour therapy is a proven effective intervention for all types of SAPs.
2. Which statement is correct about pupils with attendance problems?
   a. The majority of school refusers are female.
   b. Pupils are more likely to exhibit school attendance problems in primary school.
   c. School non-attenders generally hide their absence from their parents.
   d. School refusers are often older siblings.
   e. It is common for school refusers to experience academic underachievement, employment difficulties and increased risk of criminal offending.
3. Which statement can be described as an example of SAPs?
   a. Attendance at school under duress and pleas for non-attendance.
   b. Repeated tardiness in the morning to avoid school, followed by attendance.
   c. Complete absence during a certain period of the school year.
   d. Complete absence for an extended period of time.
   e. All of the above are examples of SAPs.
4. Which statement is incorrect about the assessment of SAPs?
   a. The views of parents and staff should be sought, but the views of the child are of limited value.
   b. Information should be gathered from a variety of different sources and methodologies.
   c. Information about areas of the pupil's life outside of school should be sought and taken into consideration.
   d. It is important to consider what the pupil is doing when they are not in school.
   e. Patterns in school attendance should be looked for and where they exist, should be explored.
5. Which statement about SAPs is correct?
   a. SAPs are the result of poor parenting.
   b. SAPs are usually motivated by a number of different factors, but it is often useful to identify a possible primary or predominant motivation.
   c. SAPs are driven by difficulties within the child and the influence of school is minimal.
   d. School refusal is another word for truancy.
   e. SAPs are solely a behavioural issue and not an emotional one.

Key References

Heyne, D., (2019). Developments in classification, identification and intervention for school refusal and other attendance problems: introduction to the special series. *Cognitive and Behavioral Practice*, 26: 1–7.

Kearney, C., Graczyk, P., (2014). A response to intervention model to promote school attendance and decrease school absenteeism. *Child Youth Care Forum*, 43: 1–25.

Maynard, B., Brendel, K., Bulanda, J., et al., (2015). Psychosocial interventions for school refusal with primary and secondary school students: a systematic review. *Campbell Systematic Reviews*, 2015: 12.

52 Addictions

Jack Groom

KEY CONCEPTS

- Around 50% of school-aged children are estimated to have used drugs.
- Addiction is generally defined as a psychological and/or physical inability to stop using a substance or participating in a behaviour, despite it causing psychological and/or physical harm.
- The scope of addiction is changing, with behavioural addictions now recognised by ICD-11 and DSM-5 alongside substance use disorders.
- Behavioural addiction is an emerging field that is poorly understood and can be difficult to untangle.
- CBT can be a useful tool to treat the cognitive distortions that are often a core component of addiction.

Introduction

When thinking of addiction in adults, we often think of alcohol, drug misuse or smoking as the big players. In children, we are currently seeing a wide range of proposed behavioural addictions alongside substance misuse, i.e. internet use, gaming, gambling, pornography, exercise, shopping and so on. The ICD-11 is even considering gaming disorder as a diagnosable condition. Where things become unclear is the exact nature of an addiction and to what extent behaviours should be medicalised.

Addiction here is defined as a chronic disorder, characterised by uncontrolled use of substances or participation in behaviours, despite negative consequences or disruption to normal functioning. These behaviours can become physiologically addictive, whereby the brain begins to crave stimulation via the substance or behaviour. It is more difficult to pinpoint the psychological component of addiction. The rituals surrounding it become hugely important and necessary for cessation of craving. The word 'addiction' is often omitted from diagnoses because of the uncertainty of its definition and negative connotations.

What behaviours should we worry about in children and adolescents? Is gaming comparable to alcohol misuse? And what can clinicians do to manage addiction? First, we must examine some common addictions and behaviours, before moving on to potential treatments.

Substance Use Disorder

Introduction

Although arguments for the popularisation of casual drug use by social media and celebrity culture are important, the use of harmful substances is deeply ingrained in our society. The number of public houses in the UK is, in itself, a testament to that. In addition, there is increasing pressure on young people to appear attractive, fun and successful on social media, plus ever more imminent worries about the environment, the economy they will inherit and their future. No wonder young people are tempted by drug use.

In a recent survey, 18% of secondary school pupils had taken drugs in the previous year, 44% of 11–15-year olds have drunk alcohol and 20% have smoked, with these figures rising as they become older (Kardefelt-Winther et al., 2017). Despite the overall trend declining, substance use is still incredibly common, but when does this behaviour move from normal rebellion and impulsivity, to a mental health problem?

Diagnosis

Substance use is not unusual among young people, but dependency and substance use disorder are relatively rare. According to the DSM-5, to diagnose a substance use disorder, several criteria must be met:

- **Impaired Control**
    - Substance is taken in larger amounts over longer periods than planned.
    - Unsuccessful attempts to decrease use.
    - Large amounts of time dedicated to substance.
    - Craving the substance when it is not being used.
- **Social Impairment**
    - Failure to fulfil obligations at school and work.
    - Interpersonal problems and tensions.
    - Withdrawal from normal activities and hobbies.
- **Risky Use**
    - Continued use despite knowledge of psychological or physical health consequences.
    - Use in situations that are physically harmful.
- **Pharmacological**
    - Tolerance – person requires increased dose or experiences decreased effect.
    - Withdrawal – varied symptoms after stopping the substance use (e.g. insomnia, tremors, nausea and vomiting, irritability).

Substance use disorder ranges from moderate (e.g. two or three symptoms present) to severe (six+ symptoms), and is usually specific to the substance being used.

Assessment

As always when assessing young people, consideration must be given both to presenting symptoms and to the wider systems the children inhabit. Necessary to the assessment of addiction are:

- **History of Drug Use**
    - Which substance; frequency; how long it has been used for; where it is being taken; with whom; how is it paid for; when/why it started.
    - Effect of the drug use on their life, i.e. psychological, financial, physical.
    - Past psychiatric history (e.g. ADHD, ODD, conduct disorder, autism, depression).
    - Developmental history (e.g. temperament, milestones, early oppositional behaviours).
- **Family**
    - Details of pregnancy. Did the mother use substances whilst pregnant?

    - History of mental health or drug misuse.
    - Family system.
- **Social**
    - School/college. Academic, social, and behavioural difficulties.
    - Peer relationships.
    - Contact with other agencies, e.g. police or social services.

Symptoms will generally follow the criteria of diagnosis, and the systemic approach to these patients is imperative as substance misuse relies not only on biological re-wiring of the brain, but on the environment these young people inhabit. Assessment of the family structure that allows this behaviour, e.g. where drugs are procured from, can help guide the choice of therapy and explain the aetiology of the mental illness.

Intervention

As always, the effectiveness of any intervention will depend on the young person's willingness to change and their ability to engage with services. From a CAMHS perspective, the young person will usually be referred to a local drug and alcohol misuse programme, whose specific services and remits are defined by the local authority. In the case of strong opioids, e.g. heroin, replacement medication such as methadone may be used. Young people who inject substances can be referred to needle-exchange schemes. If the problem lies deeper within a system of mental health issues, or underlying family dysfunction, other therapies, e.g. family therapy or CBT, may be appropriate.

Behavioural Addiction

Introduction

Behavioural addiction as a diagnosis is a relatively new concept, first discussed in 2001 (Holden, 2001) and only included officially in the DSM-5 (2013) and ICD-11 (2018 draft). This shift in category from 'Substance-Related Abuse and Dependency', to 'Substance-Related and Addictive Disorders', symbolises a shift in the way we approach addiction and mental health. But it raises many questions about the body of research behind it and the methods by which we assess behavioural addiction.

Defining Behavioural Addiction

Currently, there is no consensus as to how a behavioural addiction should be defined. DSM-5 defines 'non-substance-related disorders' as addictive disorders where no substance is ingested. However, there are some issues simply with removing the substance from the definition.

Firstly, there has been no evidence to suggest that behavioural addictions share the same aetiology, course or treatment as substance-related disorders. Currently, only gambling disorder is included in behavioural addictions in the DSM-5, and internet gaming disorder is to be included in ICD-11. This is likely due to a distinct lack of high-powered studies that investigate its roots and its course.

In addition, little work has been done to tease out the defining features of behavioural addiction when compared to normal behaviours. High-level athletes share many of the same characteristics as those relating to behavioural addiction, but these can be attributed to a lifestyle choice that many deem normal or even valuable in our society. So what exactly separates internet gaming disorder from high-level athletics in terms of the behaviours that drive them?

Questions such as these make it difficult to disentangle what is deemed 'normal' behaviour, and what is deemed 'addiction'.

One proposed working definition by Kardefelt-Winther et al. (2017) seems a sensible starting place to conceptualise these behaviours:

> A repeated behaviour leading to significant harm or distress. The behaviour is not reduced by the person and persists over a significant period of time. The harm or distress is of a functionally impairing nature.

These must include exclusion criteria however, and according to Kardefelt-Whinther et al. would *not* be considered behavioural addiction if:

- Behaviour is better explained by an underlying disorder.
- Impairment results from an activity that is a wilful choice, e.g. high-level sports.
- Can be characterised as a period of prolonged involvement that detracts from other aspects of life but does not lead to significant functional impairment.
- Behaviour is a result of a coping strategy.

Although not a perfect definition, this at least allows a framework on which to hang formulations. New additions to diagnostic manuals will prove whether this can bear weight.

Diagnosis

Currently only two disorders are recognised by diagnostic manuals: gaming disorder and gambling disorder. Here we will focus on the ICD-11 definitions of these as gaming disorder is not included in the DSM-5 and the definitions more closely align with the proposed framework above, rather than relying on tweaking substance use disorder criteria.

Gaming Disorder

Diagnosis

Gaming disorder is a newly added category in ICD-11 and relates to the use of video games in any form, i.e. mobile, games console, internet and so on. The prevalence of gaming disorder seems to vary between countries, with a recent review of epidemiological data in China placing it between 3.5 and 17%, but in Europe and the USA rates were lower, between 0.3 and 1.2% (Long et al., 2018).

It is defined as:

> A pattern of gaming behaviour characterized by impaired control over gaming, increasing priority given to gaming over other activities to the extent that gaming takes precedence over other interests … and continuation or escalation of gaming despite the occurrence of negative consequences.
>
> (Przybylski et al., 2017)

The behaviour above must be severe enough to impair personal, social, educational or occupational functioning and to have been present for at least 12 months. The difficulty with gaming disorder is, like most behavioural addictions, making a diagnosis without pathologising common behaviours.

Currently, this seems to be a clinical judgement from the assessing clinician as to the severity of the impairment caused. However, a changing landscape of leisure activities among younger generations has made placing a boundary on 'acceptable levels' of gaming difficult. For many children, online gaming is a way of socialising with friends through in-game chats and can alleviate some sense of isolation that children may feel because of living further from friends, or existing mental health conditions that can make in-person socialising difficult. These details need to be teased out through careful questioning and by understanding what is important to the child and why.

Intervention

Currently, the most commonly used treatment for gaming disorder is CBT (Stevens et al., 2019). This can be delivered individually, or in a group. Currently, the American Psychological Association favours group therapy, as it allows a closed and safe environment whereby participants can share their gaming experiences with others who understand gaming, something a clinician may not know much about, and sensitive topics can be openly discussed with others in a similar position. The evidence for medication is limited, and studies have only shown effectiveness in reducing behaviours if there is an underlying condition associated, e.g. depression or anxiety.

Gambling Disorder

Diagnosis

The main characteristic of gambling addiction or 'pathological gambling' is frequent and repeated episodes of gambling that 'dominate the patient's life to the detriment of social, occupational, material, and family values and commitments' (WHO, 2018). It aligns with the pattern seen in other addictions, such as escalating behaviour despite negative consequences, preoccupation with gambling and increasing time devoted to it. Gambling disorder has only recently been classified as an addiction, rather than an impulse control disorder.

Despite adolescents being much less likely to report gambling behaviours, reviews have found that the proportion of pathological gambling among adolescents could be three times that of the adult (National Research, 1999). Since these findings have been shown, the nature of gambling for adolescents has shifted, with much more focus placed on online gambling and gambling within video games.

Gambling within video games particularly is an emerging issue, as it is not restricted in the same way as more traditional gambling. It involves players paying money for the chance to receive in-game items or bonuses, using what are termed 'loot boxes'. This is often the case with initially free-to-play games that are very popular among young people. Huge sums of money can be spent on these 'loot boxes', and this causes significant financial strain on families, if not controlled.

Intervention

At the moment, evidence is limited for any single form of treatment for gambling addiction in adolescents. However, CBT has had some success in treating the cognitive distortions that are a prominent feature of gambling disorder. No pharmacological interventions are currently recommended.

Adolescent gamblers are hugely reluctant to seek treatment and will often not present until they have experienced significant familial, academic, social or legal difficulties. Gambling disorder often presents with co-morbidities, such as depression, that can muddy the waters. This creates a challenge in the treatment of gambling disorder itself, as most cases that present are severe, or clouded by co-morbid conditions. Referral to local addiction services is recommended first and foremost.

Summary

The scope of addiction is slowly expanding to include behavioural addictions, rather than solely substance use disorders. There is much debate as to the exact definition of behavioural addictions, let alone the proper diagnosis and management of such conditions. Adolescents are particularly susceptible to drug-taking behaviours for a number of reasons, e.g. peer pressure, family and social groups, a lack of education around drug use, a general propensity for rebellion and a healthy curiosity common to their age group. Many of the emerging addictive behaviours are aimed at young people, such as internet use or gaming disorders. Much more work is needed to untangle the bio-psycho-social underpinnings of addictions and the methods we have available to both prevent them, and treat young people struggling with this difficult set of conditions.

Case Study: James

James (16) presented to CAMHS with low mood and suicidal ideation. He had been sleeping at a friend's house for some weeks as he felt he could not be at home at the moment, due to thoughts of self-harm. School referred him due to him seeming low, falling behind on work and falling asleep in class.

After speaking with James, he told us that he has been using MDMA and ketamine for about a year and that this had become more frequent since moving to his friend's house as they tended to do this together in the evenings. James noted that his mood was lower in the morning after using the drugs, and he was aware that his tiredness and a component of his low mood were related to his drug use. He said that he began using MDMA after his parent's divorce and that he was currently living with his father, which he does not like.

James was referred to the local drug advice service where a counsellor met with him to discuss the harm of long-term drug use and the ways in which he can avoid situations that may make it more likely for him to use drugs. Some low-intensity CBT work was undertaken to help stop his use of MDMA and to raise his mood. He was referred for family therapy with the aim of exploring the family system, the issues he had about living with his father and how the family unit could be strengthened to help support him.

Multiple-Choice Questions

See answers on page 671.

1. Which of the following are features of a substance use disorder?
   a. Substance is taken in larger amounts over longer periods than planned.
   b. Withdrawal from normal activities and hobbies.
   c. Continued use despite knowledge of psychological or physical health consequences.
   d. Person requires increased dose or experiences decreased effect from substance.
   e. All of the above.
2. Which of these are listed as official conditions in the DSM-5?
   a. Internet dependence
   b. Gambling disorder

   c. Pornography addiction
   d. Compulsive shopping disorder
   e. Social media addiction
3. Medication is effective in reducing the severity of behavioural addiction.
   a. True
   b. False

Key References

Holden, C., (2001). 'Behavioral' addictions: do they exist? *Science*, 294(5544): 980–982.

Kardefelt-Winther, D., Heeren, A., Schimmenti, A., van Rooij, A., Maurage, P., Carras, M., ... Billieux, J. (2017). How can we conceptualize behavioural addiction without pathologizing common behaviours? *Addiction*, 112(10): 1709–1715.

Long, J., Liu, T., Liu, Y., Hao, W., Maurage, P., Billieux, J., (2018). Prevalence and correlates of problematic online gaming: a systematic review of the evidence published in Chinese. *Current Addiction Reports*, 5(3): 359–371.

Przybylski, A.K., Weinstein, N., Murayama, K., (2017). Internet gaming disorder: investigating the clinical relevance of a new phenomenon. *American Journal of Psychiatry*, 174(3): 230–236.

Stevens, M.W., King, D.L., Dorstyn, D., Delfabbro, P.H., (2019). Cognitive–behavioral therapy for Internet gaming disorder: a systematic review and meta-analysis. *Clinical Psychology & Psychotherapy*, 26(2): 191–203.

WHO. Gaming Disorder, (2018). World Health Organisation. [Online] September 2018. www.who.int/features/qa/gaming-disorder/en/.

53 Screen-Based Activities and Social Media

Vicki Bright and Cathy Laver-Bradbury

KEY CONCEPTS

- There are many benefits for young people in using social media in terms of information finding, accessing self-help programmes, creativity and feeling more connected to others.
- Current research points to an association between mental health problems, e.g. depression and anxiety, and social media usage. However, there is no clear causal link.
- Many young people are aware of potential online risks.
- Digital citizen programmes are being considered for 4–14-year olds to empower children and young people and to help them negotiate their way through internet use.

Introduction

The use of social media by young people is widespread and growing fast. This represents a change in society into the digital age, with children as young as three years having access to tablets. Many young people have smartphones to access the internet where they can find information and support and communicate with others in real time. Young people may have virtual relationships via social media or other apps, e.g. Instagram.

Young people are more adept at using cyber technology, i.e. accessing and using social media and evading parental controls of the internet, than their parents or CAMHS professionals. This is acknowledged (Dickson et al., 2018). Some young people have developed lucrative careers through 'YouTube' by becoming 'social influencers'. Whilst there can be many benefits in using social media for children and young people, there are many serious concerns from parents, teachers and agencies working with children and young people (CYP) about the potential impact of online experiences on CYP's mental health and well-being. In particular, excessive time spent on social media is a concern and has raised questions about the possible impact on the young person's mental health and psychosocial wellbeing.

Online activities can cause distress in young people and can be associated with risk- taking behaviour, e.g. meeting people that have made contact via a chat room. Other concerns are when a young person spends more time online than interacting socially and anger issues when being asked to stop playing online games.

Most CAMHS workers will have encountered young people referred to the service because they have been negatively affected by cyberbullying, grooming, sexting or by excessive screen time usage. These experiences can impact on young people's mental health. The Royal College of Psychiatrists has recommended that social media usage should be evaluated at CAMHS assessments, i.e. not just actual time spent on devices, but what activities the young person is involved in.

Current research studies are looking at identifying a relationship between screen-based activities and mental health outcomes and whether there is an association between screen-based activities and mental health in terms of increased risk of anxiety or depression. As yet, no causal relationship has been established (Dickson et al., 2018).

What Are Screen-Based Activities?

Screen-based activity includes any activity using a screen, on- or offline, any activity using access to the internet, social media and social networking sites (Dickson et al., 2018). Common social media applications used by young people are apps, such as Facebook, Instagram, TikTok and Snapchat. Social media can be used in a variety of ways to communicate and access information. Examples of screen-based activity might be sexting, texting, selfie-taking, gaming, generating content, posting online and searching for information, in addition to making new friends.

Benefits and Positives of Onscreen Activities

There are many positives and benefits to using screen-based activities to access information and communicate with others via the internet. Anderson and Jiang (2018) found, in their large survey of US teenagers aged 13–17 years, that 69% of young people believe that the internet helps them to interact with a more diverse group of friends. Eighty-one percent thought that the internet made them feel more connected to what was happening in their friends' lives. Young people have the technological skills to access information. Current research is being done on designing treatment packages that young people can access via the internet for common mental health conditions, e.g. anxiety disorders. There is a risk that, without clear protection by internet companies, and parental controls, young people are at risk of unintentionally accessing pornographic sites and sites that can unhelpfully glamourise mental illnesses. This could lead to young people not accessing professional help (RSPH, 2017).

Online Activity and Mental Health

Over the last few years, the amount of time spent onscreen has increased for all age groups. This has led to concerns relating to young people's psychosocial and mental health. Evidence suggests that children as young as three to four years use tablets to watch TV programmes (Dickson et al., 2018), whilst older children are more likely to use social media apps to seek out friends and participate in group chats.

Anderson and Jiang (2018), in a recent survey of US teenagers aged 13–17, showed that many of them are aware of the potential risks of using social media. Children are concerned about the levels of advertising, pornography and violence. One in five adolescents were said to have experienced something worrying and unpleasant online. Young people said that they prefer to discuss issues about staying safe online by talking to their peers, as they do not trust that their teachers are confident in their knowledge of internet use. Online self-disclosure, identity issues, fear of missing out (FOMO) and cyberbullying can be major issues for young people to negotiate.

No causal relationship between screen-based activities and mental health has been identified, but the studies do highlight that there appeared to be some association with an increased risk of anxiety or depression.

Glamourising Mental Health Problems

Some young people are aware that, in using social media, they risk accessing harmful or distressing images. They are aware of sites that have harmful content, e.g. sex or violence, pro-anorexia and self-harm sites.

Current thinking is that, for those young people who self-harm and are at risk of suicide, their problems may be related to social media. This is a major concern. Legislation and advice to the press have been given to ensure that suicides of celebrities are reported simply as deaths and that a multi-agency approach to the prevention of suicide and self-harm in young people is developed. Work is being undertaken to offer online support to young people who are at risk, and sites that can unhelpfully glamourise mental illnesses, such as the pro-anorexia sites, are being reported.

Case Study (1): Jodie

Jodie (13) had recently been referred to CAMHS, due to significant thoughts of self-harm, culminating with her putting a ligature around her neck. The triggers to her self-harm were friendship issues at school. Jodie texted her friends on the group chat, some of whom self-harm. They recommended a 'good' website to look at for self-harm. Jodie saw there how ligatures could be used and decided to use one. Jodie's mother had checked Jodie's phone and discovered that people in the group chat had been describing, encouraging and showing images of self-harm. Jodie acknowledged she had been impulsive in attempting to copy the idea.

We discussed the plan to keep Jodie safe and for her mother to monitor her social media usage. Parental controls were installed to block the sites and unhelpful people.

Case Study (2): Harvey

Harvey (14) had been sending nude, legally considered indecent, photos ('sexting') of himself to his boyfriend. His boyfriend had asked him to send them. The boyfriend shared the images to his peer group at school. This resulted in Harvey being bullied. The head teacher of the school became involved, and a referral was made to social services.

There is evidence to suggest that most young people do not engage in sexting and if they do, it is within the boundaries of a relationship. Young people are not always aware that it is illegal to send indecent pictures, if under the age of 18. The most appropriate way of managing 'sexting' by agencies is as a safeguarding issue, rather than by criminalising the young person concerned.

Safeguarding and Online Activity

It is possible for young people to access self-harm and pro-anorexia sites that can be detrimental to their mental health. They can experience 'grooming', and encounter indecent images and pornographic sites. Discussion around online activity at a CAMHS assessment offers the opportunity for a young person to talk about some problematic issues arising from social media usage that may be impacting on their mental health.

Steps (e.g. parental controls), that many internet providers recommend, can reduce the risk of accessing harmful sites. Most children's agencies recognise the need for open discussions to help children and young people understand the risks involved and how to negotiate the internet and minimise the risks.

Research into children who have been groomed online suggests that it has a devastating effect on the child and that they are often unlikely to confide in their parents or seek support or help. Young people create multiple accounts and share passwords, despite being underage. They find terms and conditions inaccessible and take too long to read and so are unlikely to be aware of the terms and conditions of using a site.

Risk Taking

Considerable work has been undertaken as to whether any specific group of young people are more likely to be at risk online. It is thought that more resilient young people may be more able to cope. Young people at risk offline are more likely to be at risk online with risk-taking behaviour.

Examining individual risks is a complex process as different vulnerabilities and risk factors can shape a young person's online experiences. This is mediated by other factors (e.g. cognitive and emotional development, social needs, peer culture and identity).

Health Promotion

Health promotion advice about screen time in relation to behavioural and sleep problems can be conflicting and confusing. In practice in CAMHS we see many young people who have sleep difficulties associated with screen time prior to and during sleep time. Many parents or carers find that their child has difficulty stopping internet activities when asked. It is acknowledged that children and young people are not adequately equipped with the skills to navigate their lives online, and work is being undertaken by Wise Kids to develop a digital citizenship task programme for 4–14-year olds.

Young people can have considerable skills in using the technology, and it has been shown that some parents are unfamiliar with how the apps work and may not realise how easy it is for young people to meet others online, whose identity is uncertain. There are now many sites available to guide parents and to encourage discussion with young people about their internet usage, their experiences and the risks involved.

Summary

Current thinking around internet safety is that education, industry, legal agencies and academia need to work together to research online risks for children and young people and then implement recommendations. The plan is that there will be a voluntary code built into all internet technology to address and encourage young people to use sites safely.

Organisations such as NSPCC, Department of Health and YoungMinds are driving the government to put safeguards in place to protect young people. It is accepted that the way to help protect young people is via a multi-agency approach involving schools, young people and parents to educate everyone about how to reduce the risks when using social media. There are many websites that can guide parents and professionals about how to identify, and protect young people from, the hazards of social media.

Open discussions with young people can help to build up online resilience and awareness. Current research is looking at the delivery of CBT interventions for young people to access any treatment they need. Davies et al. (2019) comment that there is not currently enough conclusive evidence-based research on which to base guidelines for social media or screen time so that the government can provide guidance in response to societal concerns, that takes into consideration the viewpoints of stakeholders, e.g. parents, young people, academics, teachers.

Future research is planned to see if longitudinal studies can identify the mechanism of harm. Currently there are no studies looking at radicalisation and its role within social media.

Multiple-Choice Questions

See answers on page 671.

1. What is the percentage of teenagers that have reported coming across something unpleasant on line?
   a. Approximately 50% of teenagers
   b. Nearly one in five teenagers
   c. Every teenager
   d. Nearly 75% of teenagers
2. What is 'digital citizenship'?
   a. A programme that aims to provide a way to encourage digital resilience for young people
   b. A test you have to do, to be computer literate
   c. One of the on-line interventions for mental health
   d. A new computer science

Key References

Anderson, M., Jiang, J., (2018). Pew Research Centre, Teens' Social Media Habits and Experiences .pewresearch.org/internet (accessed 13/4/19).

Children's Commissioner for England, (2017). *Growing Up Digital A Report of the Growing Up Digital Taskforce.* www.childrenscommissioner.gov.uk.

Davies, S.C., Atherton, F., Calderwood, C., McBride, M., (2019). *United Kingdom Chief Medical Officers' Commentary on 'Screen-Based Activities and Children and Young People's Mental Health and Psychosocial Wellbeing: A Systematic Map of Reviews.* Department of Health and Social Care.

Dickson, K., Richardson, M., Kwan, I., MacDowall, W., Burchett, H., Stansfield, C., Brunton, G., Sutcliffe, K., Thomas, J. (2018). *Screen-Based Activities and Children and Young People's Mental Health and Psychosocial Wellbeing: A Systematic Map of Reviews.* London: EPPI-Centre, Social Science Research Unit, UCL institute of Education, University College London.

Useful Websites for Professionals, Parents, Young People

https://learning.nspcc.org.uk
https://www.saferinternet.org.uk
https://www.thinkuknow.co.uk
https://www.childnet.com
https://wisekids.org.uk/wk/digital-citizenship/

54 Self-Harm and Suicide

Anthony Crabb (updated by Margaret J.J. Thompson, with material from Suyog Dhakras and Julie Waine)

Introduction

Self-harm in the adolescent age group is relatively common, but completed suicide is thankfully less so. The average age of onset for self-harm is 12 years old (Mental Health Foundation, 2006), and it is a symptom, rather than a cause or disease in its own right. Approximately 25,000 young people are admitted to hospital in the UK each year after deliberately harming themselves, and most of these are from self-poisoning (Fox and Hawton, 2004).

Estimates of the prevalence of self-harm in school settings were 6.9%, with participants in the survey reporting an act of deliberate self-harm in the previous year of those that met study criteria. Only 12.6% of episodes had resulted in presentation to hospital. Deliberate self-harm was more common in females than it was in males (11.2% vs. 3.2). In females the factors included in a presentation of deliberate self-harm were recent self-harm by friends, self-harm by family members, drug misuse, depression, anxiety, impulsivity and low self-esteem. In males the factors were suicidal behaviour in friends and family members, drug use and low self-esteem (Hawton, et al., 2002). In acute adolescent mental health inpatient settings, the rates have been reported to be upwards of 80% (Ougrin et al., 2012). Self-harm is four times more common in girls than boys. Gathering accurate data can be difficult due to the stigma of self-harm and access to those that self-harm.

For each of those who actually self-harm, there are many more who have thoughts about it, but do not go on to actually do it. There is widespread misunderstanding about the causes and consequences of self-harm, and a self-harming child can receive very negative responses from family, friends and professionals when self-harm is initially disclosed, reducing the likelihood of further disclosure.

KEY CONCEPTS

- Self-harm can mean a range of behaviours intended to cause pain for a young person, but NOT necessarily about suicidal intent.
- The average onset for DSH behaviours is 12 years.
- When a young person presents with DSH, it is important to take a non-judgemental approach.
- Key areas of assessment would include method, intent, previous history of DSH, precipitating events, thoughts/feelings after the event, on-going support systems.

What Is Self-Harm?

Self-harm can mean a range of behaviours that cause physical harm or pain to a young person. It can be hidden from others for a long period of time. Self-harm is usually intended to harm, not kill. According to Fox and Hawton (2004), 40–100 times as many young people engage in self-harm as those that actually complete suicide.

Self-harm can involve:

- Cutting
- Burning
- Scalding
- Banging or scratching one's own body
- Breaking bones
- Hair-pulling
- Ingesting toxic substances or objects

It can include not taking, or overdosing on, medications for illness, e.g. insulin for diabetes, in addition to drug or alcohol use (Mental Health Foundation, 2006).

Self-harm can be the presenting symptom of mental illness or distress, but sometimes it can be difficult to identify a particular trigger. Sometimes it is viewed as an active coping strategy that reduces stress or anxiety in the short term, and it can be a way of communicating distress when other forms of communication are either too difficult or have been tried without success. The relief from anxiety or tension that is provided by acts of self-harm is short lived, so that the self-harm needs to be repeated. This can set up an addictive cycle (MHF, 2006). For some young people physical pain can be easier to deal with than emotional pain (Fox and Hawton, 2004).

Some of the more common triggers of self-harm include:

- Daily stressors – schoolwork/family arguments
- Feeling isolated
- Self-harm/suicide by peer
- Low self-esteem
- Relationship difficulties
- Bullying
- Emotional/physical/sexual abuse
- Mental health problems
- Physical health problems

Self-Harm and Suicide

Although the two are closely linked, there are some differences in attempted suicide and self-harm. Self-harm can occur in the absence of suicidal thoughts, i.e. the young person is distressed and wants to relieve that distress by self-harming, but has no suicidal intent. As described above, it can be seen as a way of managing distress. Some researchers refer to non-suicidal self-injury (NSSI).

Attempted suicide is a way of ending distress and thus has different motivation. Sometimes the distinction is difficult to tease out. The group of young people who self-harm is somewhat different to those that attempt, or complete, suicide. Completed suicide is more common in males, who tend to use more violent and lethal methods. The most significant risk factor is a previous suicide attempt (30× increased risk for males and 3× increased risk for females).

Assessment

Guidelines from NICE (2011)self harm and see Kendall, T.et al, , (2011). Longer term management of self harm: summary of NICE guidance. *Bmj*, *343*, d7073. suggest:

- Adopting a non-judgemental and respectful approach
- Trying to see the young person on their own if possible
- Assessing the young person in an appropriate setting
- Respecting confidentiality within the limits of the Children Act

The assessment of young people who have self-harmed is usually undertaken in a hospital or in a community child and adolescent mental health service (CAMHS) setting. It can be very difficult for young people to admit to self-harm as they are often afraid of negative reactions from parents, friends and professionals. Although most present with a parent or guardian, some may be alone, and it is important to try to see the young person by themselves, unless they request otherwise.

NB: the majority of patients who die by suicide actually *deny* having suicidal thoughts when last asked prior to their death, or communicate their risk in more behavioural ways (rather than verbal messaging – Appleby L. et al., 1999).

Key Domains of Assessment

- Method
- Intent/perceived lethality of self-harm
- Isolation
- Precipitating events
- Previous history of self-harm
- On-going intent to self-harm
- Mental health problems
- Physical health problems
- Substance use
- Social support
- Discharge/follow-up plans

Protective Factors

- Attachments to peers
- Attachments to school
- Problem-solving skills
- Supportive family

Method

As stated above, by far and away the most common method of self-harm is self-poisoning. It is important to take a detailed and accurate description of what harm has actually been done. You may need to ask for information from a friend or family member who was present at the time. Those young people who self-harm by cutting are much less likely to present to A&E, and many instances are unreported and are not known to CAMHS or A&E. The method of self-harm is influenced by the availability of items such as tablets. The choice of method can indicate the seriousness of the intent. For example, superficially cutting one's forearm carries less risk of intent of suicide than hanging.

Intent/Perceived Lethality

It is important to find out what the perceived lethality of the self-harm was. Did the young person think that the method used was likely to kill them? Most young people are aware of the potential for harm in differing methods; however, there is a common misperception that paracetamol is safe. Conversely a self-harm episode that the assessor might consider to have little potential to be fatal may, in the young person's mind, have been likely to succeed. Subjective lethality is a better predictor of risk than objective lethality. It is impossible to be definitive about risk factors, and risk prediction is very inaccurate.

Isolation

Sometimes referred to as the likelihood of discovery, it is important to ascertain who was around at the time of the self-harm. A self-harm episode in the company of friends and family carries less risk than one done in isolation. It is important to find out who sought help following the self-harm. Was it the young person, or was it a friend or family member? How soon after the episode of self-harm was help sought?

Precipitating Events

- Were there any immediate triggers for the episode of self-harm, and are these triggers persisting?
- Can any of the triggers be modified?

Previous History of Self-Harm

Given that the most important predictor of future behaviour is past behaviour, it is necessary to obtain as much information as possible about previous episodes of self-harm.

On-Going Intent to Self-Harm

Although some young people will find it difficult to disclose on-going thoughts of self-harm, for many the desire to self-harm initially reduces after the act. On-going voiced intent to self-harm obviously increases the risk of future episodes.

The Future

Asking a young person about their plans for the future, such as college and work aspirations, can help gauge any hopes/aspirations they may have and possibly indicate a lower risk of completed suicide.

Mental Health Problems

Mental health problems increase the risk of further self-harm and may require specialist input from a CAMHS team.

Physical Health Problems

Not only does chronic illness increase the risk of self-harm, it can provide the means for unusual methods of self-harm around both the illness itself and its treatment. Some treatments can be very dangerous if taken incorrectly, e.g. insulin.

Social Support

It is necessary to ascertain what social supports a young person has. Those in foster care or temporary placements are especially vulnerable.

Discharge/Follow-up Plans

Ensure that there is a responsible adult to supervise the young person on their return home. Discuss limiting access to methods of self-harm on return home. Follow-up may need to be with a local CAMHS service.

Person-Specific Risk Factors for Self-Harm

- Previous self-harm or suicide attempt
- Mental illness
- Poor social support
- Physical illness, especially chronic illness
- Child abuse/bullying
- Substance abuse
- Social media; almost 45% of CYPs check devices at night, one in ten at least ten times a night
- Impact of contagion/media influences
- Self-harm/suicide clusters: schools; in acute inpatient units (PICUs)
- Media influences on self-harm and suicide – heightened awareness

High-Risk Groups

- Homeless/poor social supports
- Mental health problems
- Victims of abuse
- Mental health inpatients
- Those that are imprisoned
- Substance users
- Those with sexuality issues
- Where a family member or best friend has committed suicide
- Impact of self-harm clusters

Prevention/Intervention

There is no strong evidence base for specific interventions for self-harm. It is apparent that a 'one size fits all' approach cannot be taken and a tailored approach appropriate to the specific young person who has self-harmed is required.

School-based interventions, such as access to someone to talk to at school, have been cited by the national enquiry (MHF, 2006) as a possible preventative measure. Peer support schemes, anti-bullying strategies and a reduction in the sense of social isolation have all been suggested as interventions that could be helpful in reducing self-harm.

Self-help is crucial. Distraction techniques are important in addition to substitution acts, e.g. pinging a rubber band on the wrist to inflict pain or rubbing ice on skin.

Case Study (1): Jake

Jake (seven years old) ties a cord round his neck in front of his mother following an argument with her. The younger a child is at the time of self-harm, the less likely the intent is to die, as they are less likely to have a fully formed understanding of what death is. Unfortunately, this group can be very impulsive and may sustain significant injury that is unintentional. Social factors need to be considered carefully as self-harm behaviour in this age group may be learned from observing others. Although the method used carries high risk, the isolation and the perceived lethality may be low; although this would need detailed enquiry.

Case Study (2): Melina

Melina (15 years old) takes 20 paracetamol tablets at her boyfriend's place after breaking up. She does this in front of him. In this scenario it is more likely that the young person's intention is to communicate distress, rather than to die. Although the perceived lethality of the intent may be low, it is important that Melissa receives medical attention, as the risk of significant liver damage in untreated paracetamol overdose can be high.

Case Study (3): Richard

Richard (15 years old) repeatedly cuts his forearm to help 'reduce stress'. Appropriate medical treatment needs to be given for any wounds, even if they are superficial, as poor healing can lead to permanent scars that outlast any emotional distress that precipitated the self-harm. Along with an assessment of mental state, work undertaken with the boy might include the suggestion of substitute acts, such as using a rubber band on his wrist to inflict pain.

Case Study 4): Jamie

Jamie (16 years old), out of school, with depression, goes into woods alone and takes 100 Fluoxetine. This scenario is one where the perceived lethality may have been high even though Fluoxetine is safe in overdose. The degree of isolation is high, with less likelihood that Jamie would be found and help summoned. Jamie is already in a high-risk group, as he is out of school and has a mental illness. This young person would warrant a very detailed assessment and a robust safety plan following hospital treatment.

NICE Guideline on Self-Harm (2004): Key Points

All children and young people who have self-harmed should normally be admitted to a paediatric ward and be assessed the following day before discharge.

CAMHS workers involved in the assessment and treatment of children and young people who have self-harmed should:

- Be trained specifically to work with young people and their families after self-harm.
- Be skilled in the assessment of risk.

- Have regular supervision.
- Have access to consultation with senior colleagues.

Take-Home Message (NCISH, 2020)

- Increased support for young people who are bereaved (especially by suicide).
- A greater focus on mental health in colleges and universities, housing and mental health care for looked after children.
- Mental health support for young people who identify as lesbian, gay, bisexual or trans (LGBT).

Multiple-Choice Questions

See answers on page 671.

1. Which statement is correct about self-harm?
   a. Self-harm and suicide always have the same motivation.
   b. It can be triggered by relationship difficulties.
   c. Young people always report episodes of self-harm.
   d. Self-harm is due to poor parenting.
2. Which method of self-harm is the most common?
   a. Burning
   b. Cutting
   c. Overdose
   d. Hair pulling
   e. Hanging
3. Which of the following predict increased risk of self-harm?
   a. Social isolation
   b. Mental health problems
   c. Previous self-harm
   d. Substance use
   e. All of the above
4. Which of the following is true about BOYS that self-harm?
   a. They don't overdose on tablets.
   b. Self-harm is more common.
   c. They use more violent methods.
   d. They have better outcomes than girls.
   e. They don't use cutting.

Key References

Fox, C., Hawton, K., (2004). *Deliberate Self-Harm in Adolescence.* London: Jessica Kingsley.

Hawton, K., Rodham, K., Evans, E., Weatherall, R., (2002). Deliberate self-harm in adolescents: self-report survey in schools in England. *BMJ*, *325*(7374): 1207–1211.

Kendall, T., Taylor, C., Bhatti, H., Chan, M., Kapur, N., (2011). Longer term management of self-harm: summary of NICE guidance. *BMJ*, 343: d7073.

Mental Health Foundation, (2006). *Truth Hurts: Report of the National Inquiry into Self-Harm among Young People.* London: Mental Health Foundation.

National Confidential Inquiry into Suicide and Safety in Mental Health access February, (2020). https://sites.manchester.ac.uk/ncish/reports/suicide-by-children-and-young-people/

National Institute for Clinical Excellence, (2004). *Self-harm: The short-term physical and psychological management and secondary prevention of self-harm in primary and secondary care. CG16.* London: National Institute for Health and Clinical Excellence.

National Institute for Health and Clinical Excellence, (2011). *Self-harm: longer-term management. (Clinical guideline CGI 33)* http://guidance.nice.org.uk/CG133.

Part VI

Therapeutic Approaches to Working with Children, Young People and their Families

Cathy Laver-Bradbury

When making decisions with children, young people and their families around the most appropriate intervention, the primary consideration must be their ability and motivation to engage with what is offered. Although practice policy and guidance around therapeutic interventions should be and often have an empirical evidence base to support their efficacy, the values base of the individual child/young person and/or family is central. This may mean considering the use of alternative treatment approaches that may 'fit' with them. Alongside this it is important that any intervention is age appropriate for the child/young person. For example, play therapy may be more beneficial to younger children, who may not have developed the appropriate language to express their emotions, whereas a more talking therapy approach may suit older children and adolescents (although this is not always the case).

This section can be divided broadly into several 'parts': psychopharmacological, psychoanalytical, psychological, behavioural and systemic, although in reality some cannot easily fit into one category. Often approaches are used concurrently, for example individual and family approaches, or psychopharmacological and individual therapy. Therefore, we have chosen not to place the chapters under formal headings.

Part VI

Therapeutic Approaches to Working with Children, Young People and their Families

55 General Principles of Clinical Psychopharmacology in Children and Adolescents

A Practical Guide

Samuele Cortese

Introduction

Pharmacotherapy can be one important component of the multimodal, comprehensive management strategy of psychopathological conditions/disorders seen in child and adolescent mental health services (CAMHS). This chapter, addressed to prescribers at any level of expertise in CAMHS, is organised in a question-and-answer format. Practical clinical aspects, rather than theoretical issues and the neuroscience underpinning clinical psychopharmacology, are the focus.

The overarching aim here is to provide a practical guide that can support the prescriber in evidence-based decision-making and practices in the pharmacological treatment in CAMHS. This chapter deals with the general, rather than specific, issues that apply to the pharmacological treatment of any disorder in CAMHS.

When Should I Consider a Pharmacological Treatment in CAMHS?

It is commonly stated that practitioners should consider a pharmacological treatment when the disorder is impairing, and non-pharmacological strategies have proved to be ineffective. The decision on the type of treatment, pharmacological or non-pharmacological, depends on the type of outcome considered to be the target of the treatment. Different treatments may have different effects on different outcomes related to a specific disorder.

A typical example is represented by attention deficit hyperactivity disorder (ADHD), for which there is evidence that:

- The pharmacological treatment is efficacious, based on data from double-blind randomised controlled trials (RCTs), on ADHD core symptoms, i.e. inattention, hyperactivity and impulsivity (Cortese et al., 2018).
- Non-pharmacological treatments do not seem to be effective for ADHD core symptoms (Cortese et al., 2016; Cortese et al., 2015; Sonuga-Barke, 2013), but some of them, i.e. behavioural parent training programmes, are beneficial in domains related to ADHD, e.g. oppositional behaviours and conduct disorder (Daley et al., 2014).
- Pharmacological treatments are less efficacious for non-core symptoms, e.g. emotional dysregulation, than for core symptoms (Lenzi et al., 2018).

Across different disorders, there will instances where:

- Non-pharmacological treatments are the first-line or only option, e.g. for core symptoms of ASD, for which there are no currently available medications, even though a number of drugs are currently under investigation (Hong et al., 2019).

- Pharmacological options are the first line, e.g. to control psychotic symptoms (McClellan et al., 2013).
- A combination of pharmacological and non-pharmacological treatment is the most effective option, e.g. for severe depression (NICE, 2019).

The prescriber should be familiar with recommendations provided by the National Institute for Health and Care Excellence (NICE) guidelines (https://www.nice.org.uk/guidance) or other guidelines/guidance, such as the Scottish Intercollegiate Guidelines Network (SIGN: https://www.guidelinesinpractice.co.uk/home/the-scottish-intercollegiate-guidelines-network-sign/305547.article) or the practice parameters of the American Academy of Child and Adolescent Psychiatry (AACAP) (https://www.aacap.org/AACAP/Resources_for_Primary_Care/Practice_Parameters_and_Resource_Centers/Practice_Parameters.aspx).

Guidelines for a specific topic may be lacking or outdated. As such, prescribers need to retrieve the most updated evidence to inform daily clinical decision-making.

How Do I Retrieve the Most Updated and Rigorous Evidence Base to Inform Clinical Decision-Making?

A relatively quick way to retrieve relevant papers is to search the free-access database PubMed (https://www.ncbi.nlm.nih.gov/pubmed/), using the following search syntax: name of the disorder, e.g. anxiety [ti]) AND (medication* [ti] OR drug* [ti] OR pharmacological [ti] or pharmacotherapy [ti]), where * indicates a truncation term, so that, for instance, the system will search for *medication* and *medications* and [ti] will restrict the search to references containing the keywords in the title, therefore providing the most relevant papers.

The prescriber may want to limit the search to papers published in the last five years. NB: this option is available on the left side window of PubMed, to retrieve only the most up-to-date evidence. It is likely that such a search will retrieve a high number of references. To narrow down the search, it is important to limit it to systematic reviews with meta-analyses, when available, of randomised controlled trials (RCTs) using the relevant option on the left side window.

A particular type of meta-analysis, referred to as network meta-analysis (NMA), allows the comparison of the efficacy and/or tolerability of two or more treatments, even when they have not been compared head-to-head in individual RCTs. This informs the process of clinical decision-making when a specific medication needs to be chosen among a number of available ones. Prescribers should be familiar with the most updated network meta-analyses on medications of interest. A comprehensive overview of available network meta-analyses of pharmacological treatments in child and adolescent psychiatry is provided in Cortese et al. (2019).

Meta-analyses of RCTs will be informative, in general, on the short-term efficacy of medications. Due to ethical and financial constraints, the length of RCTs for mental health conditions is generally limited to some weeks/months. The so-called withdrawn discontinuation design (Matthijssen et al., 2019), where patients who have been pharmacologically treated for a long period are randomised to continue the treatment or discontinue it, is helpful on the long-term effects of medication, and prescribers should be familiar with this study design.

Finally, prescribers may want to search for another type of studies that may inform clinical decision-making, i.e. the observational case studies. A number of important outcomes that are relevant in the daily clinical practice, e.g. suicidal ideation or physical injuries, are not usually included in RCTs, due to their low frequency or to the difficulty in measuring them in an RCT.

In the case studies, the outcome of interest is measured in the same patient when they are on and off medication. As the patient acts as their own control, this removes the bias, typical of observational studies, derived from comparing the outcome in two different groups, treated and non-treated, that may differ in baseline characteristics and limit the validity of the comparison.

Am I Allowed to Prescribe 'off-Label'?

Prescribing off-label means prescribing outside the limits of the marketing authorisation or product licence in relation to one or more of the following:

- The type of disorder being treated
- The age of the patient
- The route of administration
- The duration of treatment
- It is different from prescribing an unlicensed or withdrawn drug.

Until recently, there were no statutory requirements to conduct trials in children to support the marketing authorisations in this population. This has changed due to initiatives both from the Food and Drug Administration (FDA) and European Medicine Agency (EMA), for a number of drugs data, but they are still being extrapolated from studies in adults.

There are drugs for which there is good evidence of efficacy and safety but that do not have authorisation, yet, in children/adolescents. These include Sertraline for anxiety disorders and OCD, Risperidone for psychosis/schizophrenia and Clonidine for tics/Tourette syndrome.

Prescribing within the existing authorisation does not guarantee that the medication will be safe. Haloperidol up to 10 mg/day and amphetamine are licensed in the UK, respectively, for Tourette syndrome in children and ADHD in pre-schoolers. In both cases, there is a lack of, or limited evidence on, their safety at the dose, for Haloperidol, or the population, for amphetamine, for which they are licensed. It is evident that there is often a mismatch between the licence, on the one hand, and evidence of efficacy/safety, on the other. From a medico-legal standpoint, prescribers can prescribe any drug, i.e. licensed, unlicensed or off-label, if this is supported by a reasonable body of medical opinion (UK Medical Act, 1983).

The BNF for Children states that when possible, a licensed drug should be considered, but acknowledges that a number of patients, children or adolescents, require medications not licensed for that particular use. Interested readers can find additional information, including relevant legislation, in the British Association for Psychopharmacology (BAP) position statement: off-label prescribing of psychotropic medication to children and adolescents (Sharma et al., 2016).

How Does This Knowledge Help Me in the Decision-Making?

Knowledge on the pharmacokinetics of medications is fundamental when prescribing to children and adolescents. It is important to be aware that, even though children have smaller absolute body size, the relative mass of their liver and kidney tissue is larger than in adults after adjusting for body weight. Thus, decreasing adult doses based on child weight may result in sub-optimal treatment (IACAPAP, 2019).

Some medications used in psychiatry inhibit some of the enzymes that metabolise other medications. For instance, 3A4 metabolised enzymes can be inhibited by Fluoxetine or Fluvoxamine, so that co-administration of Fluvoxamine (inhibitor of 3A4) and Quetiapine or Aripiprazole (metabolised by 3A4) may lead to higher than expected levels of Quetiapine or Aripiprazole, that may lead to prolongation of the QTc interval.

Genetic polymorphisms for these enzymes may lead to poor metabolisation. About 7–10% of Caucasians, 1–8% of Africans and 1–3% of East Asians have been reported to be poor metabolisers of CYP2D6. Whilst tests to assess the profile of metabolisation of an individual are available, they are not recommended in routine practice, as there is still limited evidence to support a significant correlation between genetic polymorphisms and blood drug levels.

The prescriber should be aware that for some medications, both the dose and the duration of treatment can influence pharmacokinetics, e.g. it has been calculated that after a single dose of Sertraline 50 mg in adolescents, the mean half-life is about 27 hours, but after repeated administration this decreases to about 15 hours. Moreover, the steady-state half-life is about 20 hours after administration of higher doses (100–150 mg). Lower doses, i.e. 50 mg of Sertraline, should be given twice a day to prevent withdrawal, while higher doses, i.e. 100–150 mg doses, can be given once a day (IACAPAP, 2019).

What Shall I Do before Issuing a Prescription?

Psychoeducation with the patient and family is key. Information on efficacy, effectiveness, frequency of possible adverse events during the pharmacological treatment and how to manage them should be clearly discussed with the patient and family. Leaflets produced by local Trusts or other organisations (e.g. Royal College of Psychiatrists: https://www.rcpsych.ac.uk/mental-health/treatments-and-wellbeing/antipsychotics)are helpful but should not replace face-to-face conversations. When discussing any specific medication, prescribers should remember that the current nomenclature of medications is being changed. The current nomenclature may be misleading and confusing for users, e.g. when an 'antidepressant' is prescribed to treat anxiety.

A number of international organisations in the field of psychopharmacology have endorsed the so-called neuroscience-based nomenclature (NbN), whereby each compound is referred to based on its mechanism of action rather than the supposed disorder it is aimed to treat. A version for child and adolescent psychiatry has been recently developed (https://nbnca.com/), with an app currently being tested.

In addition, it is crucial to discuss the specific outcomes that are the target of a medication, e.g. 'hyperactivity' and 'aggressiveness' are two distinct targets that may require different treatment approaches, the time-frame to assess them and what should be done if the medication is not effective and/or not well tolerated.

Before issuing a prescription, it is important to have a baseline measurement of symptom severity, via commonly used and validated rating scales, to track the changes in severity over time during the pharmacological treatment, alongside a baseline rating of symptoms, e.g. headache, or objective measures, e.g. weight, height or blood pressure, that are informative for the assessment of the safety/tolerability of the medication. Whilst laboratory tests are not indicated for some classes of drugs, e.g. the so-called antidepressants, they are for others, e.g. the so-called antipsychotics. Tools such as the spread sheets provided by the Canadian Alliance for Monitoring Effectiveness and Safety of Antipsychotics in Children (CAMESA) and freely downloadable may be helpful for the prescriber (http://camesaguideline.org/information-for-doctors) and for parents/patients (http://camesaguideline.org/information-for-parents).

The role of other tests, e.g. ECG before stimulants, is matter of discussion/controversy. International authorities, e.g. the European ADHD Guidelines Group (EAGG), suggest that the ECG is not mandatory before starting a treatment with stimulants, but should be performed, alongside other cardiovascular assessment, when there is increased cardiovascular risk.

How Should I Prescribe?

An interesting study (Kovshoff et al., 2013) focussing on the prescription practice in the field of ADHD, but that can be extrapolated to other disorders, showed that prescribers could be divided in different groups based on their attitudes:

- Pro-psychosocial.
- Medication focussed.
- Unsystematic.
- Response optimisers. Response optimisation (finding the best dose in terms of effectiveness and tolerability, after trialling all possible doses, is considered the best approach to achieve the best response in the long term – Coghill et al., 2019). Rather than 'being satisfied' when there is some symptom improvement, the prescriber should aim to achieve the maximum symptom improvement, optimising the dose.

What Should I Do after I Have Prescribed?

It is crucial to periodically monitor effectiveness and tolerability, based, if possible, on different sources of information, e.g. patient, parents and teachers. Guidance is available to manage the common adverse effects that may happen during treatment with medication (Cortese et al., 2013). The key concept to consider is that underestimating the side-effects of a medication can lead to harm, but overestimating them, or not knowing how to manage them, could mean that the patient may not benefit from effective medications.

'The Medication You Prescribed Used to Work Well but Now It Does Not Work Anymore': What to Do?

Prescribers hear this quite frequently. Before thinking of the possible mechanism of tolerance that may happen, although it is in in general quite rare, prescribers should consider the following:

- Is adherence to medication regular? Sometimes parents may not be aware of what should really happen with their child's prescription.
- Has the patient's symptoms severity reached a plateau beyond which it is difficult to progress, but parents would like to see more?
- Are parents referring to the outcome that is the target of the medication?
- Has anything happened, i.e. at the personal, family, interpersonal level, that may explain changes in behaviour?

When Should I Stop a Medication?

Unfortunately, guidelines are less good in highlighting when/how a medication should be stopped. They all concur in suggesting that period breaks should be considered to assess the levels of symptom severity and impairment, when the patient is off medication. This should be done during periods when the usual functioning of the patient can be assessed. Summer holidays may not be ideal to fully reflect the usual functioning/expectations.

Summary

Even though prescribing is still perhaps an art, it should be based on rigorous and updated evidence. Evidence from research studies is only one of the components that should be take into account in the decision-making process, alongside patient circumstances and preferences. Research studies provide, in general, evidence that is useful to inform the decision at the group level, e.g. medication A may be the best for children with anxiety at the group level, but some children may benefit more from medication B.

The development of individual patient data network meta-analyses (IPD-NMA) may fill this gap, providing information useful at the single-patient level (Kernot et al., 2019). This would contribute to closing the gap between research and clinical practice.

Multiple-Choice Questions

See answers on page 672.

1. What is off-label prescribing?
    a. Prescribing outside the limits of the marketing authorisation or product licence.
    b. Reading the label on the medication but using another description.
    c. Where the pharmacist gives a generic medication instead of a prescribed one.
2. What is helpful when considering using a pharmacological intervention?
    a. Searching the literature for evidence-based treatments
    b. Reading clinical guidelines and clinical case studies
    c. All of the above
3. What should a practitioner do after they have prescribed?
    a. Feel relaxed as the patient now has medication
    b. Periodically monitor effectiveness and tolerability, based, if possible, on different sources of information, e.g. patient, parents and teachers
    c. Quickly titrate the dose

Key References

Cortese, S., Adamo, N., Del Giovane, C., Mohr-Jensen, C., Hayes, A.J., Carucci, S., Atkinson, L.Z., Tessari, L., Banaschewski, T., Coghill, D., Hollis, C., Simonoff, E., Zuddas, A., Barbui, C., Purgato, M., Steinhausen, H.C., Shokraneh, F., Xia, J., Cipriani, A., (2018). Comparative efficacy and tolerability of medications for attention-deficit hyperactivity disorder in children, adolescents, and adults: a systematic review and network meta-analysis. *Lancet Psychiatry*, 5(9): 727–738.

Cortese, S., Ferrin, M., Brandeis, D., Holtmann, M., Aggensteiner, P., Daley, D., Santosh, P., Simonoff, E., Stevenson, J., Stringaris, A., Sonuga-Barke, E.J., European ADHD, Guidelines Group (EAGG), (2016). Neurofeedback for attention-deficit/hyperactivity disorder: meta-analysis of clinical and neuropsychological outcomes from randomized controlled trials. *Journal of the American Academy of Child and Adolescent Psychiatry*, 55(6): 444–455.

Cortese, S., Ferrin, M., Brandeis, D., Buitelaar, J., Daley, D., Dittmann, R.W., Holtmann, M., Santosh, P., Stevenson, J., Stringaris, A., Zuddas, A., Sonuga-Barke, E.J., European ADHD Guidelines Group (EAGG), (2015). Cognitive training for attention-deficit/hyperactivity disorder: meta-analysis of clinical and neuropsychological outcomes from randomized controlled trials. *Journal of the American Academy of Child and Adolescent Psychiatry*, 54(3): 164–174.

56 Creative Therapies (Art and Play)

Margaret Josephs, Emma House, Sarah Holden and Loz Foskett

KEY CONCEPTS

- Creative therapies involve a therapeutic relationship between the therapist and the individual, within a clinical practice framework.
- The use of visual images, art materials and objects as a medium for the development of this relationship is central.
- This allows for additional and alternative means of communication, that enable individuals to explore their emotions and the feelings related to their difficulties in a safe, facilitating and creative environment.
- Children and young people can be offered a wide range of media with which to work, ranging from play equipment, e.g. sand trays with appropriate toys, dolls, dolls' house and puppets, to art materials, e.g. clay, paint, varying crayons and pencils, to verbal communication.
- Children and young people engage and explore through the creative process or 'impulse', described by D.W. Winnicott (1971) as 'prerequisite for human development'.

Introduction

Children and young people can often have some difficulty articulating their feelings verbally. The use of play, drama and art within therapy offers a more natural non-verbal language for them to express distress or unhappiness. This chapter will focus primarily on the mediums of art and play therapy, but first will make brief comment on drama therapy.

All creative therapists, including music therapists, working within the statutory agencies must have completed a post-graduate MA or diploma pre-2004 and be registered with their appropriate professional body.

Drama Therapy

In ancient Greek 'drama' meant the thing that is acted out or lived through. It does not need to be on a stage or have costumes or props. However, it does need an individual or group of people who use action and/or speech to create a story or scene. Using drama begins at a very early age. Through imitation and experimentation, a child learns how to take on a role, e.g. imitating sounds before he or she can talk and to use objects in play. Children and young people can use drama as a way to express conflict in a safe and structured environment.

A number of key processes lie at the heart of drama therapy, illustrating how the healing potential of drama and play is realised through drama therapy. These include dramatic projection, therapeutic performance process, embodiment (dramatising the body, playing and transformation).

Art Therapy

Art therapy is a clinical practice involving a psychodynamic and psychotherapeutic relationship between the art therapist and the client, working either 1:1, dyadic, i.e. with parent/carer, or in a group setting. At the heart is the artwork, which helps to develop a trusting relationship and communication between the client and the therapist. Clients of all ages can learn to use artwork as a way to express inner thoughts, feelings and conflicts. From this creative expression, various levels of conscious and subconscious issues emerge. These can be worked with at the depth and pace that are appropriate for the client at the time, with the ratio of time spent between producing artwork and talking being the individual's choice (art therapy is usually non-directive).

The process of working with art materials, and the ensuing images, can release clients from their traditional ways of thinking and behaving. This can facilitate a new way of exploring difficult issues, promote self-awareness and increase self-esteem. Art therapy is highly adaptable so that children and young people with particular needs can access the therapy, e.g. someone who is on the autistic spectrum may be more able to interact with sensory types of art materials.

Art therapists are sometimes dual trained and might consider adapting the art therapy to incorporate other models of therapy if felt appropriate to the client's needs, such as incorporating some psychoeducation into the work.

When looking for the origins of using art in therapy, Tessa Dalley in *Art as Therapy* (1984, re-printed 1996) suggests its consideration in the context of the arts generally. 'Art is an indigenous feature in every society', she writes. Odell-Miller, Learmouth and Pembrook state that creativity is part of human problem-solving. It is used as a resource for dealing with distress and disturbance; therefore it is common sense to put creativity, through the inclusion of creative therapies, at the service of improving mental health.

Creative therapy, particularly art therapy, differs from other psychological therapies, in that it is a three-way process between the client, the therapist and the image or artifact, offering a third dimension to the process. The art activity provides a concrete, rather than verbal, medium, through which the client can achieve both conscious and unconscious expression. It can be used as a valuable agent for therapeutic change.

Art therapy is practiced in a variety of both residential and community settings, within health, social services, education and the voluntary and private sector. Clients are seen individually with their families and in groups.

Art Therapy Groups for Adolescents

Art therapy groups are useful for young people, aged between 10 and 16 years, who find it difficult to express their feelings, struggle with relationships and are not seen as fulfilling their potential, young people who protect themselves by withdrawing from the world, either refusing/not being able to go to school, not mixing with their peers or losing themselves in the care they provide for others. A high proportion of referrals have a parent with a diagnosed mental health problem, or parents who are fragile for a variety of reasons (e.g. victims of violence, or abusive or broken relationships), and who have depended on the support of their child. Some young people themselves are experiencing long-term health issues, such as degenerative loss of hearing or brain tumours.

Within art therapy groups, the group therapists are seen as the facilitators of that space. The process is intended to be collaborative and as transparent as possible, from beginning to end. Great importance is placed on engaging and negotiating what each person, their family and the referrer are hoping to gain from the young person's attendance in the group. Each group usually runs for an academic year, and meetings are held with the group facilitators, young person, family, referrer and, if appropriate, any other involved professionals, to assess their appropriateness for the group and to set outcome targets. These are reviewed and updated at further meetings half way through and when the group has finished. For art therapy groups, it is important that:

- A range of art materials are available.
- Group members are encouraged to use the art materials in a way that encourages the development of free expression.
- The amount of art work and discussion varies from week to week, depending on the needs of the group.
- The way the work is created varies, i.e. working individually, or in pairs, small groups or larger groups.

Over the years the importance of 'messy painting' has increased and noted to be significant in the development of group members' ability to emerge as individuals within the group if they can develop in ways that allow them to:

- Find their own identity through their feelings.
- Recognise themselves as separate from others.
- Recognise and relate to others and develop reciprocal relationships.

They must first go through the process of 'immersing' themselves in the materials, in a way that allows them to 'let go' of previously held pre-conceptions about themselves, giving them the freedom to explore new ways of developing as individuals.

Issues about boundaries and containment emerge. Fears of being overwhelmed can be explored through the metaphor of the paint on the paper. What happens to the messy paintings is always a matter for discussion, as they can take days to dry. The paintings are usually photographed in their original state and then stored in plastic boxes.

For many of these group members, it may be the first time they have had an experience in a group that they can relate to. Saying goodbye is inevitably challenging and can be painful. Often young people's previous experience of endings has been to withdraw themselves before the end, to protect themselves, or to behave in such an unacceptable way as to be excluded. The end result is the same, i.e. the avoidance of the end and saying goodbye. The group, therefore, spends most of the final term preparing for finishing and has developed several methods for addressing the issues around leaving.

Case Study: Sophie

A child and adolescent mental health service (CAMHS) colleague referred Sophie to the art therapy group. Sophie was described as presenting with clinical depression, frequently experiencing suicidal ideations. She complained of sleep disturbance and early morning waking. Sophie described herself as a 'psychotic neurotic'. A psychiatric assessment had been requested to discuss medication.

Both Sophie's parents had been treated for depression in the past, and she believed she would inherit it. Sophie came to our initial meeting, accompanied by the CAMHS worker. Her parents were unable to attend.

The group uses a rating system to evaluate progress. Sophie scored herself at 1 out of 10 for how she felt about herself. She said she would like to be between 7 and 9 out of 10. Her aims for attending the group were to be happier, more expressive, better at explaining things and able to go out more. Sophie spent most of her time on her computer, staying up well into the night. She was in her last year at school, where there were issues of bullying.

From the start of the group, Sophie used the materials in a very creative way, immediately painting pictures to describe how she was feeling. She described herself as 'mad'. She would often talk about being let down by other adults, including her GP, teachers and mental health workers.

Her early pictures describe being 'stuck in the dark' and 'standing on the edge looking on' (Figures 56.1 and 56.2).

'Things looking all right on the surface but not underneath'.

Sophie spoke about hitting her head on her desk when everything was too much for her and about how coming to the group and painting helped her and her school feel she was doing something about her situation. Sophie did not talk about her family until late into the group. She began to wonder out loud about being depressed, and started to show visible signs of distress, becoming withdrawn and tearful.

Sophie found it more helpful to focus on her artwork, which she found easier to share, and she joined in with the discussions about others feeling overwhelmed and overwhelming. She would describe herself as 'dead' and as needing more than anyone could offer. She was still spending much of her time on the internet, where she felt she could be herself because she could not be seen. She began to talk about arguing with her parents and resisted attempts by other group members to meet up outside the group, although she would sometimes communicate with a group member by e-mail and text.

The group was exploring issues around safety and either drew or made models of a place where they could feel safe. Sophie made what she described as a padded cell out of modelling material to which, she said, she had swallowed the key. She described being afraid of hurting others more than hurting herself, which was an issue shared by several others in the group.

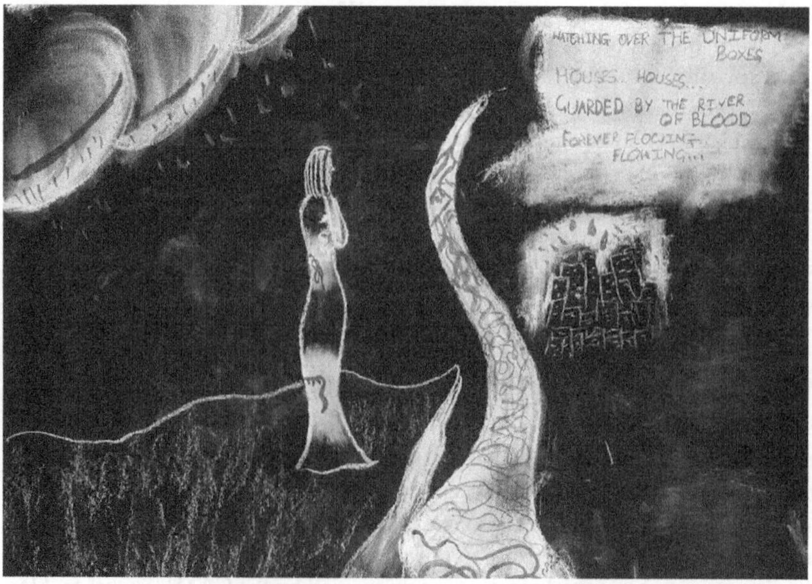

Figure 56.1 Under the Surface.

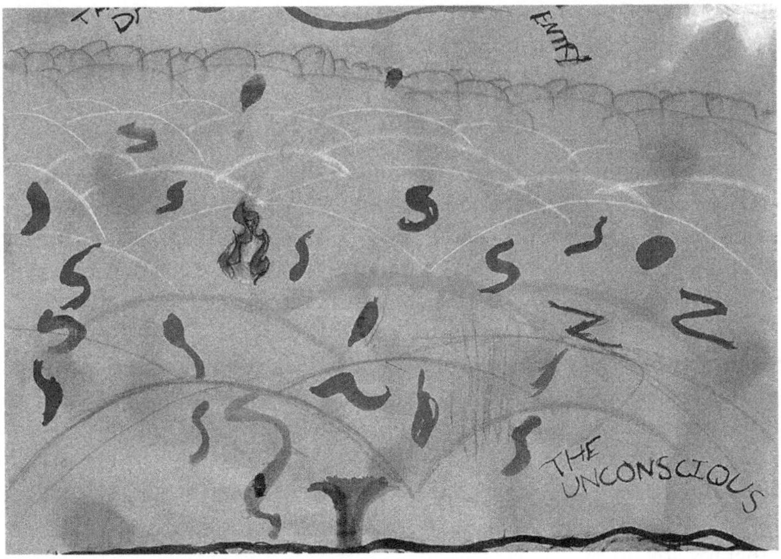

Figure 56.2 Stuck in the Dark.

The last time she could remember feeling safe was when she was seven years old, and her father was working a night shift. Then she would be allowed into bed with her mother to watch TV and have 'lots of cuddles'.

Sophie's use of the materials helped her to identify what she was experiencing, looking for and feared, in a way that could be discussed openly within the group.

Unfortunately, neither Sophie's parents nor the referrer could attend the mid-group review. This fuelled Sophie's feelings of loss and rejection. She attended on her own and was very distressed. This allowed for the issues to be addressed and then, with her permission, shared within the group.

From then onwards, Sophie became noticeably more playful and relaxed. She engaged in group discussions and used the materials much more freely. In a group discussion preparing for the end of the group, the group members described her, among other descriptions, as caring, understanding, trustworthy, serious, sensitive, funny and a good listener. This seriously challenged Sophie's previous view of herself.

Sophie's parents attended the final meeting. They were very positive about the changes they had seen in her. They described their daughter's mood as 'up'. Sophie was being more sociable, less tired, more energetic and with a much-improved sleeping pattern.

Sophie now rated herself as between 7 and 8 out of 10. She had plans to attend a local college after finishing school. She had been able to hold onto the feedback from the group and was letting go of her previous self-perceptions. There had been no incidents of self-harm since the group began.

Sophie's involvement in the art therapy group shows how the facilitation of a space where thoughts and feelings can be explored, at the client's pace and in a way that encourages exploration and development through the use of art materials, can result in a whole new way of experiencing oneself and the world. Unconscious material surfaces through images and words. It is the therapist's task to help the young person make sense of it. Clear boundaries and limits make the group a safe experience for intense and powerful feelings to be expressed and worked through. The groups are hard work and can be hectic, disruptive and angry, or thoughtful, reflective, sharing and supportive. The young people's commitment is admirable, and the feedback from parents and schools indicates the level of change that can be achieved.

Play Therapy

Play is central to human development and enables a child to express bodily activity, repetition of experience and demonstrate fantasy in preparation for life. Through play children develop motor and cognitive skills, language, emotional and behavioural responses, social competence and morals alongside coping and problem-solving skills, in the context of the ecological environment. The British Association of Play Therapists defines play therapy as

> The dynamic process between child and play therapist, in which the child explores, at his own pace and with his or her own agenda, those issues past and current that are affecting the child's life in the present. The child's inner resources are enabled by the therapeutic alliance to bring about growth and change. Play therapy is child-centered, whereby play is the primary medium and speech is the secondary medium.

Key elements of play therapy are:

- Its suitability for children aged approximately 2.5 years to 12 years and sometimes older, depending on the child's developmental stage.
- Play and toys are a child's primary form of communication.
- Materials are selected (a) to match the developmental stages of play and (b) to encourage children to express feelings.
- Change happens through the therapeutic relationship with the therapist.
- Given the opportunity children have an innate desire to resolve difficulties.
- Play therapy can help presenting problems such as aggression, impulsivity, isolation, low mood arising from, e.g. loss, trauma, abuse, neglect, illness or disability.
- Treatment can be short or long term, non-directive or with a focussed approach.
- Consistency is vital. Sessions should be with the same play therapist at a regular time and in the same place.
- Active work with a parent/carer alongside the play therapist is desirable and often essential for the best outcome from therapy.

Play therapy practice has developed in the UK over the past 35 years with post- graduate level training established around 1993. Trained play therapists can apply for full membership of two regulating bodies, the British Association of Play Therapists (BAPT) and Play Therapy UK (PTUK). Both are members of the Professional Standards Authority and run their own registers of therapists and supervisors.

Play therapy training is underpinned by theories and research that help the therapist make sense of the child's play as it unfolds. They include normal and atypical child and adolescent development (Meadows, 1992), trauma (Van Der Kolk et al., 1999), attachment theory (Bowlby, 1973), neuroscience (Panksepp, 2004; Perry 2016), theories of play therapy (Axline, 1989; Landreth, 2002; West, 1996) and sensory processing and integration (Lloyd, 2016).

Non-directive play therapy is rooted in person-centred therapy (Rogers, 1976) and developed further in the UK by, amongst others, Cattanach (2008a; 2008b), Jennings (1999) and Ryan and Wilson (2005). The recent BAPT publication ***Becoming and Being a Play Therapist*** (Ayling, Armstrong and Gorden- Clark, 2019) serves as a succinct and comprehensive precis of the process and challenges facing trainee and qualified play therapists, including the role and importance of supervision following qualification and personal therapy during training and after, as appropriate.

Who Can Benefit?

Play therapy can be helpful for youngsters of all ages and adults who might benefit from exploring their life experience through narrative and non-verbal means. It is most often used for children aged approximately 2.5 to about 12 years, whose development is delayed or arrested as a result of adverse life experiences or developmental disorders. These can lead to behavioural and emotional difficulties, i.e. the child's way of expressing a reaction to some or all of the following, because they often do not have the words to explain their feelings:

- Trauma, neglect, abuse.
- Loss through bereavement, family breakdown or separation from culture of origin.
- Witnessing or experience of domestic abuse or parental substance misuse.
- Developmental disorders that impact on their ability to express themselves through speech, e.g. ASC, ADHD. The physical aspects of play can aid regulation for those with complex disorders.

Child-centred play therapy can be particularly helpful for children in the care of the local authority. It can help them make up for the early play and developmental experiences they may have missed because of their adverse life experience. Their play in therapy tends to focus on activities to help neurosequential brain development, e.g. sensory play (Jennings, 2011; Malchiodi, C. and Crenshaw, 2014), and then moves on to help them process some of their lived experiences, that are often traumatic in nature.

What Happens in Play Therapy?

Current play therapy practice, although rooted in the non-directive approach (Axline, 1989), can be on a continuum from non-directive to focussed therapy. Those who use focussed activities, e.g. with a bereaved child, may choose a storybook with a relevant theme, a board game or a creative activity to help the child make sense of their loss. Play therapy is creative in nature, seeking to work with the child's natural likes and needs, and it always maintains a child-centred approach.

Assessment

Play therapy assessment is undertaken to ensure that it is the most appropriate form of treatment for the child and that the family/carer(s) can commit to supporting the child through therapy. The assessment will usually comment on the child's developmental level and take note of the media that help them regulate mood and affect. The child's ability to relate to the therapist and the quality of that relationship can help inform the child's attachment style, which, in turn, can aid meaningful communication and help the family/carers understand the child's emotional needs. Some children who have experienced trauma, abuse, neglect and/or multiple caregivers take a long time to build a therapeutic alliance and trust, hence the importance of the option of long-term therapy for these children. Thought should be given during the assessment as to where the therapy is best conducted to suit the individual child.

Traditionally, therapy occurs in a specially equipped room, often in a clinic setting or in the child's school. However, in the past few years the Collaboration of Outdoor Play Therapists, formed in the UK as a direct result of Alison Chown's work, has advocated the use of the outdoors in therapy (*Play Therapy in the Outdoors: Taking Play Therapy out of the Playroom and into Natural Environment*, JKP, 2014). This research arose from her observations that, when working with certain children, the confinement of the room appeared to be too much for them to tolerate, often as a result of their life experiences. Allowing the therapy to occur using the natural environment and natural materials available to the child resulted in better therapeutic outcomes for those children. This is particularly true of children in the care system, whose overwhelming need for sensory experiences sometimes means the outdoors can offer those, without the confinement of the room and the restrictions on the unconditionality of the therapeutic relationship that arises when 'mess' has to be contained. It can reduce hypervigilance and enable a child to develop a sense of how their body is designed and operates through natural sensory stimuli.

Therapeutic outcomes are usually better when another professional works in parallel with the family/carers to help them manage any issues arising from the child's sessions and offer a systemic perspective, rather than total focus being on the child, their behaviour and role within the family. Sometimes the parent/carer is trained to replicate the therapeutic play relationship after therapy ends with the child (Filial Therapy, Van Fleet and Gurney, 2003). This helps to sustain the improvement gained during the therapy.

Good communication with the wider network is important. Consistency and reliability are vital for the child to gain maximum benefit from the therapy. The sessions are usually weekly, at the same time and in the same venue, with planned holiday breaks. Depending on the referral, play therapy may be contained within –six to ten sessions or can last over a year. Regular reviews are held and endings always carefully planned.

Why 'Play' in Therapy?

Play is a vital part of child development. It promotes socialisation, gross and fine motor skills, emotional and social intelligence, empathy, reflection, problem-solving, creativity, initiative and resilience to stress. The therapy room is equipped with a variety of toys and creative art materials selected to match developmental stages of play and to encourage children to express their feelings. The child is not judged or rushed and can experiment without fear of criticism, thereby giving them control over their healing.

He or she is free to play about issues and may choose materials as symbolic representations of people and events:

- Clay, playdoh slime, sand and water encourage sensory/embodiment play, allowing the child to regress to preverbal experiences and to express emotions that are difficult to articulate.
- Art and craft allow the child to externalise and represent inner feelings.

Projective play and the use of toys such as puppets, little figures, animals and dolls help children to make up stories and offer the opportunity to explore real-life experiences at a safe distance, using metaphor and symbolism.

- Role play and dressing-up offer the chance to play out scenes and take control of the narration.
- Musical instruments are useful for all children, but particularly those with limited verbal ability or with learning difficulties.
- Carefully chosen books with themes relating to the child's own experiences can help them identify with the story and validate their feelings.

Outcomes

Outcomes will vary depending upon each child's situation, whether their living conditions are stable and the support offered in their wider environment. The aim is that therapy will lead to changes in the child's behaviour and to a more positive view of themselves, promoting self-esteem, confidence, emotional regulation, healthier relationships with others and a greater ability to problem solve, innovate and be willing to experiment. The child can try out different scenarios until they reach a healthier understanding of their experiences. This is then validated by an attuned therapist.

As with other therapies (e.g. psychotherapy and counselling), that are qualitative in nature, and the fact that positive change happens in the child's inner world and perceptions, it is difficult to quantitatively measure the success of play therapy. This is especially true since the 'unique strength of play therapy is to tap into the world of the child in the "language" of that child through play and this is often overlooked in research'. However, qualitative outcomes can be gained anecdotally from the adults in the child's network, (home and school) and the Child Psychotherapy Q-Set (Schneider and Jones, 2004) offers a validated measure of progress that has credence across therapeutic modalities. Additionally, UK researchers are building upon research undertaken by Bratton et al. (2005), which demonstrated the effectiveness of play therapy. Where trust is an issue and the child may be ambivalent about therapeutic work, progress may best be made through a child-centred approach or play therapy (Doyle, 2012). Ryan (2004) provides evidence of play therapy effectiveness in working with attachment disorders and sexual, emotional and physical abuse. Professor Mick Cooper and colleagues have published several papers that are generating an interesting evidence base regarding the efficacy of humanistically based therapies in schools (Cooper et al., 2009, 2013, 2015).

Outcome measures, on the whole, do not measure changes in the internal world of the child. However, Strength and Difficulties Questionnaires (SDQ) (Goodman, 1997), Child Behaviour Checklist (Achenbach, 1991) and the Child Global Assessment Scale (CGas) can give third-party views on the impact of the child's behaviour on the lives of the adults around them.

Case Study: Megan

Megan (eight) was referred to the therapeutic service for children in care because of her distractible, impulsive behaviour, difficulty in peer relationships at school and angry outbursts in her foster home. A psychiatric assessment had considered the presenting behaviour, alongside the traumatic early experience that had led to her being accommodated by the local authority for four years. Megan had witnessed her drug-dependent father severely abuse her mother, including cutting her face with a knife, and she had suffered long periods of neglect when she was not fed or nappy changed as a baby. A possible diagnosis of ADHD was ruled out and, with a belief that her difficulties stemmed from attachment issues and early trauma, she was referred for play therapy. During 18 months of therapy, Megan played out what she had seen and worked through the developmental stages of play, making up for what she had missed in the parental home. These experiences were witnessed, acknowledged and validated by the therapist. The first 12 weeks consisted of extreme 'messy play', mixing red paint and sand and enjoying the sensory sensation. Later Megan moved into projective play, using the dolls' houses and figures to make sense of her current situation in the foster home and her contact with her mother. Finally, she used role play, making up scenarios that she controlled and in which she directed the therapist to follow her lead.

In parallel with the therapy, the foster carers were encouraged to allow Megan's play to regress at home. They gave her regular access to sand, water and 'gunge'. Work was undertaken with the carers and school staff, to help them understand Megan's behaviour within the context of her early experiences. A gradual improvement in her behaviour at home was replicated at school, her concentration improved and she began to attend after-school clubs and to cope with the social relationships this involved. At the close of individual therapy the carer was trained to continue to offer regular play sessions based on non-directive play therapy principles.

Multiple-Choice Questions

See answers on page 672.

1. What is the primary role of a play therapist?
   a. To have fun in the playroom with the child
   b. To help the child make sense of difficult life experiences and relationships
   c. To show parents how to play with their child
   d. To find out whether a child has been abused
   e. To show a child how to use the different toys and media
2. Who can benefit most from play therapy?
   a. All children up to age 16 years
   b. Any child who has experienced trauma and neglect
   c. Children with a learning difficulty
   d. Children aged 2.5–12 years who have had difficult life experiences
   e. Children who have behaviour difficulties at school
3. Why play therapy rather than talking therapy?
   a. The play therapist prefers playing to talking.
   b. Playing helps the child feel in control.
   c. Play is the child's primary form of communication.
   d. Expecting a child to sit and talk for an hour is unrealistic.
   e. Children should have every opportunity to play.
4. What media would a play therapist make available to help the child access pre-verbal memories?
   a. Story books
   b. Sensory materials such as 'gunge' and sand
   c. Dressing up clothes
   d. Little animals
   e. Dolls
5. What were the original theoretical approaches underpinning non-directive play therapy?
   a. Many different theories
   b. Child/person-centred
   c. Psychodynamic
   d. Social constructionist
   e. Systems theory

Key References

Ayling, P., Armstrong, H., Gordon-Clark, L., (2019) *Becoming and being a Play Therapist. Play Therapy in Practice.* London: Routledge.
Cattanach, A., (2008b). *Play Therapy with Abused Children.* London: Jessica Kingsley.
Dalley, T., (1984, re-printed 1996). *Art as Therapy.* London: Routledge.
Jennings, S., (1999). *Introduction to Developmental Play Therapy.* London: Jessica Kingsley.
Winnicott, D.W., (1971). *Playing and Reality.* London: Penguin.

57 Child and Adolescent Psychotherapy

Miranda Passey

Introduction

Child and adolescent psychotherapy derives from the ideas and psychoanalytic theories first created by Sigmund Freud and later elaborated on by Melanie Klein and others, as well as attachment theory and child development research. The professional association was founded in 1949, and the first formal training was presided over by Dr John Bowlby at the Tavistock Clinic. Today, child and adolescent psychoanalytic psychotherapists (CAPPs), to give them their full title, come from several training schools and form part of the multi-disciplinary team in many children and young people's mental health services (CYPMH) settings.

What Do Child Psychotherapists Do?

Child psychotherapists aim to allow the child to express and describe his unique picture of the world and his relationships within it, by means of play, drawing, words or other behaviour in the therapy room. They believe that this internal picture of our world is not just created by our actual experiences, but that it is also altered by what we have made of them, because of the unconscious ideas (known as 'phantasies') that we have attached to that experience. Psychotherapy can bring these phantasies to light. For example, a child who has suffered the loss of a parent or sibling often secretly believes that they caused this loss or damage, because of their own behaviour. This belief can be compounded by the *even more unconscious* knowledge that he has, at times, felt full of hatred and anger towards that lost person or indeed, at times, wished, for example, that his infuriating sibling had not even been born. Once this unconscious version of events can be seen, described and shared, it can also be thought about by both therapist and child. Once it has been thought about, often over a period of time, traumatised children can slowly begin to think about themselves and their states of mind, rather than just reacting to anticipated events, or remaining convinced that their version of events is the only one, or automatically 'blocking out' the attempts of concerned adults to get through to them. In the words of Margaret Hunter (2001) they can become 'master of their own house'. This self-understanding can build long-term resilience and strength to deal with future challenges.

Because many disturbed and traumatised children cannot in fact 'play', child psychotherapists have to use their capacity to observe minute details of behaviour and shifts of feeling, in addition to interpreting the meaning of play or drawings, in a more conventional way. They often find themselves treating children who are so disturbed, e.g. autistic and severely learning-disabled children (see references), that other forms of therapy from other professionals, which rely on more traditional forms of communication, have not been helpful for them. Child psychotherapists also work with parents, families, mother–infant couples and groups, and not only one-to-one with patients. They work in other settings such as hospitals and specialised in-patient units, and also in special schools and nurseries. They participate in outcome monitoring and research projects. They offer teaching, training, support and consultations to a wide range of other professionals working with troubled children and young people.

Key Concepts in Psychotherapy

Projection and Containment

We all use projection. It is the mechanism whereby painful feelings are transferred from ourselves to others, to rid ourselves of those feelings or, sometimes, to communicate our distress in a primitive way. For example, a baby crying is projecting the feeling of distress and terror. Those hearing the cry are meant to find this unbearable and be moved to action. Similarly, in therapy, the child may project all kinds of feelings into the therapist in the hope that his experience will be received and understood. Because traumatised children may have had terrible experiences, which they have not been able to make sense of, they are left terrorised and in the grip of, often, unbearable states of mind, acute mental pain or confusion.

The therapist's task is to attempt to contain and hold in mind these feelings, whilst refraining from action. This is often extremely difficult, as with very disturbed children, projection of feelings may involve shouting, screaming or physical violence, all designed to give the therapist a taste of how it might feel to be a terrorised child. When the therapist creates a space to think, these experiences can be reflected on, and when appropriate, shared with the child. However, the first crucial therapeutic tool is this capacity to receive and contain in oneself the distress, muddled confusion or despair of the child, and *not* to set some premature 'task', goal or activity, which would serve to keep the 'message' at arm's length. The experience of being contained can be some children's first experience of someone struggling to understand and crucially give meaning to their most raw experiences. This, by itself, is therapeutic.

Transference

Unthought-about, unprocessed events that have frightened or troubled us remain with us. They emerge in unexplained fears, in nightmares or in apparently random fixed likes or dislikes. Recent important work in the field of neuroscience (Music, 2010) has helped to map the effect of trauma on the developing brain and explain how trauma impairs the capacity to think and process information. Psychotherapeutic work over time can also be shown to heal and restore some damaged connections. Important relationships will be re-enacted and repeated in the present, transferred onto the therapist and re-experienced by the child in therapy. This process is facilitated by the fact that the therapist is receptive and open to what the child brings, rather than directing what happens, telling the child how they should respond or shaping what the child chooses to do. As Hunter puts it 'the child is not jollied out of their hostility or seduced from their distrust', but instead negative feelings are acknowledged and accepted when they emerge. A child psychotherapist pays careful attention to their patient's body language, and signs that they may be re-experiencing trauma in the here-and-now relationship with them. Over time, by means of the new, constantly re-examined relationship that the psychotherapist makes with the child, the child's way of seeing the world and his expectations of it can be changed and modified.

Children who have been sexually abused, for example, will often at some time demonstrate (often with weary cynicism) that they expect to be abused in the therapy. This 'transference' can provide powerful, living evidence of the child's experiences. Faced with a child inviting her to abuse them, a therapist's task is to put into words what the child expects and fears. The therapist might find herself saying something like: 'I think you are showing me that deep down, this is what you feel all adults want from you. And you feel I am no different'. Or 'You can't imagine that there might be any different way to be with a grown-up, who is interested in you'.

It may take many months, or even years, before such a child can begin to trust, to reconstruct painful memories and experience rightful anger, outrage and sorrow. While being understood brings relief, it often brings emotional pain, as the capacity to *feel* is rediscovered. Re-visited painful experiences will show themselves in disturbances or outbursts in the therapy room. However, a child who has become more 'emotionally alive' is freed to experience life in a much richer way, e.g. to become more able to learn, to respond to parental love and concern, to take in ideas at school and to make fulfilling friendships.

Introjection

Over time, if therapy goes well, the child discovers a greater capacity to think and understand. He can struggle more and more to make sense of his feelings, put them into words and notice his different states of mind. This capacity comes from the experience of his relationship with a therapist, who has struggled to understand *him* and has not enacted his fears and expectations of relationships (e.g. that he would be misunderstood or rejected) but has given him something different. If this new experience can be introjected (taken in) the child can better use his own mind and can begin to believe that knowing about other people's minds is worthwhile. His painful experiences, once mourned, cease to have such a destructive impact on the present and can be allowed to recede to the past, allowing more room for the relationships of the here and now.

Freud described how mental pain is expressed as anxiety. This anxiety causes us to develop defences against the pain. These defences in turn can cause symptoms. A child psychotherapist may be asked to help when a child is suffering from serious emotional problems which cannot be easily understood or resolved, which are inhibiting normal healthy development and spoiling relationships. The work involves trying to understand and describe the child's defences and helping the child to become more aware of the hidden pain these defences were designed to conceal or avoid. Slowly the child can develop a greater understanding of himself and of his fears and feelings and reclaim buried experiences. The primary focus of the work is the unconscious: the hidden, inner world of feelings and experiences that lies inside all of us but is not available to conscious awareness. This inner world is usually only known to us through our dreams, and in the case of children, through their unique instrument, play.

Many of the children and young people child psychotherapists see are suffering from developmental trauma in response to deprivation, separation or loss, and many are 'looked after' children. By understanding and bringing to light buried pain and confusion and exploring the unique meanings which each child has attached to their experience, child psychotherapy can help the child to see reality more as it is. As a result, they are more able to learn and to use the support on offer from parents or other carers, because they are no longer 'locked' in the grip of their past experiences.

The Setting for Therapy

Crucial attention is paid to the setting for child psychotherapy. Children are seen in the same room, at the same time each week, over a sustained period of months or years. The room is safe and as free as possible from any of the therapist's personal possessions and with minimal 'no-go areas', to allow for exploration. There is often access to water and/or sand. Each child is provided with a sturdy box in which to keep the play materials for their exclusive use. These materials form part of the younger child's 'language' or 'tool box' for therapy, facilitating exploration and the opportunity to make sense of their experience. Older children and young people may still wish to draw, for example, if communication with words feels hard.

Typically, the therapy box will contain paper, pens and crayons, family dolls, wild and domestic animals, building blocks or Duplo, fences, small cars and trucks, string, glue, Sellotape, scissors, plasticine or playdoh and a soft ball. Whatever the child creates stays in the box. The meaning that is attached to whatever is made resides within the therapy. It may often be revisited as the child begins to change and can reflect in a different way and notice his different feelings. The room becomes a safe, private place where deep feelings can be explored and held. The therapist ensures the safety of the child and of herself: e.g. sometimes having to stop sessions until the next time, if the child's violence or fear of his feelings cannot allow him to continue within safe bounds for that day.

It is crucial for the success of therapy that there is both support for the child and regular support for his parents or carers. A child needs an ally who will help him to come for regular sessions, even when he is reluctant or apprehensive. This can also be a social worker or family support worker. Parents need to feel there is someone to help *them* to make sense of what they are feeling and what their child is going through, and to keep pace with changes in the child.

Assessment

A child will have three or more assessment sessions to establish whether this work may be of help to him and give him a taste of what psychotherapy involves. Children who come for psychotherapy will often have had previous forms of intervention, perhaps in a family context, which in itself can be a form of screening, and can help inform a decision to offer psychotherapy.

Training, Personal Therapy and Supervision

CAPPs undergo a long and rigorous post-graduate training. An MA followed by four years' clinical training and a doctorate leads to membership of the Association of Child Psychotherapists. This is the regulating body for standards and ethics in the UK. The fundamental core of the training is the trainee's own intensive personal psychotherapy. This ensures that, so far as possible, undigested issues from the therapist's own experience and history are not transferred into their work with their patients. In-depth work with deeply troubled children can stir up very powerful and primitive feelings and anxieties. Therapists have to prove over this long training that they can contain, and struggle to think about, extremely disturbing events and states of mind that their patients bring to them. All child psychotherapists have regular supervision from senior colleagues so that detailed accounts of their work can be shared and explored. This remains an essential part of good practice.

Alongside the study of formal theory and technique, the third cornerstone of the training is the Infant and Young Child Observation. This is the detailed observation, for an hour a week, of the first two years of an infant's life, within the context of his family and relationships. An under-five-year-old child is also observed for one year. Written-up observations are discussed in weekly seminars, providing a lived experience of each child's unique emotional development. Here the student also develops the capacity for in-depth detailed observation and learns a richer understanding of the unconscious meaning behind our actions and responses.

Case Example (1): Work with a School-Age Child (Tracey)

Tracey was six years old when I started work with her. The work lasted for two years. She had been left in the care of a mentally ill and sexually abused mother, when she was two and her parents separated. During this time, she was sexually abused by the maternal grandfather and left with a mother who was alternately groggy with medication or 'smothering', insisting that Tracey sleep in her bed. When the abuse and inadequate care came to light, Tracey was removed into local authority care and eventually, aged five, placed with her father, who had returned to the area, really wanting to play a part in his daughter's life. Tracey's father had severe physical health problems of his own. Tracey was referred for help because she was failing to learn at school and had inappropriately touched other children. She suffered from nightmares.

In therapy, Tracey presented a brittle, superior, almost manic façade, keeping up a running commentary 'look at me how clever I am', and being frantically busy, making imaginary meals, doing acrobatics and singing and dancing. It felt as though this was to ward off any kind of sadness, any real contact or dialogue with me, or any awareness of her own limitations. By contrast, I felt heavy and stupid, and often unable to think or follow what was happening. I wondered if I was being 'made' to feel like a drugged, mentally ill mother or like a confused, impotent and bewildered Tracey, faced with behaviour she could not make sense of.

Because Tracey had been abused and terrified as a small child, life experience had taught her to be cynical about adults and to fear any real close connection with them. She showed me that it did not feel safe to stop for a moment or relax her guard. She could not allow anything 'in' from me, because it might turn out to be abusive or dangerous. This closed-off quality accordingly severely impeded her capacity to learn. At times, I felt under great pressure to join in and admire her as a miracle 'performing child' and to forget the embracing sadness I felt when I was with her and remember that she could not read or write or even do simple sums. The painful task was to help her make more contact with her fear and terror and underlying sadness, and to remember some of the frightening and confusing experiences she had undergone. She could then be helped to differentiate between then and now and to make more use of me to help her think and become more reflective about her real needs and difficulties.

In one moving session, after many months of manic activity, Tracey made a 'bed' for herself with the rug and pillow I had provided for her. She allowed herself to lie quietly and to have an experience of being contained and thought about, as I sat at a safe distance and spoke to her gently.

As some of her past experiences could be played out, and thought about, Tracey became more able to take things in and learn at school. As she changed, her father became more aware of the real vulnerability beneath her brittle, premature grown-upness, and began to feel braver to challenge her and provide firmer boundaries, to which Tracey responded with relief. She began to heal and to be able to trust again.

Case Example (2): Parent–Infant Work (Jane)

Jane came for help because she felt depressed and overwhelmed by her six-month-old daughter who she felt cried without stopping and 'did not like her'. When she began to explore her own experience of mothering in childhood with the therapist a painful story emerged of her own depressed and overwhelmed mother, who sent Jane away to be cared for by an aunt for the first year of her life. Jane experienced her baby's gestures towards her as hostile and would flinch when her baby reached out to touch her face. Slowly the therapist helped Jane to separate out her past experience of being given up by her own mother and voice her fears about her mother's dislike of her, so that she could distinguish between these experiences and learn to 'see' her own real six-month-old daughter. Their relationship began to improve with mutual enjoyment, and the little girl began to thrive and cried much less.

Case Example (3): Work with an Adolescent (Sarah)

Sarah came for help because she was struggling with self-harm and furious outbursts at school and at home. Her parents had separated, and she could not accept her mother's new partner or find her place in two newly constituted families. With the therapist's support, she was able to come to terms with her powerful jealousy and possessiveness and to understand her wish to control everything, because of her fear of being abandoned. Gradually she could allow herself to be more separate from her mother, to develop and learn more at school, to voice her fears and worries rather than expressing them by means of cutting her arms, and her relationships improved.

Multiple-Choice Questions

See answers on page 672.

1. Child psychotherapy addresses what is going on in:
    a. The external world of the child
    b. The internal world of the child
    c. Both external and internal
2. Child psychotherapy attempts to help the child explore and change
    a. Other people
    b. Their own view of the world and relationships
    c. Learn coping strategies
3. Child Psychotherapy training lasts for
    a. One year
    b. Three years
    c. Six to eight years
4. Child psychotherapy draws on
    a. The work of Freud and Melanie Klein
    b. The work of John Bowlby on attachment
    c. Both of the above

Key References

Hunter, M., (2001). *Psychotherapy with Children in Care: Lost and Found.* Hove, East Sussex: Brunner-Routledge.

Lanyado, M., Horne, A., (Eds.), (1990). *The Handbook of Child and Adolescent Psychotherapy.* London & New York: Routledge.

Music, G., (2010). *Nurturing Natures: Attachment and Childrens' Emotional, Sociocultural and Brain Development.* London: Psychology.

Pally, R., (2000). *The Mind-Brain Relationship.* London: Karnac.

Sinason, V., (1992). *Mental Handicap and the Human Condition.* London: Free Association Books.

Sutton, S., (2014). *Being Taken In, The Framing Relationship.* London: Karnac.

For further information, contact the Association of Child Psychotherapists, CAN Borough, 7-14 Great Dover Street, London, SE1 4YR https://childpsychotherapy.org.uk.

58 Counselling Children and Young People

Jacquie Kelly

KEY POINTS

- Each young person has the potential and resources to make positive changes.
- Counsellors understand a young person's way of seeing their experiences, suspending judgements and opinions.
- A trusting relationship is created by being consistent and authentic.

Counselling Children and Young People

Although the term 'counselling' can be applied to a wide range of helping activities and many professional disciplines use counselling skills, counselling itself is a specific kind of therapy that is widely used with young people.

Counsellors are trained according to various theories that have been developed since the 1940s, and schools of counselling are usually distinguished by the theoretical approach used. Much of the counselling provided for young people in the UK is broadly humanistic in approach, using either a single model or integrating different models, depending on the counsellor's training and on what they assess will benefit the client. Humanistic approaches include person-centred, gestalt, transactional analysis and existential therapies, and integrative counsellors may use approaches from outside the humanistic tradition, such as mindfulness or cognitive behavioural techniques. There is some debate about the distinction between counselling and psychotherapy, because many practitioners use the terms interchangeably, whilst others would distinguish counselling as shorter-term work or as involving shorter training than psychotherapy.

Counselling training involves between three and five years' study, leading to qualification at diploma, BA or master's Level. Trainees are required to complete at least 100 hours of supervised counselling practice, and most courses require students to undertake personal therapy. Throughout their career, all counsellors are required to receive regular supervision for discussion of their work. Counselling children and young people is a specialised field and, as most counselling courses are designed for practice with adults, youth counsellors need to develop the additional knowledge and skills essential for working with this client group. These include an understanding of child development, familiarity with legal frameworks and the ability to maintain confidentiality whilst relating to carers and professional networks around a child (BACP, 2019).

In the UK, counselling for children and young people is predominantly provided in educational settings, e.g. schools and colleges, and in youth counselling agencies run by local authorities or third-sector organisations.

Humanistic Counselling

Humanistic approaches share a belief that clients have the resources to find their own solutions to their difficulties and to make positive changes, rather than seeing the client in terms of problematic symptoms or behaviour. Carl Rogers, the founder of the person-centred approach, saw it as the counsellor's responsibility to provide the environment for a relationship to develop in which the client can achieve their potential. He identified essential qualities ('Core Conditions') that enable the counsellor to provide it (Rogers, 1957):

- **Empathy** – understanding the client's experience, meanings and world view
- **Unconditional positive regard** – accepting and validating the client as an individual person, suspending judgments and opinions
- **Congruence** – being open, being themselves and challenging when appropriate

These conditions enable the counsellor to form a relationship with the client, based on developing increasing trust. The safer a young person feels, the more openly they can express themselves and the more effective the counselling will be in addressing their real issues. The relationship with the client is central to the therapeutic work, and interventions are designed to engage the client as a partner in that relationship.

Any therapist is in a position of power in relation to a client, and with young people there is the added dimension of being an adult relating to a child. To empower the client within the relationship, counselling sessions are driven by what is important to the young person. The counsellor's role is to facilitate exploration of their feelings and experiences.

Young people may not have control in many aspects of their lives and can lack maturity in their decision-making, but by listening carefully to their concerns and helping them to understand themselves, the counsellor can support them to make choices and find their own way forward. This does not mean the counsellor simply agrees with the young person. Being congruent may involve challenging what they have said or how they have acted. In these situations, the foundation of the relationship is crucial, because they are more likely to receive challenge in a constructive way if they feel they have power in the relationship and that they are respected and valued.

When Is Counselling Appropriate?

It is important that the client understands the counselling process, so they can take an active role. For counselling to be effective, a young person needs to attend voluntarily. It will not work if they only attend the sessions because someone else thinks they should.

For young people who find it difficult to express themselves and for younger children, counsellors often use creative techniques, art materials, toys or worksheets. This is not the same as play therapy or art psychotherapy (see relevant chapters), and it is essential to assess when one of these other interventions may be more appropriate. With young people with learning disabilities, the counsellor can adapt their approach to take account of the client's cognitive and verbal abilities, ensuring that they can take an autonomous part in the therapy.

Counsellors take a holistic approach to problems that a client is facing, and mental health issues are seen in the context of the whole person. This is particularly useful in working with children and young people where developmental and environmental issues have such an impact. It can have a destigmatising effect, because counsellors do not see young people's issues in terms of diagnoses or dysfunction.

The Counselling Process

Counselling sessions are held at a regular, agreed time, usually on a weekly basis. They last for a pre-defined time, often 50 minutes or an hour, but can be shorter for younger children or to fit in with lesson times in school. Work with young people may be short- or long-term. Many services limit the number of sessions a client can access, whilst some allow the client to decide when the sessions will end.

The counsellor begins by establishing a therapeutic 'contract' with the young person. They explain how counselling works and what to expect, including the limits of confidentiality, how many sessions are available and how the counselling will be reviewed.

Using active listening skills, the counsellor encourages the young person to tell their story in their own way and at their own pace. The counsellor tries to understand how the client sees their problems, what brings them to counselling now and what they would like to achieve. Through this exploration, the client understands themselves and their problems more clearly and is supported to make decisions about what action they want to take.

Regular reviews help the counsellor and client assess how the counselling is progressing. This will inform whether further sessions are required or whether some other interventions are indicated in addition to, or instead of, counselling. Endings are part of the counselling process, offering the opportunity to evaluate the progress the client has made and provide a positive experience of a relationship ending.

Outcomes

The goals of counselling are guided by what the young person wants to achieve, but in general would include increasing their:

- Understanding of themselves, their problems and other people
- Ability to make links between experiences, feelings and behaviour
- Ability to make decisions and take responsibility in their lives
- Development of interpersonal and relationship skills
- Self-esteem and self-confidence

These outcomes are challenging to measure, and it is important to use measures with an established evidence base, whilst ensuring that they are valid for the outcomes counselling is designed to achieve. Questionnaires can influence what a young person decides to talk about, and they need to be carefully introduced in a way that is consistent with the therapeutic process. When integrated effectively, many young people find it helpful to have explicit and tangible ways of identifying goals and measuring their progress.

Measures widely used for counselling children and young people are the Young Person's-Clinical Outcomes for Routine Evaluation (YP-CORE) for use with young people from 11 to 16 years. The version for adults, CORE-10, is used with over-16s and the goal-based outcome (GBO) tool for 0–18 years. These measures are designed for use on a session-by-session basis. There is a wide range of other measures that can be used as pre- and post-counselling measures, including the Strengths and Difficulties Questionnaire (SDQ) and the Revised Children's Anxiety and Depression Scale (RCADS) (BACP, 2016).

Case Study: Aaron

Aaron is a 13-year-old boy referred to the school counsellor by his form tutor, Mr Clarke. He was often into trouble for angry outbursts that resulted in repeated detentions, but Mr Clarke felt that counselling might be more helpful than further disciplinary measures. Aaron often came to school in dirty clothes and Mr Clarke suspected he was being bullied, although Aaron denied it.

Aaron was seen by the school counsellor, Gina. She explained how counselling works and that Aaron could talk about anything he wanted to. She would try to understand how he saw what was happening in his life. She emphasised that counselling helps people find their own solutions to problems, rather than telling them what is best for them. She showed him how he could write down what he wanted to achieve or change in his life and that they could keep track of his progress together.

Aaron spent most of the session looking at the floor and saying very little. At the end, Gina asked if he wanted to come to more sessions, but he said he did not see the point. Gina replied that she would be happy to work with him, if he changed his mind.

The following term, Aaron was referred again, following a suspension from school for hitting another student. This time, Gina was able to encourage him to tell her what had happened and how it felt from his point of view. Aaron said that the boy had taken his clothes during a PE lesson and that he had had to go to lunch in his games kit. The boy had laughed at his dirty clothes in front of the whole school. Gina helped him to talk about how that felt and to understand that he lashed out at the boy because he felt so humiliated.

Over subsequent sessions, Aaron talked more about his life, and how different he felt to other people at school. He lived with his mother, who had suffered with severe back pain all his life. He had two much older brothers, who had moved away. Aaron felt it was his responsibility to look after her. He said that, when people laughed at his dirty clothes, it reminded him that he was not doing a good enough job. Gina replied that it sounded as if he felt he was not coping with all the expectations on him.

This was a turning point in the therapy. Aaron realised that the real issue for him was not being able to manage at home. Gina helped him identify what he could do to improve the situation.

The first task was to let people know that he was struggling. Gina reflected that it had taken a long time for him to open up to her, but now that he had done that, she asked if he could choose someone else he trusted to talk to. Aaron decided to speak to his Head of Year, who contacted a young carers' group. This gave Aaron the chance to speak to other young people with similar experiences. Gina wondered if Aaron's mother could be a source of support. He was reluctant to let her know how he was feeling, because he did not want to worry her, but Gina challenged this by asking whether there was any way that his mother could help with the household chores, even if she could not do them herself. He decided to ask his mother for advice on how to do the laundry and as a result, she was able to help him be more organised about washing his school uniform.

In his final session, Aaron and Gina reviewed the progress Aaron had made since his suspension from school. He understood why he was so angry and how much he was struggling to manage the situation at home. Through talking with Gina, Aaron realised the importance of sharing his feelings and finding support.

Multiple-Choice Questions

See answers on page 672.

1. One of the counsellor's main aims is to
   a. Solve a young person's problem
   b. Advise a young person about their problem

    c. Understand how the young person sees their problem
    d. Assess what is wrong with the young person
2. A counsellor creates a trusting relationship with a young person by
    a. Agreeing with the client
    b. Being honest and being themselves
    c. Promising to keep everything confidential
    d. Giving them their mobile phone number, in case they need to talk to someone between the counselling sessions
3. Who decides on the focus of a counselling session?
    a. The referrer
    b. The counsellor
    c. The parent or carer
    d. The young person
4. Which of the following is NOT true?
    a. A young person can benefit from counselling, even if they don't know what their problem is.
    b. If a young person doesn't want to speak to anyone, they should still be made to attend counselling.
    c. Young people can benefit from counselling, even if they find it hard to express their feelings.
    d. Clients need to be able to understand what counselling is.
5. A key outcome for counselling with children and young people is...
    a. They will definitely achieve solutions to their problems.
    b. They will realise their problems are not as bad as they thought.
    c. They will have a greater understanding of themselves and their relationships with other people.
    d. Their bad behaviour will improve.

Key References

British Association or Counselling and Psychotherapy, (2016). *Children and Young People Practice Research Network (CYP PRN): A Toolkit for Collecting Routine Outcome Measures.* Lutterworth: BACP. Available at: https://www.bacp.co.uk/media/2355/bacp-cyp-prn-toolkit-for-collecting-routine-outcome-measures.pdf Accessed 5 June 2019.

British Association for Counselling and Psychotherapy, (2019). *Competences for Work with Children and Young People (4–18 Years).* Lutterworth: BACP. Available at: https://www.bacp.co.uk/media/5863/bacp-cyp-competence-framework.pdf (accessed 6 June 2019).

Rogers, C.R., (1957). The necessary and sufficient conditions of therapeutic personality change. *Journal of Consulting Psychology*, 21(2): 95–103.

59 Cognitive Behavioural Therapy

Sarah Mottram

Introduction

Cognitive behavioural therapy (CBT) is a type of talking therapy that looks at our thoughts, feelings and behaviours, and considers how each of these areas interact. CBT combines cognitive therapy (thinking about thinking) with behavioural therapy (what we do and why we do it).

KEY CONCEPTS

- CBT relies on the assumption that how people think impacts how they feel and how they behave. How an individual behaves in turn impacts on the individual's thoughts and feelings.
- Individuals can develop maladaptive thinking processes that can cause negative automatic thoughts (NATS). These are influenced by our early life experiences and the beliefs we form about our self, others and the world.
- Individuals can believe NATs are facts, and CBT aims to consider evidence for thoughts, to understand how accurate the perception and thought process is.
- CBT encourages the idea of changing the behaviours and experimenting with this change, to create further evidence to understand the thoughts.
- It is important to consider the wider support around the child and young person. CBT should include the involvement of parents and the school, where possible.

Development of CBT

Cognitive therapy was initially proposed by Beck in the 1970s for the treatment of depression in adults and focusses on maladaptive thinking. Beck believed people develop negative beliefs about themselves, the world and the future, known as the cognitive triad, based on their life experience. This can lead to maladaptive thinking patterns based on these beliefs. People interact and understand the world through their mental representation of it. If this is inaccurate, they will evaluate and perceive things inaccurately and this will impact on their emotions and behaviour. For example, if someone interprets a situation negatively as a result of these thought patterns, they are likely to experience negative feelings and, based on those negative thoughts and feelings, behave in a certain way.

Behavioural theory considers how our behaviour is shaped through reinforcement. Difficulties, such as phobias, can develop through an individual attempting to manage the anxiety. If a child feels anxious when they go to school, their natural reaction is to rid themselves of the unpleasant feeling of anxiety. To do this they ask their mother to take them home. They find when they leave school that the anxiety goes away. The behaviour, asking a parent if they can go home and leaving school, is reinforced by the reduction in anxious feelings. The individual then learns that 'if I want to feel better, I will repeat the behaviour to achieve the same result', i.e. the reduction of anxiety. Behavioural theory aims to stop the reinforcement of the unwanted behaviour and to reinforce a new, desired behaviour.

Combining both cognitive and behavioural theory incorporates both aspects and analyses both how our thinking makes us feel and how what we do affects our thoughts and feelings. CBT focusses on creating change either in how we think or in what we do and regularly monitors progress with the use of goals and measures.

CBT in Children and Adolescents

CBT is widely used in adults because of its significant evidence base for the treatment of anxiety and depression in addition to other more complex disorders. More recently, CBT has had a growing presence in the treatment of children and adolescents, with an emerging evidence base for separation anxiety, generalised anxiety disorder, OCD, PTSD, panic, social anxiety, depression and eating disorders.

Within CAMHS nationally, there is a shift in focus towards evidence-based practice. Over the last few years CBT training has been funded in CAMHS to provide both low-intensity CBT-informed work and full CBT, in line with the Improving Access to Psychological Therapies Strategy (CYP-IAPT). 2019 has seen the launch of the educational mental health practitioner role (EMHP). The EMHPs are trained in CBT-informed interventions to work in schools with a view to provide early help when problems first emerge, preventing difficulties escalating and the need for CAMHS input.

Before working with a young person through CBT, the practitioner needs to consider their suitability for this type of work.

An individual is suitable if they have:

- The ability to vocalise their thoughts and the maturity to think about their thinking, considering developmental age.
- Some flexibility in their thinking. This can be difficult with individuals who are believed to have autistic spectrum condition traits.
- Motivation to partake in making changes in their life.
- Can think about what they want to look different in their life and, with help, can formulate a goal to work towards.
- The commitment to work on things outside of the session, i.e. homework. This may require the commitment of someone at home to support them.

For CBT to be successful, an appropriate assessment is undertaken and a formulation created to capture the main problem and what is maintaining it. Goal- setting is a key aspect of keeping the sessions focussed and structured. CBT follows a step-by-step process:

- Assessment
- Formulation
- Goals
- Treatment planning
- Intervention
- Review
- Relapse prevention

Cognitive Behavioural Therapy Assessment and Formulation

Assessment and formulation are a key aspect in CBT work. It allows the CBT practitioner to understand the main problem the intervention needs to target and to capture the maintenance, i.e. what is keeping the problem going.

The practitioner should adopt a curious and open stance, using Socratic dialogue and guided discovery to help the young person to gain insight into their own difficulties.

There are several assessment tools available to assist the practitioner to understand and pinpoint the main problem:

- **4Ws** (Richards and Whytes, 2009)
  What 'What is the main problem?'
  Where 'Where is it a problem?'
  When 'When does it happen?'
  With whom 'Who is it better or worse with?'
- **FIDO**
  Frequency – 'How frequently does this problem occur?'
  Intensity – 'How intense are the feelings of anxiety?' (Often we ask children and young people to rate the intensity of their emotions on a 0–10 scale.)
  Duration – 'How long do those feelings last?'
  Onset – 'When did you first start to notice the symptoms?'
- **Funnelling and Feedback** (Richards and Whytes, 2009)
  Funnelling is the concept of asking open broad questions and following a line of enquiry, asking more specific open questions to lead to accurate identification of the problem (Figure 59.1). Funnelling requires curiosity, asking follow up questions and following lines of enquiry to gain greater insight into the problem.
  During this process, the practitioner will summarise and feedback their understanding of what has been said, in addition to seeking clarification that it has been understood correctly. This process ensures that the young person feels heard, builds rapport and trust and ensures that the information has been correctly understood by both parties. The

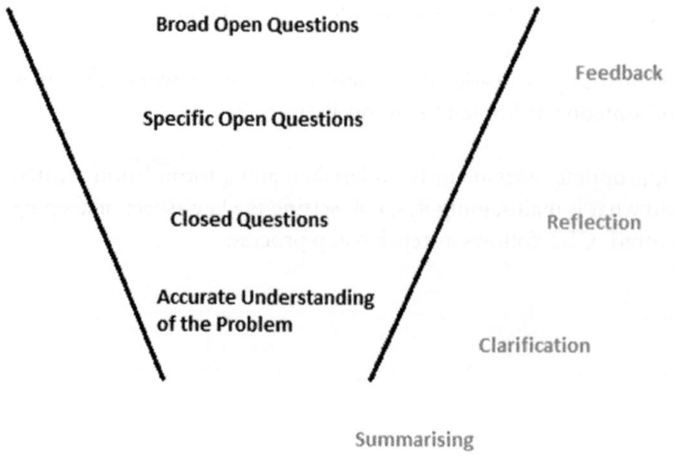

Figure 59.1 Funnelling.

information is gathered and fed back and leads to further lines of questioning to create another specific question, leading to further depth of understanding.

- **Routine Outcome Measures**

  Progress is measured throughout assessment and treatment using several different tools, gaining a mixture of both quantitative and qualitative data. Routine outcome measures (ROMs) are commonplace in work with children and young people and form part of the assessment and treatment. These are age-specific but are often used across therapeutic modalities.

For young people over the age of 16, CBT-specific adult measures can be used which are disorder-specific. These include the Patient Health Questionnaire 9 (PHQ9), Generalised Anxiety Disorder 7 (GAD7), Social Phobia Inventory (SPIN), Impact of Events Scale Revised (IES-R) and Obsessive Compulsive Inventory (OCI).

Formulation

Cognitive behavioural formulation creates a diagram of the information gathered in the assessment phase. It allows joint understanding and presents the information succinctly. It aims to capture both how the problem occurs and what keeps the problem going. This captures a reference point representing the young person's presentation at the beginning of therapy and gives an idea of what maintains the problem. The formulation is a blueprint of therapy that guides the planning of specific interventions that are individual-specific, yet protocol driven.

There are many different ways to formulate, either using a generic model or a disorder-specific model. The 5 Areas Model (Padesky, 1986) or 'hot cross bun', is a common generic formulation (Figure 59.2).

This model captures the relationship between thoughts and feelings and the impact this can have on our physiology and emotions. For instance, if an individual is anxious about the judgement of others, a trigger might be an invitation to a party (Figure 59.3). This could trigger thoughts around 'what if I wear the wrong thing?' 'people will laugh at me'. This could lead to anxious feelings and potentially trigger the fight/flight response. With the thoughts appraising the situation negatively and leading to unpleasant symptoms, it is likely that the individual will do something to stop the anxious thoughts and symptoms (e.g. avoiding the friend who invited them to the party or making excuses not to go).

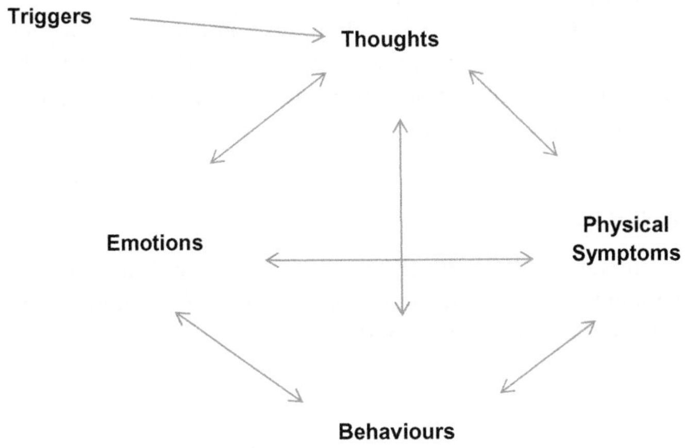

Figure 59.2 The 5 Areas Model.

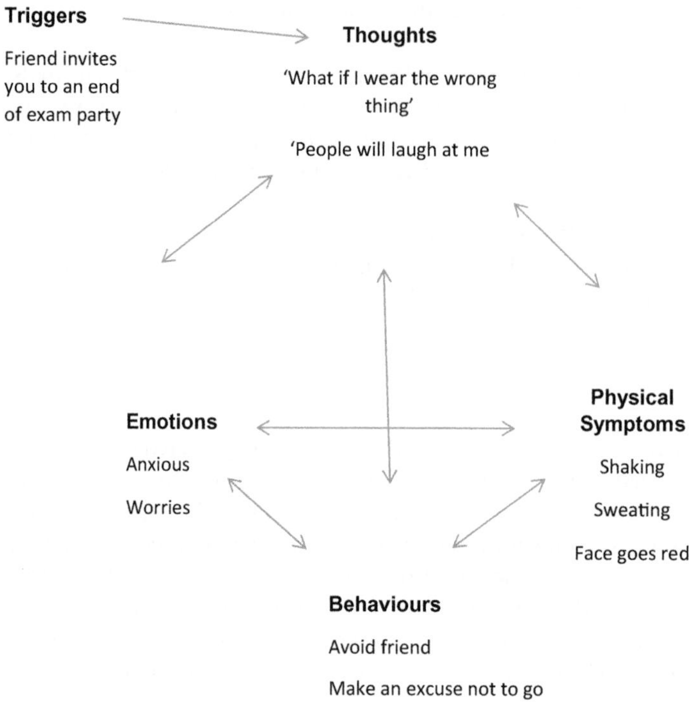
Triggers
Friend invites you to an end of exam party
Thoughts
'What if I wear the wrong thing'
'People will laugh at me
Emotions
Anxious
Worries
Physical Symptoms
Shaking
Sweating
Face goes red
Behaviours
Avoid friend
Make an excuse not to go

Figure 59.3 Using the 5 Areas Model in Formulation.

This leads to a reduction in the intensity of anxiety, and the physiological symptoms will reduce. We are no longer worried about other people laughing if we do not attend the party. The reduction of symptoms reinforces the behaviour through operant conditioning, increasing the likelihood that if they were faced with the scenario again, the individual is likely to repeat the same behaviours, i.e. avoiding the friend or making an excuse not to go. This creates the vicious cycle an individual finds themselves in. Despite feeling better in the short term, long-term the anxiety still exists if a trigger arises. If someone is often anxious around others, they will face this trigger frequently at school or socialising with friends. It can have a significant impact on their lives.

It is important that the individual understands how their thoughts and behaviours impact the problem and that each area is linked. For younger children, this can be adapted creatively to help aid understanding. Alternatively, the formulation can be created with the parent and allow parents to be co-therapists in the child's treatment.

Cognitive Behavioural Treatment

Interventions for treatment are based on the collaboratively created formulation. It may consist of one intervention or several techniques as part of a disorder-specific protocol. Each intervention aims for change in the cognitions, the behaviours or both.

Common CBT Interventions

- **Graded exposure** involves creating a hierarchy, working towards the fear by taking gradual steps towards it. When conducting graded exposure, it has to abide by four conditions:

graded, prolonged, repeated and without distraction. Several variations exist in other disorder-specific work, e.g. exposure and response prevention in OCD.

- **Cognitive restructuring**: a technique looking at the evidence for and against a specific thought, challenging the individual's belief. The process includes rating their initial belief, considering the evidence in support of and against the thought, reconsidering the belief rating and considering an alternative thought that agrees with the evidence.
- **Behavioural experiments** consider creating alternative evidence to test out the accuracy of a thought, often orchestrating a situation and manipulating the variables to see what happens, somewhat similar to a scientific experiment.
- **Problem solving**: a technique to look at solving problems encountered. Often individuals suffering from mental health problems will have low problem- solving ability. Unsolved problems generate excessive worry and lead to a sense of helplessness.
- **Behavioural activation**: a specific protocol to help with depressive symptoms. Based on the idea that depressed individuals often withdraw from social interaction and suffer anhedonia. Behavioural activation aims to build up activities to change the way one feels from engaging in pleasurable activities that offer a sense of achievement. This approach only focusses on behaviours. Cognitions are viewed specifically as rumination, and ruminating is a behaviour to be targeted.
- **Behavioural reward systems** are used to condition and reinforce new desirable behaviours in children. The target behaviour is rewarded with something the child deems desirable. This could range from stickers, tokens or choosing a film to watch or what to eat for dinner. Rewards must be age appropriate.

For children under 12 years old, the evidence suggests that parent-led CBT is most effective. One of the most common programmes is 'Overcoming your child's fears and worries' (Creswell and Willetts, 2019) which focusses on empowering parents with cognitive and behavioural techniques, guided by a practitioner, that they can implement at home with their child.

Relapse Prevention

CBT aims to make the child or young person 'their own therapist', giving them the tools to build resilience and to know how to tackle future problems they encounter. Part of this involves creating a strong relapse prevention plan. This should include approaches that the therapist and child or young person have used together and that have been found useful, including the sheets or workbooks used. It can be helpful to consider what has helped to create change and how they might implement the same approach on their own. Sharing with others helps the individual gain support and helps others to understand the best way to encourage them.

Key Elements of Relapse Prevention

- What has been helpful and why was it helpful?
- What do I need to keep doing to stay on track?
- What should I do if I have a wobble?
- Who should I ask to support me?
- What are the signs and symptoms if things are getting worse?
- What do I need to do if I have a relapse?

It is good practice to set up one or two review dates to monitor progress and give an opportunity to correct any lapses before they become relapses.

Case Study: Jonathan

Jonathan is a 14-year old referred for symptoms of low mood. He described feeling low for the last two years since his parents' separation. As a result of their divorce, he moved schools approximately a year ago.

Jonathan's parents have noticed that his grades have been dropping. During the assessment Jonathan stated, 'I don't care about school anymore', and when followed up he said, 'what's the point, I'm no good at anything anyway'. He reports struggling to make friends since joining his new school and often spends break and lunchtimes on his own in the library using the computers. As a result, he often does not eat his lunch and has lost weight. He insists he does not feel hungry.

Jonathan's parents report that when he is at either his mother's or at his father's house, he stays in his room and is reluctant to spend time with his family. Jonathan does not have friends over to his house and does not spend time with friends after school.

More recently, his mother has noticed Jonathan has been sleeping more than usual, struggling to leave his bed in the mornings and will often sleep when he comes in from school. He reports that he feels tired all the time and cannot be bothered with anything.

When discussing spending time with friends, Jonathan said that he does not have any friends. When his mother suggested that he could contact his friends from his old school, he replied 'they don't want to see me anymore, they don't care'.

Case Analysis and Discussion

From the timeline of Jonathan's story, it is clear he has had a couple of difficult and disrupting events that seem to have clear links to the onset of his symptoms.

- **Trigger**: from the case study, it can be inferred his low mood is present most of the time. School and friendships seem to be a trigger, and Jonathan reports struggling with friends and with schoolwork. The historic trigger appears to be his parents' divorce that led to Jonathan moving schools. The impact of not seeing his usual friends every day and starting at a new school would be understandably anxiety-provoking to anyone, but it appears Jonathan has particularly struggled to settle and the situation has become progressively worse in the last year.

It would be interesting to know if Jonathan is an only child and if he has any siblings, how they are managing the divorce and subsequent changes.

- **Cognitions**: Jonathan reports thinking 'I don't care about school anymore', 'I am no good at anything', 'They don't want to see me anymore', which fit the concept of negative automatic thoughts. This could lead to further negative emotions and to his disengagement with friends and school.

There is little presented in the case study around Jonathan's view of the problem and his thoughts towards the divorce. It is important that the child's view is captured as often the wider network makes decisions on their behalf without listening to the individual. Collaboration is a key concept in the CBT process and ensures a fair power dynamic.

- **Behaviour**: Jonathan appears to be isolated, spending time on his own, both at school and at home. This means he has time to dwell and ruminate on his position, leading to more negative cognitions.

His behaviour appears to be avoidant, and more exploration is needed to uncover what he is trying to avoid. Often avoidance is understood in the context of anxiety, so it could be that Jonathan is anxious about something and is avoiding people, i.e. suffering from social anxiety. Avoidance can be characterised within depression as a relief from burdensome activities. People suffering from depression avoid social activities, as they struggle with tiredness and motivation and often lose the enjoyment they might otherwise have felt. Jonathan is over-sleeping and reports a loss of appetite, both of which fit the DSM-5 and the ICD-11 for diagnosis criteria of depression.

Working therapeutically with Jonathan, it would first be important to understand what he would like to achieve from the sessions. This could establish some goals to give a focus to the sessions. When working with depression, the practitioner aims to inspire hope and motivation as a way to engage the individual in making changes.

There appears to be some established negative thinking maintaining the problem. These NATs may lead Jonathan to a distorted view of himself, others and the world, that contributes to his presentation. One route of intervention is to consider challenging these cognitions by considering the evidence. Jonathan's presentation of withdrawal and avoidance may be maintaining his presentation, allowing him endless time to think. Activity scheduling could be a solution, encouraging him to do more activities that might lead to a more positive mood.

CBT is constantly evolving, and the underlying principles are used to underpin some newer 'third wave' psychotherapies. These include dialectic behavioural therapy (DBT), acceptance and commitment therapy (ACT), mindful-based CBT (MBCBT) and compassion-focused therapy (CFT).

Multiple-Choice Questions

See answers on page 672.

1. What are NATs?
   a. Negative automatic thoughts
   b. Not always thinking
   c. Negative adapted thought
   d. Not adapted thoughts
2. What is CBT unpinned by?
   a. Cognitive theory and schema theory
   b. Behavioural theory
   c. Medical model
   d. Cognitive theory and behavioural theory
3. What is not a common CBT intervention?
   a. Graded exposure
   b. Behavioural activation
   c. Transference interpretation
   d. Cognitive restructuring
4. What do the five areas consist of?
   a. Thoughts, behaviours, anxiety, situation, people around
   b. What, where, when, how, why
   c. Trigger, thoughts, behaviours, physical symptoms, emotions
   d. Situation, NATs, anxiety, heart racing, avoidance
5. What would be recommended for children under 12?
   a. Individual one to one
   b. Cognitive restructuring
   c. Parent-led CBT programme
   d. School involvement

Key References

Fuggle, P., Dunsmuir, S., Curry, V., (2012). *CBT with Children, Young People and Families.* London: SAGE.

Richards, D., Whyte, M., (2009). *Reach Out: National Programme Student Materials to Support the Delivery of Training for Psychological Wellbeing Practitioners Delivering Low Intensity Interventions.* Rethink Mental Illness.

Williams, C., Chellingsworth, M., (2017). *CBT: A Clinician's Guide to Using the Five Areas Approach.* Boca Raton, FL: CRC Press.

60 Cognitive Analytic Therapy (CAT)

Sally Gray and Di Glackin

Introduction

The one shared understanding within all approaches to psychotherapy is of the value of the therapeutic relationship as a way of understanding a person's inner world. It is within this confidential relationship that psychological and emotional wounds reveal themselves in relation to the therapist and have the opportunity to heal. The structure of CAT offers important contributions to this potential healing journey through the relationship: the shared description of learned patterns of relationship, known as reciprocal roles in CAT, and how these patterns of relationship will almost inevitably be experienced in the relationship between the client and the therapist. This is called 'enactment' in CAT and can be a powerful learning experience for the client and the therapist. The therapist recognises and names these difficult relationship patterns as they occur. This process is then shared and explained in a mutual and respectful way.

KEY CONCEPTS

- In CAT the process of change comes from naming, experiencing, sharing, recognising and understanding these patterns. In acknowledging these patterns and bringing awareness to them, a new healthier relationship pattern can develop.
- The relationship between the client and therapist itself models this more accepting and respectful way of relating.
- CAT tries to focus on what a person brings to the therapy, i.e. 'target problems', and the deeper patterns of relating that can underlie them. It is less concerned with traditional psychiatric symptoms, syndromes or labels.
- CAT recognises that people are so much more than their identified problems or diagnoses and helps each individual find their own language for what appears to go wrong in addition to setting manageable goals to bring about change.
- CAT therapists work with people with a variety of disorders, e.g. eating disorders, addiction problems, obsessional problems, anxiety, depression, phobias, psychosis and bipolar illness.
- CAT therapists can work across age groups and with people with learning difficulties and work in a variety of settings, e.g. CAMHS, forensic and addiction services.
- CAT is usually offered to individuals, but it can be used effectively with couples, in groups and to help teams understand the 'system' in which they work.

The Origins of CAT

Dr Antony Ryle, a GP and trained analytical psychotherapist, developed cognitive analytic therapy. In his research as an analytical psychotherapist, he noticed, when looking at transcribed sessions, that many of the difficulties were mentioned in the first sessions but took a long time to resolve in traditional approaches. CAT evolved as an integrative therapy based on ideas from cognitive and analytic therapies, but took less time as an intervention.

CAT was influenced in part by George Kelly's constructivism. Kelly developed personal construct theory and the repertory grid method. Kelly's approach to therapy 'offered a model of nonauthoritarian practice' that Anthony Ryle found appealing. Ryle proposed a shorter, more active form of therapy that integrated elements from cognitive therapy practice, e.g. goal-setting and Socratic questioning, into analytic practice, i.e. a very clear formulation of the problems experienced by the patient and then sharing this formulation with the patient to engage them in psychotherapy as a joint approach.

CAT in Practice with Adolescents

Before starting an individual CAT therapy with an adolescent, it is important to remember that a young person is always surrounded by some system of care, usually their family. Initial assessment should always include this system, as the young person may be showing difficulties because of their reaction to problems in this system. There may be marital relationship problems, parental illness or parental substance misuse. It might be better to target these problems rather than offer individual therapy to the young person. At the same time, a CAT therapy for the young person may help them to develop resilience to these problems, if they cannot be resolved.

It is important to offer both the young person, and their main carer, an explanation of the CAT model and information about how the therapy may progress. The therapist must think about how the carer can be included in reviews of progress and given information about anything they may be able to do to help. Confidentiality should be discussed, and the young person reassured that it will be their choice how much of the work they want to share.

One model of CAT therapy with an adolescent might be a joint initial assessment and explanation of the therapy with both the young person and their carer, followed by eight individual sessions and then a joint review, followed by a further eight individual sessions and then a follow-up joint review. In some circumstances, it may be appropriate to offer therapy using a CAT model to a young person and their carer together, where the relationship between the two seems to be the most pressing problem. Another model might be to offer family therapy and, at the same time, individual CAT therapy to the young person. Where the family is attending family therapy, it may be appropriate for the young person to share either their reformulation letter, or their diagram, within the family therapy at some stage.

Anyone offering CAT to adolescents should have experience of working with this age group or be supervised by someone with such experience.

Factors that would make one believe that an adolescent might make good use of CAT would be:

- Their ability to self-reflect and be aware that some their own behaviour may be unhelpful.
- An acknowledgement, by the young person, that early experiences and relationships have had an impact on them and the way they feel.
- A willingness to talk about early life experiences in therapy.
- The ability to form a good collaborative relationship.

We are beginning to see evidence that CAT therapy is acceptable and helpful for adolescents. An audit carried out in a UK CAMHS found that the tools of CAT, the reformulation letter and the diagram, were helpful to adolescents. The average rating out of ten for how helpful the therapy had been was eight (Jenaway and Mortlock, 2008). Young people often find it difficult to persevere with a course of therapy, and dropout rates for CAT are similar to those for other types of therapy, at around 40% (Jenaway and Mortlock, 2008; Wierzbicki and Pekarik, 1993).

Research groups in Australia have compared CAT with intensive outreach standard care for young people with early signs of personality disorder (Chanen et al., 2006). They found that CAT was as helpful as the standard care and seemed to work more quickly. Denis Ougrin in the UK has developed a form of therapeutic assessment for young people who self-harm. The assessment is based on a CAT model, the development of a diagram for the young person and thinking about alternatives to self-harm. They found that the young people who had the CAT-style assessment were significantly more likely to engage in the follow-up treatment that was offered than those who had a standard assessment (Ougrin et al., 2008).

Case Study: Edward and Charlie

Edward, known as Charlie, was referred to CAMHS following a self-harm assessment at the local General Hospital. Charlie had not been known to CAMHS prior to his admission. Family and friends reported no signs that he was suffering with his mental health. Charlie had been spotted in a tree with a ligature round his neck by a passer-by and had told them that he was planning to hang himself. Following an urgent CAMHS assessment, Charlie was allocated to a CAMHS clinician to manage the risk, whilst awaiting a course of cognitive analytic therapy.

Charlie's risk had reduced whilst he awaited CAT. This was attributed to the level of containment provided by the CAMHS team. Charlie and his family had been supported by the CAMHS duty service alongside regular face-to-face meetings with a CAMHS clinician.

Reformulation

At the start of therapy, Charlie was self-harming by cutting to his thighs and experiencing distressing internal voices, assessed as a representation of his internalised critical thinking and his extreme anxiety as a result of traumatic experiences. This left him feeling criticised, judged and frightened. The voices were abusive and threatening, instructing Charlie to harm himself.

Prior to CAMHS involvement, Charlie had been observed by others to be a quiet and charming young man, with an impeccable behaviour record at home and at college, a high achiever and popular with his peers. Charlie himself identified feelings of self-hate, worthlessness, with troublesome thoughts and a frightening repertoire of voices in his head. Charlie described two distinct aspects of self, 'Superman' aka Charlie and the 'Hulk' aka Edward; both positions left him fearing judgement, abandonment and exposure.

Sixteen sessions of cognitive analytic therapy were planned and during the goal- setting meeting Charlie identified the following goals for therapy: to rid himself of Edward 'the Hulk', to rid himself of the voices and to feel as though he had a life worth living. Charlie was not sure if he wanted to give up self-harming by cutting, as he could not identify a more effective way of managing his emotions.

Historical Information

Charlie's family background was reportedly very unsettled. He was adopted as a baby, but when he was three years old his adoptive parents had a biological child who tragically died within six months of his birth from a genetic disorder known as Edward's syndrome.

Reflection

Charlie said he had always known that he was adopted although he could not recall this ever being spoken about by his family. At age 16, Charlie came across documentation in his parents' study relating to his adoption. His biological parents were young Irish Catholics who conceived him out of wedlock. Charlie's maternal grandfather insisted on either adoption or expulsion from the family. His parents were 17 years of age at the time, and it is understood that they had brought great shame to the family and to their religious community.

The death of Charlie's younger brother was never discussed, although Charlie noted that home was always an unhappy place and he could smell the sadness in the air and sense it in the pit of his stomach. At some point, Edward became known as Charlie, his middle name. He often wondered if his parents could not tolerate his first name due to the link to his brother's death, and this left him feeling guilty and ashamed. During the initial sessions, Charlie completed a family genogram, glossing over the difficult parts, as if reading from a textbook or talking about someone else.

Recognition

Target problem (TP) and target problem procedures (TPPs) in the form of:

Traps, Dilemmas and Snags...

Charlie completed the CAT psychotherapy file that highlighted the following target problems and target problem procedures. Charlie described the **trap** of trying to be perfect and pleasing others and being anxious that he would be rejected or abandoned in relationships. As a result, Charlie felt taken advantage of in relationships; feeling unimportant and unworthy left him overwhelmed by angry feelings. This gave him the **dilemma** of either cutting off from unmanageable feelings and becoming 'Superman' or allowing his feelings and becoming the 'Hulk'. His main fear was that of risking loss and abandonment for the second time in his young life and, either way, these limited choices left Charlie's needs unmet and came at a cost.

Charlie had developed two distinct aspects of self that left him with polarised choices, the less objectionable of the two being 'Charlie', seeking acceptance, love and belonging by striving for approval from others, in contrast to 'Edward' cutting off from others and explosively expressing deeply hidden, hurt and angry feelings, leaving him fearful of abandonment and ravaged by terrifying voices.

Early reformulation by way of a map, i.e. a sequential diagrammatic reformulation (SDR), was introduced to Charlie, to help him recognise patterns in relationships and to trace links between past experiences and current thinking and behaviour. Unhelpful procedures, i.e. his coping strategies, were highlighted and linked back to patterns in relationships by way of the reciprocal roles.

Charlie's early life experiences could be summarised as a pattern of 'lonely coping' in relation to 'abandoning, hurting and ashamed'.

Charlie's own 'limited' options may have served him well as a young child, when trying to stay safe and make sense of his experiences. However, his core belief, **snag**, that he was not worthy of love and belonging, made him split off perceived 'good' and 'bad' aspects of the self into two halves. Charlie identified with either feeling intense extreme and uncontrollable emotions or a blanked-off state where he remained in control, but distant from others.

The voices seemed to articulate Charlie's deep emotional pain, feelings he had not developed a language for, processed or resolved.

Charlie received his map well. It was followed by a reformulation letter. When I finished reading his letter, he simply asked how I knew so much about him. We reflected that I was merely providing the emotional scaffolding, guidance and support for Charlie to work things out for himself and that I only knew what he had told me. The reformulation letter sets out reasons for coming to therapy, exploration of family history and the 'roots' of the problems by way of traps, dilemmas, snags and unstable states that had been the means to cope with chronically endured pain, but that actually reinforce the false beliefs and the pain itself.

Possible transference invitations were included through reference to the reciprocal roles. Predictions were made for what may be possible in therapy and potential therapy-interfering behaviours, e.g. placating the therapist to avoid possible rejection or abandonment. The collaborative nature of therapy was explored and Charlie's metaphors used throughout, i.e. the 'Hulk' and 'Superman'. Charlie declined an invitation to make any amendments to his letter or to write a reply that was discussed using the map, to explore possible enactments of TPPs in the therapy room.

The Work of Therapy

The map was placed on the table between us week by week. Charlie and I were able to give new meaning to his experiences, make links between past loss and trauma and his core pain and to recognise and revise ways of coping that were unhelpful.

Work involved reintegrating the split-off aspects of self by showing compassion for 'little Edward' and for his family in the context of grief and loss, by acknowledging and accepting his emotional pain and anger in the context of his life experiences. By seeking a middle ground where Charlie could learn to tolerate all aspects of the self, 'good' and 'bad', finding more balance in relationships, including the relationship with his voices.

An important part of therapy was to explore Charlie's core belief that he was not worthy of being kept by his biological parents. We did this by considering their actions in the context of the culture and the time and acknowledged their limited choices. It was important to provide a containing relationship where Charlie could speak of the 'unspoken' and in doing so, challenge some deeply ingrained beliefs. Charlie worked hard in therapy to explore patterns in relationships. He acknowledged that he always felt as though love and care were conditional and that he must only let others see the 'good' in him. He recognised that his mask 'Superman' had been useful to a point, although he understood that it had become his own, self-built prison where even he could not recognise his own needs or wants or name his emotions. This all left him feeling unreal, exhausted and fearing exposure.

As therapy progressed, Charlie worked hard to make sense of the voices, and with help, he was able to acknowledge them as a meaningful response to traumatic life events. The voices provided insight into emotional distress, and Charlie was encouraged to make sense of the messages being carried by the voices, rather than believing them to be a literal truth. The turning point for Charlie was in recognising that the most menacing of the voices represented the most deeply hurt part of him and carried overwhelming messages in relation to unprocessed, deeply buried unresolved emotions and thus needed the most kindness and care.

Revision

As we progressed to the final part of therapy, Charlie began to revise unhelpful coping strategies and to add them to his map as exits from traps, dilemmas and snags. Charlie's main exits involved asserting himself in relationships, including with himself, challenging his thoughts, taking control by choosing to accept or reject them and to actively put the 'positives' in by using affirmations, making the unfamiliar familiar and by collaborating, communicating and setting boundaries for the voices and learning to tolerate his distress until it passed, rather than acting on urges to harm himself.

The map (SDR) provided a visual formulation of his difficulties and helped Charlie to recognise early on in the cycle when he was becoming caught up in unhelpful patterns of thinking and behaving, thus giving him time to take exits.

Ending

The goodbye letter gave a brief summary of the reasons for coming to therapy and agreed goals, using Charlie's words and metaphors. Reference was made to the therapeutic relationship/alliance and how this developed, including threats and ruptures to the relationship. The letter included an acknowledgement that Charlie had experienced some forced and difficult endings in his young life and how ending therapy in a planned way could provide an opportunity to experience a more controlled, contained and predictable ending.

Reference was made to the analogy used during therapy, where we likened Charlie's deeply painful feelings and memories to a wardrobe, full of clothes, all crumpled up and shoved in with the door shut tight, i.e. unprocessed emotions. Through therapy, we sought to empty out the wardrobe and take a look at each and every garment, make sense of it together and hang it up and put it away again, in the hope that small triggers would not lead to the entire contents of the wardrobe falling out, i.e. huge reactions.

Charlie chose not to write a goodbye letter, but he did draw a single picture of one boy named Charles Edward, in order, he said, that I could hold him in mind until the follow-up session.

Follow-up at Three Months

Charlie and his parents attended the follow-up appointment prior to him leaving for university. As a family, they reported progress in 'having difficult conversations', something they acknowledged they had all tried to keep at bay for fear of the consequences. Charlie reported that he had sometimes had a return of negative thoughts that life was just too hard, and on one occasion, shortly after ending therapy, his mother found him curled in the foetal position softly crying.

His mother held him until he settled and, together, they were able to ride the waves rather than drown in them. Charlie reflected that he could not make sense of his feelings at the time, but what he did know was that they would not last and that he was safe.

Throughout the course of therapy and follow-up period, Charlie had not acted on any urges to harm himself or end his life through suicide.

Multiple-Choice Questions

See answers on page 672.

1. Who was the founder of CAT?
   a. Anthony Ryle
   b. George Kelly
   c. Denis Ougrin
2. CAT can be used with
   a. Individuals
   b. Groups
   c. Couples
   d. All three

3. TPP in CAT stands for
   a. Talking personal problems
   b. Tackling policies and procedures
   c. Target problem procedures
   d. Top problem people

Key References

Chanen, A., et al., (2006). A randomised controlled trial of psychotherapy for early intervention for borderline personality disorder. *Acta Neuropsychiatrica*, 18(6): 319.

Jenaway, A., Mortlock, M., (2008). Service innovation, offering CAT in a child and adolescent mental health service. *Reformulation*, 30: 31–32.

Ougrin, D., Ng, A.V., Low, J., (2008). Therapeutic assessment based on cognitive analytic therapy for young people presenting with self-harm. *Psychiatric Bulletin*, 32: 423–426.

Ryle, A., Kerr, I., (2002). *Introducing Cognitive Analytic Therapy.*

Wierzbicki, M., Pekarik, G., (1993). A meta-analysis of psychotherapy dropout. *Professional Psychology: Research and Practice*, 24: 190–195.

61 Dialectical Behavioural Therapy

Laura Nisbet

KEY CONCEPTS

- Dialectical behavioural therapy was developed to help individuals manage overwhelming distress and dysfunctional behaviours.
- It uses the biosocial model to understand emotional dysregulation.
- It helps individuals to cope with their emotions without losing control and acting destructively or making their situation any worse and helps them to create a life worth living.
- It combines an acceptance approach with behaviour change.
- It places importance on the relationship between the therapist and individual to actively motivate change.
- It teaches emotional regulation, distress tolerance, interpersonal and pro-social skills that the individual has not so far been able to develop.

Introduction

Dialectical behavioural therapy was developed by Marsha Linehan in the 1970s. It is an intervention for individuals with borderline personality disorder (BPD) where treatment has been ineffectual to treat severe and chronic symptoms including suicidality, non-suicidal self-injurious behaviours (NSSI), e.g. cutting or burning, and emotional dysregulation. NSSI behaviours are dysfunctional coping strategies for extreme emotional distress. These impulsive behaviours risk rapid escalation to an unintentional suicidal act. Linehan found that individuals with chronic emotional distress and hopelessness, and who wished to be dead, did not possess the skills to develop a 'life worth living', a key concept in DBT (Miller et al., 2007).

Previous approaches to treatment would focus on change that would invalidate the experience of the individual, leading to over-arousal or emotional shutdown. Other attempted approaches validated experiences but were insufficient to direct the individual towards change. Individuals would feel that his/her needs were not met, which would increase the potential for further distress and result in dropping out of therapy (Ritschel et al., 2018).

Based on cognitive behavioural therapy principles, DBT developed a new approach that created behavioural change and encouraged the therapist to integrate acceptance and problem-solving-based strategies. The aim is to validate the individual's emotions and experiences whilst gently moving them towards change.

Since its development, DBT has been empirically accepted as reducing the distress and dysfunctional coping strategies in these individuals. It has been recognised as being applicable across a broad number of conditions where emotional dysregulation is evident (Ritschel et al., 2018). There is now evidence to support the use of DBT with eating disorders, substance misuse, post-traumatic stress disorder, aggression and impulsive behaviours and adolescents (Groves et al., 2011).

Biosocial Model in DBT

The biosocial model is the theory of how symptoms arise and are maintained. In DBT, it is the underpinning of understanding emotional dysregulation (the core symptom). **Emotional sensitivity + invalidating environment = pervasive emotional dysregulation.** This model believes that emotional sensitivities are inborn. These individuals are naturally highly sensitive and reactive to intense emotional responses and take a long time to return to their regular emotional baseline. This can be across both negative and positives, and they will have impulsive emotional reactions/behaviours in response to their feelings (Rathus and Miller, 2015), but this alone is not enough to cause difficulties. An invalidating environment is any environment where the individual does not fit. This does not necessarily have to be an abusive environment. An invalidating environment is when an individual's private and emotional experiences are not recognised as valid responses to events.

In turn, the individual may feel ignored, punished, trivialised and that they are accused of overreacting in certain circumstances. An invalidating environment reinforces the person's emotional sensitivity, creating an individual who is unable to label or regulate their emotions, cope with distress or believe in their own emotional responses. Instead they turn to their environment and others for cues as to how to act and feel.

Over time the combination of the two results in situations where the individual responds to heightened arousal by either ignoring their emotions or by reacting with extreme behaviour displays, potentially causing harm not only to themselves but to their relationships (Rathus and Miller, 2015).

Dialectics

Dialectic is when two opposite beliefs are known to be true at the same time. It is not a search for right or wrong but an endeavour to develop understanding. Dialectics in DBT are not only about recognising others' perspectives in order to find common ground but about finding a balance between the individual accepting themselves, their emotions and behaviours as valid and recognising that they may be unhelpful and in need of change (Miller et al., 2007). By doing so they can begin to learn to cope with their emotions in a different way.

Criteria for Treatment

Individuals meeting the criteria for DBT will display high levels of pervasive dysfunction in daily activities and frequent threats to their lives, for instance, repeated accident and emergency admissions through suicide attempts or NSSI, non-attendance at school or work, breakdown in family or friendship relationships and risky and out-of-control behaviour (Rathus and Miller, 2015; Linehan, 1993). They have heightened emotional responses and express feelings of worthlessness and hopelessness and are unable to imagine any future.

Stages Of DBT

- **Pre-treatment stage**
- **Orientation, commitment to treatment and goal-setting**

The first few sessions are important in developing the therapeutic relationship between the individual and therapist and in cementing their decision to work reciprocally together. In these sessions the therapist will carry out a full assessment of needs, take a detailed history and undertake a behavioural analysis of the targeted behaviours, in addition to setting goals. The individual and therapist would discuss and agree their expectations from one another and understanding of the therapy, its duration and reasonable outcomes. The therapist would introduce the concept of team-working to the individual and place an emphasis on skills training and practice in order to decrease harming behaviours and develop a life worth living (Rathus and Miller, 2015; Miller et al., 2007).

Stage 1

The primary target of DBT is to bring behaviour under control. It is assumed that an out-of-control life is unbearable. An individual is unable to work on any emotional issues until they are skilled enough to manage their emotions without harmful coping strategies and are committed to therapy (Linehan, 1993; Rathus and Miller, 2015).

Stage 1 addresses life-threatening behaviours first, i.e. suicide attempts, suicidal ideation or communication and NSSI, before moving on to quality-of-life interfering behaviours, e.g. high-risk behaviours, alcohol and drug misuse, low self-esteem, co-current mental health disorders, sleep and appetite issues, to name a few.

In this stage, the therapist will work with the individual in targeting therapy-interfering behaviours, i.e. not attending sessions or attending but not engaging, walking out of sessions and dropping out. The therapist themselves might bring therapy-interfering behaviours, e.g. not being dialectical, focussing too much on either change or validation, becoming too rigid or too flexible with the individual or by being disrespectful and patronising towards the individual (Linehan, 1993). In DBT, individuals are encouraged to challenge their therapists on any behaviours that they find therapy-interfering. This opportunity empowers, shows respect and validates their experiences and feelings in a way that they may not experience in other situations (Rathus and Miller, 2015). The individual will begin group-based skills work at this time to learn positive coping strategies to replace current dysfunctional behaviours.

Stage 2

Stage 2 targets emotional experiences, previous traumas, faulty belief systems and maladaptive thought patterns. This may illicit strong emotional responses in the individual and can only be targeted once their behaviour responses are under control. The length of time in Stage 2 can depend on the severity of the trauma and the individual's resilience, behavioural and social coping skills to manage this part of the therapy process (Linehan, 1993).

Stage 3

Stage 3 overlaps the first two stages. Up until now the individual will have developed some dependence on the therapist, having moved from mistrust in the first stage through to relying on the therapist to help solve problems. Stage 3 develops the individual's ability to trust their own emotions and experiences, develops problem-solving skills, taking them out of the therapy room and into everyday life situations, increasing happiness, positive experiences and building trust, values, self-respect and achieving their set goals (Rathus and Miller, 2015).

The DBT Approach

DBT has four components:

Individual Therapy

In individual therapy, the sessions are usually weekly but can be increased to twice weekly at the beginning of therapy and in crisis. This is usually time limited. During these sessions, the therapist creates an environment that validates rather than blames and encourages positive behaviours from the individual, rather than harmful. The therapist's role is to reinforce skill-based training and positive behaviours so much for the individual that they continue with the positive behaviour and stop the harmful ones (Linehan, 1993). The therapist needs to possess warmth, compassion, sincerity, commitment, patience and persistence and a belief in the therapy that will withstand the individual's mistrust, questioning and disbelief.

The therapist validates the individual's emotions and experiences, eliciting their strengths and playing to these. Linehan (1993) states 'the therapist both believes and believes in the patient'. In addition to validation and problem-solving, the therapist uses metaphor to aid understanding of situations, suggest solutions to problems and reframe situations, 'devil's advocate' by using a more extreme example of an individual's dysfunctional belief and in turn, moving the individual to the opposite approach from their original belief, a more therapeutic approach (Miller et al., 2007) and 'extending', i.e. taking an individual's belief to the extreme in order to challenge and move them to a more therapeutic stance.

Telephone Consultation

The telephone consultation is an important coping mechanism in DBT. It provides the opportunity for individuals to ask for help outside regular therapy sessions, provides support to generalise the skills learned in the group into their everyday lives and offers coaching and additional support in times of crisis. The telephone consult gives an opportunity to repair client/therapist relationships if there has been a conflict in session, rather than waiting until the next session (Linehan, 1993)

Skills-Based Group

Skills groups provide cognitive, emotional and behavioural skills that the individual does not possess or is unable to use effectively (Rathus and Miller, 2015). There are three functions of the group skill attainment: (a) instructing, modelling and advising, (b) skill strengthening, i.e. practicing, role-play and feedback and (c) skill generalisation, applying skills outside the therapy session, phone call coaching and homework practice. Skills groups can run for a duration of up to one year. The skills groups are usually run by clinicians who are not the young person's individual therapist, to prevent any interference in therapy.

There are five skills taught within the group:

Mindfulness

Mindfulness is based on the Zen practice of Buddhism. Often when individuals are dysregulated, they focus on past events and/or worries about the future. Mindfulness practice helps to centre a person in the here and now, focussing on what is happening in the present. This introduces the concept of three states of mind, emotional mind, rational mind and wise mind (Figure 61.1).

When experiencing dysregulated emotions, the individual oscillates between extremes of emotion, moving between opposites rapidly. Others may switch all feelings off completely because they are too painful to bear. When we are in 'emotional mind' we believe our feelings to be fact and act in response. When we are in 'reasonable mind' we act based on fact, logical reasoning and ignore our emotions. 'Wise mind', the third state, balances the two and helps us to recognise the emotions we are experiencing but to think about the situation in a logical manner, e.g. what would be the most effective way for me to act right now (Miller et al., 2007)?

To be in 'wise mind' takes a great deal of practice. Linehan describes the brain as 'like a naughty puppy that needs to be trained to act and think the way that we want it to' (Rathus and Miller, 2015). Individuals practice mindfulness in the skills group by learning two skills: the 'what' skills (observe, describe and participate) and 'how' skills (non-judgmentally, one-mindfully and effectively). Mindfulness and recognising states of mind are important underpinnings in DBT and in targeting emotional dysregulation. It is practiced within its own module and at the start of every group session.

Emotional Regulation

Emotional regulation explains the function of emotions, to identify and label them correctly, understand the physiology within the body with each emotion and begin to link how our thoughts and feelings, physiological sensations and behaviours influence each other. It teaches basic self-care, looking after our physical health and the effect this has on mood and self-esteem.

Using the PLEASE skill, it encourages group members to make sure they have enough sleep, are eating and drinking properly and taking physical exercise. It teaches building mastery, doing one thing every day that you are truly good at and setting value-based goals (Linehan, 1993; Miller et al., 2007).

This links to the idea of wise mind, recognising our emotions, looking after ourselves and building more positive experiences in our lives. This module introduces the idea of seeking

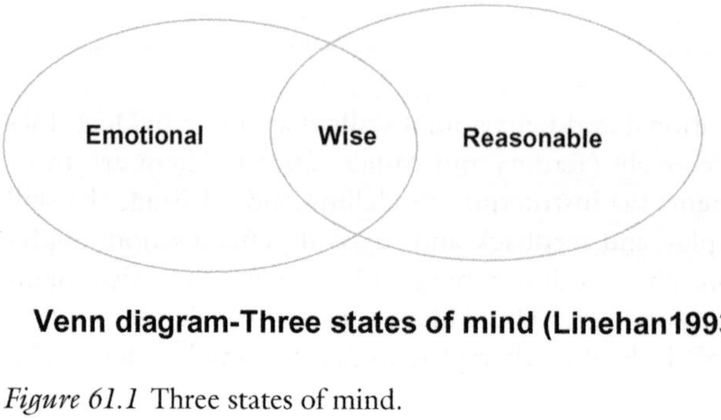

Figure 61.1 Three states of mind.

out pleasant events and asks that group members plan enjoyable activities into their day, increasing positive experiences, positive emotions and moving the individual closer to their life worth living.

Distress Tolerance

Distress tolerance practices techniques for coping in an emotional crisis. Some individuals experience extreme physical and emotional distress more frequently and forcefully than others. When experiencing these intense emotions, they believe that they will never go away, and these individuals are unable to cope with the high level of distress they are experiencing (Mckay et al., 2007; Miller et al., 2007). In such situations impulsive behavioural urges come into play, often their emotional mind sets in and harmful unhelpful behaviours are carried out to rid the person of their distress as quickly as possible. Often these impulsive behaviours are followed by further emotional and physical pain and lead to prolonged suffering (McKay, 2007).

This module provides skills to endure emotional pain and suffering, to temporarily distract the individual from their feelings and create time to think about the best way to cope in the situation, using 'wise mind'. Distress tolerance skills include temperature, intense exercise, paced breathing and progressive muscle relaxation (TIPP), quick ways to change our body chemistry to calm body and mind when we are unable to think clearly about what skill to use. Distraction with ACCEPTS, various distraction suggestions using cognitive and physical activities, shows that distraction can be effective in the short term. Self-soothing with six senses is an essential skill in surviving a crisis since emotionally dysregulated individuals find it difficult to self-sooth when highly aroused.

The idea is to consider previous impulsive actions and the effect of these both positive and negative alongside the skills they have learnt in the group in order to IMPROVE the moment, changing the way you think about a situation or yourself or by focussing your mind in a helpful way, e.g. with imagery (Rathus and Miller, 2015).

Walking the Middle Path

This module was developed especially for the DBT adolescent approach and is designed to develop an understanding of balancing validation and problem-solving skills in addition to addressing unhelpful behavioural patterns (Miller et al., 2007). It targets changing distressing emotions and unhelpful coping strategies and balancing these with acceptance of themselves and their feelings and behaviours.

This module introduces the idea of dialectics to the group. Often adolescents and their caregivers can end up at polar opposites in their viewpoints. 'Walking the middle path' can help to understand others' perspectives and inform decision-making on how to behave whilst acknowledging the validity of both sides (Rathus and Miller, 2015). Beginning to have a more systemic understanding of situations and behaviours can have a positive impact on interpersonal relationships. By learning about behaviour modification (e.g. positive and negative reinforcement), the individual can begin to self-modify their behaviour and that of those around them.

Interpersonal Effectiveness

Interpersonal effectiveness is a people-skills module. It develops strategies for keeping healthy relationships, reducing conflict, asking for what we need and saying 'No' in a way that keeps our self-respect and values in the relationship. Emotionally dysregulated individuals often fluctuate between avoiding conflict and extreme confrontation and often end relationships quickly from fear of rejection, anxiety, distress or inability to improve the situation. The skills taught in this module are to maximise the chances of the individual's needs being met without damaging their relationships. Using **D**escribe, **E**xpress, **A**ssert, **R**einforce, **M**indful, **A**ppear Confident, **N**egotiate (DEAR MAN), as well as **(be) G**entle, **(act) I**nterested, **V**alidate, **(use) E**asy Manner (GIVE) and **(be) F**air **(no)A**pologies, **S**tick to values, **(be)T**ruthful (FAST) skills, the group learns and through role-play practices how to balance assertiveness, stating their needs with being gentle and validating others' feelings and desires, how to negotiate and learning to 'agree to disagree' (Linehan, 1993).

Case Consultation Meeting

Case consultation meetings are obligatory for all clinicians who are taking part in DBT therapy. Working with dysregulated individuals can be stressful and demanding, and if they are not careful, clinicians can experience burnout. In addition to the individual's progress in therapy, risks or therapy-interfering behaviour, the consult provides space to examine the client/therapist relationship and any current challenges, and indeed the clinician's own behaviour (Linehan, 1993).

Consideration for Adaptations for Adolescents

In 1995 Miller and Rathus developed dialectical behavioural therapy for adolescents (DBT-A). This was in response to an increasing rate of adolescent suicidality and a growing evidence of NSSI. The factors that put adolescents at risk of suicidal behaviours overlap those of BPD and are predominantly previous suicide attempts, mental health disorders such as, but not exclusive to, depression and anxiety, substance misuse, coexisting disorders, gender issues, wider systemic family issues and parental suicidal behaviour, ethnicity and socio-economic status. Evidence has shown that through DBT intervention dysfunctional coping strategies in adolescents were reduced and they were hospitalised less frequently (Groves et al., 2011).

Considerations for adaptation for adolescents should include shortening the duration of therapy, in particular skills-based group, from one year to a more condensed 16-week programme to facilitate commitment and attendance (Miller et al., 2007). Adapting the paperwork to be more adolescent-friendly and the inclusion of family members should be considered so that they can provide coaching for the adolescent, to identify and work on any family therapy-interfering behaviours and because they, parents or caregivers, often have deficits themselves (Rathus and Miller, 2015).

Case Study: Emma

Emma (16) was referred to CAMHS with symptoms of depression, anxiety and hearing voices. She was self-harming by cutting her arms on a regular basis and experiencing a strong desire to end her life. She had been admitted to A&E on two occasions because of taking an overdose of over-the-counter medication, and she often did not take her prescribed medication. At the time Emma was referred for DBT she had not been in school for over six months because of her high levels of anxiety. She was barely leaving the house.

Emma found attending the orientation and commitment session difficult. She was reluctant to engage and became distressed when the topic of goal setting was introduced. She stormed out of the session abruptly and the therapist followed her, encouraging her to return. A tearful Emma explained that she saw no point in setting goals as she 'had no future, couldn't change and nothing could help'. Her therapist validated her distress and how her experiences so far had brought her to this belief and then, using 'devil's advocate', pointed out to Emma that she had attended the session that day and so maybe a small part of her did want things to be different and how, with the support of the therapist and the skills learnt in group, they could work together to create that change for Emma.

Emma identified the following aims:

- To stop life-threatening behaviours, i.e. not to take any overdoses or to self-harm during therapy.
- To decrease therapy-interfering behaviours, i.e. to attend sessions, not to walk out and to engage.
- Decrease quality of life-threatening behaviours, i.e. to reduce not taking prescribed medication, letting the voices take control, lack of motivation, self-harm, self-loathing and impulsive behaviour.
- Increase behavioural skills – aim to attend group and learn positive coping strategies.

Emma initially found attending the group difficult. She was acutely anxious, hyper-vigilant and seen to be watching the exits in the first few sessions. As she became more familiar with the other young people she began to relax and became more involved. She was able to identify that she was always in 'emotional mind' and reacted impulsively to most events. By practicing mindfulness and awareness of the wave of emotion, she was able to sit with her anxiety of being in busy environments and attend a concert that she had previously missed because of her mental health a few years before.

She began to take her medication regularly and change her sleep patterns. Emma learned from having more awareness of her emotions and the physical sensations that accompany them. She was more able to identify when she was becoming anxious. She was able to use distraction and self-soothing techniques to cope, so that the voices were less distressing, and she no longer acted on her urges to self-harm. She began to spend more time painting and playing guitar, hobbies that she had enjoyed previous to becoming unwell and which had a positive impact on her self-esteem and quality of life.

Multiple-Choice Questions

See answers on page 672.

1. Which symptom is the main underpinning for DBT therapy?
   a. Self-harm
   b. Emotional dysregulation
   c. Worthlessness
2. Name three of the five modules in the skills group.
   a. Mindfulness, behaviour modification and self-soothing
   b. Emotional regulation, walking the middle path and distress tolerance
   c. Interpersonal skills, telephone consultation and devil's advocate
3. What would be classed as therapy-interfering behaviours?
   a. Walking out of sessions, turning up late and not engaging
   b. Self-harming, low self-esteem and not attending sessions
   c. Therapist being patronising, calling therapist outside sessions and not engaging
4. What adaptions could be made for DBT-A?
   a. Longer session times, parents attending group and no individual sessions
   b. Shorter group duration, family members attending group and adapted paperwork
   c. Adapted paperwork, telephone consultation and shorter session times

Key References

Linehan, M.M., (1993). *Cognitive Behavioral Treatment of Borderline Personality Disorder.* New York: Guildford Press.

Miller, A.L., Rathus, J.H., Linehan, M.M., (2007). *Dialectical Behavior Therapy with Suicidal Adolescents.* New York: Guildford Press.

Rathus, J.H., Miller, A.L., (2015). *DBT Skill Manual for Adolescents.* New York: Guildford Press.

62 Theory and Practice of Behaviour Modification

Hannah Kovshoff and Jayne Muldowney

KEY CONCEPTS

- Understand what is causing and maintaining the child's behaviour.
- Give short and clear messages when something has to happen.
- Anticipate difficult situations and give warnings.
- Work hard to use positive ways of helping him/her to increase self-esteem.
- Positive praise for good things that have been achieved will encourage good behaviour.
- Stay calm, mirror image, model appropriate behaviour.
- Avoid confrontation.
- Use distraction and try to diffuse situations early.
- 'Time-out' procedure.
- Remove the child from the situation in which he/she is creating a problem, then return him/her without comment.
- Children are less difficult to manage if the regime offers them consistency, predictable routines and clear boundaries.

The Behavioural Model

Every behaviour has a function. The consequence of a behaviour can increase, decease or leave unchanged the likelihood of the behaviour occurring. By changing the environment, you can alter the **antecedent** (the event, situation or trigger) that leads to the occurrence of the **behaviour** and **consequence** (the response to the behaviour and changing the behaviour itself).

A	B	C
(Antecedent)	**(Behaviour)**	**(Consequence)**

Functional analysis provides valuable information about possible antecedents, consequences and sources of reinforcement for behaviours.

Functional Analysis

A functional analysis aims to identify what purpose a behaviour serves and identify the context and behaviours that are maintaining that behaviour. When initiating a functional analysis, it is important to identify the predominant inappropriate behaviour. Behaviour modification is most effective when a limited number of behaviours are targeted at any one time. A functional analysis can be most informative when the targeted behaviour is complex and the function is not easily identifiable.

Typical functions of maladaptive behaviours include:

- Escape/task avoidance
- Initiation of social interaction
- Gaining attention, desired activities or sensory stimulation

The target behaviour might serve multiple functions. Whilst one function might be dominant, it is important to acknowledge any other lesser functions served by the behaviour to maximise the benefit of intervention.

Identify Behaviour

The identification of those behaviours most in need of change can be done through formal assessment or discussion with parents, teachers and significant others. Assessment should always include direct observation of the individual displaying the behaviour. The maladaptive behaviour must be identified clearly and a desirable outcome agreed upon. Outcomes must be realistic and achievable. By producing an accurate definition or description of the behaviour, the effectiveness of the intervention is maximised and the propensity of accurate and consistent measurement of the behaviour is increased.

Recording

It is important to identify any potential internal cause(s) of the behaviour to ensure that it is not a direct result of, e.g. medical conditions and/or medication effects, disrupted sleep patterns, emotional responses to traumatic events, etc. Behaviours that are attributable to internal causes are not appropriate for behaviour modification (e.g. when a child is experiencing symptoms of depression following a bereavement or following early childhood traumatic experiences). It is helpful to identify whether the behaviour is pervasive, i.e. that it manifests itself in all aspects of the individual's life, or whether there are situations in which it is more *likely* to occur.

To establish an accurate function of the behaviour, observe and record the frequency, intensity and duration of each episode and the antecedents and consequences of each episode. When recording behaviours, be as creative as is necessary to gain the relevant information, e.g. discuss the behaviours informally with teachers, parents or caregivers and significant others. ABCC charts can be completed either by the practitioner, caregiver or by a significant other. It is important to record the time and date, the location of each incident, who was present when the behaviour occurred and the antecedent, behaviour and consequence, to identify any significant patterns or trends.

Ideally, the behaviours targeted for behaviour modification/intervention should be observed on a number of separate occasions and in as many situations and contexts as possible. There is no specific length of time recommended over which to conduct these observations. Recording should continue until a clearer understanding of the behaviour has been obtained. Behavioural assessment must include ascertaining the views of the child, plus an assessment of the child's skills, particularly those adaptive skills which do, or might with encouragement, serve the same function for the child as the problem behaviour, by achieving similar results.

Establishing Function

Once a satisfactory amount of observation data has been recorded and the child has had an opportunity to reflect on and share their own views regarding their behaviour, look for trends in the frequency, intensity and duration of the target behaviour. Explore whether there are any consistent antecedents and/or consequences – do temper tantrums regularly follow a demand made by the parent to the child? Are the child's 'temper tantrums' controlled by the removal of any demands? Once a hypothesis has been developed, informal discussion with the child, if appropriate, and the child's significant others can be helpful in reaching a consensus. Meetings attended by professionals involved in the case can provide an opportunity to discuss the formulation with those who know the child well.

Avenues for Intervention

Methods for Increasing Appropriate Behaviour

One of the most frequently observed methods of modifying behaviour involves the use of reinforcement. By definition, reinforcement is any consequence which, when it follows a behaviour, strengthens the probability of that behaviour re-occurring. Reinforcers can be primary, secondary or social. A primary reinforcer is an immediate, tangible reward (e.g. food, drink, toys and so on). A secondary reinforcer is a 'means to an end' form of reinforcement whereby the individual 'earns' tokens or money that can be exchanged for primary reinforcers. Social reinforcement includes smiling, praise and positive attention.

When selecting a reinforcer for use in an intervention programme, it is critical that it is done in collaboration with the individual to design a realistic and meaningful reward system. The reward used in the intervention programme must be meaningful to the individual to maximise its reinforcing potential. A reward that has little significance or value to the child will be ineffective in producing the desired change in behaviour and results will be negligible. The reinforcing value of a particular reward may vary over time. Reinforcers will need to be modified and updated frequently.

Positive Reinforcement

When a positive consequence (e.g. praise, toy) is provided, the behaviour is strengthened. Examples of practical applications of positive reinforcement in the modification of maladaptive behaviours include differential reinforcement of other behaviour programmes (DRO, see below), praising in front of others and token economies.

DRO Programmes

These intervention programmes involve the positive reinforcement of a more appropriate response to antecedents or consequences, that would ordinarily have pre-empted the undesirable behaviour. For example, if a child has previously learned that a 'temper tantrum is effective in gaining attention from a teacher', the implementation of a DRO programme would often involve the 'planned ignoring' of temper tantrum behaviour and the positive reinforcement of a more appropriate method of gaining attention (e.g. raising a hand).

Token Economies

These programmes involve rewarding the child for appropriate behaviour during pre-arranged time-periods. Using the information gathered in the functional analysis regarding the frequency of the behaviour, an action plan can be developed to divide a task into manageable segments appropriate to that child, e.g. if a child displays a challenging behaviour on an hourly basis, it would be appropriate to provide a small reward for the child for each hour in which the behaviour was not displayed. These small rewards are effective in maintaining the child's attention and focus on withholding the inappropriate behaviour. To maximise the effect of intervention it is useful to provide a larger reward, achievable following the successful completion of the token economy schedule. The number of tokens the child must earn before a larger reward should start small and work up to larger numbers. Common practical resources involved in intervention programmes using the positive reinforcement principle include pasta jars, marble jars and star-charts that serve as secondary reinforcers, recording progression towards achieving a pre-defined goal.

Methods for Decreasing Inappropriate Behaviour

'Talk-down Time'

Talk-down time, similar to time-out, can be used in two situations as a method of reducing inappropriate behaviour. It can be used specifically to target one behaviour or when a child's behaviour becomes overly counter-productive, aggressive or difficult to manage. Then, it is often appropriate to select a safe and comfortable area of the room, free of any distractions, where the adult can help the child reduce the problematic behaviour to an acceptable level. This can be achieved through the use of distraction techniques or other calming strategies.

Talk-down time must not be used when the child is attempting to escape demands or in an unwanted situation, because avoidance is often the function of maladaptive behaviours. An effective functional analysis of the behaviour would hopefully have identified this. In these situations, the time spent calming down should be used proactively to identify alternative ways for the child to deal with the situation.

Extinction

This strategy is similar in principle to DRO techniques, but whereas DRO aims to reduce a target behaviour by replacing it with another, extinction is based on the theory that the target behaviour will automatically decrease, following the removal of the consequences that maintain it. The essential difference here is that extinction does not support the development of alternative behaviours, e.g. in the classroom example given earlier, an extinction strategy would aim to reduce temper tantrums by simply taking no notice of such behaviour.

Extinction strategies often result in an 'extinction burst' whereby the strength and frequency of the behaviour temporarily increases whilst the child becomes frustrated that a previously reinforced consequence no longer produces the desired outcome.

Developing Interventions

Preparation

All professionals involved with the child should be made aware of the behaviour modification programme. Professionals should decide upon the length of the programme based on the frequency and intensity of the behaviour. Programmes are generally implemented for a minimum of two weeks. Ensure that all members of the team involved in implementing the programme are fully briefed in its employment. This will ensure the programme's consistency and maximise its efficacy.

Execution

The recording process initiated in the functional analysis should continue throughout the programme to record progress and identify any areas requiring revision, e.g. rewards initially identified as desirable by the child may gradually lose their potency. If this happens, discuss with the child and agree upon a more meaningful reward.

Review

At the end of the allocated period of time, the team should gather to review the effectiveness of the programme. If the desired changes have not been achieved at this point, the programme may be refined and reactivated.

Case Study: Kate

Kate (eight) has a history of emotional and behavioural difficulties, including temper tantrums, inappropriate use of language, disturbed sleep patterns and poor eating habits. Kate's father, Paul, does not live in the family home and has irregular contact with Kate and her younger brother, Joseph. This is the first time that Kate's mother, Janet, has sought help for her daughter's behaviour, following a referral from her GP.

Whilst problematic at home, Kate's school does not report similar behaviours. However, Jane remains concerned that Kate's behaviour will lead her into difficulties at her new school when she begins there in September.

Through discussion, the most problematic of Kate's behaviours would be identified and, in this case, her temper tantrums were targeted for intervention. Recordings of her behaviours revealed that 90% of her tantrums occurred when Joseph was occupying Janet's full attention. The functional analysis revealed that Kate's temper tantrums occurred regularly throughout each day, at least one every two hours. When Janet was not present, incidences of Kate's inappropriate behaviour were significantly fewer. It was hypothesised that Kate's temper tantrums were a means by which she could gain attention from her mother, whenever her brother was around. The functional analysis revealed that Janet would intervene, thereby providing Kate with the attention she wanted. Giving attention was observed to reinforce the tantrums.

The intervention was designed to reduce Kate's temper tantrums by removing Janet's positive reinforcement of the inappropriate behaviour. Janet and Kate discussed the programme and agreed a reward that Kate could earn for improving her behaviour, a trip to a swimming pool where Janet and Kate could spend some quality time together without the distraction of Kate's younger brother.

A DRO programme was subsequently developed. In practice, this meant that Janet was asked to ignore Kate's temper tantrums and move to safe space or another room with Joseph. When a more appropriate method of initiating contact with her mother was displayed, Kate would be rewarded with praise. A star-chart was used to record Kate's improved behaviour and maintain her motivation and interest. For every two-hour interval, where no tantrum-like behaviour was displayed, Kate would receive a sticker on her star-chart. Kate and Janet agreed that when she had earned 25 stickers, they would go on their special trip together.

The behaviour modification programme was successful for several weeks, during which Kate and Janet went on four trips to the swimming pool. But then, Janet reported she had recently noticed a gradual increase in the tantrums. Talking this through with Kate, Janet learned that Kate no longer wanted to go to the swimming pool as much as she did when the programme started. Kate now would prefer the quality time she spent with her mother at the pool to a trip to the café for a hot chocolate. With a renewed interest in the programme and regular changes to the reward, Kate's inappropriate temper tantrums reduced at a consistent rate, until the behaviour became infrequent.

Multiple-Choice Questions

See answers on page 673.

1. Behaviour is shaped and maintained by:
    a. Antecedent stimuli
    b. Parents and caregivers
    c. Its consequences
    d. Establishing operations
    e. The environment
2. A comprehensive behavioural assessment must provide:
    a. Details about the A-B-C contingency
    b. How establishing operations affect the behaviour
    c. Measurable and operational information about the target behaviour
    d. Information about the context in which the behaviour occurs
    e. All of the above

Key References

Cooper, J., Heron, T.E., Heward, W.L., (2007). *Applied Behavior Analysis* (2nd Edition). Upper Saddle River, NJ: Prentice-Hall.

Kearney, A.J. (2007). *Understanding Applied Behavior Analysis: An Introduction to ABA for Parents, Teachers, and Other Professionals.* London: Jessica Kingsley Publishers.

Williams, B.F., Williams, R.L., (2011). *Effective Programs for Treating Autistic Spectrum Disorders: Applied Behaviour Analysis Models.* New York: New York Publishing.

63 Social Stories™

Liz Smith

Introduction

Social Stories™ support the exchange of information between parents, professionals and the target individual. The goal of a Social Story™ is not to change an individual's behaviour, but it is hoped that improving the child's understanding of social events and expectations will lead to more effective responses (Gray, 2015). The visual presentation of social rules is thought to be less confusing, compared to other methods of teaching social skills, e.g. social skills groups, where children may struggle with the high verbal demands (Rust and Smith, 2006). Social Stories™ are tailored to each individual child in accordance with their level of understanding, relate to a particular area of difficulty that they are experiencing and can incorporate themes and characters that chime with their interests. The idea is to increase the child's level of interest and motivation.

KEY CONCEPTS

- A Social Story describes a situation, skill or concept in terms of relevant social cues, perspectives and common responses in a specifically defined style and format (Gray, 2015).
- Social Stories are short personalised stories designed to teach children how to manage their own behaviour during a particular social situation that they find challenging or confusing (Gray and Garand, 1993).
- The story describes the context of a specific social situation and includes detail relating to where the activity takes place, when it will occur, who will be participating, what will happen, how other people may be feeling and why the child should behave in a given manner.
- A Social Story is written from a first- or third-person perspective and uses positive language.
- A set of specific criteria, outlined by Carol Gray, guides story development and delivery to ensure the emphasis is on sharing descriptive, as opposed to directive, information. (Please see www.carolgraysocialstories.com for up-to-date guidance.)

Story Structure and Sentence Types

Each Social Story™ has a title and is made up of three sections. The title and first section (introduction) clearly identify the topic. The main body of the story adds the detail, and the conclusion summarises and reinforces the key points. According to Carol Gray's criteria, there are seven sentence types that can be used within a Social Story™. These fit within two categories.

Category A: Sentences That Describe (Four Types)

- Descriptive sentences: describe the facts relating to the situation in a manner that is free of opinions or assumptions (e.g. 'Everyone needs to see the doctor from time to time').
- Perspective sentences: describe people's thoughts, feelings or beliefs (e.g. 'When I try my best my mum feels very proud of me').
- Affirmative sentences: positive phrases that enhance the meaning of another sentence or reinforce a key point (e.g. 'this is okay' or 'this is very important').
- Partial sentences: incomplete sentences used to establish or check the child's level of understanding (e.g. 'I need to wash my hands after I have been to the toilet because…').

Category B: Coaching Sentences (Three Types)

- Sentences that describe or suggest an appropriate response (e.g. 'I will try to put my hand up when I want to speak to my teacher').
- Sentences that suggest a response for the caregiver (e.g. 'Mrs X can help me to use the soap dispenser when I am washing my hands').
- Sentences that are developed by the child (e.g. 'I can draw in my special drawing book if I am feeling sad').

You do not need to include all of the seven sentence types within the story. It must contain at least one descriptive sentence, with an option to include one or more of the other six sentence types. The key is to have more sentences from Category A (sentences that describe) than Category B (coaching sentences).

Writing a Social Story

Step 1: Picture the Goal and Identify the Target Behaviour

The author translates social information into meaningful text and illustrations, describing abstract concepts and ideas with visual, concrete references and images. The priority is to share relevant social information in a meaningful way.

Step 2: Gather Information

This includes when and where the situation occurs, who is involved, how events are sequenced, what occurs and why. This information can be gathered through direct observation and/or discussions with school staff and parents.

Step 3: Tailor the Text

The author customises the text and images to the learning style, needs, interests and abilities of the child. Some generic stories are available (see key references below), and these can be a helpful starting point covering a range of topics such as sharing, going to the hairdressers and so on.

A Social Story™ has the following key characteristics:

- Aims to share accurate social information.
- Answers 'wh-' questions, including who is involved, where and when a situation occurs, what is happening, how it happens and why.
- Has an emphasis on providing descriptive information as opposed to giving direction/instructions.

- Written from a first- or third-person perspective.
- Written in positive language. If a reference to negative behaviour is made, it is done with caution and from a third-person perspective, e.g. 'sometimes people may unintentionally say something that hurts another person's feelings. This is a mistake'.
- Includes more sentences that describe (Category A) than coach (Category B).

Example

My teacher talks a lot.
Sometimes she talks to me.
She gives me directions and helps me with my work.
Sometimes she talks to other people.
She might talk to other children about their work.
She might talk to another adult.
It is okay when she talks to other people.
When my teacher talks to other people I can keep working or playing.
This will make my teacher happy.
I will try to keep working or playing when my teacher talks to other people.

Phrases such as 'I will try', 'sometimes' and 'usually' are good to use in stories.

Social stories are good because they:

- Are visual
- Provide a consistent, concrete message
- Are permanent
- Are individualised
- Are practical
- Provide an opportunity for children to practice skills before attempting the real situation

How to Use Them

Identify an appropriate focus, and then create a social story. Make them individualised, and think about yourself in the child's shoes. Make them visual if necessary, by using illustrations or any symbols the child is using. Technology can be used to enhance engagement and provide support for both story writing and delivery. A number specific Social Stories™ apps have recently been developed.

Try reading the story once a day, if possible, immediately before the situation in question.

The use of the story should be reviewed after about two weeks. Do you think it is working? What are you going to look for to tell you if it is? If it has not been working, do you have the right focus for the story? Will you keep using stories with a particular child? What might be your next focus? How will you store the stories and celebrate achievement?

Multiple-Choice Questions

See answers on page 673.

1. Which of the following is NOT one of the seven common sentences types used in social stories?
   a. Perspective
   b. Affirmative
   c. Cathartic

   d. Descriptive
   e. Coaching
2. Which of the following is NOT a defining characteristic of social stories?
   a. Answers 'wh-' questions.
   b. Written in the first or third person.
   c. Written in positive language.
   d. Must include all seven different sentence types.
   e. Uses a smaller ratio of coaching sentences compared to sentences that describe.

Key References

Linehan, M.M., (1993). *Cognitive Behavioral Treatment of Borderline Personality Disorder.* New York: The Guildford Press.

Miller, A.L., Rathus, J.H., Linehan, M.M., (2007). *Dialectical Behavior Therapy with Suicidal Adolescents.* New York: The Guildford Press.

Rathus, J.H., Miller, A.L., (2015). *DBT Skill Manual for Adolescents.* New York: TheGuildford Press.

64 Family Therapy Models and Practice

Monica Roman-Morales and Christine M. Hooper

KEY CONCEPTS

- Using a family therapy approach, a family member's symptoms are that person's response to their environment and the environment's response to the symptoms.
- An assessment is made as to how the family interact together, both in the here and now, and over time. Family trees are drawn up and discussed with the family to identify patterns, family values and belief systems that will all influence how the family see the difficulties and how they might respond to professional intervention.
- Any intervention must 'fit' with the family's own beliefs and values.
- 'Joining with the family', using their language so far as is possible and trying to enter into their experience and understand it, is seen as a crucial tool in the work.
- Family members are the therapists' partners in the resolution of the problems.

Innovative Practitioners in the Field

Salvador Minuchin

Salvador Minuchin became Director of the Philadelphia Child Guidance clinic in the USA in 1965. He was an Argentine-born psychiatrist and psychodynamic psychotherapist. He worked with families living in poverty and often with only one parent at home. In 1967, he published *Families of the Slums.* Salvador Minuchin introduced several new techniques, and focussed on establishing a hierarchy of 'executive system' and 'child sub-system' in the family. His approach became known as **structural family therapy**.

Main Structural Techniques

- Joining with the family, i.e. establishing rapport.
- Establishing an executive sub-system of adult(s) and, perhaps, older children.
- Enactment, i.e. encouraging acting-out in the session of how the family interact around the problem behaviour.
- Intensification, i.e. 'turning up the heat' on the problem so that the seriousness is appreciated.
- Unbalancing, i.e. allying with different family members in the session to allow each family member to have a voice.

- Identifying alliances, i.e. where two family members are particularly close. This was seen as a problem, even dangerous, if such closeness crossed generational boundaries.
- And identifying coalitions, i.e. where two or more family members are allied against another family member.

Key Structural Ideas

- **Boundaries**: problems emerge when the boundaries of the family are not functioning well.
- **Disengagement**: Minuchin noticed that sometimes a child had to take their behaviour to an extreme before the other family members took notice. These families were known as 'disengaged'. This meant that the boundaries were so rigid that a family member could be isolated.
- **Enmeshed**: by contrast, some families rally enthusiastically around a minor difficulty, sometimes involving extended family or neighbours. These families were known as '**enmeshed**'. Boundaries here are too permeable so it is difficult to differentiate the individual views and beliefs of the members of the family.

Structural family therapy came to be seen as somewhat 'masculine' in approach, problem-solving, rather than problem-understanding, and it fell out of favour as feminism swept in during the 1970s. Many of the techniques are still used and found most helpful for families with younger children. A structural family therapist takes charge of the conduct of the session and, by implication, of the outcome.

Mental Research Institute Team at Palo Alto in California, USA

This team were influenced by the work of Milton Erikson that emphasised a lifelong process of socialisation, adjustment and learning within families. Difficulties within families were identified as associated with transitional stages in the family life cycle, e.g. when children begin school, a new child is born, adolescents leave home, parents separate, bereavement. Over time, several important therapists, Jay Haley, Don Jackson, Gregory Bateson, John Weakland and Paul Watzlawick among them, worked with the team. Gregory Bateson introduced the idea of looking at a family as a 'cybernetic' system, governed by unwritten rules of interaction. These ideas became known as **Strategic Family Therapy**.

Key Strategic Ideas

- Use of warfare language: tactics, planning and resistance.
- 'Uncommon solutions'. Each family was seen as unique and each intervention tailor-made to their situation.
- Family behaviour patterns were expected to be resistant to change, and often paradoxical solutions were proposed. Direct interventions are 'compliance-based', whereas paradoxical interventions are 'defiance-based', i.e. if the family were to follow the advice given, the outcome would be the opposite of what is desired.
- 'Feedback' shapes and maintains social relationships over time.
- 'Complementarity' is an interactional pattern whereby the parties to the interaction respond to one another with opposite behaviour, e.g. if one person is aggressive, the other is passive. 'Symmetry' is an interactional pattern where if one person is aggressive, the other is equally, if not more, aggressive. Either pattern results in 'runaway', if unchecked.

Strategic family therapy has been criticised for its assumption that the family will be resistant and devious means are needed to change behaviour. **Brief solution-focussed therapy** evolved from the ideas of the strategic family therapists.

Milan Associates

Cecchin and Boscolo, Selvini-Palazolli and Prata. These four Italian psychiatrists and psychotherapists initiated a mode of family session, whereby two of the team would talk with the family, whilst their two colleagues watched the session behind a two-way screen. The observer therapists were distanced from the family because it was believed that the interviewing therapists could not help being ‘pulled into’ the family system. The observer position was known as ‘second order cybernetics’. The Milan group took family therapy in a new and more sophisticated direction.

Key Milan Ideas

- Hypothesising – constructing an informed guess from information already available about the family dynamics that might be maintaining the problem behaviour. This hypothesis is then tested out in the session.
- Curiosity – letting questioning flow freely as more information is revealed. This is called the ‘feedback loop’.
- Neutrality – the therapist does not reveal any particular position vis-à-vis the problems.
- Re-framing – finding an equally valid frame for the difficulties that would ‘fit’ with the family relationships system, rather than the difficulties belonging to the ‘symptom-carrier’.
- Positive connotation – acknowledging each family member’s contribution to the resolution of the difficulties.
- Circular questioning – asking one family member to comment on the behaviour of two other family members, the idea being that that person can be more objective if they are not under the spotlight themselves. A picture of the family dynamics can be drawn up in view of these different responses.
- Italians are traditionally seen as remaining close to their extended family, and the Milan group made particular use of family trees to throw light on generational family patterns.
- The ‘invariate prescription’ – a standard intervention of directing the parents to go out together once a week.
- Messages – sessions ended usually with a message to the family, sometimes written down, sometimes read out. The message could prescribe a family ritual or contain a paradoxical intervention.

The Milan group’s work became known as Milan-systemic therapy. Many of their ideas are part of the more eclectic family therapy approach now, notably hypothesising, the use of family trees, circular questioning and re-framing.

Case Study (1): Timothy

Timothy (five) has just begun primary school, but he is reluctant to attend. He clings to his mother’s legs and cries when she tries to leave him. Once in school, Timothy does settle, but he is often aggressive to other children if they try to share his activity. Timothy’s father left home when Timothy was three years old. His mother has a new partner now and there is a new baby.

His maternal grandfather, whom Timothy was close to, died recently. Timothy has no health problems and is of average ability. He reached all his developmental milestones on time. He was not difficult to manage before the birth of his baby brother.

- Remember to draw up a family tree, so that you are clear about who is important in this family.
- Think about Timothy's family. What do you need to know to help you make a hypothesis?

Analysis

Timothy's father had been violent towards his mother. Timothy did not witness the violence, but he did feel afraid of his father. Whenever Timothy is aggressive at school, or towards his baby brother, his mother believes he has inherited his father's angry temperament and she feels powerless. Timothy does not have contact with his father.

At the back of his mind, Timothy wonders if his mother will be safe with this new partner. He would prefer to be at home with her. He is jealous of the new baby at home with his mother all day, when he has to be at school. Timothy's mother was depressed after Timothy was born, and it was difficult for him to gain her attention. He found that if he was aggressive, she took notice of him. Timothy's grandfather spent time with Timothy, trying to compensate for him not having a father around. Timothy misses his grandfather. So far, Timothy's 'step-father' has not made much effort to forge a relationship with Timothy. Timothy thinks inside that he prefers his own new baby. When other children take Timothy's things at school, it reminds him of his little brother and it makes him feel upset.

Possible Interventions

Structural: a small daily reward for Timothy separating more calmly from his mother in a morning might help, especially if this involved the new partner, e.g. a bedtime story with him or some time playing football in the park.

(NB you would want to know something of the new partner's history first…) It would be important that Timothy's mother and her partner were consistent in their way of managing Timothy's behaviour and acted as an 'executive system'.

Strategic: this is a complicated transitional stage for Timothy and for his mother. They are adjusting to two new family members, the partner and Timothy's half-brother. Timothy has just started school. Think about how Timothy's mother reacts when Timothy is angry. Does she feel personally vulnerable, even though he is only five years old? Maybe some story work with Timothy and the family would be helpful, looking at fairy tales that mention step-fathers and half-siblings, or kind grandfathers, or the therapist might make some up as a vehicle for exploring how this all feels to Timothy.

Milan-systemic: it would be important to move away from the idea that Timothy is a replica of his natural father. It is rather a linear concept and does not suggest a way forward. The interactions around Timothy's behaviour would be examined to highlight the family dynamics. It might be suggested that Timothy's mother and partner go out together once a week to show their commitment to one another as a couple ('the invariate prescription'). There might be some attention to the generational patterns of how new family members have been absorbed into existing family structures or, even, how the family see the behaviour of boys in contrast to girls. Milan-systemic therapy is usually more explorative and less prescriptive.

Case Study (2): Jennifer

Jennifer (15) lives with her biological parents and a younger sister, Joanne. Jennifer has been losing weight for the last six months. She has not had a period for the last two months now, although menstruation was well-established previously. Jennifer has decided to become a vegetarian and has been preparing her own food and eating it in her room. A friend has told Jennifer's mother that she has seen Jennifer throwing away her school lunch. Jennifer has started going running in the evenings, with her father. Jennifer is a high achiever academically and expected to achieve very good GCSE results.

NB family therapy is considered to be the best approach where anorexia nervosa is suspected in children and young people up to 18 years of age. In these cases, it is most important that the therapist works closely with a medical colleague, either the family GP, a child and adolescent psychiatrist or a paediatrician.

Analysis

Both Jennifer's parents felt they had been emotionally neglected by their own parents. Her father had been unhappy at his boarding-school. Her mother's family are wealthy and had engaged a nanny for her. They had agreed, early in their marriage, that they would spend as much time as they could with their children, taking an active, possibly even intrusive, interest in their education and hobbies. They seldom go out together, sacrificing their own relationship to be with the children.

Jennifer attends a highly regarded school, out of catchment. She adores her parents and wants to do well to please them. To keep up with her peer group, she has to work really hard. She is desperately worried about letting her parents down. GCSEs are on the horizon now. She would like to go to a university that specialises in sports science. A boy at school has said nastily that she is 'too big' to think she could ever be any good at sport.

- Remember the family tree and use it to explore the family's belief systems.
- Look at pre-disposing, precipitating and perpetuating factors.

Interventions

Structural: the parents insist that Jennifer eats with them, and both sit with her until she has finished her food. There would be a structured reward system for eating and sanctions for refusing to eat. Jennifer would be weighed regularly and the rewards and punishments tied in to her weight. Her parents, encouraged by the therapist, would take charge of her eating. The parental (executive subsystem) is reinforced by working calmly but firmly towards addressing the eating disorder.

Strategic: the symptoms are looked at as a metaphor for what Jennifer is trying to escape from by making herself 'invisible', e.g. disappointing her parents over the exams. Or Jennifer is encouraged to envisage anorexia nervosa as the enemy within, that she can overcome. Or narratives are used to explore Jennifer's feelings about her family and their expectations. All these can be used in family meetings.

Milan-systemic: the medical aspects of the illness are managed by a medical professional, leaving the therapist to explore family myths and beliefs about gender issues generally, how women are perceived in the family, in society and in the media. Jennifer's younger sister may know more about Jennifer's 'inner world' than either of their parents.

NB in practice, anorexia nervosa is often a very difficult condition to treat, and any of the ideas from the different models might be tried during treatment.

Multiple-Choice Questions

See answers on page 673.

1. Which family therapy approach is associated with Salvador Minuchin?
   a. Strategic
   b. Milan-systemic
   c. Structural
2. Hypothesising, curiosity and neutrality are associated with which family therapy approach?
   a. Strategic
   b. Narrative
   c. Milan-systemic

Key References

Burnham, J., (1986). *Family Therapy: First Steps towards a Systemic Approach.* London: Tavistock Publications Ltd.

Carter, B., McGoldrick M., (1989). *The Changing Family Life Cycle: A Framework for Family Therapy* (2nd Ed.). London: Pearson.

Dallos, R., Draper, R., (2000). *An Introduction to Family Therapy: Systemic Theory and Practice.* London: Open University Press.

65 Brief Solution-Focussed Therapy

Jonathan Prosser

Introduction

Brief solution-focussed therapy (BSFT) has evolved from the earlier family therapy models. Here, individuals and families are encouraged to change the way they think about and talk about their problems, and to avoid 'problem-saturated' talk.

KEY CONCEPTS

- BSFT is a structured and focussed approach to problem-solving.
- Attention is paid to the client/family's strengths and resources.
- The therapist encourages 'problem-free' talk.
- Attempts to 'understand' the problem are not seen as necessarily helpful.
- It is assumed that the client is 'doing some of the solution some of the time'. The aim of the work is to encourage 'more of what works'.
- Small achievable steps in the right direction promote resolution of the problem.
- Unless there are statutory considerations, the client is seen as the best judge of when the problem is resolved.
- BSFT has a specific style of questioning.

Key Techniques

Goal Setting

It is important to be clear with the client what the goals are, so that both therapist and client recognise when they have been achieved. Goals are written down at the start of the therapeutic work. Here are some typical questions to encourage goal setting.

- How will you know at the end of the session that it was worthwhile coming to see me today?
- When will your social worker/health visitor/community psychiatric nurse know that it is okay for them to stop worrying?

BSFT has introduced a special question known as the 'Miracle Question'. The Miracle Question is often asked in this way:

> Let us imagine that while you are asleep tonight, a miracle happens and the problems that have brought you to see me are all resolved. You do not know that the miracle has happened because you are asleep. What will be different when you wake up in the morning that will tell you that a miracle has happened? What might you be doing that is different and what will other people around you be doing that is different, that will tell you that a miracle has happened?

And then:

> What would be the very first thing that you would notice?

This line of questioning should be pursued until a well-explored and concretely describable scenario has been generated. The Miracle Question helps the client to visualise a problem-free future and to identify the small steps that will be needed to achieve it.

Exception-Finding

Exceptions are those moments, hours or days when the problem is not happening. There must be some. No child is oppositional all day and every day. The client can be encouraged to recognise the particular circumstances in which the problem behaviour occurs and to take some control over it.

Typical exception-finding questions would be:

- Tell me about those times when the problem is not happening.
- When does the problem bother you less?
- When do you resist the urge to…? (smack…shout…cry…have a drink…)
- What are you and the other people around you doing differently at those times when the problem seems not to be happening?

Measuring Change

Scaling questions are a very important tool in brief solution-focussed therapy. They are used to measure the client's perception of change and to enhance the sense of moving forward. Scaling questions can be used at each session.

Typical scaling questions would be:

- On a scale of 0–10, with 0 being the worst possible case scenario and 10 being how you would like your life to be, where are you today?
- So, if you are on 3, how will you know when you have reached 4?
- What have you done to move from a 3 to a 4 this week?
- What will life look like when you reach 10?

Building on the Client/Family Strengths and Coping Strategies

BSFT always looks out for the client or family's own resources and highlights them. It is assumed, and it is true, that everyone has both strengths and weaknesses. The strengths are what are needed to resolve the difficulties. The weaknesses are not dwelt on.

Typical strength-building/coping strategies questions would be:

- When you have been in this kind of situation before, how did you manage to resolve it?
- What other really difficult situations have you managed to come through?
- What is it that helps you to get through?
- What gives you the strength to get up in a morning?
- What are you doing to stop things getting worse?

Helping Clients to Re-Assess Their View of Themselves

The individuals and families who find their way to the helping agencies have sometimes had to wait for a referral and then for an appointment and may have seen several other professionals along the way. They may have sought help from family, friends and neighbours, that has not made any difference. Their self-esteem has taken a battering. It is crucial that this is restored to give them optimism that they can influence their own lives and have a happier outcome.

Typical re-assessment questions would be:

- What do you know about yourself now that you did not know last week?
- What have you learned from how well you have managed things recently?

When our lives seem to be problem-saturated, the past can be over-shadowed by the present difficulties, so that only the more negative experiences from the past are recalled. It is possible through careful questioning to bring out memories of happier times. The idea is for the client to re-examine their life experience in the light of achievements, rather than failures.

- Have you always been a survivor or did you learn the hard way?
- Describe a time when you made the right choice of what to do.
- Who do you know who will be really surprised to hear about the difficulties you have overcome?

Constructive Feedback

The therapist needs to pay attention to constructive feedback and to avoid any shift back into hopeless and helpless thinking. Any progress towards the agreed goals should be emphasised. Other behaviour should, whenever possible, be ignored, unless there are statutory or child-protection considerations.

Typical questions would be:

- Who was the first person to notice how much more determined you are now to get on with your life?
- How are people treating you differently now they can see the change in the way you are managing the difficulties?
- Who will be first person to congratulate you on how well you are doing?

The client/family decides, where possible, the frequency, timing and ending of the therapy sessions. Each session is potentially the last one. This keeps both client and therapist focussed on change.

The goals may not necessarily have all been achieved when the therapy stops, but hopefully the client should feel confident that they have the skills and resources to reach their desired outcomes.

When the therapist's employing agency has an agenda about what changes are not only desired, but compulsory, e.g. for a child to be allowed to continue living at home, both the client's goals and the agency's goals must be openly shared and negotiated. Follow-up sessions at intervals are recommended to focus on how the improvements are being maintained. The temptation might be for clients to assume that follow-up is an invitation to explain that the difficulties are either worse or not improved and this has to be resisted.

Case Study: Liam

Liam (ten) was referred to the clinic because of occasional spells of school refusal. He attends school generally, but there are times when he misses a week or more. Liam explained that he often felt ill, with headaches and stomach-aches. Liam's mother works full-time, and his father is in charge of the home and child-care. There is an older sister, Claire. Claire is a high-achiever and expects to go on to university. Liam has moderate dyslexia and struggles at school.

Liam's parents both attended the appointments. Liam's father was inclined to be more lenient with Liam. He said he knew him well and believed Liam would not say that he was ill, if he wasn't. Liam's mother was more confrontational. She was afraid Liam would not make a successful transition to secondary school.

With careful questioning, it was clear that Liam's school refusal was initially in the context of his mother either working from home or going to work later in the day. Once he was out of the routine of school, it was difficult to persuade him to return. When Liam was reluctant to go to school, his parents found themselves arguing about it and, sometimes, Claire would try to help out by supporting her mother's position. It was as if Liam had three parents all saying different things.

Liam's mother's answer to the Miracle Question was that she would like Liam to bring her a cup of tea in bed, already dressed for school. It was important for Liam's parents to decide and agree how they would handle Liam on those days when he was not keen to attend school. They were obviously able to negotiate and had done so when they had to choose which of them would work outside the home. Liam's answer to the Miracle Question was that he would wake up on a Saturday and learn that he would be spending it with his mother and without his sister, Claire. With further questioning, he was able to describe exactly how he would spend that day. Liam's father wanted his wife to respect his instincts about the children and to make time to go out with him once a week, rather than prioritising her work. This would help Claire to recognise that her parents were in charge of decisions about Liam and she could relax her own position with regard to helping her parents deal with him.

Liam began secondary school in the September term. He has attended regularly and now has special help for his reading and writing difficulties, and a school mentor.

Multiple-Choice Question

See answers on page 673.

Brief solution-focussed therapy focuses on…

a. Finding the cause of the problem
b. Using 'problem-free' talk and the Miracle Question
c. Exploration of past events

Key References

De Shazer, S., (1992). Doing therapy: a post structural re-visiting. *Journal of Marital and Family Therapy*, 18(1): 71–81.

George, E., Iveson, C., Ratner, H., (1990). *Problem to Solution: Brief Therapy with individuals and Families*. London: Brief Therapy Press.

Nylund, D., (1994). Becoming solution-forced in brief therapy: remembering something important we already knew. *Journal of Systemic Therapies*, 13(1): 5–12.

66 Narrative Therapy

Andrew O'Toole and Anne Brewster

Narrative therapy emphasises the importance of listening to the story.

> There are those who think a story is told only to reveal what is known in this world. But a good story also reveals the unknown.
>
> (Griffin, 1992, cited in Weingarten, 1998)

KEY CONCEPTS

- Narrative therapy is based on the supposition that in large measure people are the stories they tell themselves and that are told about them.
- Stories shape our lives rather than reflect them back to us.
- According to this position, the process of therapeutic re-authoring of personal narratives is constitutive of identity (Carr, 1998).
- The foundation of clinical practice is based on collaborative understanding and re-authoring of meanings.
- One of the tasks is to help people make sense of their lives, which is a far different project from explaining or diagnosing their behaviour.
- An important difference of the narrative approach is shifting the attention from what the therapist thinks about what the clients are saying, onto trying to understand what the clients think about what they are saying.
- Seeing oneself in relation to a problem, instead of having or being a problem, creates the possibility of imagining oneself in a different relationship to the problem.

What Is Narrative Therapy?

Narratives can occur at different levels of social functioning. There are social and cultural narratives, interpersonal narratives and intra-personal narratives. The narrative approach rests on the assumption that narratives are not representations of reflections of identities, lives and problems. Rather narratives constitute identities, lives and problems. Our stories are embedded in, and influenced by, a wider social and cultural context.

One of the central ideas of narrative theory is the idea of 'discourse'. Discourse relates to the idea of concepts that have negotiated and accepted meanings. A possible discourse might be 'fatherhood'. When a man becomes a father, the story he will tell about being a father will be influenced by the wider accepted meaning and language about fatherhood present in his contemporary society and culture. It will be influenced by personal experiences of fatherhood or its absence, interpersonal relationships and internalised models of such relationships. The discourse on fatherhood does not exist discretely, but is influenced by other discourses, e.g. patriarchy, motherhood, sexuality, power. Whether we are aware of a discourse or not, it can powerfully influence the stories we can tell and the stories we can hear.

Discourse can be described in terms of:

> Historically, socially, and institutionally specific structures of statements, terms, categories and beliefs that are embedded in institutions, social relationships and texts. (Carr, 1998)

Narrative Assessment Process

- The goal of assessment is to encourage the development of a narrative, a telling and re-telling of events in a way that allows new understanding and meaning to emerge.
- What traditionally may have been regarded as information, leading to a diagnosis and intervention by an expert, is instead used to facilitate the child and family in a conversation of understanding.
- The object is not to explain but to understand, giving meaning to the child's presenting problem.
- To assess a child is to have a desire to hear his or her story, whilst therapy concerns fostering this desire in all family members.

Key Narrative Strategies

Re-Authoring

- Privileges the person's lived experience.
- Adopts a collaborative co-authoring position.
- Encourages a perception of a changing world through the plotting or linking of lived experience, through the temporal dimension.
- Helps clients view themselves as separate from their problems by externalising the problem.
- Helps clients pinpoint times in their lives when they were not oppressed by their problems, by identifying 'unique outcomes'.
- Helps clients develop new stories based on the unique outcomes.
- Links unique outcomes to other events in the past and extends the story into the future, to form an alternative and preferred self-narrative, in which the self is viewed as more powerful than the problem.
- Invites significant members of the person's social network to witness this new self-narrative.
- Documents new knowledge and practices that support the new self-narrative using literary means.
- Allows others, who are trapped by similar oppressive narratives, to benefit from their new knowledge.

'Externalising' is a concept developed by Michael White and David Epston (1990). Externalising conversations separates persons from problems and blocks the fusing of the person with the problem. Seeing oneself in relation to a problem instead of having or being a problem creates the possibility of imagining oneself in a different relationship to the problem.

Externalising the problem:

- Decreases unproductive conflict between individuals, including those disputes over who is responsible for the problem.
- Undermines the sense of failure that has developed for many individuals to the continuing existence of the problem, despite their attempts to resolve it.
- Paves the way for people to cooperate with each other, to unite in a struggle against the problem.
- Opens up new possibilities for them to take action to retrieve their lives and relationships from the problem and its influence.
- Frees individuals to take a lighter, more effective and less stressed approach.
- Presents options for dialogue, rather than monologue, about the problem.

Case Study: Nick

White and Epson (1990) describe the case of Nick, a six-year old brought by his parents. He had a very long history of encopresis. They describe how Nick had made the 'poo' his playmate, smearing and streaking it, rolling it into ball and flicking it behind cupboards and wardrobes. The family was asked how the 'poo' was influencing their lives, i.e. its sphere of influence. They outlined a number of ways. For Nick, it isolated him from his peers and prevented him from being seen for who he was. For his mother, the 'poo' was creating misery, forcing her to doubt her capacity to be a good parent. She felt overwhelmed by it. Nick's father was deeply embarrassed by the 'poo' and felt that it isolated him and the family.

White and Epston develop the assessment in this way. It is made clear that the 'poo' is a 'sneaky poo', because it claims to be Nick's friend, but it causes so many problems. The encopresis becomes externalised as 'sneaky poo'. The process then begins to look for unique outcomes, times when the 'sneaky poo' has not been allowed to have a negative effect. Battle is then waged against 'sneaky poo' until its sphere of influence is reduced. Each member of the family can reclaim their lives through the telling of new stories about how they live in a world controlled by them and not by 'sneaky poo'.

There are always alternative stories to the ones currently dominant in a person's life. It is helpful for both the storyteller and the listener to be mindful that this is only one version of the story, the current version. One strategy for generating alternative stories is the identification of 'unique outcomes'. A unique outcome is when something happens that disconfirms the current story and allows alternatives, i.e. new meanings, to be seen. These unique outcomes might be historic, current or potential, i.e. future.

Not Knowing or Suspended Knowing

One of the difficulties of the narrative approach is how the professional might be able to contribute expertise, without disempowering the client narrative. Empowerment, from a narrative perspective, is related to one person experiencing another person as accepting and elaborating what they have to say, without challenging its basic integrity. A response to this dilemma is the strategy of the 'not knowing' stance or 'suspending knowing'. Here the professional keeps professional knowledge in the background, in order to privilege the client's story. Once the story has unfolded, an exchange of meaning and ideas can take place.

Repositioning

A further key idea in narrative theory is the notion of 're-positioning', i.e. taking up a different position in relation to the young person and/or the problem. 'Externalising' and 'suspending knowing' would both be examples of re-positioning.

Noting the Characteristics of the Story

The narrative task is to help people tell those stories whose effects on their lives are preferable to the stories they are currently telling. In doing this, paying attention to the characteristics of the story is important. Weingarten K. (1998) identifies three important features of the story:

- **Narrative coherence**: narratives can be more, or less, coherent. Coherence is established by the inter-relationships between plot, characters roles and themes. In attachment narratives, the degree of the coherence of the narrative is a predictor of secure attachment. Coherence has been linked to well-being ('salutogenisis').
- **Narrative closure**: Occurs when a story is told that seems to have only one way to understand it.
- **Narrative interdependence**: Refers to the relationship of one person's narrative to another's. The stories we tell ourselves almost always create 'positions' for those we speak about, some of which are more desirable than others.

Crossley M. (2000) offers further strategies for exploring the story:

- **Narrative tone**: a pervasive feature of a personal narrative conveyed both in the content and the manner in which the story is told. The tone might be, e.g. predominately optimistic or pessimistic.
- **Imagery**: look out for the unique way in which imagery is employed in the story. It might be helpful to look at the origin of such imagery. Is it embedded in early experience or in the wider dominant discourses of the society the storyteller lives in?
- **Themes**: what are the dominant themes or patterns of the story as it unfolds? What are the motivational themes behind the story? Love and power have been suggested as common themes in human stories. Power is seen both in terms of a sense of agency, self-efficacy and love and in terms of the desire for connection and dependence.

Perhaps an easy way to begin thinking about the narrative process is to consider your own narrative. Crossley offers a detailed structure for exploring our life narrative. One exercise can be done fairly quickly and helps to illustrate narrative ideas.

Exercise

Take some time to consider your life narrative. Begin by thinking of your life as a book. Each part of your life composes a chapter in the book, clearly as yet unfinished. Select at least two or three chapter headings for your story or at most seven or eight. Give each chapter a name and describe the overall contents for each chapter.

When you have done this, you could address a number of questions.

1. In choosing to talk about what you did, what might be some of the untold stories?
2. If you had done this exercise five years ago, or in five years' time, how might things be different?
3. How have you ordered the narrative and why that order?
4. Are there discernible themes?
5. What is the overall tone so far?
6. How about your use of imagery?
7. If you were telling this story to different significant people, how might the story change with each listener?

Summary

It is unlikely that many practitioners will use a purely narrative approach. However, narrative offers an interesting dimension to the process of assessment and treatment. Perhaps the most significant element is the privileging of the client story over other forms of knowing about and describing the problems the family have. Such a strategy is likely to enhance trust, respect and engagement. Some narrative strategies, e.g. 'externalising', could be used very effectively, alongside other therapeutic processes.

Multiple-Choice Question

See answers on page 673.

Narrative therapy…

a. Encourages the development of a narrative, a telling and re-telling of events in a way that allows new understanding and meanings to emerge
b. Involves the therapist telling stories
c. Encourages people to stick to one story

Key References

Carr, A., (1998). Michael white's narrative therapy. *Contemporary Family Therapy*, 2(4).
Crossley, M.L., (2000). *Introducing Narrative Psychology: Self, Trauma and the Construction of Meaning*. Buckingham: Open University Press.
Weingarten, K., (1998). The small and the ordinary: the daily practice of a post-modern narrative therapy. *Family Process*, 37: 3–15.
White, M., Epston, D., (1990). *Narrative Means to Therapeutic Ends*. London & New York: WW. Norton & Company.

67 The Open Dialogue Approach

Cathy Laver-Bradbury and Monica Roman-Morales

This is a systemic approach developed in Western Lapland in the 1980s and used in the treatment of psychosis in adults. It is gaining some momentum for its use within CAMHS.

The Systemic Theories That Informed the Approach

Bakhtin was a Russian philosopher (1895–1975). He developed the theory in a context where the government was seen to be telling the 'truth'. He talked about the importance of many dialogues in order to hear many voices, none of which were considered to be the truth, but each held importance irrespective of whether they were positive or negative. He believed that it is the dialogue itself which eventually leads to a consensus.

Marcelo Pakman (2000) is a psychiatrist from Buenos Aires, where he was working as a psychotherapist. He referred to poetics and micropolitics; poetics referred to the language and communication practices that occur in face-to-face encounters. Micropolitics referred to larger institutional practices where 'expanded models of dialogue can address both the poetics of the interview room and the larger bureaucratic politics that can constrain and deaden them'. Bateson (1962) discussed double-bind communication, an idea that came from a theoretical attempt to imagine the kind of context to which 'psychotic speech and behaviour would seem adaptive'. In their writing, both Bateson and Pakman indicate the professional struggle with issues of chaotic, procedure-driven managed-care environments.

At the same time, the Milan team described a technique of the 'Counter Paradox' to untangle paradoxical communication, offering a new logic of positive connotation, or a new ordering of behaviour, in the form of a ritual. They took a psychoeducational family approach. Michael White's (1995) narrative practice of externalising the problem places symptoms as outside of the person rather than as an inner experience.

Initially the Open Dialogue approach began with a treatment meeting prior to therapy. This evolved into open meetings. This was in contrast to family therapy sessions where the person and their family decide who will attend. The addition of the reflecting team and the Galveston group's (Anderson, Goolisham and Pulliam) collaborative language systems approach became the framework for the Open Dialogue approach developed by Jaako Seikkula (2003) and his team.

A Convergence of Approaches: The Open Dialogue

- The idea is that neither the patient or family are seen as either the cause of the psychosis or an object of treatment but as competent or potentially competent partners in the recovery process.

- Narrative practice of externalisation, i.e. psychosis seen as outside the person rather than seeing it as a manifestation of inner experience.
- The importance of the dialogue from all participants, whether this is affirming or not.
- Psychosis is adaptive to the person and the understanding of this is important to others.

What Is the Open Dialogue Approach?

Tolerance of Uncertainty (Anderson and Goolishian, 1992)

- 'What shall we do? is kept open until there is a collective response. There is no hypothesising and no preliminary definition of the problem, in the hope that the dialogue itself will bring forward new ideas and stories.
- The meetings can happen daily if needed, so that the family does not feel alone in the crisis. Scheduling includes the possibility of meeting daily for 10–12 days initially. Uncertainty can only be tolerated if the therapy is experienced as safe.

Dialogism

- Reducing isolation by constituting a dialogue built around a communicative relationship with the patient and the persons involved with him or her.
- 'Psychosis is a temporary radical and terrifying alienation from shared, communicative practices. A "'No Man's Land"' where unbearable experience has no words and thus the patient has no voice and no genuine agency'.
- The idea of listening is more important than interviewing. No theme is decided in advance.
- The speaker and listener are intimately joined together in making sense of the psychotic episode.
- Creative participation that attends both to what people say and to the existing feelings and sensuous responses that flow between them. 'Language for suffering may be born that can give the suffering a voice'.

Polyphony

- Multiple subjects forming a polyphony of multiple voices.
- The team no longer focuses on the family structure, but instead on all the individuals involved, allowing the 'system' to be created in every new dialogue. The conversation itself constructs the reality, not the family rules or structure.
- The questions or reflections of the professional should not interrupt the ongoing dialogue, unless what they say fits in with it.
- Then professionals can comment either by asking another related question or by starting a reflecting dialogue about it with the other professionals.
- Reflections are more impromptu, and can occur during the most stressful moments with the aim of promoting a sense of emotional reassurance.
- There is no right or wrong thinking. The goal is to generate joint understanding rather than a consensus.

Practicalities

- Primarily seen at home, but can be seen elsewhere.
- No waiting time. Whoever takes the call co-ordinates the care.

- Day and night access.
- Sitting together to understand more. Open Dialogue has no expert or solution focus. The purpose is to have dialogue and from that find the solutions.
- The work is shared all the time. The thoughts are in movement all the time. Thoughts and reflection happen all the time.
- There are usually two therapists.
- Or even three, if working with a family.

Principles

- None-secretive and non-hierarchical.
- Therapists work in reflecting teams that are open. Ideas can be bounced with other therapists and other families.
- There are meanings in the discussion.
- There is the opportunity to listen to each other and reflect on issues. This is therapeutic in itself.
- The therapist(s) are viewed as visitors in people's lives. It is more important that the person is understood by the significant others in his/her life.
- Psychosis is seen as an answer to a very difficult life situation.
- The therapist is more interested in the stories that seem crazy.

Do They Use Diagnosis in the Approach?

- They might, but not often.
- It can be a metaphorical way of speaking about something they have not been able to speak about, i.e. a dilemma in their personal life.
- It is conceptualised as a problem in relationships, not in the individual.
- If there is risk of suicide, the patient stays in their home with support, avoids hospitalisation and has more opportunities to talk.
- Treatment meetings can be every day and continue for as long as needed.

Medications

- Seldom use medications.
- Sleeping tablets sometimes, maybe four or five days' worth.
- Medication neuroleptics can be used, but only small doses and for a short time. Approximately 35% of patients are offered them.
- Therapists question each other about why they are prescribing medication and what they hope for; this happens in front of patients.
- Other ways to help are discussed, e.g. diet, sobriety, yoga, meditation, journaling, music, nature, exercise, work friendships, supplements and art.

Micropolitics

Implementing an Open Dialogue approach requires an organisational change, both in terms of service delivery and in terms of professional contexts. All staff need to be trained in the approach, and all must be able to work in teams. The approach challenges mental health perspectives, and the work is organised around the person and the family's needs, not the professional context. It commits the team to work with the family when there are problems or challenges. The team is together during the entire course of treatment to guarantee psychological continuity.

Application in CAMHS

The Open Dialogue has been applied mainly in the adult mental health services (AMHS) but has begun to be implemented in the work with children and adolescents by CAMHS and social care. It works well when families have several different agencies and services involved.

The 'Anticipatory Meeting' is a variation of the Open Dialogue that provides a clear co-ordination of the roles and responsibilities of the team members involved, including family members (Seikkula and Arnkil, 2006). The main principles of the Open Dialogue are followed in the Anticipatory Meeting with an emphasis on working collaboratively with families. One of the outcomes of this type of meeting is the reduction of anxiety in the family and the network system, as it offers a clear structure to the network, following the main hopes and wishes, regarding the concerns voiced by the family.

Multiple-Choice Question

See answers on page 673.

The Open Dialogue Approach...

a. Involves working with the individual
b. Is the convergence of several systemic approaches working with the individual and the family to gain multiple views of the difficulties
c. Does not need to have consistency in professionals

Key References

Anderson, H., Goolishian, H., (1992). The client is the expert: a not-knowing approach to therapy. In S. MacNamee, K. Gergen (Eds.) *Therapy as a Social Construction* (pp. 54–68). London: SAGE.

Clement, M., Mc Kenny, R., (2019). Developing an open dialogue inspired model of systemic social work assessment in a local authority children's social care department. *Journal of Family Therapy*, 41(3): 421–446.

Seikkula, J., Arnkil, T., (2006). *Dialogical Meetings in Social Networks (Systemic Thinking and Practice)*. London: Routledge.

Seikkula, J., Olson, M. (2003). The open dialogue approach to acute psychosis: its poetics and micropolitics. *Family Process*, 42(3): 403–418.

Useful Website

http://opendialogueapproach.co.uk

68 The Group Process

Stuart Gemmell and Cathy Laver-Bradbury

Introduction

Groups can be a significant therapeutic tool and a particularly helpful approach for young people. Where possible, the group should be time-limited and closed. There should be co-workers running the group, and they must identify a supervisor. The co-workers must ensure that they are freed by their employing organisation to ring-fence the group work time. Where possible, the group should be of mixed gender. A common unifying need for the group must be identified. Group members must be willing to explore new skills and coping mechanisms in a group setting.

There is a clear step-by-step approach to identify and act upon to ensure effective group work. Anything short of this process and the group itself becomes at best unmanageable and, at worse, counter-productive to the group members' needs and well-being.

Key Principles

- Step One: Identify need for group
- Step Two: Identify co-workers
- Step Three: Co-worker planning and identifying a supervisor
- Step Four: Advertise group
- Step Five: Referral stage
- Step Six: Individual assessments and plenary session
- Step Seven: Group up and running
- Step Eight: Group ending

Step One: Identify Need for Group

> Many emotional problems involve difficulties in relating to others ... Although the therapist can help to work out some of these problems, the final test lies in how well the person can apply the attitudes and responses learned in therapy, to relationships in everyday life. Group therapy permits clients to work out their problems in the presence of others observe how other people react to their behaviour and to try out new ways of responding when old ones prove unsatisfactory.
>
> (Edward et al., 2000)

Atkinson's notion that groups can act as a training environment for the individual to 'practice' new coping mechanisms is supported further by Doel and Sawdon (2001) who state, 'Groups can provide a more effective environment to experience empowerment because they can be used to replicate or simulate the larger society: in many respects they are microcosms of the wider society'.

Evidence-based group interventions in specialist CAMHS can involve children and young people (CYP), e.g. dialectical behaviour therapy (DBT) groups, mindfulness and anxiety groups, or can involve the parents supporting their child or young person, e.g. the New Forest Parenting Programme for parents of children with ADHD (Thompson et al., 2009) or non-violent resistance groups for parents who are helping their child or young person to learn to self-regulate.

The number of group inventions available and the evidence base have been developing in recent years. Group interventions might be considered more cost- effective in under-resourced services, but this is not always true depending on how the intervention was researched and the requirements of translating the research into clinical practice. Despite this, their popularity has grown in services, and most services regularly offer them.

Step Two: Identify Co-Workers

There are many benefits to co-working, i.e. the ability to enhance practice, learn new interventions from another professional, receive instant feedback on the delivery of an intervention and share an experience that is all too often lost in individual work. However, Doel and Sawdon (2001) caution that:

> Co-working a group can be a bit like parenthood; as a twosome everything has been going fine, but when the children come along you suddenly discover you have very different views about how to raise them!

Step Three: Co-Worker Planning and Identifying a Supervisor

Planning

The organisational background of the group is important. Facilitators need to ensure there is enough support from colleagues and management to allow the group to take place. The objectives of the group need to be made clear so that all stakeholders, including potential group members, are aware of the functions and expected outcomes of the group.

Details of group composition, size (6–12 is ideal), timing, accommodation and transport are to be flagged up at this stage of planning, plus any requirements for special facilities, materials and equipment (Doel and Sawdon, 2001). Dedicated time should be allocated for co-worker reflection and supervision.

There is a practical, stress-reducing exercise co-workers should consider undertaking at this stage of the planning, i.e. spending time individually to create a 'What If' list in relation to scenarios that may arise in the group.

e.g.

What if ...	I can't make it one week, will you run the group alone?
What if ...	I don't agree with a statement you make in the group?
	Do I challenge you there and then or wait for wash-up time or supervision?
What if ...	I plan to go on holiday during the timespan of the group?
What if ...	I have different attitudes to you? Say, about swearing?

The more 'What If's' that are raised, the more preparation and contingency plans are identified, thus reducing anxieties should any arise.

Supervision

A supervisor is vital for the well-being of the co-workers. The supervisor should have previous experience of group work and appreciate the 'marriage of convenience' the co-workers have entered into. A supervisor does not need to be an 'expert' in a particular group theme, but their supervision skills should be sought due to their understanding and experience in such areas as systems theory, co-working and recognition of the dynamics that operate within groups.

Supervision can help to:

- Resolve any difficulties in the complex co-leadership relationship
- Manage the anxieties and demands of group work
- Discuss issues raised within the group
- Monitor the effectiveness of the work
- Develop the skills and knowledge of the workers
- Share responsibility for the group

Step Four: Advertise Group

Groups do not exist in a vacuum and largely rely on the wider community or organisation giving the identified group validity and sanction.

Thus, the first task facing the co-workers is the engagement of the organisation and wider community, ensuring that:

- Individuals are supported outside the group by the organisation, often by a key worker.
- The organisation openly supports the group's aims and objectives.
- The organisation recognises the boundaries of the group in a practical manner, i.e. a dedicated room that will not be interrupted by other staff or visitors.
- The co-workers are given protected time for the organisation and planning of the group.

Advertising

There are a variety of ways to advertise the group, including:

- Presentations to the organisation, including the aims and objectives, practical matters and protocols, that will include a referral form
- A written memo or flyer to each relevant organisation member detailing the points highlighted above

Step Five: Referral Stage

Once the group has been advertised, referrals should begin to reach the co-workers, and they may consider the following:

- There are identified criteria for the group, and each co-worker should be satisfied that every referral meets those criteria.
- Making themselves available to possible referrers to talk through appropriate referrals.
- Visualising the referred individual in the group setting.
- The composition of the group in relation to age, gender, race and presenting difficulty. It is unrealistic to expect a single female or male to attend a group of six or seven members

of the opposite gender. This is not a criterion for exclusion, but rather the need for that particular individual to be made aware that they might be the only male/female.

A letter is often the first contact between the co-workers and the individual referred. It is essential that the letter is clear, concise and friendly. The letter should include a brief statement regarding the aims of the group and include practical statements with regard to the frequency and timing of the group.

Step Six: Individual Assessments and Plenary Session

Individual Assessments

The whole notion of holding individual assessment interviews allows both the referred person and the co-workers the opportunity to explore the viability of working together. It is important that the individual being interviewed voices their own perceived benefits and concerns about attending this group. It is vital that practical considerations are highlighted, e.g. how the person is to travel to the group.

One aspect the co-workers may consider voicing at the initial interview is that they are not expecting the interviewee to commit to the group until they have experienced the plenary session.

Self-Evaluation Forms

There are many ways to evaluate group work, but probably the most rewarding is a self-evaluation form that group members use to monitor their own sense of development. Despite being a self-assessment tool, the by-product may be used in auditing the effectiveness of the group.

Outcome Measures

Whilst self-evaluation is rewarding for group members, outcome measures are increasingly required to demonstrate that an intervention is doing what it set out to achieve. Developing the evidence base for clinical interventions is important, especially in translational science. There is a range of outcome measures recommended for use in CAMHS services. These can be found on the Child Outcomes Research Consortium's website (CORC). Outcome measures can be used at the start of a group and repeated throughout or used at various time points. Independent measures by others, e.g. school teachers, not involved in the intervention, can help to demonstrate the efficacy of an intervention.

Plenary Session

The function of the plenary session is to achieve three distinctive goals:

- To give prospective group members a 'taster' of the group the co-workers hope to run.
- To give all those attending the plenary meeting the opportunity to familiarise themselves with the other group members.
- At the end of the plenary session individuals 'sign up' to the group. This allows the formation of the group and group trust to be initiated through a sense of ownership.

Step Seven: Group up and Running

Members have a right to expect that the co-workers will have a clear plan of how the group will run and operate, in terms of content and style. Time spent by the co-workers before and after each group will allow negotiation of changes to take place so that the material, methods and pace of the group can be constantly adapted to suit the needs of its members.

Such meetings can reduce stress on the partnership by highlighting worker differences, the allocation of group tasks, e.g. who opens or closes the group, who introduces what and when in the group and the administration and record-keeping for the group.

Step Eight: Group Ending

> The best way to achieve a concerted closure is to ensure that everybody knows when that is.
>
> Doel and Sawdon, 2001

The ending of a group is as crucial as the beginning and should be planned by the co-workers and group members well in advance.

The following is a list of useful considerations when planning the end of the group:

- Ensure that the group ends in the same environment as it began.
  This will enable the members to say goodbye both practically and, just as importantly, psychologically.
- Ensure that any graphics or written work produced by the group is on display. This will help with the group evaluation process and encourage individuals to recall the journey they have undertaken in the group's lifetime.
- That, whilst the co-workers hope that the members may keep in contact with one another for on-going support, the group itself is ended and will not be repeated in this format.

Group Evaluation

It is important to recognise that whilst members remain individuals, they, including the co-workers, have shared a unique experience and will need to validate and evaluate that experience as a group. Evaluating the group as a whole permits all the membership to grasp the uniqueness of the group's experience.

Exit Interviews

When the group is ended, the co-workers and individual group members meet up for one last time to consider the progress the individual has made in relation to the group experience. At this interview, the self-evaluation form is again completed and reviewed, alongside the earlier pre-group form. It is important for the individual to identify what has changed for them and how this change has occurred.

The co-workers should be aware that many individuals find it difficult to attend the exit interviews, regardless of how positively, or even negatively, they have viewed their own participation in the group.

One way of maximising the potential for this final exit interview is to arrange exit interviews in the final group session. In the final interview, it is important that the co-workers make reference to the participation of the individual and express openly and with conviction that the uniqueness of the group was down to the participation of that individual being present in the group.

Case Study: Sarah

Sarah (13) is young carer who lives with her disabled mother.

As a result of bullying, Sarah had become more and more isolated and suffered from considerable anxiety at the thought of attending school. The school referred Sarah to the specialist CAMHS, due to her non-attendance and with growing concern about her mental health, both in terms of anxiety and low mood. Both her mother and the school reported that Sarah is an able student but that her anxiety was compromising her ability to attend school and that, at times, she appeared very low in mood.

Outcome

Through an individual assessment with the group's co-workers, Sarah was offered a place in the dialectical behaviour therapy (DBT) group. Sarah attended all 12 sessions. Through direct interventions on issues, e.g. anxiety management, self-esteem and emotional regulation, Sarah was able to 'practice' new ways of challenging, managing and sharing her worries, reducing both her anxiety and low mood. The outcome was rewarding both for Sarah and for her fellow group members. She became more open to discussing her fears with her mother and with her peers. Sarah is taking her GCSEs and now attends school regularly, receiving on-going support from the Young Carers Association. Her mother has a support worker.

Group Work for Parents of Children with ADHD: The New Forest Parenting Programme

Key Ideas

- Group programmes for parents whose children have ADHD should target the neuropsychological deficits seen in ADHD.
- The group should include psychoeducation about ADHD, and this should be tailored to the individual child.
- Groups can provide welcome support for parents whose child has ADHD.

The New Forest Parenting Programme (NFPP) group programme has been developed over a number of years with the help of many parents and professionals. It aims to improve the parents' knowledge of what ADHD is and how it affects their child and to give them a toolkit of ideas to help them to help their child. Helping parents understand ADHD is fundamental to the programme, as is targeting the particular areas of difficulty their child has.

The group allows parents to highlight the special areas of difficulties they recognise in their child and often provides specific, in addition to general, ADHD knowledge. The programme can be used alone or with media productions, e.g. the DVD 'Living with ADHD' (Thompson M., Laver-Bradbury C., Weeks A., Sonuga-Barke E., Chen W., University of Southampton Media Services, 2009). PowerPoint slides or online resources are particularly useful for those parents who have difficulty with literacy or whose learning style is visual. It is worth asking parents discreetly whether they need any help with reading. Experience tells us that often parents with literacy difficulties will have someone whom they trust to read important information to them. If this is not the case, then alternative arrangements need to be identified.

The benefit of a PowerPoint or of video clips is that they provide a focus for discussion and can be shown in sections each week to reinforce the strategies being discussed. On Week One, when parents can be nervous at attending the group and speaking out, they can give a visual reinforcement that they are not the only ones experiencing difficulties, as parents talk about their children on the online resource/PowerPoint. Handouts can be given and shared with partners or grandparents unable to attend the group to provide a consistent approach for the child.

Evidence Base for the NFPP

This group programme has been developed from the New Forest Parenting Programme, a one-to-one home-based intervention (Sonuga-Barke et al., 2001; Thompson et al., 2009), for use in a group format. The benefits of a group intervention are to enable parents to support one another, to share concerns and importantly, for parents to realise they are not the only ones having difficulties. Parents whose children have ADHD are often isolated and feel under-skilled as parents. The group aims to raise the self-esteem of parents, to empower them in being their child's advocate in a variety of settings and to increase their knowledge and understanding of ADHD. This approach has been subject to evaluation (Laver-Bradbury and Harris, 2008).

Age Appropriateness of the NFPP

The NFPP-group programme is not age-specific, although it is most widely used by families of under 12-year olds. The core ADHD characteristics often remain similar after pre-school up until adolescence and arguably into adulthood. The main difference in adolescents is that the hyperactive symptoms in the child reduce and the young person is seen as fidgety and internally restless, rather than hyperactive. Understanding the characteristics is crucial to helping either a younger child or a teenager with ADHD.

Both children and teenagers need to understand themselves, and their good and less good attributes, in addition to learning to problem-solve for themselves. The strategies that parents of adolescents can use are similar, if not the same, as for younger ADHD children, but they need to be adapted to fit the teenage years, i.e. in how the strategies are initiated. Humour can be used to allow the adolescent to understand their difficulties, without feeling humiliated or ridiculed. There should be more of a focus on independence and the skills needed for them to learn to manage on their own.

From experience it is often valuable to have mixed-age groups of children whose parents attend the group and, so long as they are not the only one with a teenager, it seems to work well. This does depend on the young people having ADHD but without conduct disorder. If the adolescent is exhibiting conduct difficulties, it can be worrying for parents of younger children to hear that teenager's problems. It is best to be mindful of this when organising the group. It may be better to run a group specifically for those parents whose children have both ADHD and conduct disorder, as their needs will be different.

Length of the NFPP

The NFPP group programme is a minimum of six, and preferably eight, weeks. It is designed that the weeks can be interchanged to meet the specific needs of the group of parents in the programme. At the beginning, it is important for parents to tell the group leaders what they are hoping to gain from the group. This helps parents feel that they are being listened to and that their concerns are being taken seriously, rather than a 'this is a programme for parents of ADHD children' approach.

Our experience has been, when running the groups, that those parents, when asked, say they want to know how to manage their child's temper outbursts and their own, how to keep calm and how to deal with outside pressures. They appear to have some understanding of the characteristics of ADHD, but have difficulty in recognising these characteristics in their child's behaviour. Exploring and highlighting the characteristics of ADHD throughout the sessions, as parents offer examples, appears to enhance their understanding and allows them to identify what are ADHD characteristics and what are not and then to learn how to deal with difficult issues.

Practicalities

Each week of the programme has an outline of what should be covered. This is based on the NFPP-Step-by-Step, *Helping Your Child with ADHD* (Laver-Bradbury et al., 2010 that is given to parents at the beginning of the group. There is some flexibility in how the sessions can be arranged. The order of the weeks depends on the group requirements, and those can be ascertained in Week One. The outline of the contents of the next five weeks can then be completed and linked to the manual, and a copy given to the parents so they have a rough outline of what will happen each week. This helps the group leaders to remain focussed. Additional problems can be discussed as the group progresses or extra sessions can be added. We have found that review groups approximately six to eight weeks after the end of six-/eight-week programme allow the group to meet up again and support each other and serve as a reminder of the strategies. We use a simple question-and-answer paper for parents as a starting point for discussion.

It is expected that group leaders will have in-depth knowledge of the NFPP and familiarise themselves with the contents, prior to running a course. The group programme is set out in weekly sessions with handouts included for each session. Basic evaluation measures are undertaken at the beginning and end of the group.

Multiple-Choice Questions

See answers on page 673.

1. What is the ideal number of individuals to have in a group setting?
   a. 4–5
   b. 5–7
   c. 6–12
   d. 8–14
   e. 0–16
2. Which of the following is not an essential consideration when setting up a group?
   a. Identifying the need for a group
   b. The group identifying a common need once established
   c. The group co-workers identifying a supervisor
   d. The group and co-workers being of the same gender
   e. The group co-workers having time away from their organisation to facilitate the group
3. What considerations should be considered when running a group for parents?
   a. How to teach parents
   b. Parents' learning style
   c. Making sure everyone agrees
   d. That it is short

Key References

Doel, M., Sawdon, C., (2001). *The Essential Group Worker in Teaching and Learning Creative Group Work* (2nd impression). London & Philadelphia: Jessica Kingsley.

Edward, E., Bem, D.J., Nolan, H., Smith, S., (2000). *Hilgard's Introduction Psychology* (13th Ed.). San Diego: Harcourt College Publishers.

Laver-Bradbury, C., Harris, H., (2008). *Advanced Nurse Practitioners for Attention Deficit Hyperactivity Disorder (In) Department of Health, New Ways of Working in Child and Adolescent Mental Health.* London: Department of Health.

Laver-Bradbury, C., Thompson, M., Weeks, A., Sonuga-Barke, E., Daley, D., (2010). *Step by Step Help for Children with ADHD.* London: Jessica Kingsley.

69 Theoretical Underpinnings of Parent-Led Interventions to Treat Psychopathology in Children

Catherine Thompson, Margaret J.J. Thompson and Cathy Laver-Bradbury

Introduction

Using parents as an agent for change to improve childhood behavioural disorders has been a feature of psychiatry and psychology for over 70 years. This is a prominent method of treatment for the following conditions:

- **Disruptive behaviour disorders** (DBD), e.g. oppositional defiant behaviour, aggressive/socially inappropriate/conduct disorder behaviour and attention disorder hyperactivity disorder (ADHD)
- **Emotional disorders**, e.g. anxiety, school refusal, phobias and obsessive-compulsive disorders (OCD)
- **Autistic spectrum disorders** (ASD), **the** main difference is the use of operant behavioural methods to produce change in ASD versus the use of social rules and natural consequences, though these can be included in children with more developed theory of mind
- **Trauma/abuse/neglect**, e.g. family death/illness, emotional/sexual abuse or early institutional care with physical neglect
- **Learning difficulties**, to support the families
- **High family risk**, e.g. areas of high demographic risk, first-time mothers, poor early parental role model, parental substance abuse or learning difficulties
  See Early Intervention Foundation Guidebook, https://guidebook.eif.org.uk/. **NB** this lists only evidence-based programmes.

Here we look at the role of these programmes in:

- Changing parental attitudes, their understanding of their child and any relevant pathology.
- Parenting styles/behaviours related to effective parenting.
- Relationships between the parent–child dyad and other family members.
- How to structure their child's learning and acquisition of life skills in the context of disrupted behaviour pathology. This will be defined as abnormal levels or severity of socially inappropriate behaviour that cause significant morbidity for individuals, families and society during childhood.

Disruptive Behaviour Disorders (DBD)

Disruptive behaviour disorders in this context refer to any behaviour expressed by children that is deemed socially inappropriate, according to their age/developmental level, and causes them or others significant negative consequences.

Changing child behaviour by adapting parenting approaches or teaching parents to use specific strategies and more positive alternatives has been around for at least 60 years. Table 69.1 shows the origins and psychosocial and developmental theories underpinning current available interventions.

Despite being able to diagnose disruptive behaviour disorders, we are still not consistently identifying and treating them effectively. (Sonuga-Barke et al., 2013). This is reflected in outcomes, e.g. increased family stress in families living with ADHD (Barkley, 2013, poor academic achievement and future employment prospects (Mannuza et al., 1993), social and romantic relationships failure and levels of ADHD in incarcerated young people (Faraone, Biederman and Mick, 2006) comparable across studies. Three issues appear to prevent researchers reaching clear, consistent and translational results (results that can be directly used to improve diagnosis, treatment and prevent long-term problems) from these conditions:

- Large individual variation in genetic risk and key environmental processes and how these interact across time.
- Inconsistent ways of measuring these in different studies, often due to problems around power and sample size, resulting in different variables being included and measurements not being comparable across studies.
- Differences in the way DBD conditions are diagnosed, treated and followed up over time, e.g. trying to compare medication treatment with parent-led behavioural interventions, when some are interventions are eight weeks long and others continue for up to two years.

What Is the Role of Parenting in the Presentation of DBD and the Short-/Long-Term Prognosis in Children?

Here we use the word 'parenting' to bring together any aspect of the way the parent feels, behaves towards and interacts with their child. This can be extended to how two parents/carers, if present, work together or differently, in terms of how they 'hold the child' through to adulthood. Siblings, other carers and academic settings become increasing relevant as the child grows older and can have both positive and negative impacts on the child in terms of DBD problems.

As with all aspects of assessing, treating and monitoring psychopathology in children, clinicians will have to develop their own framework to manage each individual. The following sections show the evidence of how different parenting elements may come together to produce a certain pattern of behaviour. Understanding these processes and their relative role in a family can help clinicians identify possible lines of treatment and prioritise them (genetic risk of presenting with externalising behaviour at a pathological level (Leve, 2007)).

Oppositional defiant disorder (ODD), conduct disorder (CD) and ADHD have a high level of genetic risk attached to them (Thapar et al., 2001).

Genetic risk can be thought of as the baseline chance at conception/birth one child has of ever showing DBD at a problematic level during their lifetime compared to another. There is increasing evidence from behavioural genetic studies for a role of genetic influences in the aetiology of CD/ODD, with 40–50% of variance in these conditions explained by heritable factors and a relatively large contribution of shared environmental factors relative to other psychiatric disorders (Rhee and Waldman, 2002) and for ADHD (Plomin et al., 1994; Chen and Taylor, 2006).

The high level of genetic heritability behind externalising behaviour and specific diagnostic criteria such as ADHD could suggest that changing parenting and/or environment in the early years might not be a useful avenue of treatment. Twin studies, combined with adoption and

Table 69.1 Origins of Parenting Programmes

Behavioural Parent Training, Hanf 1969 Social learning theory Operant conditioning direct to mother–child dyad ('bug in ear') Family systems theory Life skills					**PMT-Oregon Model**, Patterson 1982 Coercive-cyclical processes Causal model and factors behind severe CD
Parent–Child Interaction Therapy, Eyberg	**Defiant Child**, Barkley	**Helping the Non-Compliant Child**, Forehand and Mahon	**Incredible Years**, Webster-Stratton	**COPE**, Cunningham	**Adaptions for specialist groups**
Closest to original Hanf model **Attachment** theory and use of **play**	**ADHD targets** **Group learning** vs. individual **School** vs. home consistency	**Generalising** to non-home environments	Natural and **social-based consequences** and response cost **Video-based** examples with parents **role playing in groups**	**Video examples** with problem-solving parenting in **large discussion groups**	**Foster care** (Chamberlain, 1994); **Substance abuse** (Dishion and Kavanagh, 2003); **Single-mothers** (Forgatch, 1994); **Stepfamilies** (Forgatch and Rains, 1997) **Risk for conduct disorder**, e.g. abusive environments (Ramsey, Antoine, Kavanagh and Reid, 1992a, 1992b)
New Forest Parenting Programme, Thompson, Laver-Bradbury and Weeks		**Attributions and the effects** on parent–child relationship and behavioural analysis		**Triple P**, Saunders	
ADHD-specific psychoeducation **Adaption** of behavioural strategies and play **for ADHD neurocognitive deficits**		Holding the parent through change: **i.e. managing deeper cognitions and schema** without drifting into other therapeutic roles		**Use of resiliency and child positive** attributes. **Role of larger social systems** in making change at population level in antisocial behaviour	

surrogacy, show that adding in non-shared genetic and environmental influences in development and outcome from DBD lowers the impact of genetic influences significantly. Given the large impact of DBD on individuals and society, neglecting to address these factors is not an option (Leve et al., 2007).

The Role of Positive and Negative Parenting on the Pathology and Severity of DBD in Children

The second source of evidence for the role of parent-led treatment in DBD is the clear link between parenting behaviours or styles that lower the child's level of genetic risk for DBD problems and those that increase the likelihood they will show significant problems (Thompson et al., 2002; Kaminski et al., 2008). Parenting behaviours that affect the development, severity and long-term problems from DBD in children are shown in Table 69.2.

The conclusion from cross-sectional and longitudinal data is that the behaviour a parent shows to their child or the style they use to parent them significantly changes their child's externalising behaviour over time as expected (Reid and Patterson, 1989). But these studies and meta-analyses show that a child who expresses significant levels of DBD results in a parent showing less positive behaviours/parenting style and more negative/less protective ones. This bi-directional effect is found for parental responsiveness/warmth, good positive behaviour control, an authoritative style, harsh/negative control and psychological control. This gives some indication for the type of behavioural strategies that may be effective in parent-led behavioural interventions to treat DBD.

Other Processes between Parent–Child and Family that Add to the Child's DBD Genetic Risk

These behaviours as measured on a questionnaire or observation do not directly suggest the process by which the parenting behaviour/style causes improvement or worsening of the child's behaviour. It is worth looking briefly at different aspects of the parent–child interaction and relationship that are potentially processes by which parenting links to DBD in the child. This will lead into the strategies used by most parenting programmes currently available.

Table 69.2 Parental Style or Behaviour

Parental Behaviour or Style	This increases/decreases the chances of a child developing and having adverse effects from EB problems
Harsh/negative control Including physical or verbal punishment	Worsens...
Psychological control i.e. negative emotional manipulation, e.g. humiliation	Worsens...
Good positive behaviour control e.g. clear, consistent *boundaries*	Protects against...
Parental responsiveness/warmth e.g. sensitivity and positive comments	Protects against...
Autonomy granting i.e. encouraging independence without over-intrusiveness	Protects against...

Parent–Child Emotional Relationship

The first process by which parenting and associated environment can protect against or worsen the chances of a child having significant DBD in older years is the parent–child emotional relationship. The psychosocial and behavioural theories that provide explanations as to why this could worsen a child's emotional and behavioural self-regulation are attachment, positive reciprocal parent–child interaction and social learning theory.

Attachment

- Attachment status is linked to significant levels of DBD in children. Studies show that attachment status of any insecure type significantly distinguishes between children with and without DBD.
- Disorganised versus secure attachment is more strongly linked to DBD.
- Gender moderates the effect of attachment status to levels of DBD in both the associations.
- Having a (presumed) higher severity of child DBD can change the relationship between attachment status and DBD pathology.
- Socioeconomic status does not affect the relationship between attachment and DBD in children (Rutter et al., 2009).

Positive Reciprocal Parent–Child Interaction

This, although not a named theory historically, is based on the work of Reid and Paterson (Reid and Patterson, 1989) around coercive parent–child interactions and the role this has in antisocial behaviour pathology. Using traditional behavioural theories of reinforcement (Pavlov) and conditioning (Skinner) (McLeod, 2007) these authors noticed the role of positive reinforcement of negative behaviour in maintaining a cycle of non-constructive discipline between parent and child.

Positive parenting practices that have been shown to protect a child against problems from DBD pathology are those that epitomise positive reciprocal parent–child interaction and the negative consequences from less positive parenting are the reciprocal effects the child can show back to the parent (Miller-Lewis et al., 2006). The degree of positive versus negative parent–child interaction tends to be quantified using scoring systems applied to observed interaction of the parent and child during a structured play situation, e.g. working together on a puzzle.

Social Learning Theory

The work of Bandura and colleagues (Bandura, 1978) outlines the fact that children learn by observing repeatedly over time how others handle certain social, emotive and behavioural situations, not only by trial and error. This, in the context of DBD pathology, is most significant in how children learn and apply social rules to fit into society.

'Social rules' is a term that incorporates systems theory and cognitive sociology to explain how children develop a framework for what is, and is not, appropriate in expressed emotions and behaviour. Negative parental behaviours and environments that worsen DBD pathology in terms of social learning theory are those that are inconsistent, e.g. rule setting between parents, those for which the enforced rules with the child are not modelled by the parents, e.g. mutual respect for others, psychological/emotional manipulation and physical abuse and the influence of wider systems, e.g. religion, influence of local neighbourhood support networks or negative influences, morality and criminality.

In conclusion, many parent-led interventions focus mainly on behavioural change and do not identify and work on matters around the parent–child emotional relationship. The following are important foundations for a child to gain from their emotional experiences in early childhood, if the parent is to be influential in managing the DBD child's behaviour (Grych et al., 2001):

- Self-esteem – so that they feel they are a good enough person inside.
- Self-belief – that they think other people think they are a good enough person and that others need and want them around.
- Self-efficacy – that, within reason, if they try hard and keep going, they can succeed in what they want to achieve.

Behaviour Resulting from the Child's Behavioural Self-Regulation and Effortful Control

In the context of DBD pathology and more specifically ADHD, this is an important process by which parenting and associated factors can protect or worse a child's genetic risk of long-term DBD sequelae.

Aspects that are less controllable in the child are:

- **Temperament**
- **Emotionality** – how quickly, how fast and how much a child physiologically responds to emotional triggers. High emotionality, with high/over-sensitivity and minute-to-minute fluctuations, is a feature of people with ADHD.
- **Reactive control** – the child's internal capacity for holding that emotion and coping with it until it recedes with time, without needing to externalise it as behaviour that might have negative consequences.
- **Effortful control** – bottom-up control that is driven by the emotional system.
- **Inattention** – whether a child is aroused enough and maintains that arousal high enough to remain alert to changes in their emotional and physical environment.
- **Impulsivity** – how aware a child is of the link between their sensory systems, sub- and fully conscious thought processes and behavioural reactions so they can stop themselves reacting without thinking beforehand.

This is the only area in which medication management may need to be prioritised over parent-led behavioural treatment. If a child has such poor attention that they are not receiving the cues they need to learn to self-regulate effectively or are so impulsive that they cannot prevent showing behaviour with negative consequences, medication is indicated, especially for inattention.

More learned and strategy-dependent aspects of self-regulation are:

- **Effortful control – top down**: this incorporates how a child uses goal-directed behaviour in combination with potential consequences of their behavioural choices to maintain long-term family, social, work and romantic relationships.
- **Motivation and effort** including using long-term rewards versus short-term rewards and how strong the reward is. Children with ADHD have abnormal delay-reward curves (Marco et al., 2009).
- **Social rules**.
- **Mood and anxiety influences** including the child attributions and experience of stigma around their own DBD problems, as they age.

Strategies for lowering ADHD/impulse- or inattention-led behaviour are mainly to do with:

- Identifying the child's triggers to poor self-regulation and minimising the effect of these (e.g. planning ahead, quiet time).
- Encouraging the child to understand the way emotions affect the body and to spot the times at which they might be about to react impulsively, i.e. 'stop and think' before they do in addition to talking about feelings and asking for help.
- Rewarding positive behaviour and ignoring, as far as possible, negative behaviour.

Prevent or Stop the Cycles of Coercive Behaviour between the Parent and Child

Externalising behaviour is worsened by negative patterns of parent–child interaction around boundary-setting and enforcing rules. This is especially relevant in children with oppositionality- or callous/unemotional-type personality traits.

Impulse- and inattention-led behaviours that cause unwanted consequences are more likely to be managed by good organisation and planning, structure and routine, boundary-setting and consistent parenting by everyone involved in the child's care. Children with oppositionality and those with less empathy and motivation to think of others are more likely to stick to their own goal, even if that means they affect their emotional relationships in the short and long term.

From the parent's point of view, children who are always resisting their authority, and not necessarily open to positive reward and praise to choose positive ways of achieving their goals, are difficult to live with. The parent may be left feeling less satisfied with their parenting and as having less positive, relationship-building times with their child. In addition, they need more emotional energy and support to manage even the smallest everyday exchanges that can increase the likelihood that they will struggle to self-regulate their own behaviour.

In parent-led interventions, whether individual, or group-based, most therapists/facilitators will use 'episodes' in the family's day-to-day life to illustrate areas and strategies for change. Coercive cycles can be identified using the framework of antecedents, behaviour and consequences (ABC), and this framework is often used in the context of carrying out 'functional analysis' of goal-driven behaviours (Hastings, 2000).

Once the parent and therapist/group facilitator have identified the cycles they wish to break, they need to know what the replacement behaviour or strategy is going to be for the longer term. The parent needs to know why they are using this strategy, e.g. quiet time as a positive reinforcer for the child's environment control versus time-out when they finally lose control, and how that strategy will make their lives easier in the long run.

The parent needs to find the right motivation for the child to successfully apply the strategy and have the energy and skills to 'hold the child through change' whilst they achieve it.

Parent–Child Working Relationship and Its Role in Prevention or Intervening in DBD Problems

Parent child working relationship is a term used to refer to the way a parent works with their child to help them learn how to learn, i.e. trial and error and learning by observation. The role of a parent changes as the child ages, in terms of modelling and structuring their development and learning. This change involves balancing sensitivity and supporting and addressing the child's needs with encouraging independence and allowing the child to exert their autonomy, as they discover the person they want to be. Several theories exist in the teaching literature about how children learn. Behaviourally structuring a child's learning in all aspects of development is known as 'scaffolding'.

Scaffolding and the Zone of Proximal Development

Scaffolding theory in learning terms (Fani and Ghaemi, 2011) looks at the role of an expert supporting a novice in learning essential skills. It involves repeating the steps in Figure 69.1 repeatedly until the child has fully mastered the task.

The Zone of Proximal Development is the area between what the child can do now with no support and the next step that they cannot do yet independently. These are difficult concepts to relay to parents. The principles of breaking down learning into steps, modelling the skills and explaining the relevant concepts to the child, helping the parent to identify the relevant strategies and supporting them as they trial them, are fundamental and achievable in practice.

This is especially important when using parent-led interventions for children with ADHD for two reasons. First, the child themselves may have problems with executive functioning and with issues around motivation, delay/reward, attention and secondary effects of failure. Second, the parent may themselves have ADHD and all these cognitive sequelae and they need to be taught how to structure their own lives and to problem-solve if they are to model these skills for their child. Self-regulation and impulsivity in the parent can be expressed as frustration

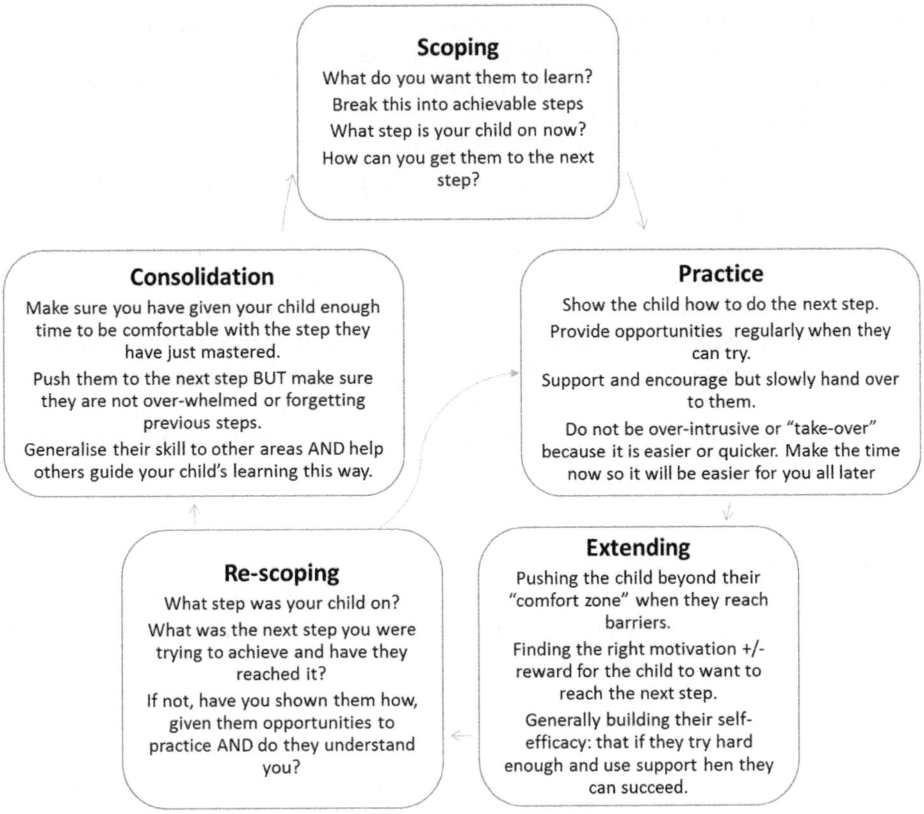
Scoping
What do you want them to learn?
Break this into achievable steps
What step is your child on now?
How can you get them to the next step?
Practice
Show the child how to do the next step.
Provide opportunities regularly when they can try.
Support and encourage but slowly hand over to them.
Do not be over-intrusive or "take-over" because it is easier or quicker. Make the time now so it will be easier for you all later
Extending
Pushing the child beyond their "comfort zone" when they reach barriers.
Finding the right motivation +/- reward for the child to want to reach the next step.
Generally building their self-efficacy: that if they try hard enough and use support hen they can succeed.
Re-scoping
What step was your child on?
What was the next step you were trying to achieve and have they reached it?
If not, have you shown them how, given them opportunities to practice AND do they understand you?
Consolidation
Make sure you have given your child enough time to be comfortable with the step they have just mastered.
Push them to the next step BUT make sure they are not over-whelmed or forgetting previous steps.
Generalise their skill to other areas AND help others guide your child's learning this way.

Figure 69.1 Scaffolding and the Zone of Proximal Development.

and impatience with the child and are often barriers for the child to achieve independence and gain effective learning skills.

Systems Theory: Consistency in Parenting within and beyond the Family Unit

Systems theory originates from engineering. When applied in the field of sociology, it takes the form of family therapy. The concept is that the 'difficulty' is not based within the individual, but in the reciprocal interactions, that can be with another individual or a wider system. The belief is that the 'difficulty' is serving a purpose for the system or the relationship.

One of the theories used within family therapy is to observe the behaviour in the context of the family and to help parents become aware of patterns of interactions that are maintaining the behaviour and, should they choose, take steps to alter them. The therapist can explore a parent's knowledge of a particular mental health condition and think about the effect this narrative has on the individual and on the family. This can help their understanding of their child and the possible purpose behind a behaviour.

By examining the behaviour with the parents, and perhaps with the teachers, in the particular setting or context in which it occurs, an understanding of the cause and maintenance of the behaviour can be explored. In particular, a focus on the parenting system, if in couple relationships, can be useful in order to explore different attributions.

The role of wider systems in parent-led interventions mainly comes in after the therapist/facilitator has worked with the parent to promote understanding of the child's problems and helped them to identify which of their child's behaviours they wish to change. Putting strategies in place to make these changes with the parent and child dyad is the next step. Once the parent is proficient and confident in making the changes they feel they can, need and want to make, other parties can be brought in.

The second parent/carer, if present in the child's life, is one of the main targets for consistency in how the child is managed. Barriers to encouraging the parent and child to work together in using parenting to change DBD are, e.g. different attributions as to why the child behaves the way they do, different levels of acceptability of the child's behaviour and whether they agree it needs to change, practical issues like time available to learn strategies and practise them with the child, emotional issues around fitting their role into that of their partner's and lacking confidence in discussing differences of opinion and finally that second parents/carers in a family unit rarely attend the parent-led intervention sessions with their partner, not necessarily by choice. They may be discouraged from doing so. Siblings, extended family, social networks, e.g. religious gatherings, support groups and/or school are the other systems that can be fundamental in achieving effective and long-term change.

A therapist/facilitator works with the parent to discuss if and how they could ensure others are working to manage their child's DBD in the same way as they are. It is important to remember that the parent themselves may need to compromise in some aspects and may find that other people or places have had more success, using a different approach. Unfortunately, the short nature of most parent-led interventions and the lack of provision for repeated courses or supportive follow-up prevent this in many cases.

Key References

Sanders, M.R., (1999). Triple P-Positive Parenting Program: towards an empirically validated multilevel parenting and family support strategy for the prevention of behavior and emotional problems in children. *Clinical Child and Family Psychology Review*, *2*(2): 71–90.

Sonuga-Barke, E.J., Daley, D., Thompson, M., Laver-Bradbury, C., Weeks, A., (2001). Parent-based therapies for preschool attention-deficit/hyperactivity disorder: a randomized, controlled trial with a community sample. *Journal of the American Academy of Child & Adolescent Psychiatry*, 40(4): 402–408.

Webster-Stratton, C., Reid, M.J., (2018). *The Incredible Years Parents, Teachers, and Children Training Series: A Multifaceted Treatment Approach for Young Children with Conduct Problems.*

70 Parenting Programmes

Cathy Laver-Bradbury

KEY CONCEPTS

- Different parenting programmes target different difficulties and can be underpinned by different theoretical models.
- Choose the programme most suited to the child's difficulties and the parent's needs.
- Remember that parents often need 'top-ups' post-parenting programme in order to maintain progress.
- In the absence of support nationally over the last ten years there has been an increase in the commissioning of private providers to meet the needs of the parents.

Background

Programmes to support parents in raising children have been around for a number of years. However, the evidence for their long-term effectiveness is limited. Various governments have invested in both preventative and intervention programmes. A high-profile example of this was the establishment of 'Sure Start' (1998) areas, in which a variety of services are available for families to support their parenting. These were often found in areas of deprivation and poverty, both factors known to be associated with behaviour problems in children. The change in government, and with this different priorities, has seen the demise of many of the Sure Start centres over the years with few remaining.

In 2007, the National Academy of Parenting Practitioners (NAPP) received government funding for a number of functions that included listing and evaluating the parenting programmes being used in practice in England. The academy was funded to commission the training of practitioners able to deliver parenting programmes to ensure that there were trained staff in each area to support parents in need of help.

NAPP produced a Tool Kit for commissioners to provide information about these programmes. NAPP researchers rated the programmes on a number of factors. One of these was that the research evidence available for the programmes indicated their suitability for different age groups and presenting problems. Higher ratings were given to those programmes evaluated in randomised controlled trials.

The Tool Kit allowed commissioners access to the programmes with the most robust evidence. A significant amount of training for practitioners was commissioned throughout the UK. Predominantly, these were the Incredible Years Programmes imported from the USA, that help children with conduct disorder (Webster-Stratton, 1991; Jones et al., 2007) and the

Triple P Parenting Programme from Australia (Bor et al., 2004). Both of these have demonstrated evidence in improving children's behaviour problems.

NAPP encouraged training on a smaller scale, for a number of other programmes aimed at specific groups such as Mellow Parenting for parents with relationship problems with their children (Puckering, 2004) and the New Forest Parenting Programme (Sonuga-Barke et al., 2001; Thompson, M.J.J. et al., 2009), an early intervention parenting programme for pre-school children presenting with ADHD difficulties. These programmes were seen as specialist programmes targeting specific difficulties, rather than a more general 'catch-all' approach.

NAPP's work ceased in 2010 and has been replaced by the Early Intervention Foundation (EIF), https://www.eif.org.uk. This is the organisation currently providing information about parenting programmes. The EIF produces a guidebook that provides information on a range of parenting interventions, the evidence for their effectiveness, the delivery model, the age group they target and where the intervention takes place, in addition to the child outcomes and cost rating. It looks at the availability of these across countries.

In 2011 the Department of Health publication 'Delivering Better Mental Health Outcomes for People of All Ages' (DH, 2011) discussed the use of parenting interventions for young people presenting with mental health difficulties.

In 2017 the government again looked at parenting programs in terms of the Social Mobility framework. The Global Social Mobility Index, published again in 2020, outlines why economies benefit from fixing inequality. It discusses the five determinants of social mobility, i.e. health, education, technology access, work opportunities, working conditions and fair wages and, finally, social protection and inclusive institutions. Social mobility is seen as an important factor for economic growth and in this context, parenting was further explored. The literature review by the Social Mobility Commission looked at the extent to which public policy levers can influence what parents do and what those policy levers might be.

The advisory group produced a report, 'Helping Parents to Parent', and found the following:

- There is evidence to demonstrate that public policy can have an impact on parenting behaviours.
- The most successful parenting interventions appear to include a focus on equipping parents with a greater understanding of child development.
- Research suggests that parenting advice has a significant influence on developing parental confidence in their role and reducing stress and tension within the family.
- Some governments are beginning to approach universal parental support as a public health issue. Although there is a lack of robust evaluation for many 'universal' parenting interventions at present, it appears that this approach is beginning to normalise the concept of support for parenting, leading to success in engaging parents.
- To reduce the stigma associated with parenting interventions and to encourage parents to seek the help and support they need, the interventions delivered 'targeted' services under the umbrella term 'universal'. This resulted in enhanced parental participation. A localised approach can help to enhance parental engagement in parenting programmes.
- Home visiting programmes, alongside services delivered to groups of parents, appear to have moderate to high levels of success. Highly trained and skilled practitioners are crucial to the successful delivery of parenting interventions. Some successful interventions recruited practitioners from a broad range of professionals, e.g. nurses, social workers and teachers, to deliver parenting support.
- There is a lack of longitudinal and follow-up studies in the evidence. This limits long-term findings. Much of the assessment of the success of parenting interventions is based on their short-term gains. The government should commission further research to address

the gaps in this evidence, and a robust and consistent tool for the evaluation of parenting interventions is needed.

For the full details, see https://www.gov.uk/government/publications/helping-parents-to-parent.

Summary

Different governments have shown an interest in parenting over several years. Different departments of government have different reasons for their interest, e.g. raising educational attainment, Dept. of Education; the impact on children's mental health, Dept. of Health; and most recently, the link to economic growth. All in their own way have recognised the important role of parents in helping children.

Consistent government policies supporting parents across government departments do not appear to be co-ordinated or well evaluated in the long term.

This is in part likely to be due to the frequent changes in government and their changing focus on parenting policies and support for them. There is the question of what the evaluation of programmes is trying to achieve. Most programme developers target specific outcomes based on the aim of the programme and its usefulness for parents. They are not focussed on what effect their programme has in 30 years' time on the economic wellbeing of the child.

Which Parenting Programme?

There are several parenting programmes available for families. These range in cost, length of delivery and the age group of the children to whom they apply. They can be delivered on an individual basis or in a group setting. Both approaches are facilitated by voluntary workers, in addition to members of the statutory services, e.g. social workers, health visitors, school nurses, educational psychologists and teachers.

More recently private organisations can bid for a role as providers of parenting programmes. Some are well-recognised organisations, e.g. Barnardo's. Others are less recognised nationally, but known locally (Pentecost, D., 2000).

Alongside the research in the parenting programmes there is some significant research regarding which attributes in parents may make accessing a parenting programme difficult, e.g. parental ADHD (Sonuga-Barke et al., 2002), and what support is needed to maintain engagement and motivation (Green, 2006; McCurdy, K. et al., 2006; Routh et al., 1995; Kazdin et al., 2006).

Theoretical Background

Parenting programmes can make use of different theoretical backgrounds.

- Some parenting interventions might use a psychodynamic understanding of parenting in order to promote 'attachment' behaviours between a parent and child. This approach is often used for children who have experienced developmental trauma and/or abuse and for those children who are fostered or adopted.
- Others may use a more biological basis especially if linked to a diagnosis, e.g. using psychoeducation to help parents understand their child's difficulties, e.g. children with ASD or ADHD.

- Cognitive theories in a programme might target the attributions of a parent and child and their meanings. The programme might choose to explore those attributions that are helpful and challenge those that are less so. This approach can be useful for young people experiencing anxiety or depression.
- The behavioural model is often seen in parenting programmes, and parenting programmes can be developed around this model. Parents are seen as the prime agents of change and are encouraged to look at and analyse the underlying problem. They are helped to understand that behaviour is learned and can be changed and to target trying to change the child's non-compliance. Techniques are taught around shaping behaviour, ignoring bad behaviour in order to lead to extinction, using clear commands especially 'do' commands rather than 'don't' commands, 'catching the good', using alpha and beta commands, i.e. alpha commands are positive and aim to increase a child's compliance. Beta commands do not allow a child a clear opportunity to respond, using the 'five second rule' so as to give the child time to respond, use of house rules and clear behavioural expectations. This approach is often used in children with oppositional behaviour or conduct problems (Forehand, R. and Long, N., 1996).
- Systemic approaches to parenting remove the focus of the difficulty as perceived as belonging to the child to one where it is viewed as something that has arisen to serve a purpose for the system that they are in. It looks at the interactive relationships within a family and explores their meanings and function to the family, or school, system. This approach is often used in children and young people with eating disorders but can be used with a range of difficulties.

Whilst I have separated the theoretical models out, in reality most of the parenting programmes use a variety of models in their development, e.g. the New Forest Parenting Programme, that was written to support parents of children displaying features of ADHD, incorporates all the theoretical models (Thompson et al., 2017; Thompson et al., in preparation).

What to Consider When Recommending a Parenting Programme

It is important for the therapist to have the knowledge and experience of a programme and its theoretical underpinnings, in addition to understanding the particular problems the child has, before recommending a parenting programme to a family. This means the therapist is able to outline to a parent why a particular programme could help the parent and her child and what she would gain from attending.

An assessment of the parent's particular parenting style would be useful, e.g. if a parent has a very authoritative parenting style then a programme primarily aimed at discipline may not be helpful. Equally a programme based on play, for parents who already play with their child, may not bring about a change in behaviour or the willing participation of the parents.

As a professional choosing how to deliver a parent training programme, it is important to consider whether this is best done on an individual basis or within a group setting. Sometimes, a combination of both approaches helps parents. Initially seeing a parent at home may help the parent transition to a group if she has already met the professional who will be running the group.

Group Delivery of Parenting Programmes

Advantages

- Positive interactions between parents.
- Parents can learn from each other.

- A chance to socialise.
- Can facilitate programme delivery to a large number of parents at once.
- Possibility of fewer distractions.
- Possible use of crèche.
- Can be fun.
- May provide additional encouragement for both parents to attend.

Disadvantages

- Better to work with a co-therapist, so more expensive and requires planning and discussion.
- Finding a suitable venue, with appropriate equipment and chairs.
- Cost of venue.
- Staff to run crèche.
- Possibility of being side-tracked.
- Managing different views within the group.
- Reliant on people attending regularly.
- Confidentiality for group members.
- Location of venue may not suit everyone, and times of sessions may be inconvenient.
- Reliant on advertising for group members.
- Too many in a group.
- Parents may be intimidated by other group members.

Individually Delivered Parenting Programmes

Advantages

- Could be in family home.
- Chance to 'model' some of the interactions with the child.
- More personalised approach.
- Appointments can be tailored to the family's schedule and may mean parents are more likely to attend.
- A chance to practise advice in own situation.
- Easier to 'hold' through change.
- Can begin the sessions immediately with no need to wait to make up numbers for a group.

Disadvantages

- Staff travel time, if in family home.
- Less chance of learning from others doing same programme.
- Can be difficult, if child is present, especially if parent is being negative.
- Less in control of environment, e.g. visitors, TV, safety factors and so on.
- There may be less commitment from parent.
- The professional must consider what is the purpose of offering a parenting programme.
- Has the parent approached you for help or is it that you feel they may benefit from some of the advice available? This can affect compliance. Is there an education aspect to the programme?
- Are you aiming to offer support rather than advice? Which do you feel may be more effective at this time?
- How do you assess whether the programme is having the desired outcomes? For you? For the family? For the child?

Research confirms that group-run parenting programmes are effective (Webster-Stratton, 1991; Jones et al., 2007). But even the best researched parenting programmes have a drop-out from the intervention offered, sometimes as high as 50%. This implies that for 50% of families, it was unhelpful. There have been a number of reasons given for this. These include parental factors and child factors, in addition to some of the disadvantages listed above.

Why Parenting Programmes May Not Work

Parent Factors

- Often only one parent attends the session, so the approach taken may be inconsistently applied. There may be a lack of partner support for the parent attending.
- Parental depression.
- Parental ADHD.
- Wrong timing for parent emotionally, e.g. too much else going on to focus on changing behaviours, e.g. domestic violence, divorce.
- Lack of motivation.
- Dislike of having to do 'homework'.
- Parental attributions.
- Physical illness in parent/s.
- Mental illness in parent/s.

Child Factors

- Parenting advice may not suit temperament of child.
- Undiagnosed developmental disorder, e.g. ADHD, autistic spectrum disorder, speech and language disorder.
- Emotionally sensitive child.
- Physical illness in child.
- Mental illness in child.

Reflection and Evaluation

After each session, it is important for the practitioners to reflect on how the session went. This can be done with the parent(s) and alone, and can be done in a number of ways. Reflecting back to the parent acts as a summary of what has been said and offers an opportunity for the parent to say if she thinks something has been particularly helpful. Often written information is used to back up what has been said, as people absorb different amounts of information.

Using diaries to monitor behaviour can be useful, especially if the diary is designed with a 'how did you resolve this?' type question. This can often demonstrate how the parent has interpreted the advice given and checks their understanding. Personal reflection can be very useful, especially if you are able to recognise what may be transference or countertransference occurring in the group. Understanding and recognising emotions that may not originate with the practitioner can be a vital skill when working with parents. It enables emotions to be brought into the room, that can be explored with parents before strategies can be used.

There is often a grieving period for parents for the child they wanted, often a quiet compliant one, as opposed to the child they have, e.g. a busy 'into-everything' one. This may happen half-way through a programme and needs to be acknowledged. There is no quick fix for most behavioural changes.

Parenting advice is based on helping the parent accept the child they have, with their particular temperament, in order to find a way to work with the child to change behaviours. This includes acknowledgement of the child and the role the parent has with that child. This may be difficult and can cause a variety of emotions within the parent.

Questionnaires can be used at the beginning and end of the whole programme as a way of evaluating its effectiveness. Consideration should be given to how these are used. Is the parent to complete them in the presence of the professional? This could have an influence on how the parent completes them. Ideally, the evaluation should be given or sent, after the parenting programme intervention, with a stamped addressed envelope provided for return and parents' anonymity assured, This may allow for more freedom in the information received. The return rate for questionnaires is often very low. The compromise is to give the parents the questionnaire, to complete anonymously and then place in a sealed envelope.

If you want to measure change from the beginning to end of an intervention, then using a colleague, who was not involved in the delivery, who can give the parent a unique number identifier only known to this colleague and thus when analysed the confidentiality of a questionnaire is maintained from the beginning to the end of the course, and can then be evaluated without identification of participants

If working with a colleague, it is possible to review each other's parent or group. This could involve a possible focus group or interview, to explore with the parent what she gained from the intervention. This gives parents a chance to say what may have been more helpful or what they would have liked more of, without offending the professional involved in the work.

The outcomes described above, and generally used, are focussed on the here-and-now, i.e. has the programme helped you to help your child? Independent measures of the child's behaviour can support the view that it has been helpful, i.e. from the child's school, but are rarely available in clinical services.

Long-term follow-up is rare as is the collation of evidence on a national basis, so that long-term effects could be reviewed. This would have significant cost and analysis difficulties given the number of programmes available and would require significant policies and financial support.

To some extent the IAPT programme that has favoured the USA's Incredible Years Programme (Webster-Stratton, 1991; 2011; Jones et al., 2007), for children with oppositional and conduct problems, has been trying to address this in its training of IAPT parenting practitioners, with close supervision of practitioners and analysis of their results.

Webster-Stratton has follow-up studies on her cohorts of children treated approximately 12 years after treatment. The original intervention was at between ages three and eight years, and the follow-up demonstrates some lasting effects.

Multiple-Choice Questions

See answers on page 673.

1. What should you consider when recommending a parent to attend a parenting programme?
    a. Suitability of the programme to meet the parent's needs
    b. The location
    c. The parental motivation
    d. All of the above
2. The Early Intervention Foundation was preceded by
    a. The NHS
    b. Education
    c. The National Association for Parenting Practitioners
    d. Social services

3. When trying to find information regarding the evidence base for parenting programmes, what is the best place to look?
   a. https://www.eif.org.uk
   b. Commissioners
   c. University libraries
   d. Private companies

Key References

Clarke, B., Younas, F., (2017). Helping Parents to Parent Crown copyright 2017 https://www.gov.uk/government/publications/helping-parents-to-parent.

Delivering Better Mental Health Outcomes for People of all Ages' (DH, 2011). the Early Intervention Foundation (EIF) https://www.eif.org.uk.

Kazdin, A.E., Whitley, M., Marciano, P.L., (2006). Child–therapist and parent–therapist alliance and therapeutic change in the treatment of children referred for oppositional, aggressive, and antisocial behavior. *Journal of Child Psychology and Psychiatry*, 47(5): 436–445.

McCurdy, K., Daro, D., Anisfeld, E., Katzev, A., Keim, A., LeCroy, C., ... Park, J.K., (2006). Understanding maternal intentions to engage in home visiting programs. *Children and Youth Services Review*, 28(10): 1195–1212.

Part VII

Making Sense of Available Services

Christopher Gale

This final section broadens the view of support for children, young people and their families. Whilst identifying the specialist mental health provision with CAMH services, it also outlines the support offered by partner agencies in the statutory and voluntary sectors to promote positive mental well-being. How this looks across the United Kingdom will vary by geographical area, so the chapters here reflect some of the key provisions within a county in the south of England.

This section can be divided broadly into several 'parts': early access (health, education and social care) and specialist services (health, education and social care).

71 Early Access

Self-Help for Children, Young People and Families with Mental Health Difficulties

Melissa McKimm and Christopher Gale

Introduction

The National Institute for Health and Care Excellence (NICE, 2011) in its guidance *Common mental health problems: identification and pathways to care*, describe three main areas of self-help for mild to moderate mental health difficulties across the age spectrum (individual non-facilitated self-help, individual facilitated self-help and group-based). The aim of this guidance was to offer a viable alternative to the use of psychotropic medication, particularly in primary care settings. If a child or young person is referred to specialist CAMHS, self-help interventions should only be introduced as part of an agreed plan of care with the child or young person and their family/carers (NICE, 2019).

KEY CONCEPTS

- **Non-facilitated self-help,** sometimes known as pure self-help or bibliotherapy, often involves the provision of written or computer-based materials that are informed by age-appropriate cognitive behavioural therapy (CBT). In specialist CAMHS, practitioners would have limited involvement in this process. The child or young person would be advised to work through the materials with the support of a parent, as appropriate to age, usually over a period of six weeks. This could be supported within Tiers 1, 2 or 3 of the Stepped Care model (NICE, 2019), depending on the structure of local service provision.
- **Individual facilitated self-help interventions**, sometimes known as guided self-help or bibliotherapy, often involve the practitioner utilising a range of resources such as books, self-help manuals or computerised material, again informed by age-appropriate CBT. A practitioner with the appropriate level of training would support this process, e.g. introducing the material during a face-to-face session, then review progress at the next session before setting further 'homework'. It is recommended by NICE (2011; 2019) that facilitated self-help via telephone or in face-to-face contact takes place over approximately 6 to 8 sessions, completed over a 9–12-week period, with review at a later agreed date.
- **Group-based self-help** can be facilitated in a group environment, such as a group-based peer support programme. A group of young people with similar difficulties might be brought together to share their experiences, thoughts and feelings in a 'safe' space. Practitioners can facilitate this process by monitoring attendance, facilitating group discussion and reviewing agreed goals and outcomes. NICE (2011;

2019) describe this typically as a weekly 1-hour session over a period of 8–12 weeks. It is advised that families and carers are encouraged to attend self-help groups either facilitated by CAMHS or within the community, where appropriate.

Digital Self-Help

In a time where young people are more engaged with digital technology than ever before, digitised CBT programmes are increasingly employed within the NHS. The type and availability of these programmes within the NHS can depend on locality and the variance in commissioning. NICE (2019) identifies common themes within digital CBT programmes as:

- Psychoeducation
- Relaxation techniques and mindfulness
- Analysis of behaviour and behavioural activation
- Basic communication and interpersonal skills
- Emotional recognition and dealing with strong emotions
- Problem-solving skills
- Cognitive restructuring, i.e. identifying thoughts, challenging unhelpful/negative thoughts
- Relapse prevention strategies

SilverCloud is an example of a digital self-help programme provided locally in Hampshire by iTalk (italk.org.uk). This programme is categorised as computerised cognitive behavioural therapy (CCBT), available for people from the age of 16 and over who are experiencing symptoms of mild to moderate depression and/or anxiety. It can be accessed via a mobile phone, tablet or computer. A young person can work through the content at their own pace. It includes interactive modules, videos, quizzes and case studies. An individual is allocated an online practitioner who reviews messages that are left and monitors progress every two weeks. When logging into the programme, an individual is asked to complete an online questionnaire that tracks symptoms and changes.

Effectiveness of Self-Help

Moore et al. (2019) carried out a review of the uptake and effectiveness of a computerised self-help programme (BRAVE) for children and adolescents experiencing anxiety. Referrals to this programme came from primary care, i.e. GPs and schools, within New Zealand. Out of 1,361 original referrals, around 500 young people completed 4 sessions. Young people who completed more than four sessions reported lower levels of anxiety. Progress mainly occurred following the third or fourth session. The review concluded that the computerised self-help guide (e-therapy tool, BRAVE) was acceptable and effective when applied in the 'real world' via primary care and as part of a stepped care model for young people experiencing anxiety.

Musiat et al. (2014) carried out a study, using an advisory group, to explore attitudes and expectations towards computerised treatment, including smart phone applications, and comparing those to face-to-face treatment. The results showed that computerised treatment options did not meet most of participant expectations based on helpfulness of intervention, ability to motivate users, intervention credibility and immediate access. They did score higher when the convenience of access to the intervention was considered. It was recommended that policy makers create change in the perception of computerised interventions, but not how this might be done.

Within child and adolescent mental health services (CAMHS) the effectiveness of self-help has many variables for consideration, e.g. the degree of emotional intelligence, motivation to create change, learning style, cognitive ability, available support network, level of priority within the young person's life and the degree and impact of clinical symptoms on levels of functioning and psychological flexibility.

Case Study: Daisy

Daisy (eight) was referred to CAMHS after a six-month period of experiencing increasing anxiety. She initially reported 'butterflies' in her stomach when leaving the house for school. These later developed into recurring stomach aches and refusal to attend school. At home, Daisy's parents have been going through relationship difficulties, resulting in jointly deciding on a trial separation. Her father is sleeping in the spare bedroom and currently looking for alternative accommodation.

An anxiety workbook was used as a tool to facilitate self-help for Daisy with the support of her mother. Daisy's mother had accessed the book *Helping Your Child with Fears and Worries* (Creswell and Willetts, 2019), increasing her own understanding of how parents/carers can support a child experiencing anxiety. The workbook provided weekly topics with activities to explore Daisy's individual anxiety symptoms and techniques for managing and reducing them.

Week 1

- Why do I feel anxiety?
- Identifying physical symptoms using a body map.
- Can anxiety hurt me?
- What if my anxiety feels out of control? The Worry Hill.
- Practice task. Identifying the examples of the Worry Hill in their day to day life.

Week 2

- Why is breathing important?
- How do I change my breathing?
- Relaxed breathing.
- Am I breathing deeply enough?
- Practice task. Square breathing.

Week 3

- Why are muscles important?
- Progressive muscle relaxation.
- Practice task. To practice progressive muscle relaxation at least twice during the week.

Week 4

- What does an anxious mind look like?
- How can I stop these racing thoughts?
- The 54321 exercise.
- The pencil case exercise.
- The A–Z exercise.
- Practice task. Pick one activity to practice once every day.

Week 5

- What is a positive automatic thought?
- What is a negative automatic thought?
- Types of negative thoughts.
- What can I do about negative thoughts?
- Practice task. To challenge two automatic negative thoughts by finding evidence for and against, considering alternatives and then concluding.

Week 6

- What is a tricky situation?
- What role do negative automatic thoughts play in tricky situations?
- How do negative thoughts create tricky situations?
- How challenging thoughts can prevent tricky situations?
- Practice task. Practice thought challenging.

Daisy completed all six weeks of this workbook with gaps between sessions of one or two weeks, allowing time to practice. Having her mother involved in the sessions supported Daisy to maintain attention, provide alternative ways of engaging in the activities, bringing in evidence from day-to-day that Daisy could not recall and instilling some fun.

The feedback following these self-help sessions was positive. Daisy subjectively reported to be challenging her anxiety and using less avoidant behaviour (school refusal), that would serve to maintain the anxiety. Her mother reported increased self-awareness of physical symptoms of anxiety and more readiness for Daisy to challenge her negative thinking. Daisy's mother felt more able and confident to support this process in order to create change for her daughter.

Self-Help Material for Young People, Parents/Carers and Professionals

Although parents can play an important role in supporting an older child or young person, they are potentially less likely to require the level of supervision in engaging with self-help materials that younger children may. This is dependent on the young person's degree of functioning as a result of their mental health difficulties. Useful resources are listed and summarised below:

Websites

- NHS Choices Moodzone (https://www.nhs.uk/conditions/stress-anxiety-depression/). This NHS website is not specifically designed for young people, but provides useful information, self-assessment tools and mental well-being audio guides for a range of common mental health issues.
- Moodjuice (https://www.moodjuice.scot.nhs.uk/) is run by NHS Scotland and, like Moodzone, provides a range of self-help resources for a wide range of mental health issues, including suicidal thoughts.

Books

- *Instant Workbooks for Teens.* A series of books recommended to use with counsellors, covering most mental health difficulties experienced by young people, in addition to broader issues, e.g. self-esteem and body image.

- *Helping Your Child with Fears and Worries* (Creswell and Willetts, 2019). This is the second edition of *Overcoming Your Child's Fears and Worries* by the same authors and is designed to equip parents to give their child useful support.

Mobile Phone Applications

- Calm Harm (https://calmharm.co.uk/). Available on both Apple and Android platforms and uses the basic principles of dialectical behavioural therapy (DBT) to help users manage, and resist, the urge to engage in self-harming behaviours.
- SAM (https://sam-app.org.uk/). Available on both Apple and Android platforms. SAM stands for 'Self-Help for Anxiety Management' and has been developed by the University of the West of England (UWE). The app employs CBT techniques to help people of all ages with symptoms of anxiety.
- Headspace (https://www.headspace.com/headspace-meditation-app). Available on both Apple and Android platforms. Headspace guides the user through a series of mediation and mindfulness exercises on a daily basis.

Key References

Creswell, C., Willetts, L., (2019). *Helping Your Child with Fears and Worries: A Self-Help Guide for Parents* (2nd Ed.). London: Robinson.

Moor, S. et al., (2019). 'E' therapy in the community: examination of the uptake and effectiveness of BRAVE (a self-help computer programme for anxiety in children and adolescents) in primary care. *Internet Interventions*, 18(2019): 1–8.

Musiat, P., Goldstone, P., Tarrier, N., (2014). Understanding the acceptability of e-mental health, attitudes and expectations towards computerised self-help treatments for mental health problems. *BMC Psychiatry*, 14(109).

National Institute for Health and Care Excellence, (2011). *Common Mental Health Problems: Identification and Pathways to Care Clinical Guideline [CG123]*. London: NICE.

National Institute for Health and Care Excellence, (2019). *Depression in Children and Young People: Identification and Management: NICE Guideline [NG134]*. London: NICE.

72 Early Access: Feel the Fear and Do It Anyway

Setting up a Volunteer Support Group

Gill Waring

I've never thought of myself as a volunteer, which might seem strange considering I've spent the last four years doing exactly that! I am the mother of three children. My middle child has been diagnosed with autism, ADHD, anxiety, depression, hyper-mobility and psychosis. His needs meant that I had no choice but to give up my career in teaching. Our lives became incredibly limited, dominated by his needs and my attempts to meet them. Friends fell away as my focus had to be on him and his sisters. I became very isolated and lonely.

In the spring of 2015 I was introduced to someone who had been running a support group, outside the city where I live, for families with a child with autism. She asked me if I would be interested in running one myself, as there was nothing similar locally. I was sceptical. I had never attended a support group as I felt the needs of my son did not fit the mould. The idea of sharing our tumultuous life filled me with dread! However, I found it impossible to say no, and the idea of making something positive out of something negative took hold.

I had no idea where to start, but by asking around, I found it reasonably easy to find places that were willing to help. I wanted a safe space away from any professionals, with good parking and easy access. It would obviously help if it could be near to my house, so I could be there easily! I approached the local church, although the only link I had with it was that my children had attended pre-school there. They agreed to give us a room for free as part of their community work and before I knew it, the group had become a reality! It was important to me that we never charged families for attending or for refreshments. We wanted the group to be accessible for everyone.

Choosing a name was almost impossible! We spent hours trying to find the perfect name that was not too twee and was easy to remember. My husband finally came up with Re:Minds and it just felt right...and frankly a relief to have thought of something suitable. We created a tagline to explain our group, 'Re:Minds is a parent-led support group for families who have children with autism or mental health issues', and we were set. My first job was to create a Facebook page and then begin to send the word out. Again, I did not know where to begin, but I sent an email to the local newspaper, contacted local radio and shared information about the group to various Facebook pages that fitted our remit. To my amazement, the local BBC Radio station asked to come and interview my son and me. A few weeks later, we were perched on the sofa talking into a microphone about why we had set up the group. It felt a world away from teaching, and I continued to feel completely out of my depth. I have learned to live with that feeling, as it has never gone away.

The woman who had asked me to set up the group gave me some excellent advice. She suggested providing leaflets to put out on a table so that, as people arrived, they had something to look at rather than standing about feeling nervous. She recommended welcoming each person as they came in, putting the chairs in a circle and going round the group inviting people to tell us why they had come. Her best advice was that I would probably not like everyone I met and that many of the parents would be battling their own issues and I needed to be ready for that!

In September 2015 our radio interview aired all morning. It was the lead story in the news (perhaps it was a slow news day). As I put out the leaflets and laid out the cakes, I was convinced no-one would turn up. But they did, each person as nervous as me, and slowly we ended up with 12 people. The two-hour meeting flew by and despite my reservations, people did want to share their experiences. Meeting people who understood what life was like was an amazing and empowering experience.

As the meetings progressed we began to find speakers, who would come along to talk about topics relevant to us. Initially, these were local charities only too keen to tell people about what they did. We would spend an hour listening followed by a Q & A session, and then another hour chatting to each other – and always drinking coffee and eating cake! I would take notes, share them with parents unable to attend and ask questions on their behalf. One of the best aspects of it was that we never pretended to be experts, just other parents, but between us we knew so much. I soon learnt which members were happy to chat and asked them to greet new members, if I was busy. Over time, I was able to direct people to those who had been through something similar or could offer advice about a subject. I am proud to say that two of them now help to run Re:Minds, while many others are happy to step in and help run the group, when needed.

After a year, we were running out of speakers and numbers were steady at about ten each session. I knew something had to change. I contacted my son's psychiatrist and psychiatric nurse to ask if they could help. They both agreed to come and speak. I went all out to advertise the talk on anxiety given by the psychiatrist and on the day we had almost 50 people. Sadly, he was unable to attend at the last minute and I was faced with a room full of people who were not overly impressed! A few of us shared our own strategies and encouraged others to do the same and we made it through. It was difficult but I learnt a very big lesson, to always have a back-up plan. Other speakers have occasionally failed to attend or cancelled at the last minute. Luckily it is rare, but it does happen. I make a point of warning people to check if our speakers are still on, just in case, and I always have a back-up plan.

During the second year, I decided to set up another group, a pop-in group without any speakers. I thought it would be good to have a chance to chat informally to other families. I arranged this on a different day of the week and sat and waited and waited...and no-one came, I felt such an idiot! I could not bring myself to hold another one for a year! When I tried again, this time only two people turned up, but we had such a lovely time chatting about our lives that it felt like a success! I realised that it does not matter if only one person comes, if you can help them, that is what is important. Slowly, the group grew and now it is one of our busiest meetings. To hear 20 parents, laughing together, crying together and offering advice from their own personal experiences is such an incredibly empowering feeling. It is my favourite meeting now. We give parents the confidence to ask for help and to fight for what their children need, and in addition, we help them form incredibly strong friendships. Of our various meetings, it is this one that makes me feel that all the hard work is worth it.

Three years in, trying to find speakers became no easier and I had reached the point of forgetting about speakers altogether and cutting down the groups to one a month, when a new CAMHS manager arrived. She was the first manager who understood what we were trying to do, and she realised that if CAMHS and Re:Minds worked together, everyone would benefit. Within months, she offered to provide us with speakers and regularly attended the meetings herself. With her support, we finally managed to start drop-in clinics during Re:Minds meetings, where parents could book 15-minute appointments with a CAMHS specialist for advice about anything they were worried about. This was especially useful given the length of the

CAMHS waiting list and that many families were not even open to CAMHS services, but desperately wanted advice. This began taking some of the pressure off the CAMHS staff and helped many parents to feel calmer, knowing they could obtain advice as/when they needed it. Many clinicians were nervous about coming to speak, as they were aware that some parents could be angry, because they were so desperate for help. Occasionally, when a parent becomes frustrated, we step in to diffuse the situation and offer the chance to speak to a clinician privately. This is very rare and our members know that our ethos is all about working together with CAMHS to try to improve things, not blaming individuals. We hope families learn that it is not a case of 'them' and 'us' but that we are all in it together, trying to make the best of an under-funded system.

Under the new manager, our information became part of the pack sent to parents when they were referred to CAMHS. This signified a huge change in our group, and numbers began increasing rapidly. Within a few months, we had over 600 local members and each day, we have new people joining.

CAMHS have now begun giving us copies of the books they recommend to parents. We add these to our own library of books that parents can borrow. This has proved really popular and, as many of the books are expensive, it means parents can access them without having to worry about the cost.

The expanding numbers meant we could see how much more there was to do, and this led to a meeting with the Clinical Commissioning Group (CCG). I put together an action plan of the different aims we would like to achieve and how much each might cost, before meeting with them to pitch our ideas. I was incredibly nervous and, as always, felt out of my depth, but I told them what we did and the difference we wanted to make. Amazingly, they offered to fund two new groups for a year. It was not a huge amount of money, but it was a start! In 2019, we opened an evening group for parents who were unable to attend meetings during the day and another group for families whose children were turning 18 and leaving CAMHS. The CCG funding changed the dynamics of the group and for the first time, we are now accountable and have to create reports, but it has given us more ways to help others. We have learned that starting a new group is a gradual process, numbers take time to build, but our aim is to always be there when families need us. Slowly but surely, the new groups are building, and we are already planning to link in with adult mental health services to invite their staff to come to speak and to offer drop-in advice clinics.

One of the hardest things is limiting the group. There are so many families who need help and so much to be done that we would have to set up 50 groups to meet everyone's needs. Our action plan has helped us to keep focussed and spurred us on to seek funding from other sources for more new groups. We are even looking into becoming a charity to access other types of funding, so that we can continue to support families.

Apart from the groups, we represent our parents at meetings with CAMHS and the local authority. We have helped to give a parent's perspective during clinical interviews, new assessment pathways, staff training and inspections. We are now helping to plan a Parent Carer Mental Health Conference. We accompany parents to school meetings to act as an advocate, help with EHCPs and other forms. It feels as if we are a team with CAMHS, trying to make a difference that will benefit everyone.

Alongside the groups and meetings, our Facebook group has benefitted hundreds of families. It is a closed group, just for families and not professionals. We work hard to keep it a safe place where people can seek advice or rant or celebrate their lives. Before a person can join the group, they have to answer some questions to prove, so far as possible, that they really are family members, not professionals. We advertise each meeting on Facebook and people post questions they would like asked, if they cannot attend. We share minutes from the meetings, links to useful information and keep in touch with each other. We know it is difficult for many parents to come to the meetings, so this is a useful tool. It keeps us in touch with one another, helps lessen the feelings of isolation and if someone is desperate for advice, we can offer that, at any time of the day or night. For those not on Facebook, we send out dates and newsletters about what has been happening. We are in the process of setting up a website, so that we can post information for professionals, as well as for parents.

We have a Twitter account where we advertise meetings, although this does not meet our needs as easily.

Group Member Testimony

> I can quite easily say that Re:Minds saved me. I was desperate and flailing in a system designed to help, but that actually was not offering me any solutions or help. In my darkest hour, I considered ending it for both of us. I came to that first meeting at Re:Minds full of trepidation, I didn't know anyone else there and talking about my daughter's fragile mental health seemed a daunting thing, but I knew that we were in danger of losing her if I didn't find a way to help her myself.
>
> The group were so welcoming and Gill opened up by putting everyone at their ease and talked about her own son and his mental health. All of a sudden, I was in a room full of friends. I can say with certainty that some of these people are now friends for life. I am understood, supported, befriended and most of all I'm not on my own struggling with this scary condition.
>
> You never know when you are going to walk in these shoes and I didn't know how many people were walking in them with me. The group has gone on to make alliances with CAMHS and is well respected by parents and professionals alike. I've had training, borrowed books, drunk coffee, cried with others, and I hope helped out others along the way. Quite simply without this group, I have no doubt things could have ended up very differently.

When I began Re:Minds I had no idea of the difference it would make. With every new group we begin we gather evidence from families about what is not working for them. We take this back to professionals, not to blame anyone, but to try to find a way to change a system or make things better. We feel as if we are slowly chipping away and helping professionals to see the positives of working with parents and carers. For the first time, parents feel empowered, that they are not shouting into a black hole of desperation.

Our group has inspired other groups, and now there are four new support groups for local families in the city. Our members say that we have given them the confidence to believe in themselves. Some have returned to work; others have become volunteers themselves. When we started, I thought the group would run for a few months and then fold. I had no idea that this would become a full-time job and a passion. The group has seen me through some of the darkest times and given me friendships for life. We really have turned something negative into the best possible positive.

73 Early Access

Overview of Third-Sector Support for Children, Young People and their Families

Christopher Gale and Alice Mooney

This brief chapter provides an insight into some of the services local to the city of Southampton and county of Hampshire in the UK. Their inclusion in this book is designed to give the reader non-exhaustive examples of such services that will exist in other parts of the country.

Home-Start In Hampshire

Home-Start (www.home-start.org.uk) is a national charitable organisation that operates a number of services across Hampshire, providing a menu of programmes to support parents/carers and their children in the early years. The support and programmes on offer include:

- **Help to Access Services**
  Home-Start volunteers support families to access other local support services in their area, such as children's centres, citizens advice bureau, GP and dentistry services, housing and financial advice.
- **Home-Talk**
  A coaching programme for parents of children from birth to three years of age. Trained volunteers support families in their own homes to increase their communication and interaction with their child to ensure they offer them the best start in life.
- **Home Visiting**
  Home-Start volunteers help families facing isolation, the effects of post-natal illness, disability or mental health issues, bereavement, multiple births, poverty or financial difficulties and a whole range of other challenges.
- **Supporting Young Mothers**
  Home-Start has been running a project to help tackle loneliness by running groups for young mothers under 25 to gather, chat and redevelop their confidence.

No Limits

No Limits (www.nolimitshelp.org.uk) is a third-sector Hampshire-based young people's information, advice, counselling and support service (YIACS) providing free and confidential services to children, adolescents and young adults under the age of 26. The core service is an advice centre on Southampton High Street, open six days a week for young people to come for support. No appointment is necessary.

The service runs weekly drop-in sessions at schools and colleges in the Southampton area, reflecting similar projects across the Hampshire region.

Of the 2,247 children and young people supported through the No Limits Advice Centre in 2018, 35% were either at risk of or already experiencing mental health problems. The service offers a range of therapeutic and youth work interventions that support young people's mental health and emotional wellbeing Including:

- **Drop-in advice centre**: the 'front door', with information, advice and support offered by a qualified youth worker and trained volunteers.
- **Therapeutic groups**: youth workers can provide one-to-one support and 'signpost' on to our therapeutic groups, e.g. drug/alcohol support, Safe House for those experiencing anxiety, Young Carers.
- **Counselling**: children and young people can be referred to our professional counselling service meeting the BACP guidelines, delivered by appropriately qualified staff.
- **Primary mental health workers**: No Limits Primary Mental Health Workers practise in the community and schools across Southampton as part of a CAMHS-funded early intervention service. They will take referrals from No Limits advisory staff and the local single point of access (SPA) service for children and young people who present with anxiety, low mood and a range of other emotional difficulties, but who do not meet the threshold for specialist CAMHS. The PMHWs can support children and young people who have already accessed specialist CAMHS, as part of a step-down package of support. Typical provision may include time-limited therapeutic interventions, that could include guided self-help, solution-focussed therapy, anxiety management, interpersonal therapy and cognitive behavioural techniques.

Fairbridge

Fairbridge (www.princes-trust.org.uk) has a long history of supporting teenagers and young adults (16–25 years) on the central south coast of the UK and is now part of the Prince's Trust. Based in the centre of Southampton, the organisation offers people the opportunity to develop their confidence and work towards personal goals through a range of programmes from sports to drama and photography to cooking. In order to access the programmes, all young people must complete a five-day access course, during which they engage in outdoor activities and a residential trip. Young people have access to other Prince's Trust programmes that will develop employability skills.

NSPCC (Southampton) 'Letting the Future In' Service

'Letting the Future In' (www.nspcc.org.uk) is recommended nationally by the National Institute for Health and Care Excellence (NICE) (NICE, 2017) for its work with children and young people, aged 4–17, who have experienced sexual abuse. Using creative ways of expression, e.g. storytelling, writing, art or messy play, young people are encouraged to express feelings that cannot easily be put into words.

The programme support begins with an assessment of the child or young person's needs over three to four weekly sessions, with the most appropriate intervention selected from a practice guide. The programme usually continues for approximately a year and offers individual or joint support with parents or carers.

The service in Southampton has been running since 2015.

Barnardo's

As one of the UK's largest children's charities, Barnardo's (www.barnardos.org.uk) offers a range of services in the Southampton area, including:

- **Miss-U**: this service offers information and support to young people under the age of 18 who go missing, in some cases on multiple occasions. The service will arrange to undertake an assessment with the young person and their family or carer to determine if extra support is needed. They will then work to reduce the number of missing episodes and associated risks and work to prevent the breakdown of the home situation.
- **U-turn**: This service specifically targets young people at risk of or being sexually exploited.
- **Family support**: Offering help to parents, carers and families in the community and in diverse cultural circumstances. Guidance and advice aimed at supporting vulnerable children and their families.

Autism Hampshire

Running since the 1960s, Autism Hampshire (www.autismhampshire.org.uk) offers a range of services to children, young people and their families, including free information and signposting to other support services, local social groups and family support groups.

The services introduced here, alongside many other non-statutory organisations, provide invaluable support that can complement or provide a viable alternative to that offered by specialist CAMHS, where there is sometimes a time lapse between referral, assessment and treatment.

Key Reference

National Institute for Health and Care Excellence, (2017). *Child Abuse and Neglect (NG76)*. London: NICE.

74 Early Access

Health Visiting Service

Naomi Pang

KEY CONCEPTS

- Every family with a child aged between zero and five years is offered the Health Visiting Service.
- Health visitors are Specialised Community Public Health Nurses offering a service to improve health outcomes for children.

Every experience, every trauma, every relationship and every action have the potential to be detrimental or positive to a child's long-term health. Health visitors are an integral part of the Universal Service offered to families with children aged zero to five years. All registered health visitors are qualified nurses or midwives who complete further study to obtain a Specialist Community Public Health Nurse certification. This gives them the skills to lead and drive forward the Department of Health's 'Healthy Child Programme: Pregnancy and the First Five Years (HCP) (2009). The HCP (DH, 2009) was written as a policy paper in response to the National Service Framework for Children, Young People and Maternity Services (DH, 2004) that emphasised the need for professionals to have national standards for children's health and social care. The HCP (DH, 2009) focuses on improving outcomes for every child by working in conjunction with the 4,5,6 Approach for Health Visiting and School Nursing (PHE, 2018):

- **Four** levels of service: Community, Universal, Universal Plus and Universal Partnership Plus
- **Five** health reviews: antenatal, birth, between six and eight weeks, one year and two years
- **Six** high-impact areas: parenthood and the early weeks, maternal mental health, breast-feeding, healthy weight, minor illness/accidents and being school ready

The levels of service offered are determined as in Table 74.1.

Using a targeted universal approach allows health visitors to support and empower parents and caregivers to make healthy choices for their whole family. Working holistically, the health visitor will weave the overarching four Public Health Outcomes Framework (Public Health England, 2016) into their everyday practice. Improving these outcomes will enable a child to fulfil the potential for optimum health in adult life.

The Four Public Health Outcomes Framework (PHE, 2016):

- The wider determinants of health
- Health improvement

Table 74.1 Levels of Service

Level of Service	*Service Offered*
Universal	Five core contacts covering the six high-impact areas
Universal Plus	Five core contacts covering the six high-impact areas plus a targeted health visiting service offering more intervention
Universal Partnership Plus	Five core contacts covering the six high-impact areas plus a targeted service offering more intervention within a multi-disciplinary team. All safeguarding will be under Universal Partnership Plus

- Health protection
- Health care and premature mortality

As a 'jack-of-all-trades' practitioner, the health visitor will tailor their support for a family based on their assessment of need. Early help intervention is often determined on social need. The benefit is that interventions are led and delivered in the home by a health care professional with clinical training and experience. Despite the clear advantages, health visitors are often overlooked within the public health domain and the potential for providing service.

Their value in early help can be largely ignored by commissioners, perhaps because of the difficulty of evaluating the influence of health visitors within a short time frame. Commissioners want results and fast. The role is so variable in nature, changing and evolving to keep up with the dynamism of NHS agendas, that what one NHS Trust will offer may be very different to their neighbour.

The health visitor service was merged into the total local authority public health budgets in 2015.As public health funding is nationally reduced in the name of reforms, money for health visitors is not ring-fenced. This paints a dismal future for the HCP (DH, 2009) and forces the approach to health care into a reactive rather than proactive service.

Ironically, preventing illness is a financial investment for the future. A recently published longitudinal study (Caspi et al., 2016) has supported this theory and found that the children with lower neurocognitive status at 3 years of age were most likely to be the highest cost of economic burden 35 years later. The HCP (DH, 2009) aims to promote the highest potential neurodevelopment growth through good attachment, reducing later cost to public health resources.

The HCP (DH, 2009) aims to provide a universal health service for under fives by promoting partnership across different agencies. The core values are to give the child the best start in life and to let them reach their fullest potential. With the decentralisation of NHS commissioning to local authorities, the concern is that this universalism will soon become undervalued as other neoliberal agendas could become paramount.

Neoliberalism has many parallels with the new conservative government, i.e. cost cutting for efficiency, putting the onus of health care on the individual rather than public good and the privatisation of services. It seems that the NHS organisation and most likely the implementation plan of the HCP (DH, 2009) are already on par to follow these ideological values. Change is almost certainly imminent.

Case Study: Jenna

Jenna was 24 years old when she became pregnant with her first baby. She was visited by a health visitor at 32 weeks pregnant. Using a Family Health Needs Assessment, the health visitor built up a picture about what the unborn baby's life would be like in the early years. Jenna confided that she did not have a happy upbringing, often arguing with her mother, and that she had not seen her father since she was two years old when he was imprisoned. Clearly, Jenna did not have a healthy parental relationship modelled to her as a child. She admitted that she often argued with the baby's father, using negative language to describe him during the visit.

Their relationship had broken up three months before, and Jenna was facing motherhood as a single parent. The health visitor considered whether her ex-partner was supportive and how this would play out once the baby was born. Jenna felt excited about the baby, despite the unplanned pregnancy but did not want to sing or talk to the unborn child, saying it felt silly. The health visitor discussed attachment and stressed the importance of early neurodevelopment with Jenna. Standard health promotion was discussed with regard to feeding, safe sleep and immunisations.

The health visitor identified that Jenna would need more support as a parent. This was reviewed at the new birth visit.

Jenna had a difficult birth experience, resulting in an emergency caesarean section. She described this as 'scary' and that she felt like she had 'lost control' during the labour. Jenna was tearful during the visit, describing how she felt unsupported by her ex-partner and exhausted. She felt that she did not have any support, other than her mother, whom she felt was interfering. The health visitor noted that Jenna ignored the baby when he showed feeding cues and insisted on following a four-hour feeding regime. Jenna appeared awkward when holding him and did not comfort him when he was crying. This indicated Jenna's low self-esteem and confidence as a new mother.

The health visitor returned a week later and realised that Jenna's relationship with her son had deteriorated. Jenna did not hold her baby during the visit and complained of his excessive crying. The health visitor considered medical reasons for an unsettled baby against Jenna's perception of motherhood. Any possible medical condition was ruled out, and it was decided that monitoring over the next few weeks would be the best course of action. In the meantime, the health visitor contained Jenna's emotions in the hope that Jenna would be able to contain her son's emotions to help enable stable attachment. Using a supportive and non-judgemental approach, Jenna and the health visitor were able to build up a relationship that meant important messages about health promotion and neurodevelopment could be delivered and received.

During the time that Jenna received visits from the health visitor, agendas were matched and the health visitor delivered early help interventions, including finances, social support, infant development and mental health. Jenna eventually learnt the importance of self-efficacy and where to access support services on her own, leading to a better future for herself and her son.

Multiple-Choice Questions

See answers on page 673.

1. Which are the four levels of service offered by health visitors?
    a. Public, Universal, Universal Plus, Universal Partnership Plus
    b. Community, Universal, Universal Extra, Universal Partnership Extra
    c. Public, Universal, Universal Plus, Universal Collaborative Plus
    d. Community, Universal, Universal Plus, Universal Partnership Plus
2. What are the five core health reviews?
    a. Antenatal, new birth, three to four months, one year, two years
    b. New birth, six to eight weeks, one year, two years, three years
    c. Antenatal, new birth, six to eight weeks, one year, two years
    d. Antenatal, new birth, 3–4 months, 18 months, 3 years

3. What are the six high-impact areas?
    a. Parenthood and the early weeks, maternal mental health, breastfeeding, healthy weight, minor illness/accidents and being school ready
    b. Parenthood and the early weeks, employment, maternal mental health, breastfeeding, healthy weight and toilet training
    c. Social networks, employment, breastfeeding, healthy weight, minor illness/accidents and being school ready
    d. Parenthood and the early weeks, maternal mental health, behaviour, sleep, breastfeeding and minor illness/accidents
4. Which of the following statements is *true*?
    a. Health visitors are Specialist Community Public Health Nurses
    b. Health visitors are Specialist Community Allied Health Professionals
5. Which of the following is supported by health visitors to improve infant neurodevelopment?
    a. Toilet training
    b. Attachment
    c. Stable finances
    d. Employment

Key References

Department of Health, (2009). *Healthy Child Programme: Pregnancy and the First Five Years of Life*. London: TSO.

Public Health England, (2016). *Public Health Outcomes Framework, Improving Outcomes and Supporting Transparency*. London: Department of Health.

Public Health England, (2018). *Overview of the 6 Early Years and Schoolaged Years High Impact Areas. Health Visitors and School Nurses Leading the Healthy Child Programme*. London: Department of Health.

75 Early Access

Family Nurse Partnership: A Southampton Model

Diane Henty and Kirsteen Anderssen (updated by Andrea Thwaites)

Introduction

The Family Nurse Partnership (FNP) has been running in Southampton since September 2008. The FNP is an evidence-based, licensed home-visiting programme that improves the health, well-being and self-sufficiency of low-income young first-time parents and their children. The FNP is strength-based, comprehensive and cost-effective (Isaacs, 2007). The FNP is underpinned by three main theories, and these are thoroughly woven into practice.

KEY CONCEPTS

- The programme is underpinned by three basic theories: human ecology, attachment and self-efficacy.
- The programme goals are to improve the health, well-being and self-sufficiency of low-income young first-time parents and their children.
- The programme is delivered by highly skilled family nurses, from early pregnancy until the child is two years old.

Brofenbrenner's **theory of human ecology** looks at a child's development within the social contexts of his or her immediate family/community environment and their interactions with the larger environment, including cultural values, customs and laws (Bronfenbrenner, 1979).

John Bowlby's **theory of attachment** holds that the earliest bonds formed by infants with their caregivers will have a lasting impact throughout their life. Attachment behaviours serve to keep the infant close to its mother, thereby promoting its chance of survival (Bowlby, 1988).

Self-efficacy theory is part of social cognitive theory and describes a person's belief in their own ability to succeed in specific situations. A person with high self-efficacy is someone who believes that they can perform well and who is more likely to view a difficult task as one that they can master, rather than avoid (Bandura, 1997).

Parents recruited onto the Family Nurse Partnership programme in Southampton are aged 24 years or under and expecting their first baby. All young parents under 16 years of age expecting their first child are offered the programme, and those 17–24 years expecting their first child are triaged by using a vulnerability score.

All care leavers within this cohort are offered the programme. The majority are recruited at around 16 weeks of pregnancy and are visited by the family nurse (FN) every week for the first 4 weeks after recruitment, then every 2 weeks until the baby's birth. They are visited every week for 6 weeks following the birth and then every 2 weeks until the baby is 21 months old and then each month until the child is aged 2. Family nurses follow a comprehensive programme that uses multiple intervention strategies to help mothers develop the knowledge, skills and self-efficacy to:

- Improve pregnancy outcomes by engaging with antenatal care.
- Improve diet and reduce use of cigarettes, alcohol and illegal drugs.
- Improve child health and development by providing more responsible, competent and sensitive care for their child.
- Improve economic self-sufficiency by developing a vision for the future, planning subsequent pregnancies, continuing in education and/or gaining employment.

Family nurses use a psychoeducational approach within a therapeutic relationship with the aim of supporting clients to move towards positive change. They work in a trauma-informed way with an awareness of the potential impact of adverse childhood experiences (ACEs) on clients' behaviour and health outcomes (Felitti et al., 1998). Since 2016 the FNP National Unit have been undertaking a research project along with Dartington Service Design Lab to look at building on and adapting this offer in light of changing local and national agendas to personalise the offer more closely with clients' level of need, whilst adhering to the evidence-based License Agreement.

Ten FNP sites around England are involved in Accelerated Design and Programme Testing (ADAPT) FNPNU (2018) which is focussed on five high-impact areas:

- Neglect
- Breastfeeding
- Smoking cessation
- Maternal mental health
- Healthy relationships to prevent intimate partner violence (IPV)

Work is ongoing in developing new clinical materials within these areas, personalisation and dialling the offer up or down according to client need with the aim of improving outcomes for young parents and their children. Results of the study are due to begin being shared and rolled out at the end of 2019.

Case Study (1): Julie

Julie was 16 years old when she was recruited onto the programme. She had a history of sexual abuse by her step-father, who was no longer living at home. When she became pregnant she was living with her mother, who physically abused her. She was no longer in a relationship with the father of her baby, but she had a new partner with whom she frequently argued. Julie was a heavy smoker and drank alcohol at weekends.

The Programme

It was important for the family nurse to establish a trusting relationship with Julie and to establish an attachment relationship with her. It became apparent over time that Julie had an insecure avoidant attachment pattern, having learnt to be a 'grown up' and not show her feelings from an early age. She did not anticipate that other people would be able to respond to her needs. She 'acted out' this attachment pattern with her partner, and they often argued.

The family nurse observed that arguments between the two would become louder and louder as each competed for the other's support and understanding. Neither of them achieved their goal and the situation would escalate. The family nurse engaged in working with the couple to help them to understand each other better.

Using worksheets, role play and motivational interviewing techniques, the couple were able to explore and improve their communication. By understanding the needs and wants of the other more fully, a blueprint was created that could be transferred to their relationship with their unborn child. They were then able to consider the impact that their behaviour, i.e. arguing, smoking, drinking, might have on the baby, something they had been unable to do before. This helped create a healthier attachment with the baby once he was born.

Towards the end of pregnancy, Julie's relationship with her mother broke down. She had wanted Julie to stop working with the family nurse. The family nurse had become aware that Julie was being physically abused at home. Social services were involved and Julie was moved into her own flat. The family nurse helped maintain the tenancy. When complaints were received about noise, drinking and smoking in the flat until the early hours of the morning, the nurse was able to reflect with Julie about the impact of her behaviour on her baby. In this way, Julie found the motivation to change her behaviour by prioritising her son's need for a safe, stable home environment.

Case Study (2): Lisa

Lisa had been 'looked after' by the local authority since she was five years old, because of severe neglect and abuse. She was 15 when she was recruited to the FNP. She had been excluded from school due to several violent interactions with staff and students. Lisa had left school with no qualifications. She had a difficult relationship with her social worker and other health care professionals, but demonstrated a high level of self-efficacy.

The Programme

Although Lisa was only 15, she wanted to live with the father of her baby. Historically, Lisa had always made her own choices, so the family nurse's challenge was to find a compromise that gave Lisa some of what she had decided upon, yet would protect her and her baby. The compromise suggested was that Lisa would stay in a mother-and-baby foster placement until her baby was six months old and if all went well, at that point, she would be supported to find accommodation for herself, her baby and her partner. Lisa reluctantly agreed. A placement was identified where Lisa and Jamie could live in an apartment in the garden of the foster parent. This suited Lisa well. She could have her independence but with the safety net and support of the foster parent. When Jamie was six months old, Lisa was supported in finding and maintaining a tenancy for her family.

Extensive work was undertaken around attachment and 'tuning in' to the baby's cues, as Lisa found it very difficult to interpret Jamie's behaviour, often thinking he was trying to manipulate her and be naughty, when he was only a few weeks old. Lisa and her partner were very responsive.

When it was time for Jamie to be weaned, Lisa found multiple reasons why she could not do it. She reported that Jamie refused to take solid food, choked on lumps and projectile vomited. At nine months of age, after being seen by the GP and by the local hospital where no physical problems were discovered, the family nurse decided to open up a discussion with Lisa about what it meant to her for her child to grow up and not be a baby any more.

It became clear that for Lisa it was dangerous to grow up, because it was when she was a toddler, that her abuse and neglect began. Subconsciously, she was trying to keep Jamie as a baby, so that she could protect him from the experiences she had had. Once this was explored with Lisa and she understood the meaning of her misgivings about Jamie growing up, she was able to allow him be weaned.

Lisa's high level of self-efficacy was used to encourage her to join a local project called Learning Links. She studied for a literacy and numeracy certificate, which helped her to gain a college place. It had been Lisa's 'heart's desire' to become an actress, and she is currently enrolled at college on a performing arts course.

Multiple-Choice Questions

See answers on page 674.

1. Attachment behaviours...
   a. Apply only to the specific bond between a mother and her baby.
   b. Are absent in premature babies.
   c. Promote interaction between caregivers and their infants to promote survival.
   d. Cannot be learnt.
   e. Are only present in the first month after birth.
2. The Family Nurse Partnership (FNP) programme...
   a. Is designed for children with attachment problems.
   b. Is a home visiting programme for families from birth until the child is five years old.
   c. Consists of family nurses who work in the same way as social workers.
   d. Works with vulnerable young parents to promote attachment and child development.
   e. Consists of family nurses who prescribe medication and therapy to treat mental health disorders in young parents.

Key References

Bandura, J., (1977). *Social Learning Theory.* Englewood Cliff, NJ: Prentice Hall.

Barnes, J., Ball, M., Meadows, P., Belsky, J. (2011). *Nurse-Family Partnership Programme: Wave 1 Implementation in Toddlerhood and a Comparison Between Waves 1 and 2a Implementation in Pregnancy and Infancy.* London: DCSF.

Bowlby, J., (1988). *A Secure Base: Clinical Applications of Attachment Theory.* London: Routledge.

Bronfenbrenner, U., (1979). *The Ecology of Human Development.* Cambridge, MA: Harvard University Press.

Family Nurse Partnership National Unit, Dartington Service Design Laboratory (2018). FNP ADAPT Interim Report.

Felitti, V.J., Anda, R.F., Nordenberg, D., Williamson, D.F., Spitz, A.M., Edwards, V., Kitzman, H.J., Olds, D.L., Cole, R.E., et al., (2010). Enduring effects of prenatal and infancy home visiting by nurses on children—follow up of a randomised trial among children at age 12. *Archives of Pediatrics & Adolescent Medicine*, 164(5), 412–424.

Koss, M.P., Marks, J.S., (1998). Relationship of childhood abuse and household dysfunction to many of the leading causes of death in adults: the adverse childhood experiences (ACE) study. *American Journal of Preventive Medicine*, 14: 245–258.

Jewell, D., Tacchi, J., Donovan, J., (2000). Teenage pregnancy, whose problem is it? *Family Practice*, 17: 522–528.

Macmillan, H.L., Wathen, C.N., Barlow, J., Fergusson, D., Leventhal, J.M., Taussig N., (2009). Interventions to prevent child maltreatment and associated impairment. *Lancet*, 373, 250–266.

Olds, D.L., (2006). The nurse-family partnership: an evidence-based preventative intervention. *Infant Mental Health Journal*, 27(1), 5–25.

76 Early Access

Primary Mental Health in the Community

Margaret J.J. Thompson and Roy Smith

Background

A recent mental health survey found that 12.8% children and young people aged 5 to 16 years will have an emotional or behavioural problem at any one time, causing them, or others, concern for their functioning or well-being (The Mental Health of Children and Young People (MHCYP) survey, 2017). Yet the same survey found that, at most, only one in four of these children and young people will be known to the specialist child and adolescent mental health services (CAMHS).

Many children with such problems will be known to staff in schools, teachers or educational psychologists, school nurses or community paediatricians and other primary care staff (general practitioners or health visitors). Following a review of services, the authors of the NHS HAS report ('Bridge over Troubled Waters', 1986) suggested that services for children and adolescents should be available in the community, in the hope that this would prevent the need for further referrals into CAMHS.

Documents from the Department of Health at that time and over subsequent years until confirmed the need to further develop the skills of primary care teams in the care of mental health.

This acknowledged the fact that professionals in primary care were more numerous than those in specialised CAMHS and were well-placed to identify and hopefully intervene sooner when a child presented within their sphere of influence. This would mean that problems could be assessed and treated sooner, or referred on as appropriate, to prevent problems spiralling out of control.

Better partnership between the primary care sector, education and social services, and with secondary care colleagues, e.g. paediatricians and child psychiatrists, was encouraged. Money was released from the Department of Health to forward this work.

The staff in primary care needed support and more training. The Departments of Health and Education began introducing more support for health visitors, school nurses and teachers.

Most specialist CAMH services (SCAMHS) began working more in the community, usually 'out reaching' from their Tier 3 service, e.g. running workshops for health visitors on behavioural strategies for pre-school problems, e.g. sleep, pre-school ADHD and maternal depression (Stevenson, 1990; Stallard, 1995) and for GPs (Bernard et al., 1999). The staff began to work more closely with schools and voluntary adolescent support teams in the community.

A consultation model was developed whereby professionals from CAMHS would meet with GPs, health visitors or schools and discuss clients that were of concern. Names were only mentioned if the family had consented. This model is described by Appleton (2000), and Thompson (2005).

Some professionals began to work at Tier 2 (in the community, delivering services by up-skilling professionals). Two examples are the Parent Advisor training (Davis and Spurr, 1998) and the Flintshire model (Appleton and Hammond Rowley, 2000).

What started as an exciting way forward has become more difficult with the curtailing of the roles of health visitors, school nurses and social work services, as they have been drawn more into child protection work. In addition, there has been a change of role for educational psychologists.

The concept has changed direction with 'Transforming Children and Young People's Mental Health Provision: A Green Paper' (2017), indicating the need for services in the community to work together, especially schools and CAMHS clinics. Money has been released by the government for two specialist roles:

(a) To train counsellors to work in schools and colleges to assess and offer initial treatment to children with emotional problems.
(b) CAMHS staff are being trained as CYP IAPT practitioners to provide low- intensity CBT, systemic therapy and parenting programmes in the CAMHS setting.

The professionals attend a training course for two whole days a week for a year at various HEIs. Professionals are seconded by their organisations to undertake courses in CBT, systemic family therapy and parenting programmes, usually the Incredible Years programme. Outcome measures are collected. SCAMHS are expected to offer supervision to these staff (Shafran et al., 2014; Fonagy et al., 2017).

> More recent models, such as THRIVE, focus on the needs of children and young people, include a systems-wide framework and consider how support can be delivered by a range of different practitioners and agencies, including the role of parents and carers. Thrive www.thriveapproach.com. The THRIVE definition of a mental health intervention covers a child's needs rather than a diagnosis.

The THRIVE categories are needs-based groupings (Wolpert et al., 2015). The THRIVE framework conceptualises five needs-based groupings for young people with mental health difficulties and their families.

A Primary Mental Health Worker (PMHW)

A primary mental health worker (PMHW) is a professional who works in the community, reasonably independently of other colleagues and on a variety of tasks. It is a role well-developed in the adult services, usually by community mental health nurses. It was developed by CAMHS services following the introduction of the HAS Document, 1995. The aim is that the worker will operate within the community.

In 1995, the Department of Health released money to improve CAMHS (DoH modernisation funding, 1995), and primary mental health workers were appointed in many areas within a variety of models. In addition, money was released to set up a MSc pathway for modular training for these new professionals. These have now been integrated into mental health nursing courses. Different models operated around the country (e.g. some PMHWs were spending about 35% of their time in primary care, offering consultation and training to primary health care workers, rather than engaging in direct work with children and families). The service has subsequently changed to take referrals of families from their primary health colleagues and to have active caseloads. The management is now integrated into the SCAMHS. This has reduced the waiting list.

Most services would agree that the PMHW should be a senior mental health worker able to convey skills to professionals in the field and be able to determine which families can be dealt with in the community and which should be referred on into specialised services.

Primary Mental Health Work within a Specialist CAMHS Team (Roy Smith)

I am a registered social worker employed for four years as a primary mental health worker (PMHW), alongside colleagues within a 0 to 14 years SCAMHS team in Hampshire, UK. In 2004, the National Committee for Primary Mental Health Workers defined the role as 'to act as an interface between universal first contact services for children and families (Tier 1) and Specialist CAMHS'. Nationally, many PMHWs work within stand-alone Tier 2 teams, but in 2007, we chose to provide an integrated Tier 2 comprehensive and Tier 3 specialist CAMHS service, from within our Tier 3 team.

An integrated model was important in terms of our team providing a coherent and effective service, across the tiers, for the local population. The model made efficient use of limited staffing resources, but importantly, it enabled practitioners to access regular specialist clinical supervision, assessments and interventions across the tiers within the one team.

In addition to developing and reviewing the service, my specialism as a PMHW was to act as a prompt initial contact with families, providing clinical assessments and therapeutic interventions. Monthly group consultation with the local Tier 1 network was established, and as an integrated locality team, we provided circumscribed assessments and interventions for existing longer-term cases held by colleagues. In this way, families were able to quickly access specialist nursing, psychiatric, PMHW, OT, therapist and clinical psychology specialisms during their time with us.

Example from Roy's Practice: Oren (11)

The clinical case below is representative of the work undertaken within our integrated model. Names and additional details have been changed to ensure confidentiality.

I was initially the lead worker responsible for assessment and case management until we entered into more formal therapeutic sessions, as part of the care plan.

At that juncture, a colleague joined the system as case holder, providing a link to the professional network, family and to the rest of the team. This enabled us as a practitioner/family system to work in as clear a context as possible. The initial care plan included a referral for a formal autistic spectrum (ASD) assessment. This expansion of the assessment process marked a transition into Tier 3 and enabled a coherent context for a change in roles.

Our family sessions considered family members' understandings of one another, how to develop resilience in relation to external 'judgements' regarding the family and considered the significance for the family of a possible ASD diagnosis for Oren. In addition, the issue of sexual identity and acceptance was explored. The parents initially told us that family work would be a waste of time as Oren needed 'sorting out so that he could be more like us'.

The quality of relationships at commencement of family therapy is illustrated in Figure 76.1. Oren was the focus for many problematic narratives and was on long-term exclusion from school for an incident from some months previously.

Oren presented as a cheerful child with some idiosyncratic social skills, who wanted to be accepted and liked and was struggling with his position as a demonised individual locally

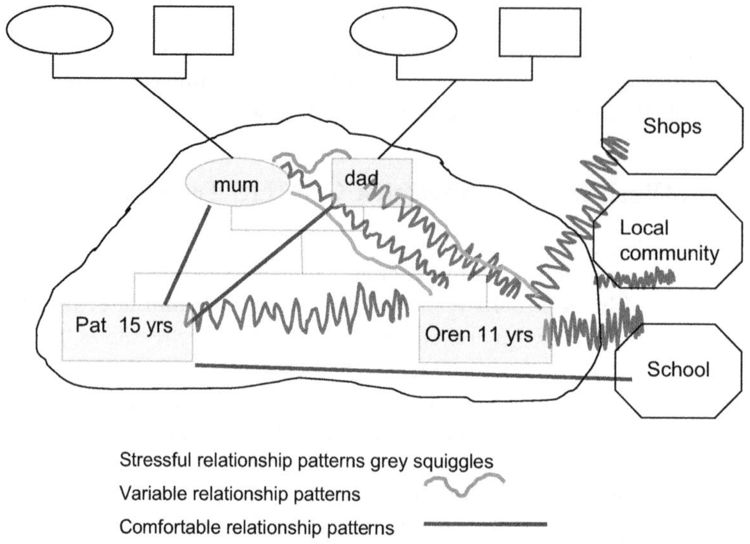

Figure 76.1 Quality of relationships at commencement of family therapy.

and within his family. His parents were bemused, irritated and protective of their son and his behaviour.

I worked with the family to consider problem-saturated stories in context of the 'shy' stories that they might relate to. My therapeutic position was informed by my training in systemic psychotherapy and my experience of receiving psychodynamic supervision over a number of years. Flaskas and Perlesz (1996) noted 'Systemic therapy has as its central focus an interactional perspective and its theory has developed recursive ways of understanding patterns in relationships'.

Strong emotions permeated our sessions. I used psychodynamic theory to inform my thoughts and my questions, these then being framed in systemic ways. Arundale (2011), writing about analytical therapy, noted 'emotional and mental events must be alive in the present moment, in exchanges between the patient and the analyst, in order for there to be psychic change'. It was clear that Pat, Oren's older brother, was particularly distressed by his relationship with Oren. We wondered what he hoped their relationship could be like, and examples were already evident within their lives. His distress and frustration linked to his love, hope and fear for his brother. He was the first family member to articulate such insights.

Our initial hypotheses included the family's belief that attending the first session was a step to achieving an ASD diagnosis, this being the 'safe, certain' explanation for a range of difficulties involving Oren (Mason, 1993). Linked to this was that the family may hold cultural beliefs because our team is part of a wider medical system. Thus, we were believed to be able and tasked to 'fix' Oren.

In the light of some reported behaviours, we wondered about sexuality and what hopes, fears and prejudices this might trigger for the family, myself and the wider system. We wondered about how did it happen that the boys had 'good' and 'bad' polarised positions. Did this link with wider social values, to disappointment? What roles were they being positioned into, how, why, who else in the family, past or present, has held such positions? What meanings were in such roles?

All the family were able to express and reflect on strong emotions and enrich their narratives regarding their need for an autism assessment. The emergent narrative linked to the bolstering of their belief in their efficacy as parents and the development of resilience to challenge the stories held about them locally. Pride became an important emergent theme.

Oren listened carefully to what was said in the sessions and increasingly added considered reflections, including challenging other family members when some 'blame' narratives were used. He had a playful approach and was aware that this could cause him problems, when other people might perceive his staring as provocative or his frankness as rude.

We acknowledged when both parents began to challenge Pat, when he berated his brother for 'not growing up'. Their challenges contained an increasingly robust position that Oren being 'different from them' was something they perceived as important for them to accommodate, rather than push for significant change in him.

Sexual identity emerged as an important theme in our sessions. We moved towards this topic via generalised conversations around unconditional support, highlighting this important value within the family. I asked if, in the future, either of the boys were to 'come out' as gay, how would he know they were supported? Oren immediately said 'I'm gay' and then laughed, saying he was 'only joking'. Both boys heard that their parents would love them in all circumstances; the biggest drawback regarding homosexuality related to the possibility of a lack of grandchildren. It was apparent that this type of affirmative reflection had not previously taken place. Links with sexuality and the boys had been negative and blaming in relation to the family defending Oren's 'name' in wider contexts. We noted how all the family were already acting to support each other, especially in the face of local hostility.

More generally, we created a range of diagrams as we mapped similarities, differences, strengths of emotions and so on, in sessions. This technique enabled Oren to actively participate in what could have been largely talk between 'the grownups'. In choosing this approach, I was being informed by my wider experience of working with children who might be on the autistic spectrum and their general preference for visual aids in discussions.

Oren was able to return to school, itself a remarkable step given the potential for hostility he faced. He experienced his family articulating and enacting acceptance, compassion and pride, and he was able to show that he was happy with who he was.

The PMHW role changed during our teams' time with the family. I was initially the case holder and formulated a care plan that remained largely unchanged over the 18 months the family worked with us. An ASD assessment was completed and a diagnosis of Asperger's syndrome made. I had left the process by this stage and the change from my case-holder role meant I could take on a new family.

During my time with the family, my role developed to provide a therapeutic intervention in line with the care plan. It was appropriate for me to provide this role directly given the circumstances and my skill base. I would have recommended a different worker if I had become an active member of the professional network. The role change occurred prior to our team stepping into the wider network in substantial ways.

Having worked for three years in separate Tier 2 and Tier 3 teams, I believe that an integrated local approach provides a more coherent service for families. Importantly, the diversity in what can be provided by the team is greater than when the tiers are separated.

For practitioners, internal referrals for additional resources are, in my experience, significantly less stressful than the external referral process between different teams. Strong working relationships based on co-working developed, and this respect was mirrored in our supportive and consultative roles within the wider professional network. I believe integrated working is worth considering as a way of delivering primary mental health work in the UK and longer-term interventions, if needed. PMHW can provide support in different ways, not limited to but including solution-focussed interventions, guided self-help, group work and one-to-one sessions.

Through this service, children and young people may be seen within school, at a No Limits base or in the community. Interventions are tailored to the needs of the individual and work with the following concerns: anxiety, self-harm, suicidal thoughts albeit without attempting or making plans to commit suicide, low mood, consistently becoming angry, being withdrawn from others, body image, self-esteem, self-worth and bullying. These interventions can help to minimise the impact of negative life experiences.

Summary: Research and Practice Issues from Working in Primary Care

- Primary mental health workers should be working within SCAMHS and be managed from within that service.
- They should have dedicated time to work in the community.
- These workers should be skilled practitioners with extra training and with on-going supervision from colleagues in CAMHS. Ideally, they should work in both settings to improve skills, especially therapeutic skills.
- They should be locality based, e.g. to populations of 50,000 (10,000 0–16-year olds).
- Consultation and training should be part of the task of a PMHW, in addition to hands-on work.
- The focus should be on high-quality work with built-in outcomes.
- Packages with proven efficacy should be used, e.g. re: Parenting, Webster-Stratton (1985); Sonuga-Barke et al. (2001); Thompson et al. (2009); Weeks, Laver-Bradbury, Thompson (1999); and re: behaviour work, Forehand and McMahon (1981).
- If families need to be referred into community CAMHS, the SCAMHS worker should 'culture carry' across to prevent parents not attending at the next referral point.
- Work in schools can include drop-in clinics run by school nurses, jointly run parenting groups and nurturing groups with colleagues from education.
- Remember primary care staff want to develop their skills, but these strategies need to be tailored to their confidence level, time commitment, i.e. seven minutes for a GP (Bernard et al., 1999), classroom needs for teachers, health visitors and school nurses.

Key References

Appleton, P., Hammond-Rowley, S., (2000). Addressing the population burden of child and adolescent mental health problems: a primary care model. *Child Psychology and Psychiatric Review*, 5: 9–16.

Arundale, J., Bandler Bellman, D. (Eds), (2011). *Transferrence and Countertransference. A Unifying Focus of Psychoanalysis.* London: Karnac.

Bernard, P., Garralda, E., Hughes, T., Tylee, A., et al., (1999). Evaluation of a teaching package in adolescent psychiatry for general practitioner registrars. *Education for General Practice*, 10: 21–28.

Davis, H., Spur, P., (1998). Parent counselling: an evaluation of a community child health mental service. *Journal of Child Psychology and Psychiatry*, 39: 365–376.

Department of Health, (2008). *Children and Young People in Mind: Final Report of the National CAMHS Review.* London: DOH.

Flaskas, C., Perlesz, A., (1996). *The Therapeutic Relationship in Systemic Therapy.* London: Karnac.

Fonagy, P., Pugh, K., O'Herlihy, A., (2017). The Children and Young People's Improving Access to Psychological Therapies (CYP IAPT) Programme in England In. D Skuse H. Bruce L.

Dowdney_(Eds),. *Child Psychology and Psychiatry: Frameworks for Clinical Training and Practice.* Chichester: John Wiley & Sons 429–435.

Gale, F., Vostanis, P., (2005). Case study the primary mental health team—Leicester, Leicestershire and Rutland CAMHS, pp. 439–444. In *Child and adolescent mental health services: strategy, planning, delivery, and evaluation* edited by Williams R and Kerfoot M Published by Shafran, R., Fonagy, P., Pugh, K., Myles, P., (2014). Transformation of mental health services for children and young people in England. In *Dissemination and Implementation of Evidence-Based Practices in Child and Adolescent Mental Health* (Vol. 158). New York, NY: Oxford University Press.

Mason, B., (1993). Towards positions of safe uncertainty. *Human Systems*: 4; 189–200

The National Committee for Primary Mental Health Workers in CAMHS and National CAMHS Support Service, (2004). *The Role of the Child Primary Mental Health Worker.* Department of Health, www.camhs.org.

Sadler, K., Vizard, T., Ford, T., Marcheselli, F., Pearce, N., Mandalia, D., Davis, J., Brodie, E., Forbes, N., Goodman, A., Goodman, R., McManus, S., Responsible Statistician: Dan Collinson, (2017). *The Mental Health of Children and Young People (MHCYP) Survey.* NHS Digital (accessed January 8th 2020 at https://digital.nhs.uk)

Thrive www.thriveapproach.com.

Wolpert, M., Harris, R., Hodges, S., Fuggle, P., James, R., Wiener, A., ... Fonagy, P., (2015). THRIVE elaborated.

77 Early Access

The Development and Practice of ELSA

Sheila Burton

Development of ELSA

The emotional literacy support assistant (ELSA) intervention had its inception in the Southampton Psychology Service in 2001, with the employment of five learning support assistants to work peripatetically in local primary phase schools. The author was charged with the recruitment, training and supervision of these first ELSAs. It quickly became evident that schools greatly valued the input of trained personnel to support individual children's emotional development, providing feedback that staff with such a role were needed permanently within schools. The school-based ELSA model was developed by the author in 2003 in Hampshire, with the educational psychology service providing centre-based training to nominated teaching assistants from schools within a small area of the New Forest. After the initial pilot project, the intervention was extended to include secondary schools and introduced in stages across all areas of the county. The reason the training has been targeted to teaching assistants is sustainability, these members of the school workforce being more likely to be allocated time for regular individual support to children.

The intention behind this initiative is to build capacity within schools to cater for a wide range of emotional needs that are evident in the school population. This is done by equipping and supporting teaching assistants, who often have a different quality of relationship with pupils than do teachers, to develop and deliver individualised programmes of support matched to pupil needs. The approach adopts an interactionist perspective, recognising that any individual characteristics present in children are affected by environmental and social experiences. Many pupils across their educational career will experience emotional challenges that can be ameliorated by the sensitive support of a trusted adult. Through the application of psychological theory, ELSAs are encouraged to consider the underlying needs behind presenting behaviours. If these needs are accurately identified, appropriate programmes can be developed to equip pupils to cope with and better manage the challenges they face. ELSAs work to develop pupils' intrapersonal and interpersonal awareness (recognising, understanding and managing their own emotional responses, while learning to recognise, understand and respond effectively to other people's feelings).

From its earliest beginnings, the demand for this training has not waned. On hearing about the work, educational psychology services in other local authorities expressed a wish to introduce it in their own areas. To facilitate this, the ELSA Trainers' Manual (Burton, 2009), comprising information, guidance, the original training materials and other resources, was published. The original training included modules on emotional awareness, self-esteem, understanding and managing anger, social and friendship skills, loss and bereavement, active listening and communication skills. Educational psychologists are adapting the training over time to reflect needs. This now often includes guidance on attachment needs, solution-focussed approaches and motivational interviewing. The modules include a combination of underpinning psychological theory and practical guidance on intervention approaches. They are delivered in one-day units across one or two school terms, allowing time within the training period for ELSAs to begin applying their learning to their school practice.

Following completion of training, which has now been extended to six days in most places, ELSAs are allocated to small supervision groups (maximum eight ELSAs) that are expected to meet for two hours each half term, led by an educational psychologist. It is the ongoing provision of professional supervision that has marked ELSA out as a unique intervention approach. Educational psychologists, with their knowledge of psychology and child development, together with their experience of the education system, are ideally placed to guide ELSAs' development. Supervision covers the three functions highlighted by Hawkins and Shohet (2007), namely developmental (developing the supervisee's skills and competence), qualitative (safeguarding the children they work with by improving the quality of the supervisee's work) and resourcing (sustaining and supporting the supervisee). An evaluation of the impact of supervision on ELSAs (Osborne and Burton, 2014) analysed the responses of 270 practising ELSAs. There was strong evidence that ELSAs experienced group supervision as a useful mechanism for discussing cases, sharing ideas and problem-solving. They felt better able to support pupils as a result of the support they received.

To promote the ELSA model of intervention, the author established the ELSA Network with its accompanying website (https://www.elsanetwork.org). This incorporates a closed forum to facilitate professional communication between trainers. Educational psychology services delivering ELSA training and supervision are encouraged to register with the Network, which provides them with support and encourages fidelity to the practice model. At the time of writing, there are over 140 educational psychology services across England and Wales providing ELSA training and supervision, with 85% registered as members of the ELSA Network. This work has also attracted interest beyond the UK.

ELSA Practice

When signing up a teaching assistant for training as an ELSA, schools are asked to ensure each person is allocated the equivalent of one day per week for the role, given an appropriate space to work in and allocated a small budget for resources. Their remit is to deliver bespoke programmes of support to children demonstrating emotional needs in school. It is recognised that unless these needs are addressed, pupils will be unable to benefit optimally from the education on offer in school. A key text for ELSAs is *Emotional Wellbeing: An Introductory Handbook for Schools* (Shotton and Burton, 2018, 2nd edition). Its chapters provide a clear overview of each topic from training, underpinned by the latest research in educational psychology, descriptions of vulnerabilities, case studies and suggestions for practical intervention activities.

ELSAs are expected to deliver proactive interventions rather than reactive support. This entails developing time-limited programmes that have clear and achievable aims. The programme develops as it proceeds, one session building upon another according to how the child responds, with a specified objective for each session. It has never been the intention for ELSA support to be an open-ended, long-term intervention for children. The approximate guidelines are for programmes (usually weekly sessions) to last normally between 6 to 12 weeks. This does not preclude pupils from receiving further targeted support programmes but recognises the need for them to have time to consolidate and apply their learning in the context of classroom and playground. In some cases, the planned programme may be followed by a period of less regular and more informal support to assist in the generalisation of new skills.

Implicit in the ELSA model is recognition that emotional literacy is modelled rather than taught. A key difference between an emotional literacy and a behaviour management programme is that the former would be reflective (exploring the child's thoughts and feelings, helping them make informed choices and set their own goals) while the latter would be directive, based on rewards and sanctions (telling them what to do and what will happen if they do or do not achieve an imposed target). ELSA support is about empowerment. Helping a pupil to make informed choices is more powerful and enduring than coercion. To that end, ELSAs are encouraged to develop some basic counselling skills including empathy, genuineness and unconditional positive regard towards those with whom they work. The programme content needs to be distinct from classroom learning experiences and inherently interesting, encouraging experiential learning through enjoyable activities, including well-chosen games and tasks that allow for creative reflection. Feedback from pupils in evaluation studies highlights two key factors of paramount importance for children – quality of relationship and respect for confidentiality. They value the development of a special relationship with a trusted adult, in which they are free to express their thoughts and feelings, knowing that the ELSA will respect the privacy of their conversations. When ELSAs believe it would be helpful to liaise with others, the child is part of the decision-making regarding this; within the normal safeguarding constraints, their wishes are respected.

Although ELSA has been conceived of as primarily individual support, there is scope for group work where appropriate. The development of social interaction skills can be assisted by having a small group context in which to try out new skills and explore their impact. Sometimes a pupil may benefit from an individual programme before embarking upon group work. If each participant has the skills and commitment to engage within a group context, there are some potential additional benefits. New friendships may be formed. Peer influence increases with age, so affirmation from peers can be very powerful in consolidating change. Pupils can also find reassurance in discovering that others have encountered similar challenges to their own. Therefore, groups focussing on anxiety, family break-up or self-esteem may be powerful interventions for some children.

Some challenges with a published and fast-growing intervention approach are maintaining fidelity to the original model and promoting safe and effective practice. The author recognised, through her own experience and contact with numerous other educational psychologists, that many questions present perennially within training and supervision, duplicated across local areas. It has also been noticeable that ELSAs are being expected to support some increasingly complex needs, not least in response to a shortage in other services. Following many years of leading in the field of ELSA, the author produced a best-practice guide for ELSAs, schools and educational psychologists alike, *Excellent ELSAs* (Burton, 2018). The guide comprises guidance in response to these frequent practice issues.

Outcome Measures

Most local services conduct their own evaluations of impact early in the implementation process using a range of measures, often including teacher, parent and pupil rating scales.

Additionally, schools and ELSAs are encouraged to measure the impact of individual pupil interventions. At the simplest level this can be whether programme aims have been achieved or not, but some use a range of rating scales reflecting social and emotional measures, such as the Boxall Profile (available at https://www.boxallprofile.org), an assessment tool for social, emotional and behavioural difficulties for children and young people, or the Southampton Emotional Literacy Scales (available at https://www.gl-assessment.co.uk/products/emotional-literacy/), a standardised assessment of children's emotional literacy.

Case Study (1): Molly

Molly (seven years old) found it difficult to accept adult direction in school, with her behaviour causing difficulties both in the classroom and playground. She often cried on arrival, reluctant to part from her mum. Jan, one of the school's ELSAs, began to greet Molly on arrival and take her to her classroom, using this opportunity to build a special relationship with her. Sometimes she would settle her by sharing a book together or playing a short game. Once a week Molly would have a half hour planned ELSA session with Jan. Having observed Molly in class, Jan realised that some of Molly's resistant behaviour occurred at independent work times. Although Molly's achievements were in the average range, Jan suspected a lack of confidence leading to anxiety. Remembering the training she had received on Borba's building blocks of self-esteem, Jan referred to the behavioural indicators and hypothesised that Molly had unmet needs in the area of security. She also wanted to help Molly find ways of reducing her anxiety. Her programme aims for Molly were for her to separate readily from her mum in the mornings, and to be able to say when she felt worried. During a reflective activity using miniatures, it became clear that Molly had found it difficult having to share mum's attention when her two younger siblings were born. Jan's consistently positive approach to Molly helped her look forward to her special times of attention. Jan helped her identify the many things she had learned to do since starting school. In the games they played, Jan would occasionally make deliberate mistakes that they could laugh about together. Molly gradually learned that making mistakes is safe and they help us learn. Jan used practical activities to demonstrate how worries grow when we focus our attention on them (illustrating this by blowing into a balloon to inflate it; when air is gradually released the balloon begins to deflate). They coloured salt and filled layers in a tiny bottle, each one representing a happy, comforting memory for Molly. She kept this in her pocket so that when she became worried, she could re-focus her thoughts on positive experiences, which helped her relax. Molly's confidence grew noticeably over the term. She came into school more readily and began to ask for help when she was unsure about her work. Molly started to relate to another girl in her class, and they began to play together at break times.

Case Study (2): Sam

Sam (13 years old) had difficulties managing frustration and presented as unpredictably volatile, both at home and school. His older brother had been permanently excluded from school for persistently challenging behaviour including aggressive outbursts. Teachers saw Sam as following in his brother's footsteps. Dan, one of the school's ELSAs, was asked to work with Sam to help him learn to regulate his anger. When he invited Sam to attend weekly sessions with him, Dan was unsure of Sam's interest in changing his behaviour. He decided to apply what he had learned during training about the motivational interviewing approach. He used a set of personal characteristics cards, asking Sam to sort them into categories of like him/unlike him. Dan then asked him to pick the five cards most typical of him, revealing that Sam was aware of his own challenging behaviour. Together they made a chart, using graphical recording, to think first about the benefits to Sam of his angry reactions. When the apparent advantages had been exhausted, Dan began to enquire about any downsides to the choices Sam was making. Dan was open and interested to all Sam's thoughts, avoiding any personal judgements about his behaviour. In their second session, Sam was able to acknowledge that life at school could be better if he were able to moderate his anger. He then accepted Dan's offer to help him explore the nature of anger, his triggers, underlying thought patterns and potential alternative responses. Asked how he would know if Dan's support had been helpful, Sam suggested he would be sent out of lessons less, not get into fights and would be completing his classwork. These became his programme aims. Sam was especially interested in the Assault Cycle showing the normal pattern of escalation and recovery in an angry outburst, recognising how this fitted him. Over the next weeks Dan used the firework model to help Sam understand the triggers to his outbursts and how his thinking patterns sustained angry feelings. Dan supported Sam to work out his own strategies for managing frustrations in different contexts. By the end of ten weeks Sam was achieving his own goals and was proud of the positive reports his parents received from teachers at the end of term parents' evening, which was a completely new experience for him.

Summary Questions

What Is the Theoretical Perspective behind the ELSA Model?

ELSA is an educational psychology-led intervention and, as such, takes an interactive perspective on emotional development and wellbeing. Any individual child's characteristics are contributed to and influenced by environmental and social experiences. It does not require diagnosis of conditions, but rather looks at potential factors influencing the children receiving intervention. A core principle is to seek to understand the underlying needs communicated by presenting behaviours and develop an intervention reflecting those individual needs.

What Is the Aim of ELSA Intervention?

The aim is to facilitate the development of coping strategies in children for those elements in their situation that they cannot change and empower them to take responsibility for those things that lie within their personal control. This is achieved through reflective activities and conversations that increase pupils' self-awareness. Planned programmes of support aim to help children develop new insights and skills, encouraging them to find their own solutions to challenges they face.

What Is the Role of Supervision?

Those undertaking the role of ELSA in school receive only five to six days of training from educational psychologists. From the outset it was recognised as professionally responsible to ensure they then receive ongoing support to build their knowledge and competence as practitioners. The importance of this has been underlined by the increasing complexity of cases brought to supervision, arising in part from a shortage in availability of more specialised services. Supervision helps to ensure ELSAs work within their professional competence and that they receive the personal support they need.

What Is the Expected Duration of an ELSA Programme?

The duration will vary according to need and pupil factors, but interventions should be time-limited and usually deliverable within one school term. This requires the identification of small, achievable targets. The planned sessions may sometimes be followed by lighter touch support to help the pupil maintain and generalise newly acquired skills. A pupil may later receive further programmes as deemed appropriate, but the intention is to help them develop their own competence rather than create dependence upon an ELSA.

Is ELSA Intervention Always Delivered Individually?

Because the development of a trusting relationship, in which a pupil can talk openly about their perceptions and circumstances, is key to the success of ELSA, most programmes will be individual. There is, nevertheless, legitimate scope for some carefully planned groupwork, where the ELSA–child relationship may be less personal but is compensated by the development of positive peer relationships.

Key References

Burton, S., (2009). *ELSA Trainers' Manual*. London: Optimus Education.

Burton, S., (2018). *Excellent ELSAs*. Poole: Inspiration Books.

Osborne, C., Burton, S., (2014). Emotional Literacy Support Assistants' views on supervision provided by educational psychologists: what EPs can learn from group supervision. *Educational Psychology in Practice*, 30(2): 139–155.

Shotton, G., Burton, S., (2018). *Emotional Wellbeing: An Introductory Handbook for Schools* (2nd ed.). London and New York: Routledge.

78 Early Access

Emotional Literacy and First Aid in Schools

Helena Hoyos

KEY CONCEPTS

- Emotional literacy is a key skill which children and young people need in order to develop as successful learners and happy, productive adults who are able to function well within society.
- Schools have a responsibility to identify children and young people who are struggling with their emotional development and to provide early intervention and support. This may take place through initiatives such as emotional literacy support assistants and/or emotional first aid.
- Emotional literacy support should ideally be part of a whole-school ethos as well as focussing on individual development. Staff emotional literacy and wellbeing are of great importance as well as those of the children in their care.

In November 2018, the Department for Education published non-statutory guidance on 'Mental Health and Behaviour in Schools'. This highlights the fact that 'schools have an important role to play in supporting the mental health and wellbeing of children by developing whole-school approaches tailored to their particular needs, as well as considering the needs of individual pupils'. This guidance is underpinned by the 'Special Educational Needs and Disability Code of Practice: 0-25', jointly published by the Department for Education and Department of Health in January 2015, which highlights the general importance of early identification of any areas of need, and stresses a key role for 'the development of good mental health through universal services, so that effective use is made of Child and Adolescent Mental Health Services (CAMHS)'.

Together, these documents indicate that schools are key providers of identification and support for children and young people who may be experiencing difficulties with their emotional development, which could have a long-term negative effect on their mental health. It is recognised that some children and young people may develop a degree of need which goes beyond the level of expertise available in schools. However, even these children and young people may take the first steps towards emotional health with the support and guidance of school staff. The members of staff who work with these children often do so through the use of programmes focussing on the development of emotional literacy, or through the application of approaches such as emotional first aid.

Emotional Literacy

Many schools have chosen to address the emotional needs of their children and young people through the use of emotional literacy as a framework for supporting individuals and for developing a whole-school ethos which promotes emotional wellbeing for pupils and staff. The term 'emotional literacy' was first introduced by Claude Steiner in 1984. However, for many years key writers and researchers in the field, such as Daniel Goleman, Howard Gardner, Peter Salovey and Jack Mayer used the term 'emotional intelligence'. In his writings in the 1990s, Goleman was one of the first to publicly champion the importance of meeting children's emotional needs in order to enable them to learn effectively. His work was very important in popularising the idea of emotional intelligence as a crucial factor in helping children become successful learners, especially within a social context such as a school. Since that time, within schools, the term 'emotional literacy' has been more widely adopted. It is likely that a key reason for this is to present a challenge to the idea of a fixed and unchanging state which is often associated with the concept of 'intelligence'. We are all familiar with the idea that 'literacy' can be taught and learned, and therefore the concept of 'emotional literacy' suggests that emotional skills can also be developed over time.

The following definition was first applied to the idea of emotional intelligence by Mayer and Salovey in 1997, but works equally well as a definition of emotional literacy: 'The ability to monitor one's own and other's feelings and emotions and to use this information to guide one's thinking and actions'. This can be broken down further into:

- The ability to perceive accurately, appraise and express emotion
- The ability to access and/or generate feelings which facilitate thought
- The ability to understand emotion and emotional knowledge
- The ability to regulate emotions to promote emotional and intellectual growth

In other words, emotional literacy is about learning to understand and talk about how we feel, to reflect on our emotions and how they are affecting our thinking and behaviour and to manage our emotions and those of other people in a productive way. All of these skills are central to our ability to function effectively in social groups, such as classrooms. They can also have a significant impact on our resilience and ability to open ourselves up to the possibility of making mistakes which is fundamental to the learning process.

Emotional literacy is now actively promoted in many schools. The Education Endowment Foundation identifies three main areas where this typically takes place, under the framework of Social and Emotional Learning, and provides guidance as to the effectiveness of approaches. These include universal programmes which generally take place in the classroom, more specialised programmes which are targeted at students with particular social or emotional needs and school-level approaches to developing a positive school ethos, which also aim to support greater engagement in learning.

Approaches aimed at supporting individual children and young people often involve training specific members of staff to work with children who are experiencing difficulty in recognising and managing their emotions, which is impacting on their learning and behaviour. One of the most widely recognised programmes in this field trains emotional literacy support assistants (ELSAs) to work with individuals and groups, and provides ongoing group supervision for the ELSAs whilst they are working in this way. ELSA is a preventative intervention which aims to build the capacity of schools to support pupils' emotional/social needs from within their own resources. This programme was first developed in 2004 as a pilot study in the Hampshire area by Sheila Burton, Educational Psychologist. The training and supervision are still provided by educational psychologists.

Emotional First Aid

Another very popular programme of emotional support for children and young people in schools is the emotional first aid approach, first developed in 2008 as a training course in

Southampton by Stuart Gemmell, Dave Smith and Jacquie Kelly. Training is available to adults working with children and young people within universal services, including school staff, who may be in a position to offer support to children and young people experiencing emotional distress. It is an early intervention approach which aims to give staff the skills they need to work alongside young people with emotional difficulties, enabling them to express their emotions and develop helpful strategies which will enable them to cope and move forward with their lives, without going on to develop a mental health problem. As with emotional literacy, emotional first aid also has an emphasis on supporting the wellbeing of adults working with children and young people experiencing emotional distress, as well as the children and young people themselves. It may sometimes build on emotional literacy development already made available to children and young people through a whole-school approach, individual or group sessions, which will have aimed to give the children and young people the tools they need to think about their emotions with a supportive adult.

What Might Emotional Literacy Support Include?

Emotionally literate people are able to understand and talk about their feelings and manage those feelings effectively, so that they do not overwhelm their capacity to think. They tune in to the feelings of other people and work co-operatively and sensitively with them, functioning well in groups as well as individually. These abilities are very important for children and young people developing their skills as learners. They are increasingly encouraged to have a 'growth mindset', which challenges them to tackle negative self-perceptions and believe in their own potential, and emotionally literate children and young people are likely to be more able to do this successfully.

There are several components to supporting the development of emotional literacy skills which make this possible. The detail and complexity of the work will vary according to the age and developmental level of the child or young person.

Conscious Awareness and Communication Skills

We all need to learn to be aware of how we are feeling and to develop a vocabulary which allows us to reflect on these feelings and communicate them appropriately to other people. This is often the first step for those working with children to help them develop their emotional literacy. In the early stages this can be as simple as helping children recognise and label the feelings that they and other people have, often through the use of resources such as 'feelings faces' and related scenarios. The use of puppets can also be very helpful as part of this process.

Understanding the Links between Thoughts, Feelings and Actions

As children learn how their thoughts, feelings and actions may be linked, their behaviour can increasingly be guided by reasoned choices, rather than being based on impulse. In the early stages this may involve working with children on the differences between thoughts and feelings and how to distinguish between them.

Managing Feelings

As children learn more about the types of feelings they are experiencing and what triggers these feelings, they are more able to recognise when the feelings are starting to get in the way and take steps to manage both their feelings and responses. They learn that we are able to control our responses and have our needs met, without our feelings overwhelming and blocking us. In the early stages this often involves helping children recognise if they are becoming angry or anxious, so that they can tell an adult and/or practice calming techniques they have learned, before the feelings become too strong for them to manage successfully. An important part of this work can be helping the child or young person attribute their emotions correctly so that they don't, for example, react angrily in one situation because they are still experiencing that emotion from something that happened earlier in the day.

Managing Conflict

As children gain increasing emotional awareness they gradually become more able to manage conflict effectively. The work often begins with helping them to recognise the triggers that make them angry and the signs that their anger is building, which are often felt in the body's reactions. This increased awareness gives them the choice to avoid the conflict before it escalates beyond their control. This is of clear benefit to the child or young person, but may also have particular relevance for those working with children and young people, who can sometimes experience their own emotional control being challenged by the emotions triggered by their work.

Understanding Groups

As we become more aware of our own feelings and reactions and those of other people, we become more able to share attention, take turns and recognise the strengths and needs that we and others bring to any situation. This helps us co-operate and communicate much more effectively in groups. Emotional literacy work often involves playing specially developed scenario-based games which help children and young people practice important skills such as turn taking, as well as giving them an opportunity to consider how they and others might think, feel or react in a range of different situations.

Case Study: Mandy

Mandy's behaviour at school has changed recently in Year 4. For the last few weeks, Mandy has often experienced strong emotions at school which don't feel good. She knows she does not feel good, but her only way of describing this is to say she feels 'bad'. She does not have the vocabulary to distinguish between different types of emotions which feel 'bad', which might include 'angry,' 'sad', 'scared', 'guilty', 'ashamed', 'frustrated', 'embarrassed', 'worried', 'confused', etc. Mandy has started reacting to feeling 'bad' by behaving in a way which challenges her teachers, such as refusing to work, being rude to her teachers, kicking the classroom furniture and destroying other children's work. Mandy often misses playtime because of her behaviour, which increases how 'bad' she feels.

Mandy's teachers are concerned about her and arrange for her to meet regularly with the school's ELSA, who Mandy knows and trusts as she has been a teaching assistant in Mandy's class. Through her work with the ELSA, Mandy starts to be able to recognise and label how she is feeling more precisely. She tells the ELSA that her mother has been ill for several weeks and Mandy worries about her when she is at school. She can't concentrate because she is worried, and then can't do her work, which makes her feel upset and embarrassed, so she refuses to try it. She feels sad, frustrated and helpless about her mother's illness, and sometimes lashes out because of this. Her friends know her mother is ill and try to support her, but she often misses spending time with them because she is kept in at playtime.

Due to Mandy's work with the ELSA, her teachers now have a very different understanding of how she is feeling and what support she needs to help her through her mother's illness. Her behaviour can be viewed and managed very differently when it is seen as a reaction to a very stressful situation and the emotions she feels in response to this. Time with her friends can be viewed as a priority, as well as help to address any gaps in her learning. Available support during the day for Mandy's mother may also be explored, so that Mandy can relax at school and know that her mother is cared for when she is not there.

So Why Is Emotional Literacy Important?

As a responsible society, we have a duty to help children develop and reach their potential as well-rounded, emotionally healthy individuals who can play a full and active part in the society of their future. The development of emotional literacy is at the heart of how we can do this, in our homes, schools and all aspects of our lives.

Key References

Department for Education, *Mental Health and Behaviour in Schools*, November 2018.
Department for Education and Department of Health, *Special Educational Needs and Disability Code of Practice: 0–25*, January 2015.
Goleman, Daniel, *Emotional Intelligence: Why It Can Matter More Than IQ*, Bloomsbury, 1995.

79 Early Access: A CAMHS' Single Point of Access

Nottingham City's Whole System Model

Anna Masding

Introduction

In this chapter we will consider:

- The benefits of a multiagency approach to screen and process referrals for child and adolescent mental health services (CAMHS), namely a **single point of access (SPA)** based within a **multiagency safeguarding hub (MASH)**; promoting a range of timely and effective preventative interventions for child and adolescent mental health needs.
- A case vignette, when responding to SPA referrals for higher risk groups, using a **Joint Protocol model**, to jointly assess and manage self-harm/suicidality and safeguarding concerns.
- Other essential components of an integrated SPA:
  a. Children, young people and parent/carer's participation
  b. Data monitoring and quality assurance processes

A CAMHS Single Point of Access (SPA) Based within a Multiagency Safeguarding Hub (MASH)

A single point of access, often referred to as an SPA or an SPO within a CAMH service, is a model or pathway where referrals and contacts into the service come into **one single point** and are screened in order for an outcome to happen. This is often referred to in health services as 'triage', a medical term to decide the order of treatment of numerous patients.

The Nottingham City model that is described in this chapter differs from other models; as this particular CAMHS SPA is embedded within the local authority (and not the NHS), it sits within a **multiagency safeguarding hub** known as a 'MASH'. This is a group of professionals who work collaboratively in an integrated way, often co-located, gathering and sharing vital information. The Munro Review of Child Protection, along with numerous serious case reviews, highlighted the failures of agencies to work together to safeguard children and young people. As such in 2011 the first MASH was developed in a response to this.

The MASH that is described here has input from social care, health, early help/targeted family support services, the police and probation, the Fire Service, NSPCC Protect and Respect, Women's Aid and many more, and it is also co-located with the CAMHS SPA.

The city SPA is an integrated model of emotional and mental health services that come together as one team (including virtual components), to offer a range of support and treatment options for children, young people and their families where there are concerns around a child/young person's emotional and mental health. This includes counselling services (both online and face to face), early intervention support for neurodevelopmental disorders, evidence-based therapeutic approaches and access into more specialist mental health treatments, such as the eating disorder service, CAMHS Crisis, psychology and psychiatric services. An SPA protocol was devised to ensure that referrals are processed as quickly and safely as possible, and that decisions are made swiftly with access to as much relevant and critical information as possible. This ensures that the decisions and outcomes are based on accurate information that is available to the services; as such access to the partner agencies' data systems is essential.

This model also means that if referrals are limited in their detail, instead of them being rejected (meaning children and young people have to wait longer for support), the service can source information from the range of data systems, or can contact families to gain the information that is essential for the screening processes. In 2018 only 6% of the total number of referrals into SPA were rejected and sent back to the referring agency for more information (Nottingham City Council, 2019).

Mind the Gap! families have told us that 'it is often hard to know what services are out there, and how to access them', and there has been much criticism that tiered models of approaches mean:

- Children are expected to fit into service, rather than services fitting to changing needs of the child.
- Confusing barriers between services.
- Confusing model for non-professionals.
- Embedding service divisions and fragmentation of care.
- Possible 'passing the buck' between services/tiers and commissioners.

(Public Health Suffolk, 2015)

The integrated SPA model offers one large front door for Nottingham City families, allowing the professionals to help them to navigate a system that historically has been complex and hard to find their way into. This ensures the right help, at the right time, in the right place for children, young people and their families. It is a model that recognises the importance of easy access, and that both early intervention and prevention are key in the support and treatment of child and young people's emotional and mental health. Its philosophy is that the emotional health and wellbeing of children and young people should be considered and understood in the broader context of their current individual circumstances, their family context and their history as opposed to a purely clinical/medical model of their presenting mental health symptoms/disorders. Moreover, a child or young person's emotional wellbeing often exists within a complex ecology of many inter-relating and determining factors that will often impact their emotional wellbeing daily, in many different and challenging ways. Thus ensuring that referrals are screened and considered within this context helps to make sure that they receive the service that is most likely to support their presenting needs, and that if a child or young person accesses a service that isn't what they need, or that is not right for them, they can easily access what is.

This model is also advantageous financially, as in 2018/19, of the SPA referrals that required CAMHS input, 92.5% remained within targeted CAMHS that were able to support them within their local community (traditionally known as Tier 2 services), with only 7.25% needing to be sent onto more specialist services. Of those accepted for treatment at targeted CAMHS, 91.3% were seen and discharged without any need to be stepped up to a supplementary specialist CAMH service, with only 8.7% stepped up either following assessment or treatment (2.1% following assessment and 6.6% following treatment) (Nottingham City Council, 2019). This means that children and young people only need to be escalated into more specialist and costly provisions when it is essential. This is a 'good news story' for commissioners and local authorities, as it means that their investments into child and young people's mental health provision not only promote a model of early intervention/prevention but are also more cost effective.

Consideration of High-Risk Groups

Nottingham ranks fourth most deprived of the Core Cities in the UK (Nottingham Insight, 2019, Indices of Deprivation); consequently, the MASH and SPA are managing various daily referrals for children and young people who are presenting with higher risk behaviours and who have been, or who are, subject to safeguarding concerns/procedures. In the safeguarding chapter we have already learnt the importance of a "*Think Family*" approach when safeguarding children and young people, and how it is essential to work smarter in order to minimise the adverse effects of abuse and neglect. There are ever-increasing numbers of referrals into SPA where self-harm behaviours and suicidality in children and young people, alongside safeguarding issues, are significant risk factors.

Prevalence Data for Self-Harm and Suicidal Behaviours

The analysis of data from *The Intentional Self-Harm in Adolescence: The Health Behaviour in School-Aged Children (HBSC) Survey for England, 2014*, identified prevalence rates at 22% for 15-year olds in England. Nearly three times as many girls as boys reported that they had self-harmed, 11% of boys compared to 32% of girls. The majority of those young people who were self-harming reported engaging in self-harm once a month or more, and it was found that the majority of people who self-reported self-harm are aged between 11 and 25 years. However, self-harming behaviours are most likely to occur between the ages of 12 and 15 years, and in those children and young people who have adverse childhood experiences (ACE) the rate of self-harm is increased. ACEs are defined as:

- Domestic abuse
- Parental abandonment through separation or divorce
- Parental mental health difficulties
- Being a victim of abuse
- Being a victim of neglect
- Living in a household where the adults are experiencing drug/alcohol use difficulties
- A member of the household being in prison

(Public Health England, 2013)

A study published in the *International Journal of Environmental Research and Public Health* found that there was clear evidence that ACEs are associated with repeat self-harm, with exposure to multiple ACEs being reported by more than 79.1% of those in the repeat self-harm group in their study (*International Journal of Environmental Research and Public Health*, 2018).

When safeguarding children and young people we know that the most effective models are those that enable professionals to make timely, appropriate and analytical decisions about the information they have. This case vignette describes how the integrated SPA model responds to such referrals using the **Joint Protocol model**. This Nottingham City model was developed in partnership with the safeguarding hub, and this response can be activated by the MASH team (which includes SPA), by either the MASH social workers, or the SPA CAMHS team. This example describes a joint risk assessment and a safety planning approach to ensure that there is a shared understanding and accountability of the levels of risk and need for a young person.

Case Study: Gemma

Gemma (aged 17) was referred into SPA by her GP, following her accessing help alone for her low mood, self-harming behaviours (by cutting her arms), intrusive thoughts of sad images and upsetting events, along with low self-esteem and a negative body image. Gemma felt that she was at the root of most arguments at home, and should be punished for them. Her relative had completed suicide a year ago, and her mother's view was that this was 'attention-seeking' and had told Gemma that she thought the same was true about self-harm. Thus, Gemma felt unable to talk to her parents about how she was feeling and had requested that any correspondence from CAMHS be sent to the GP surgery, and not to her home address. There were no previous concerns, or indicators of abuse.

From further contact with Gemma she disclosed that she had a plan and intent to end her life. At this point it was decided that CAMHS needed to work with Gemma and her parents, to ensure that she was supported to tell her parents how she was feeling, to allow them the opportunity to help to safeguard her. Work was completed with Gemma to help her understand why her parents needed to be involved in order to help them to understand what was happening for her and how she was feeling at home. The Joint Protocol was explained and reassurance was given to Gemma, and she agreed that this visit could go ahead, as long as she could have her trusted friend present.

A Joint Protocol home visit was completed with Gemma, both her parents and Gemma's trusted friend. On the visit Gemma was supported to share how she was feeling with her parents and her friend. Her low mood, current self-harm, her thoughts and plans of suicide were all assessed jointly. Gemma was able to share that her mother had been making negative comments about her self-harm and her weight, and that, as her mother was a health professional, she had told Gemma that if she shared information about her self-harm with other professionals she may lose her job, and this had made Gemma become very secretive at home. On the visit, mother was able to be reassured that this would not be the case, and that the opposite was true in terms of the importance of hearing and understanding how Gemma was feeling and that seeking support to help her daughter was crucial. Mother was able to share that she had witnessed the tragic suicide, and that this trauma had impacted on her ability to contain and support Gemma, as she needed to shut this out of her mind. Parents were also able to share that since the suicide of the relative, they had both had some challenges around alcohol misuse and this had been causing arguments between them both and Gemma. Parents were able to recognise that open communication, family time and planning things for Gemma to look forward to would all be important elements of Gemma's recovery. Information was given to the family, including a safety pack to support young people with low mood and self-harm behaviours. Social Care planned to visit the family again to complete a full family assessment focussing on the family dynamics, family relationships and alcohol misuse, to ensure that Gemma was safeguarded at home and supported with her mental health needs. Parents were offered the local self-harm parent group called 'SHARP 4 Parents', where they could talk safely about their traumatic experience of a family suicide, and to get advice and support about how to listen, help and support their daughter.

On the visit Gemma was able to share that she didn't have any current plans to end her life, but had fleeting suicidal thoughts and that she just wanted and needed to be heard and understood. The risk assessment concluded that there was a medium risk of self-harm and high risk for suicide. The clinical measures RCADS and SDQs were completed and a safety plan was developed with Gemma, her family and her trusted friend. Gemma agreed that she would like support from her college counsellor and that she would like all of the information, including the safety plan, to be shared with them. CAMHS liaised with college to share information and to arrange the counselling for her. It was agreed that the local CAMHS Crisis team would be alerted, and they agreed to complete 'check ins' with Gemma over the weekends when she didn't have access to her counsellor. A College Welfare Support liaison was arranged with CAMHS whilst a referral to adult mental health was initiated, to ensure a smooth transition happened for Gemma when she turned 18 in 2 months' time.

Questions to Consider

1. What are the main presenting concerns in this case?
2. Why and how did the Joint Protocol approach benefit the young person, family and the services involved?
3. What are some of the barriers or limitations in this approach?

Analysis

As you will have gained from the case vignette, this model allows for timely risk assessment and safety planning of a child/young person who would otherwise have been subject to two separate assessments by two separate services and professionals, through a 'single lens' approach. One service is trained and working extensively in the management of safeguarding concerns of abuse, neglect and harm, and the other trained and working with mental health conditions, therapeutic approaches and self-harm/suicidality. Bringing these services together in a *joint response* to the concerns about a child/young person, within their ecology and at the earliest opportunity (a home visit undertaken within 48 hours of the referral(s) being received), ensures that a holistic assessment is quickly completed, taking into account the safeguarding concerns, as well as the self-harm behaviours, their presentation and the current levels of risk. Safety plans are developed jointly so both the professionals and the family can agree on how to support and safely manage the child/young person's needs and behaviours.

The HBSC survey for England (2014) suggests that 'Recent investigations have stressed the importance of good communication with parents for better health and social outcomes in adolescence' (Moreno et al., 2009). The self-harm protocol encourages this at the earliest opportunity, in an attempt to reduce self-harming behaviours/suicidality, and to increase the awareness and understanding of the family in order to help keep the child/young person safe, whilst also addressing any presenting safeguarding concerns. If, however, on the home visit it is concluded that either the mental health risk is too high to implement a safety plan at home, or that the safeguarding concerns meet the threshold for Section 75 procedures (or both), then processes to safeguard the child or young person can be implemented immediately.

Essential Components of an Integrated CAMHS SPA

Children, Young People and Parent/Carer's Participation

NHS England guidance on participation sets out two types of participation in health care services:

1. People's involvement in decisions about their own health – *individual participation.*
2. People's involvement in the design and delivery of health services they use – *public participation.*

(Public Health England, 2013)

These are critical components to any effective health and social care service model, as regularly gaining the views and feedback from the children, young people and their parents/carers ensures that the service provides the support that is helpful for the child/young person and their family and that the service develops how the users would like, and not simply how professionals think it *should be.* An example of this is described here, in how the engagement of parents/carers has changed practices within the integrated city SPA.

A participation group was developed in Nottingham called '*Parents in Mind*'. The purpose of this group is for parents to come together to support each other, and to share their voice about their local CAMH service. '*Parents in mind*' gave clear feedback that accessing a CAMH service left them feeling quite worried, not knowing what to expect or what to do while they waited. They told the service that the first letter sent out to them offering an assessment appointment was not helpful, as it used unfamiliar and complicated language. As a result, the parents themselves rewrote the letter and the SPA has since implemented their approach and the revised format is now used for all the appointment letters sent to families. The parents also co-developed the idea of a new concept called '*Open Door*'. This is an open drop-in monthly session within the community where parents/carers can come to meet with their CAMH service *before* their first assessment appointment. This allows them to meet with a CAMHS professional and 'put a face to the service'. It allows them the opportunity to learn what to expect from the service, to ask questions and to get some support, advice or self-help materials whilst they wait for their first appointment. This also allows them the opportunity to understand if the service is right for their son/daughter, or if they need a different form of support instead, or in addition to CAMHS.

Understanding the parent/carers' voice in this way means that it is now more likely families will engage from the start and that parents/carers will feel able to support their son/daughter to access the right help. This in turn helps to reduce the numbers of missed appointments, meaning that the service will be more efficient. These two simple examples of how the parent's voice has shaped service delivery would have been missed opportunities had parental participation not been considered in the SPA's service development.

Data Monitoring and Quality Assurance

The SPA implements a weekly monitoring process that calculates the wait times weekly in the service for all of the assessments, consultations and the therapeutic support that are offered. This allows the service to see where there are any pressure points and to respond to these quickly by moving resources to respond to this more immediately. For instance, if there is a longer wait for consultations, but limited waits for assessments, then practitioners can offer more consultations than assessments, until the waits are cleared. Analysing the data and responding to these regularly allows for more frequent strategic service re-modelling, by way of responding to the ever-changing needs of our communities. Weekly monitoring also ensures that the service continues to offer support to families within the agreed commissioned expectations, and where there are new pressures for the service, this can be quickly identified and openly highlighted to commissioners.

Quality assurance SPA audits are completed 6-monthly with 20 randomly selected cases. This is to ensure that the SPA protocol is being followed, timeframes are monitored and that outcomes for children, young people and their families are helpful, safe and with as quick and easy access as possible. This audit process produces clear recommendations and allows for developments to the service model. These reviews have helped to shape new innovations within the SPA; an example of this is the recent development of an SPA Early Intervention Worker. This is where current vacancies for more traditional family support roles in the service have been re-modelled to allow for another 'treatment arm' to be introduced in SPA. Early Intervention Workers make telephone contact with young people and families quickly and directly, to complete mini and full assessments, clinical screening measures and to offer evidence-based self-help materials to support them while they are waiting to be seen for the most appropriate treatment or support. This again helps regulate waits, by ensuring that young people and families are contacted and offered support as quickly as possible, and that those who do not require face-to-face support are discharged with support, and for those where there are higher risk or immediate self-harm/suicidality and safeguarding concerns, the Joint Protocol can be initiated. This also ensures that if a child/young person is re-referred into the service, having already had contact with an SPA Early Intervention Worker, then they can be offered a face-to-face intervention without the wait for another full assessment.

A Summary of the Key Learning Points for the Screening and Management of Child and Adolescent Referrals

- The importance of an integrated multiagency model that allows for the gaining and sharing of accurate information for safe and informed decision-making in a timely way.
- The importance of helping children, young people and families to navigate their local services with referrals not being 'rejected' but information being sought to find them the right service to meet their needs.
- The importance of responding swiftly and in an integrated way, for children and young people who present with high-level/complex needs, or who may be living in situations of harm/abuse/neglect and who may have ACEs.
- The importance of listening to families' feedback and supporting them to co-produce and co-develop services that work for them.
- The importance of data and quality assurances processes to continue to effectively develop models of inventions, such as the SPA and JP approaches described in this chapter.

Key References

Brooks, F., Chester, K., Klemera, E., Magnusson, J., (2017). *Intentional Self-Harm in Adolescence: An Analysis of Data from the Health Behaviour in School-Aged Children (HBSC) Survey for England*, 2014., PHE by the HBSC England., PHE publications gateway number: 2016713.

Centre of Excellence for Information Sharing, (2018–2019). *Multiagency Safeguarding Hubs* [Online]. Available at: http://informationsharing.org.uk/wp-content/uploads/dlm_uploads/2017/03/COEIS-multi-agency-sharing-hubs.pdf (Accessed on 06/10/2019).

Cleare, S., Wetherall, K., Clark, A., Ryan, C., Kirtley, O.J., Smith, M., O'Connor, R.C., (2018). Adverse childhood experiences and hospital treated self-harm. *International Journal of Environmental Research and Public Health*, 15: 1235.

Moreno, C., Sánchez-Queija, I., Muñoz-Tinoco, V., De Matos, M.G., Dallago, L., Ter Bogt, T., Rivera, F., (2009). Cross-national associations between parent and peer communication and psychological complaints. *International Journal of Public Health*, 54(2): 235–242.

Munro, E., (2011). *The Munro Review of Child Protection: Final Report. A Child-Centred System.* London: Department for Education.

Nottingham City Council., (2019). *Joint Protocol.*

Nottingham City Council., (2019). *95% Referral Data.*

Nottingham City Council., (2019). *Nottingham Youth Justice Service Youth Justice Plan 2017–20: 2019–20 Update*, pp. 3.

Nottingham Insight, (2019). Indices of deprivation [online]. Available at https://www.nottinghaminsight.org.uk/themes/deprivation-and-poverty/indices-of-deprivation-2019/ (Accessed February 19th, 2020).

Public Health England, (2013). *How Healthy Behaviour Supports Children's Wellbeing* [online]. Available at: http://www.gov.uk/government/uploads/system/uploads/attachment_data/file/232978/Smart_Restart_280813_web.pdf (Accessed 15th–16th August 2019).

Public Health Suffolk, (2015). *Suffolk County Council. A Review of the Evidence on: Whole System Model/Approaches to Addressing and Preventing Emotional, Behavioural and Mental Health Difficulties in Children and Young People and Single Point of Access.*, page 4 [Online]. Available at: https://www.westsuffolkccg.nhs.uk/wp-content/uploads/2013/01/APPENDIX-5C-Whole-System-Model-Single-Point-of-Access.pdf (Accessed 29/10/2019).

80 Specialist Services

Child and Adolescent Mental Health Services (CAMHS)

Cathy Laver-Bradbury

KEY CONCEPTS

- Specialist CAMHS teams are made up of a variety of health and social care professionals and, sometimes, professionals from education.
- Recruitment and retention are major issues within CAMHS.
- The model through which a professional explains why a child or young person is behaving as they are can vary, and specialist CAMHS workers need to understand all of their colleagues' different approaches.
- Team discussions, supervision and flexibility are important when considering how first to formulate, and then plan, treatments that may need to be multi-faceted.

CAMHS is used as a term for all services that work with children and young people (CYP) experiencing difficulties with their emotional or behavioural wellbeing. These services can be from the statutory, voluntary or school-based sectors, e.g. an NHS trust, local authority or charitable organisation. They often work in a variety of settings to enable quick access at a place familiar to the young person. These interventions may be time limited.

Specialist CAMHS is a term used to describe a multidisciplinary team of clinicians who work within a health setting. They accept referrals from other services and from parents who are asking for an explanation about the CYP behaviour in relation to the child's mental health. Specialist CAMHS is usually accessed when other services or family members remain concerned about a CYP. They may or may not have accessed CAMHS support in the community for the child or young person prior to a specialist CAMHS referral. Whilst this chapter will focus on the specialist CAMHS team and the professionals who work in it, it is useful to understand the changing context in which all CAMHS services are currently working.

Context

The most recent of several national reviews of CAMHS took place in 2019 (CQC, 2019). There were two aspects within the review: Phase 1 looked at what was happening nationally, and Phase 2 reviewed ten services in depth and made recommendations. The key findings were:

- More children and young people have mental health problems than in the past.
- The availability and quality of services vary, as does the way different parts of the system are commissioned, funded and overseen.

- Heavy workloads, difficulty in recruiting and retaining staff and gaps in knowledge and skills all contribute to services missing opportunities to support children and young people's mental health and delays in identifying mental health issues.
- Many children, young people and their families or carers struggle to find timely and appropriate care when they first try to access help for a mental health problem.
- The availability of services provided by schools, local authorities, voluntary and community organisations varies from one part of the country to the next, depending on what is commissioned locally, and there are gaps in our understanding of the quality and availability of some of these services.

The review found great examples of services with caring and dedicated individuals who put children and young people at the centre of what they do. These people are often working long hours, within limited budgets and an increasing demand for their services, a situation that cannot be maintained in the long run. The structure of specialist CAMHS can vary across the country, although most follow a similar structure.

Pathway Delivered Care

Ring-fenced funding for the eating disorders pathway in specialist CAMHS services was introduced in 2014 and revised in 2019/20 with the government laying out guidelines for eating disorders (Children and Young People's Eating Disorder Access and Waiting Time Commissioning Guide, published August 2015). This was established to ensure that young people presenting with an eating disorder were seen quickly by specialist services. Services were advised on how these should be structured, and specific staff quotas were given. Financial oversight was included to ensure that the allocated money went to this pathway. This was the only pathway where funding was specified, and no further specifically allocated funding was suggested, as the other conditions were considered as being provided for within a specialist CAMHS setting.

Following the introduction of the eating disorders pathway, the structure of many specialist CAMHS changed and what emerged were services structured around the pathway model of care, but without the specific allocation of funding. These are largely in line with the NICE pathways, i.e. the autism pathway, the ADHD pathway, crisis pathway, depression and anxiety pathway and trauma pathway, in addition to the eating disorder pathway. There is often an overlap with disorders and transference of care between the pathways, depending on the needs of the young person and their family. This can mean that children and young people move from one pathway list to another depending on the resources within a service.

It is within this context that most specialist CAMH services are currently structured, and the staff are often recruited into both the generic and the specialist roles. The difficulty with this approach is that it is around diagnosis and many of the young people seen may not meet the criteria for a diagnosis, or want one, or may have overlapping disorders. The pathway model has its limitations.

The staff working within specialist services has changed with the introduction of IAPT workers, trained in low- and high-intensity CBT or parenting, forming part of the workforce (IAPT 2019, NHS Digital). Responsibilities in the teams have changed from the higher banding given for expertise now linked to working with crisis in many services, rather than in their expert role.

Specialist Staff Working in CAMHS

Management

The complexity of the needs of a multidisciplinary workforce, combined with the complexity of the children and families seen, means that careful management with a clear strategic vision is necessary for the specialist CAMHS team to function successfully. The role of the manager within a specialist CAMHS service has changed over recent years, and greater emphasis has been given to developing a close working relationship between commissioners and NHS trust management, in addition to working with other partner agencies. A crucial role of the manager is to ensure the seamless care of CYP needing to access services from a potential variety of providers.

Developing a shared vision between partner agencies is key, with clear expectations about which service is best able to meet the needs of the CYP and their families, when further care is needed and how it can be accessed.

Shared visions develop with an understanding of what an agency is able to provide and what it cannot. This is a tension for all providers and families.

The resources available within a specialist mental health team dictate what interventions are available, and these have largely evolved through research over time about what works. These resources are very limited, with most specialist CAMHS teams struggling to meet the demand.

Managers work with the clinical team in regard to treatments but have to hold the balance of what resources/interventions/staffing are available to meet those needs.

Specialist CAMHS managers can come from a variety of backgrounds. Often, they have been clinicians trained in management techniques. They work hard to lead the services whilst ensuring that both the needs of the CYP and their families, and those of the staff and organisation are met. Management is most effective when there is a strong management team made up of clinicians representing the specialist CAMHS workers alongside managers, in order to understand the complexity of the services and where the teams see themselves as learning organisations.

Consultant Child and Adolescent Psychiatrists

Consultant psychiatrists are doctors who have completed their medical training and undertaken extensive training in adult and child and adolescent psychiatry via a specialist programme. They have considerable expertise and knowledge about all childhood psychiatric disorders. Many may specialise in specific areas of child psychiatry, e.g. eating disorders or forensic psychiatry, or may have additional qualifications in specific approaches, e.g. psychotherapy or family therapy.

Associate Specialists, Specialist Registrars and Staff Grade Doctors

These are qualified doctors who have a special interest in child and adolescent psychiatry, who may be training to become consultants, i.e. specialist registrars, or have worked within the speciality for a number of years.

Social Workers

The British Association of Social Workers (BASW) expressed concern about the lack of mention of the role of specialist social workers in the green paper Transforming Children and Young People's Mental Health Provision (2017), feeling that it ignored the important role of the social worker in both preventing, and treating CYP with, mental health problems. The role previously described by the Care Services Improvement Partnership 2005, CSIP now dissolved, does seem to provide an explanation of their role within specialist CAMHS services.

CAMHS social workers offer consultation and advice to CAMHS colleagues concerning:

- Psychosocial explanations of mental health
- Child protection thresholds and safeguarding policies and procedures, including advising the team on new arrangements under the Children Act and linking with the Safeguarding Board

- Needs of looked after children and children on the Child Protection Register
- Co-ordination of work across complex systems and networks
- Development of services accessible to marginalised groups
- Mental health legislation and use of the Mental Health Act 1983/2007/Mental Health Capacity Act 2005

And in clinical practice:

- Contribution to mental health assessments and the provision of therapeutic interventions
- Supervision of social workers employed elsewhere with specialist CAMHS roles

Interfacing with children's services:

- Developing and enabling effective links between CAMHS and the children's services
- Provision of consultation, advice and training to social care staff regarding mental health issues

Provision of social work perspective:

- Promotion of client's own strengths, interests and rights
- Mental health difficulties placed within wider social context
- Active challenge of oppressive and discriminatory processes

Social workers train in social work and then specialise in assessing and treating children and families with mental health difficulties. They may have additional training in other therapeutic approaches, e.g. family therapy.

Specialist Nurse Therapists

Nursing training has changed over the last few years. Until recently most nurses' training was completed in universities. With the demise of the bursary scheme, the applications for nurse training reduced by 29%, leaving a significant shortfall in the nursing workforce. To counteract this, new measures have been introduced. First, a nursing apprenticeship was developed that has the potential to appeal to potential students unable or unwilling to incur the high costs of university fees and who prefer to study whilst doing the job. The second initiative is to support nurse training via universities. An additional payment that does not have to be repaid will be introduced later in 2020. This is very similar to the previous bursary scheme.

Nursing involves a three-year undergraduate training course in adult, mental health, paediatrics or learning disability nursing, plus further training, depending on the specialist area in which they wish to work. CAMHS nurses have specialised in the assessment and treatment of children and families with mental health problems. Within a CAMHS team, they may be from a variety of backgrounds, including mental health, paediatric, learning disability nurses or public health nurses. They may have additional qualifications (e.g. in CBT, parenting or family therapy), in addition to using the nursing models and theories in their assessment and treatment of children with mental health difficulties and providing support to the child and to their family.

Consultant Nurses and Advanced Nurse Practitioners

The first consultant nurse role was developed in 1999 with the DOH giving guidance in 2000 that

> the role should consist of 50% of the consultants' time working directly with patients ensuring faster, better and more convenient services. In line with the seniority of these posts, their contribution will be crucial to the development of professional practice, to research and evaluation, and to education, training and development. (DOH, 2000)

The consultant nurses' role varies within CAMHS, depending on their area of expertise. An evaluation of the impact of nurse, midwife and health visitor consultants by Guest et al. (2004) demonstrated that out of 419 respondents, i.e. 79% of consultant nurses in post, 86% were heavily engaged in leadership activities; 48% in practice and service development, research and evaluation; 43% in education, training and staff development; and 33% in expert practice. Fifteen percent reported that they were heavily engaged in all four functions, whilst 11% said they were not heavily engaged in any of them (Guest et al., 2004).

Over the last few years and with the financial constraints being placed on the NHS, some consultant posts are not being replaced or there may be a demand for the post to become that of a manager, a role that was not outlined in the DOH recommendations. This leads to frustration in the lack of succession planning for their role and the lack of progression for experienced nurses looking to aspire to this role. Consultant nurses are valuable assets to the NHS, but because of their diversity and the lack of research into their effectiveness, their value is often missed.

The advanced nurse practitioner role is currently being explored and recommendations made. Advanced practice is a level of practice, rather than a type or specialty of practice. Advanced nurse practitioners (ANP) are educated to master's level in Advanced Practice and are assessed as competent in practice, using expert knowledge and skills. They have the freedom and authority to act, making autonomous decisions in the assessment, diagnosis and treatment of patients.

Nurse prescribing can be a part of the consultant nurse role and the advanced nurse practitioner role. Since 2005, consultant nurse practitioners are qualified to prescribe, with a widening of prescribing to take in controlled medication, in 2009. Figures from the National Nursing and Midwifery Council (NMC), correct as of 1 April 2016, record a total of 73,804 qualified nurse, including midwife, prescribers on the register. This represents 10.7% of the total work force.

Dr Barbara Stuttle, CBE, chair of the Association for Prescribers, that campaigns for, and promotes, the role of nurse prescribing, reports that non-medical prescribing has been the most important development in nursing since it became a profession. It has allowed the development of new nursing roles, allowed genuine autonomy and benefitted both services and the patients we care for, by offering better access to medicines and smoother service delivery.

Psychotherapists

Psychotherapists undergo extensive training in the emotional development of children and events that may influence it. They offer individual work with the child and help explore the child's inner world and their understanding of its relationship to the child's difficulties. This is often through the medium of play. They usually train for about four years and often offer supervision to any CAMHS staff undertaking individual work with a child or parent.

Clinical Psychologists

Clinical psychologists have undertaken a first degree in psychology and then further training in applying psychological theories within a clinical setting. Clinical psychologists have a variety of skills, often including training in the assessment of children's abilities and working with cognitive behavioural therapy techniques or social stories, to help treat children presenting with a variety of difficulties, e.g. phobias, obsessive-compulsive symptoms or neuro-developmental disorders.

Family Therapists

Family therapists have an additional professional background, e.g. in social work or nursing, before undertaking further training, usually four years at MSc level, to qualify as a family and marital therapist. They train to understand relationships within families and how to change patterns of behaviour, using a family or systems approach. Different models of family therapy can be applied to bring about change.

- Family therapists are an essential part of CAMHS teams. They focus on relationships and communication between people and how they are influenced by belief systems and meanings.
- They enable families to talk about difficult emotions, thoughts and behaviours. They encourage the expression of multiple views in order to develop a shared understanding.
- Family therapists work to understand the views and needs of all members of the family and to identify the strengths and resources that will enable them to make useful changes in their lives.
- Family therapists work within a 'systemic' perspective, assessing difficulties in the different contexts in which they occur, i.e. individual relationships, the web of family relationships and interactions with the cultural and social context.
- They are interested in what influences the development and maintenance of problems. They develop ideas or hypotheses relating to the assessment, and these inform interventions with the family.

Family therapists work with families from a wide range of racial, cultural and religious backgrounds in a variety of family forms, including single parents, same-sex couples, families and extended families. They work with birth families, foster and adoptive families.

Family therapists provide consultation, supervision and training to other members of the multi-disciplinary team, students and members of other agencies working with children and adolescents. They contribute to the overall development of the service and undertake audit and research activities.

Systemic practitioners are clinicians who have undertaken two years of family therapy training, but have chosen not to pursue the MSc qualification.

Occupational Therapists

Occupational therapists are trained in helping children, especially those with developmental difficulties and motor co-ordination problems. They can assess children up to 18 years old, who face challenges within their home, community or school, to enable them to become more independent in daily living activities. This can involve using formal assessments or observing children within the nursery or school setting.

Some OTs specialise in using play as a form of assessment in order to identify the child's areas of need and ability. Others may work with children with sensory issues to help them to overcome their difficulties within a variety of settings.

Play Therapists

Play therapists work with children to allow the child to explore, at his own pace and with his or her own agenda, those issues past and current that are affecting the child's life in the present. The child's inner resources are enabled, via the therapeutic alliance, to bring about growth and change.

Play therapy is child-centred, where play is the primary medium and speech is the secondary medium. This therapy is especially valuable with children too young to express their thoughts or feelings and those with difficulty in expressing them. Play therapists often belong to the British Association of Play Therapists (BAPT) and have undertaken training in play therapy.

Crisis Workers

These are specialist practitioners who work with children and young people and their families in crisis. The intervention is time-limited with the aim of transferring their care to the appropriate agency or to an allocated specialist CAMHS worker. Generally, they will work with the family and young person for six to eight weeks to stabilise the mental health of a young person. This is a very responsive and flexible role that aims to reduce admissions to hospital and to mobilise local support services to help the young person in need.

Multi-Disciplinary Working in Practice

Given the wide variety of specialists and theories that can be drawn upon to make sense of a child's behaviour and the treatment options available, it is unsurprising that this can be confusing to staff new to a CAMHS team and indeed, to the families. Working together with the CYP and their family to bring about change is essential. The choice of treatments available to address their child's presenting problems should be carefully explained to the family.

If a treatment approach does not appear to be working, there should be flexibility in changing the approach. Discussions within the team, and with the family, should allow for the change of direction to be documented and justified. This will enable children and families to understand that the CAMHS service can reassess with them and change the treatment, should a specific approach not have been helpful. It is likely that in very complex situations several different approaches may be necessary.

There are sometimes occasions where the family are unhappy with the teams' suggested therapy or they find it too difficult to implement. The child or family may seek a different option. This can be a particularly difficult therapeutic challenge for clinicians and must be considered through team discussion and supervision. It may be possible for the parents to be encouraged to 'stay with an approach' for a while, in order to see change through.

Case Study (1): Ben

Ben (eight) is a 'looked after child', having been placed with experienced foster parents two years ago. He had been in short-term foster care on several occasions in his early years, but was finally transferred into the long-term foster care team when he was six. He had suffered physical abuse and extreme emotional abuse and was very frightened and anxious about his placement with the new family.

Ben was assessed at the foster parents' request, as he was different from other children they had fostered in the past. He was reported to be impulsive, lack concentration and experience extreme difficulties educationally.

At the first assessment, an attachment theory framework was used to explain Ben's behaviours, because of his very difficult early years' history. Ben commenced individual psychotherapy. The foster parents supported therapy during this process.

Three months later, the psychotherapist working with Ben noticed that Ben's impulsivity and concentration were impeding his ability to use the therapy she was offering and brought Ben's case to a team discussion.

As a result, a comprehensive ADHD and autism screening took place using health models to explain Ben's behaviour. Ben met the criteria for ADHD following developmental trauma, i.e. the abuse he suffered, and was subsequently treated with medication. His foster parents received help in understanding ADHD in the context of developmental trauma.

One month later Ben restarted his psychotherapy and used the sessions appropriately, finding them extremely helpful in making sense of his inner world.

His foster mother now understood why Ben needed a different style of parenting, having attended sessions about ADHD and what this meant for Ben. Liaison with his school about his difficulties in relation to his ADHD symptoms enabled his work to improve considerably and he was no longer at risk of exclusion.

This case study illustrates the importance of ongoing assessment during a specific treatment, careful supervision and good team working to ensure that other therapies are continually considered if, and when, necessary.

Case Study (2): Samantha

Samantha (14) was referred to the specialist CAMHS team at her parents' request after missing ten months of schooling, afraid of going out of the house. A home visit was necessary to undertake the initial assessment by the crisis worker. Samantha was found to be physically challenged with a very low weight and extreme anxiety about going outside, even into the garden. Her physical self-care was minimal. She had not had a bath or cleaned her teeth for months.

Several approaches were needed to manage Samantha's potentially life-threatening difficulties. A full medical assessment was instigated to ensure no underlying physical problem could account for her difficulties. This included a full blood, height, weight, blood pressure and pulse screening. A full psychiatric assessment was undertaken, including a risk assessment. Whilst initially the plan had been to work with Samantha at home, it was soon apparent that she needed hospital treatment for her severely compromised physical health. The crisis worker liaised with the hospital, Samantha and the family to enable a smooth transition to hospital care.

Admission to hospital was arranged and Samantha was treated as an inpatient for several months to help her gain weight and become less physically compromised by her mental health difficulty.

During this time, the family was offered family therapy sessions to explore how Samantha's difficulties had arisen, to prepare for the time when Samantha came home and to look at how the environment could support her recovery. When she was physically well again, Samantha was offered individual therapy sessions to explore how her difficulties arose and to work on relapse prevention. She continued with her education, which increased as Samantha's physical and mental health improved. On discharge from hospital, the crisis worker met with her regularly to help facilitate her discharge home.

A very practical health approach was necessary initially to ensure Samantha's wellbeing. Afterwards, a variety of approaches and theories have been used to ensure her continued recovery, increasing as transitions took place.

Key References

Birleson, P., (1998). Building a learning organisation in a child and adolescent mental health service. *Australian Health Review*, 21(3): 223–240.

Department of Health, (2010). *Keeping Children and Young People in Mind: The Governments Response to the Independent Review of CAMHS.* London: DoH.

Guest et al., (2004). *A Evaluation of the Impact of Nurse, Midwife and Health Visitor Consultants.* London: King's College.

Websites

http://www.bapt.info/ British Association of play therapists
http://www.nmc-uk.org/ Nursing and Midwifery council
http://www.gmc-uk.org/ General Medical council
http://www.aft.org.uk/ Association of Family Therapists
http://www.psychotherapy.org.uk/ UK Council for Psychotherapy
http://www.bacp.co.uk/ The British Association for Counselling and Psychotherapy
http://www.cot.co.uk/Homepage/ British Association of Occupational Therapists
http://www.basw.co.uk/ The College of Social Work

81 Specialist Services

Forensic Child and Adolescent Psychiatry

Suyog Dhakras, Jonathan Bigg and Alison Wallis

Forensic child and adolescent psychiatry (FCAMHS) is a child and adolescent psychiatry subspecialty. It deals with mental disorders and risk of harm to others, including criminal and offending behaviour in children and adolescents. Research into the causes of criminal behaviour in children and adolescents is a rapidly developing field. Whilst clearly progressing speedily, fCAMHS lags behind adult forensic psychiatric services significantly in terms of the research evidence, resources and development of services.

KEY CONCEPTS

- The age of criminal responsibility in the UK is ten years.
- There has been a strong policy drive away from criminalisation of young people in recent years. Caution-or-sentence rates of all kinds have diminished from over 140,000 in 2007/08 to under 30,000 in 2017/18.
- Custody rates have fallen significantly in recent years from 2,831 in 2005/06 to 894 in 2017/18. The average sentence length increased from 11.4 months in 2007/08 to 16.7 months in 2017/18.
- Of all convicted children, the proportion convicted of violent offences, e.g. assault against the person, has been increasing. Over the 10 years to 2017/18 it rose steadily to 29%. However, the actual number of violent offences in 2017/18 remained lower than in 2009/10.
- The rate of recognised mental disorders in young offenders, i.e. both offenders in custody and those in the community, is 30%, three times that in non-offender samples in the child and adolescent age group.
- Within the gradually shifting context of social policy, many highly antisocial children, i.e. under 18s, in the UK presenting very significant risks of serious harm to others are now managed outside the criminal justice services.

Studies in the UK and the USA show that rates of criminal and delinquent activity in adolescence are so high that they are statistically normative. The majority of young people who are violent/criminal in adolescence do not continue to offend in adulthood. Studies show that approximately 75–80% desist by the age of 21 years. Official crime rates in youth tend to peak at age 17 and then decline. Moffitt et al. (1996) have suggested that patterns of aggressive and violent offences follow two distinct courses:

Life Course Persistent (LCP)

- 5–10% of all young people who engage in violent offences and antisocial acts.
- Usually have other co-morbidities, e.g. ADHD, oppositional behaviour, conduct disorder.
- Early onset of criminal and antisocial activity, i.e. first arrest between 7 years and 11 years strongly associated with long-term offending.
- The tendency towards antisocial behaviour remains stable over time.

Adolescent Limited (AL)

- More common.
- Antisocial behaviour begins and ends in the teenage years.
- At least 75–80% will desist by early adulthood.
- Influence of delinquent peers is central.
- May usually maintain primary attachments and have capacity for empathy.

Gender Differences

- Males commit the majority of violent crime, although the rates in young girls are rapidly rising.
- Most risk factors for violence apply similarly to boys and girls.
- Severely delinquent girls are more likely to be placed in care than males. They may show early sexual maturation, i.e. menarche before 12.5 years and peer relationships with older aggressive peers.
- Fire-setting is seen more commonly in males. Younger boys who set fires alone are likely to have a learning disability (LD), whilst older youths may set fires as a part of group activity.

How Mental and Behavioural Disorders Link with Offending Behaviour

- High rates of co-morbidity between conduct disorder and ADHD – >50%.
- High rates of low mood and depressive symptoms are seen in young people with a diagnosis of conduct disorder: 11–33%.
- Adolescents with disruptive behaviour have a higher self-harm and completed suicide rate, even in the absence of depressive disorder.
- Early-onset mania may involve high rates of aggression.
- Psychoses are rare in children. Studies have shown that the predictors of violence are not significantly different from non-psychotic young people.
- Young people with anxiety are not prone to show violent and offending behaviour. However, rates of anxiety are higher in juvenile offenders in custody, 22–60%.
- PTSD may be the exception to the rule, when higher rates of aggression may be seen. Complex trauma, usually developmental trauma, is becoming recognised as closely related to dysregulation and externalising behaviours, in addition to historically better recognised internalising ones. Brutalised children are less likely to know how to show care or empathise with others.
- As we have seen earlier, approximately 25% of young offenders have LD, i.e. IQ <70. If we consider borderline IQ scores, this figure rises to just over 50%. Early literacy problems in boys at age seven are seen as a 'gateway' to later conduct problems. Higher rates of fire-setting and sexual offences have been noted in young people, especially males, with mild-moderate LD.
- Studies have shown that up to 15% of young offenders with serious offences may have pervasive developmental disorders (PDD). Impaired social abilities and the disruption of routines/rituals may lead to aggression. The lack of theory of mind may be perceived as lack of empathy and callousness.

- Rates of substance misuse, especially alcohol use, are likely to increase risk.
- Approximately 30% of all sexual offences against children are committed by other children and young people.
- Nearly half of youth displaying sexually aggressive behaviour leading to criminal offences began prior to age 12.

Risk Assessment in Children and Young People

- It is not helpful or useful to use the concept of 'dangerousness' to describe risks presented by a young person. It is a dichotomous concept. Children and young people are not 'dangerous' all the time. It is more helpful to consider whether the risk to other people is high in certain circumstances and low or contained in other situations.
- The interplay between the static/historic risk factors and dynamic contextual risk factors must be considered.
- Adolescence is a period of profound and pervasive changes and risk factors may not remain stable.
- It is important to consider positive/protective/strength/resiliency factors and not merely the absence of negative risk factors.
- Positive factors indicate the positive presence of a characteristic or person or circumstance, e.g. positive adult role model/confidante, positive engagement in education and other pro-social age-appropriate activity, compliance with a treatment programme, higher cognitive abilities such as verbal intelligence, that can act to reduce the negative impact of one or more risk factors or otherwise directly buffer the risk. These positive factors may be inherent to the young person or related to the development of appropriate social and family bonds, healthy normative social beliefs or clear standards of behaviour.
- There are useful tools for the multi-dimensional assessment of risk: Structured Assessment of Violence Risk in Youth (SAVRY), Borum et al., Structured Assessment of Protective Factors for Violence Risk – Youth Version (SAPROF-YV), De Vries Robbé et al., various AIM tools for the assessment of harmful and problematic sexual behaviours, www.aimproject.org.uk. Many of these promote the approach of structured professional judgement, combining best research evidence with clinical knowledge of a case's individual complexity.

FCAMHS Services

Small community-based forensic CAMHS have provisionally been commissioned uniformly across England, but not over the whole of the UK. These await national evaluation before becoming substantive. There are six centrally commissioned Adolescent Medium Secure Psychiatric In-Patient Units in England, based in Newcastle, Manchester, Birmingham, London, Northampton and Southampton.

In-reach mental health services of different design are supporting young people in secure welfare and criminal justice settings. An English national strategy, 'Secure Stairs', is commissioned to support more person-centred, emotionally, psychologically, developmentally and systemically informed therapeutic milieux for younger and more vulnerable young people, who do have to be incarcerated by the state. Such teams are highly specialist and work closely with specialist CAMHS, local authority children's services and youth offending services.

An Example of a Community-Based FCAMHS

The Hampshire and Isle of Wight Regional Community FCAMH Service started in April 2010. It consists of a 0.6 WTE consultant psychiatrist, a 1.0 WTE clinical psychologist and a

0.8 WTE administrator, covering the county of Hampshire including the unitary authorities of Southampton City and Portsmouth City, and the Isle of Wight, a total population of about two million people, about 115,000 being under 18. The model of working involves close liaison with CAMHS, local authority children's services and Youth Offending Teams and the Youth Justice System, using consultation and advice for the majority of cases and taking on direct work with a small caseload. The model involves a significant role in training other professionals and the strategic development of services.

While most cases consulted on and managed by FCAMHS do not have needs that require inpatient treatment, a small and important number do. Most of these will need care within the general adolescent psychiatric hospitals, with their risks of harm to others being manageable within open units, or occasionally within psychiatric intensive care.

An even smaller number require the inputs of highly specialised low or medium secure adolescent beds. Most of these are managed in the Nationally Commissioned NHS-England network that links up weekly to discuss assessments and admissions. Such cases require detention under the Mental Health Act, because these wards are highly secure. Risk management of such cases requires strong buildings, security and clear restrictions of many aspects of day-to-day liberty for safety and mental health reasons. If not incarcerated for criminal justice reasons, these patients often present grave risks of perpetrating serious harm towards other people and occasionally themselves.

Youth Justice System

It is helpful to have knowledge about the pathway that a young person may take when he/she becomes involved with the Youth Justice System (Figure 81.1a and b). The increasing emphasis of the YJS is to work in a preventative way to divert young people away from prosecution and conviction, if that is the most appropriate way forward.

Youth Court

- Is a section of Magistrates' Court.
- Deals with almost all cases to do with young people <18 years.
- Is a private arena. Members of public not allowed.
- Presided over by District Judges or Magistrates, i.e. panel of three, no jury.
- Less formal than Magistrates' Court.
- Court can hand down community sentences or Detention and Training Orders (DTOs).

Crown Court

- Deals with both adults and children.
- Presided over by a judge, either Crown Court Circuit Judge or Recorder.
- Is a public arena. Members of public can attend trial.
- Jury panel.
- Formal arena, i.e. judges wear robes, barristers wear wigs.
- Serious offences.

Custodial sentences may be spent in a local authority Secure Unit, a Secure Training Centre or in a Young Offenders' Institution.

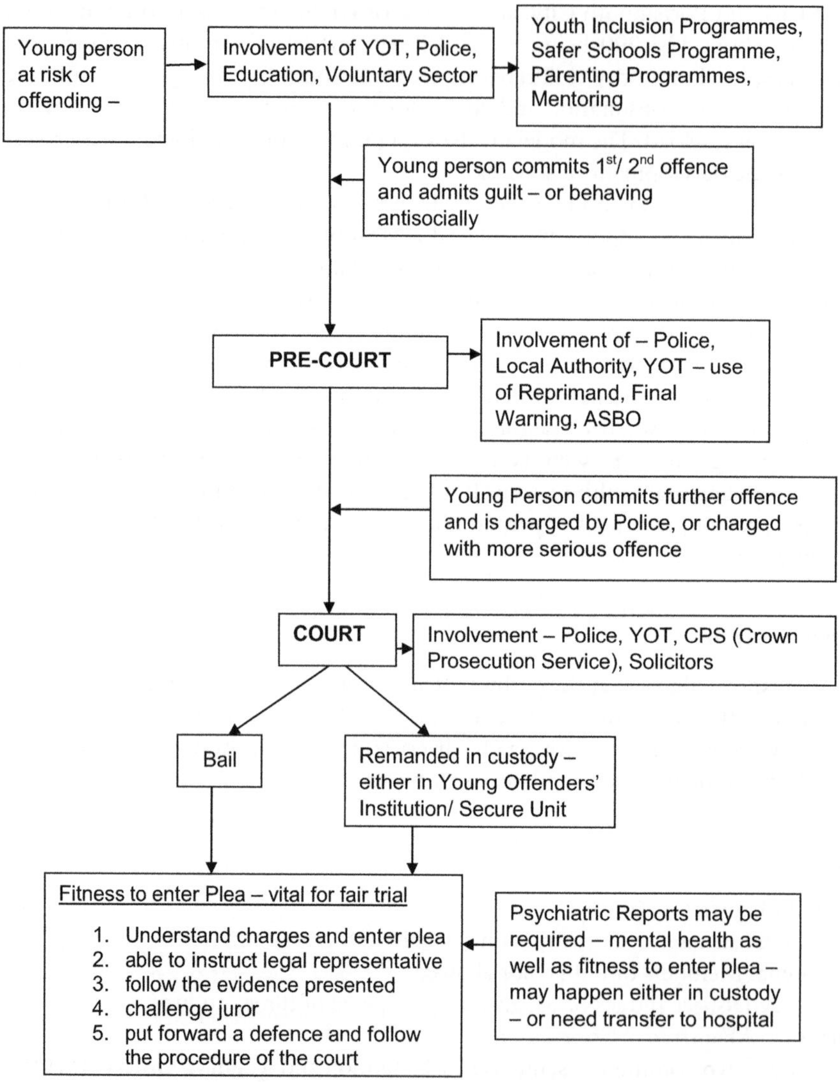

Figure 81.1a Process for young people with mental health difficulties moving through the English youth justice system.

- The annual cost per young person of custodial incarceration in government-run custody is approximately £60,000.
- The cost of incarceration for one year in a privately run Secure Training Centre is £160,000.
- The rate of re-offending within one year of release from custody is 75%.

Young people in custody are referred to the Integrated Resettlement Service. They are seen 15 days prior to release and their needs, e.g. housing, education, mental health, are assessed.

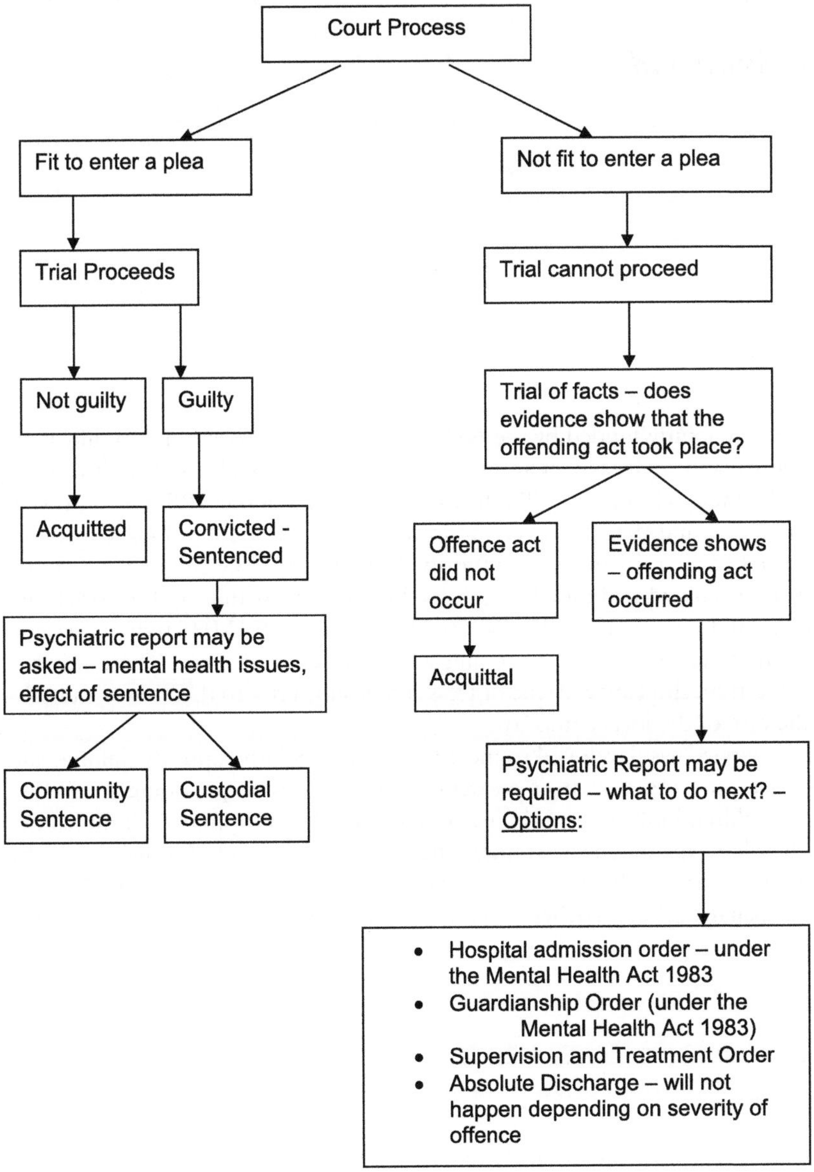

Figure 81.1b Process for young people with mental health difficulties moving through the English youth justice system.

Key References

Moffitt, T.E., Caspi, A., Dickson, N., Silva, P., Stanton, W., (1996). Childhood-onset versus adolescent-onset antisocial conduct problems in males: Natural history from ages 3 to 18 years. *Development and Psychopathology*, 8: 399–424.

Youth Justice Statistics 2017–18, (31st January 2019). Produced by Ministry of Justice. www.gov.uk/government/collections/youth-justice-statistics

Website

www.aimproject.org.uk.

82 Building Resilience and Strengths (BRS)

Michelle Simmonds

Introduction

The BRS is a local service jointly funded by the NHS and social care services. It is a fully integrated multi-disciplinary and multi-agency team, employing professionals from health, social care and education. Founded in January 2000, historically the role of the BRS was to provide therapeutic residential care and therapeutic community support for children looked after, or at risk of becoming looked after, by the local authority. In most cases, the children and young people with whom BRS worked had raised a high level of concern within health, social care and education. These children may not be best served by mainstream CAMHS services because their difficulties are the result of their social circumstances, neglect and abuse. These children were often not in education, showing extreme distress and posing a risk to themselves and others, whilst under the care of the local authority.

Over the years the service has developed to meet the needs of Southampton's children and children's social services, moving away from residential care to focus on providing a CAMHS specialising in those children looked after, aiming to understand and support their difficulties in the context of their life experiences. Therefore, attachment theory and Maslow's hierarchy of needs (as discussed in Part II), the impact of development trauma (as discussed in Part III) and a range of psychoanalytical approaches (as discussed in Part VII) have underpinned the team's ethos.

KEY CONCEPTS

- Currently BRS aims to provide an intensive, crisis intervention service for those children, young people and their families whose multiple difficulties place them outside of the local universal and Tier 3 services.
- We continue to work with the existing child or young person's personal and professional network to support therapeutic management of the case, individually tailored to the identified needs of the child or young person.
- This specialist service is accessible to all children and young people based on level of need, not only those children looked after.
- The service continues to offer a therapeutic pathway to looked after children whose needs cannot be appropriately met via mainstream CAMHS.

BRS intervention, therefore, may take many different forms, and these differences may be noted from the point of referral. All referrals will be discussed via an initial telephone triage. A referrer, i.e. a professional from health, education or social care, will contact our duty worker with consent from whomever holds parental responsibility and, where appropriate, the referred child or young person. Our duty worker will take details of the child or young person and their situation. This telephone triage will determine the immediacy of need and whether or when the BRS service should become involved.

BRS currently implements three levels of response:

- **Crisis response** is within 24 hours.
- **An urgent response**, whereby the referrer receives a decision within a week and allocation to a practitioner for work to begin occurs as soon as is practicable.
- **A therapeutic pathway** response, whereby referrals for looked after children requiring specific and possibly longer-term work are discussed at a therapeutic panel. This panel is made up of a number of universal and specialist services able to offer therapeutic input to children looked after across our city.

If a child or young person needs immediate crisis intervention from BRS this will be agreed during the call, and management oversight is sought as to the planning and implementation of an intervention within 24 hours.

All referrals go through the BRS multi-disciplinary team (MDT) meeting. These meetings occur weekly and provide opportunity for the referral, and the young person's needs, to be discussed in detail. This does not prevent the BRS implementing a crisis response between MDT meetings. If the referral is considered urgent, the allocated worker will discuss with the referrer how best to contribute to existing intervention plans. If a therapeutic response is decided upon and the child or young person's situation is considered safe enough in the meantime, the case will be referred onto therapeutic panel and decisions as to which service is most appropriate to meet the child or young person's needs will be identified at panel.

BRS intervention is underpinned by an understanding of attachment theory and of developmental trauma, and assessing the presentation of the child's or young person's difficulties in the context of their early childhood experiences.

Case Study: Jamie

In his early years, Jamie (who is now aged 11) witnessed maternal mental illness. His mother suffered from undiagnosed post-natal depression following the birth of his younger sibling. He witnessed parental drug use and sexual activity in exchange for drugs within the home, and alcohol misuse. He was physically abused by his father. In addition, Jamie experienced neglect in the form of a significant lack of boundaries and supervision and, at times, his basic needs were not met. Jamie's parents separated, and he was confused when his mother's new partner was female. This relationship exposed the children to violence and criminality.

Jamie demonstrated fight, flight and avoidant responses towards threatening situations. This often manifested in a reaction to run and climb and scale walls and buildings in the community and school facilities, placing himself at further risk. He saw no point to school but when he did attend, he appeared to live up to the negative narrative of being the 'naughty' one. His school attendance significantly decreased, and this was interpreted as a response to his increasingly volatile home environment. Jamie was unable to be safely managed, and for a while, he was unable to access any appropriate educational provision. The children were brought into the care of the local authority and Jamie was separated from his siblings. Instances of running away in the early weeks seemed to be triggered by Jamie's belief that he needed to be at home, because his mother could not look after herself. He was returned safely to foster carers on all occasions.

Jamie's first foster placement broke down after significant incidents of assault towards one of his carers. This followed supervised contact with his family. Jamie's relationship with his younger sister was particularly difficult, because she reminded him of his mother and therefore seemed to re-traumatise him. Contacts with his parents and sister were suspended, noting that this incident was a significant escalation in what had been a pattern of unsettled behaviour following contact. Afterwards it took days for Jamie to recover and settle down.

Jamie needed this interval to help him settle into a new placement and form attachments with new carers. This attachment, and thus the stability of the placement, could be compromised by traumatic contact with his parents and siblings (Schofield and Simmonds, 2011). He was transferred to a second placement and began attending a forest school on a part-time tailored timetable, far better suited to his needs than mainstream primary school.

Given the breakdown in the social care and education circumstances, along with the high levels of distress Jamie was demonstrating, BRS was the appropriate service. It appeared unlikely his presentation would be explained by a diagnosable mental illness that could be treatable with medication, and therefore, his needs could not easily be met within the mainstream CAMHS pathways.

At BRS we approach Jamie's life experiences taking into consideration not only the evident developmental trauma and its impact on the young developing brain, but considering Maslow's hierarchy of needs, identifying those basic needs that had not been met in Jamie's case and had therefore left an unstable foundation. We understand that when a parent is the source of both fear and of comfort, children are often left unable to organise their emotions and present in the disorganised style described here (Brown and Ward, 2013). For Jamie, no distance would have been a safe distance. His attempts to approach his parents for care and protection had resulted in fear and increased, rather than decreased, his anxiety. Too near and he risked being harmed, too far and he risked being neglected.

We worked to develop a new narrative around Jamie's presentation, not one of him being the problem child but one whereby, in the context of his life experience, his behaviour served a function, that function being to maintain his safety by removing himself from the threat, but not intending to place himself or others in danger. His disorganised attachment led to his heightened arousal surrounding contact with his parents and/or his siblings. It is understandable that this flight response might be transferred to education and care settings, where there are unknown adults and his disorganised attachment would be apparent in his relationships with other key adults within education and care.

Superficially, Jamie presented with self-esteem, confidence and humour. However, he described himself as bad and unwanted and projected mistrust in others. Carers observed periods of anxiety and low mood, tearfulness, irritability and feelings of worthlessness. Jamie continued to have some instances of running away but the majority of these were impulsive reactive incidents to a perceived threat or injustice.

Jamie displayed controlling behaviour to allow him to feel some degree of predictability and safety. This could show itself in him being punitive toward others or insisting on self-reliance. In these moments, he was avoidant of or rejecting of nurture. At BRS, we consider the potentially destructive effect this can have on future relationships.

One aim of the intervention was to support the care placement to establish a secure base for Jamie, provided through the relationship with one or more sensitive and responsive attachment figures who understood his narrative and were able to withstand difficult incidents to continue to meet his needs. This is done predominantly by offering the intervention not to the child but to the carers, offering information on therapeutic parenting techniques, when for such a child, traditional behavioural parenting techniques are unlikely to be successful. These can be modelled during appointments in the home and supported by telephone support between appointments.

We frequently refer to PACE, an 'active interaction that responds to and reflects upon the child's affective experience' (Golding and Hughes, 2012).

- Playfulness is a light-hearted attitude that de-escalates and protects the child against experiencing shame as distinct from guilt.
- Acceptance is acknowledging and validating the child's thoughts and feelings without condoning the behaviour, offering reassurance and making the parent or carer approachable.
- Curiosity is wondering together about what is behind the behaviour.
- Empathy is sharing the emotions, connecting with the child before problem- solving or enforcing boundaries. The parent or carer responding with PACE can create and display genuine sympathy and compassion.

As a result of being attuned to his emotional needs, ensuring his safety with appropriate supervision, routine stimulation and putting appropriate guidance and boundaries in place, Jamie achieved positive attachments with his carers.

The second aim was to gradually enable Jamie to consistently access school and activities to support him in building positive self-worth and positive relationships.

In the long term the aim would be to prevent destructive loops, by achieving aims one and two, adapting Jamie's sense of self into a more positive frame from which to develop positive, adaptive future relationships.

Direct 1:1 work was not offered until Jamie was settled in his second placement. Intervention was non-directive and child-centred, i.e. Jamie chooses the agenda, and this means that, although there are agreed aims and desirable outcomes, there is no specific direction from the worker to Jamie during an appointment, at least in the initial stages.

Non-directive play sessions last up to an hour in the same play room each week. The rooms are equipped with a variety of toys and creative art materials to match developmental stages of play (sensory, imaginative, role and projective play) and to encourage the child to express their feelings. The child is given time to build trust in the worker and may need to regress to the play more typical of a younger child. Due to their early life, they may not have had the opportunity to do this and need to make up for gaps in development. The aim was to enable Jamie to make sense of his life through play. In this way, pressure is removed from the child because there is no need for them to articulate their experiences.

When a child begins to process their experiences in this way it can impact on behaviour within the home. A placement must be sufficiently stable and consistent and the attachment strong enough to contain the emotion being expressed with consistent opportunities for co-regulation of stress, emotion and impulse.

For Jamie, this work continued over four months before sessions moved into the home where his carers could join in and begin to provide this safe space, normalising the approach as a habitual way of communicating and spending time together. The sessions were reduced to fortnightly and then monthly as the need reduced. Jamie achieved full-time attendance at the forest school with a transition plan to take him into secondary school.

Jamie is a typical example of a child presenting in crisis who, once stabilised, was able to continue work within our therapeutic pathway for looked after children. BRS intervention can include either one or multiple forms of assessment and therapeutic approach.

Assessments currently undertaken to establish a child or young person's needs:

- Family day assessment (systemic)
- Neuropsychological
- Clinical psychology
- Play therapy
- Sensory
- Forensic
- Mental state examinations
- Risk

Other therapeutic approaches undertaken are:

- Play therapy
- Theraplay
- Trauma-focussed cognitive behavioural therapy (CBT)
- Clinical psychology formulation
- Family therapy

BRS frequently uses the Strengths and Difficulties Questionnaire at the beginning, midpoint and end of intervention. There are versions for self, parent/carer and teachers to complete, indicating the child or young person's progress from their own perspective where possible and of those around them, across different settings and identifying consistency or inconsistency in presentation.

Key References

Brown, R., Ward, H., (2013). *Decision-making within a Child's Timeframe. An overview of current research evidence for family justice professionals concerning child development and the impact of maltreatment.* London: Childhood Wellbeing Research Centre, Institute of Education

Golding, K.S., Hughes, D.A,. (2012). *Creating Loving Attachments: Parenting with PACE to Nurture Confidence and Security in the Troubled Child.* London: Jessica Kingsley Publishers

Schofield, G., Simmonds, J., (2011). Contact for Infants Subject to Care Proceedings. *Family Law,* 41: 617–622

83 Specialist Services

Secure Adolescent Inpatient

Oliver White

Introduction and Background

In England in 2015 there were over 1,450 young people in secure settings at any one time. Over 300 of these were in secure mental health settings; the remaining 1,100 were in either welfare secure (approximately 100) or youth justice custodial settings (approximately 1,000). Young people in all types of secure setting have clearly established significant mental health needs (Chitsabesan et al., 2006).

Secure adolescent mental health inpatient services in England have developed considerably over recent years. The government's Future in Mind (2015) document emphasised the need for 'improved care for children and young people in crisis so they are treated in the right place, at the right time and as close to home as possible'. This includes 'implementing clear evidence-based pathways for community-based care, including intensive home treatment where appropriate, to avoid unnecessary admissions to inpatient care'. The ongoing development of community CAMHS provision, particularly CAMHS crisis and outreach teams, means that many young people who would have traditionally received inpatient treatment are now supported and treated in the community. This has resulted in an increase in the overall complexity of young people who do require inpatient admission, and the resources and environment within traditional Tier 4 General Adolescent Unit ('open') inpatient units at times are not sufficient to meet their needs. This is acknowledged within the Future in Mind document, which states

> however, there is a recognition that there will always be some children and young people who require more intensive and specialised inpatient care. The key to commissioning the right type of care, in the right places is to adopt a whole system commissioning perspective ... this should address the role of pre-crisis, crisis and 'step-down' services alongside inpatient provision.

Although secure adolescent inpatient services have existed for over 30 years, the increasing demands have more recently been recognised by NHS England via the development of Service Specifications, resulting in the more coherent and consistent commissioning of services (NHS Mental Health Implementation Plan 2019/20–2023/24).

Many General Adolescent Units have High Dependency Areas within their infrastructure, where short-term enhanced care can be provided to young people who exhibit acute behavioural disturbance as part of their mental health difficulties. When a young person's risk presentation is not able to be consistently managed within a high-dependency provision, then admission to a specialist secure unit should be considered.

There are three distinct secure adolescent inpatient provisions, commissioned via different Service Specifications and operated via different security standards: Adolescent Psychiatric

Intensive Care Units (PICU), Adolescent Low Secure Units (LSU) and Adolescent Medium Secure Units (MSU). All secure adolescent mental health inpatient units provide a range of physical, procedural and relational security measures to ensure effective treatment and care whilst providing for the safety of individual young people, other patients, staff and the general public.

Assessing the incidence and prevalence of severe adolescent mental disorders requiring secure adolescent inpatient care is challenging. Prevalence is influenced by a variety of factors (social deprivation, family breakdown, learning difficulties, ethnicity, etc.), and estimates of the prevalence of specific child and adolescent mental health disorders are often broad and relate to the full range of clinical severity whereas only a minority require inpatient and particularly secure inpatient care. In addition to epidemiological factors, service factors such as gaps in service, capacity of community services or quality of 'out-of-hours' support influence the use of all CAMHS inpatient provision, including secure adolescent inpatient services.

Adolescent PICU

Adolescent Psychiatric Intensive Care Units (PICU) provide short-term management of behavioural disturbance which cannot be contained within a General Adolescent Unit, including a High Dependency Area. Specific risk behaviours requiring admission to an Adolescent PICU include a serious risk of either suicide, absconding with a significant threat to safety, aggression or vulnerability, for example, due to agitation or sexual disinhibition. Levels of physical, relational and procedural security in Adolescent PICUs should be similar to those in Adolescent Low Secure Units (see below).

Adolescent PICUs do not have the same emphasis on providing support over a long period of time. Admissions should not last longer than eight weeks; this is a key differentiator to that of Adolescent LSU (and Adolescent MSU). Any admission likely to last longer than eight weeks should be subject, by the end of the sixth week, to robust clinical review which focuses actively on alternatives to continuing Adolescent PICU provision including where appropriate transfer to either low or medium security.

The decision to admit to any Adolescent PICU should be based on a good working risk assessment and detailed consideration as to how identified risks can be managed safely within this setting and resolved in the short term. For an admission to Adolescent PICU to be deemed appropriate the assessment will need to have demonstrate that this risk cannot be managed within a non-secure Tier 4 CAMHS General Adolescent Unit.

Adolescent PICUs complement other Tier 4 CAMHS inpatient provision for young people (including the high-dependency provision within General Adolescent Units) and should ideally be co-located with other Tier 4 CAMHS units. An Adolescent PICU service for young people will serve a wider geographical area than Tier 4 CAMHS General Adolescent Unit and typically accommodates up to a maximum of 12 young people at any one time.

Individual Adolescent PICU services should form part of a regionally and nationally co-ordinated network which would ensure parity of practice and flexibility in terms of availability of inpatient beds; this is enhanced by the current development of Provider-Collaboratives ('New Care Models').

Adolescent PICU Referral Criteria

All three of the following must apply:

- The young person is under 18 years of age at the time of referral.
- The young person admitted to an Adolescent PICU will be subject to an order within part 2 of the Mental Health Act. An Adolescent PICU setting will not be appropriate for

young people subject to hospital admission under part 3 of the Mental Health Act (this includes admissions for assessment under sections 35 and 36).

- The young person cannot be appropriately and safely managed in an open inpatient or community environment. This means that the young person will either present a risk of harm to others or themselves and suffers from an acute behavioural disturbance as a result of a mental disorder that requires intensive and acute inpatient care, specialist risk management procedures and a specialist treatment intervention. (Young people may be accepted with pending criminal charges if subject to part 2 of the Mental Health Act.)

Exclusion criteria:

- Young people who are presenting with longer term behavioural disturbance, either forensic or non-forensic, who may require care in a low secure or residential setting.
- Young people who present a grave danger to the general public (which may include some high-risk young people who may have no offending history, as well as those who have been charged with or convicted of specified violent or sexual offences under Schedule 15 of the Criminal Justice Act 2003).
- Fire setting not in the context of an acute mental illness.

Care Pathways

Adolescent PICU services provide care and treatment to a variety of young people, but the predominant need for care and treatment in conditions of intensive care will be related to the young person's assessed risk of harm to self and/or others in the context of their mental disorder. The three recognised pathways into Adolescent PICU are:

- Stepping up from a Tier 4 CAMHS general purpose adolescent service.
- Direct admission from the community, including other institutional/residential settings for young people (e.g. educational/residential social care). In this case there should be an assessment first by a senior clinician, preferably a CAMHS consultant psychiatrist.
- Admission from a low secure unit.

Adolescent Low Secure Units

Adolescent LSUs provide services for young people who present with severe mental disorders that cannot safely be assessed, treated and contained in the community, other residential or custodial settings, General Adolescent Units (including HDU provision) or Adolescent PICUs, but do not meet the threshold for admission to an Adolescent MSU. This patient group requires longer term interventions and specialist risk management procedures and specialist treatment interventions not available in non-secure or PICU settings.

Adolescent LSUs provide assessment and treatment for young people with mental and neurodevelopmental disorders at significant levels of physical, relational and procedural security. This security provision is similar to Adolescent PICU, but lower than within Adolescent Medium Secure Units. The main differentiator between Adolescent PICU and Adolescent LSU is therefore the expected duration of admission; i.e. in Adolescent LSU it (often significantly) exceeds eight weeks.

Young people admitted to Adolescent LSUs belong to one of two groups: those with 'forensic' presentations involving significant risk of harm to others and those with 'complex non-forensic' presentations principally associated with challenging behaviour arising from self-harm and other vulnerabilities.

As with all secure inpatient provision, young people admitted to Adolescent LSUs must be subject to the Mental Health Act. The predominant need for care and treatment in low secure must be related to the assessed risk of harm to others and/or self in the context of the young person's mental disorder.

There are currently (2020) approximately 150 Adolescent LSU beds within England. The majority of these are provided within the independent sector. The majority of young people admitted to Adolescent LSU are female.

Since the relatively recent formal NHS England commissioning of Adolescent LSUs, an Adolescent LSU National Clinical Network has developed. This enables the development and implementation of agreed standards and good practice. Challenges within Adolescent LSU provision can also be discussed. It also enables some national co-ordination of referrals into Adolescent LSU. The Adolescent LSU National Clinical Network sits alongside the current development of regional commissioning via Provider-Collaboratives ('New Care Models').

Adolescent LSU Referral Criteria

- The young person is under 18 at the time of referral.
- The young person must be detained under part 2 or part 3 of the Mental Health Act.
- The young person is not safely managed in an open environment, does not require a medium secure setting and is assessed as having needs that cannot be managed by shorter term admission to an Adolescent PICU.

and either

- The young person has been directed to conditions of security under a restriction order by the Ministry of Justice.

or

- The young person presents a risk of harm to others or themselves or suffers from a behavioural disturbance that requires inpatient care, specialist risk management procedures and a specialist treatment intervention.

Exclusion criteria:

- Young people who present a grave risk to the general public (which may include some high-risk young people who may have no offending history, as well as those who have been charged with or convicted of specified violent or sexual offences under Schedule 15 of the Criminal Justice Act 2003). (These young people are more suitable for medium secure inpatient settings.)
- Young people with brief episodes of disturbed or challenging behaviour as a consequence of mental disorder. (These young people are more appropriately cared for in an Adolescent PICU.)

Care Pathways

There are four recognised pathways into Adolescent LSUs:

- Transfer from Tier 4 general adolescent inpatient services or (PICU or other Tier 4 low secure units).

- Stepping down from medium secure adolescent services.
- Direct admission through a criminal court process or from youth justice custodial settings subject to an access assessment by the National Forensic Mental Health Service for Young People (NFMHSfYP).
- Admission from specialist education and welfare settings including welfare secure units.

Adolescent Medium Secure Units

Adolescent Medium Secure Units provide assessment and treatment for young people with mental and neurodevelopmental disorders (including learning disability and autism) who present with the highest levels of risk of harm to others including those who have committed grave crimes. Young people who do not present with a high risk of harm to others (even if they do have high levels of harm to self) should not be admitted to Adolescent MSUs.

All Adolescent MSUs are part of the NSFMHSfYP clinical management network. The network supports:

- A single national co-ordinated referral and admission pathway into individual service settings and across the network.
- A co-ordinated national response that evidences equity of provision across services in England.

The NSFMHSfYP clinical network consider all referrals from youth justice settings (courts and custodial units) and determine the level of security required. In general, young people from these settings are likely to require medium security (there is no high secure inpatient mental health provision for young people; this need is met within medium security with enhanced care as required), and in particular:

- Where the young person with a mental disorder including neurodevelopmental disorders such as learning disability and autism presents a grave danger to the general public (including those who are high risk without an offending history, those charged with/convicted of specified violent or sexual offences under Schedule 15 of the Criminal Justice Act).
- Where the young person in custody (remand/sentenced) requires transfer to psychiatric hospital and is directed to secure inpatient care by the Ministry of Justice (MoJ) via a Restriction Order under the Mental Health Act (s.48/s.49).
- Where the young person has been sentenced by a Crown Court to a Hospital Order (s.37) that is accompanied by a Restriction Order (s.41) under the Mental Health Act.

There are currently (2020) 6 Adolescent MSUs providing approximately 80 beds within England. The majority of these are provided by NHS Trusts. The majority of young people admitted to Adolescent MSU are male.

Adolescent MSU Referral Criteria

- The young person is under 18 at the point of referral.

and

- Liable to be detained under part 2 or part 3 of the Mental Health Act.

and

- Presents significant risk to others with one or more of the following:
  - Direct serious violence liable to result in injury to others
  - Sexually aggressive behaviour
  - Destructive and potentially life-threatening use of fire

and

- There is clear evidence prior to referral that serious consideration of less secure provision has been made and/or tested and discounted as the young person's needs/risk exceed the threshold for and ability of those services to manage.

Care Pathways

There are four recognised pathways into adolescent medium secure services:

- Direct admission through a criminal court process or from youth justice custodial settings.
- Stepping up from low secure adolescent services.
- Admission from Adolescent PICU, from the community or a non-secure adolescent inpatient service.
- Admissions from non-criminal justice and welfare settings including welfare secure units and specialist educational settings.

Common Features across Adolescent Secure Inpatient Provision

Multi-disciplinary working and the Care Programme Approach (CPA) process underpins service delivery within all secure adolescent inpatient units. Each service should provide the following:

- Care that involves young people and their families and carers.
- Adherence to the Care Programme Approach in accordance with best practice guidance, involving the young person, family, carers, community CAMHS and other relevant stakeholders.
- Provision of care in line with welfare principles from the Children Act and the Mental Health Act Code of Practice.
- Comprehensive risk assessment and management resulting in proactive (rather than reactive) management of risk of harm to self and others.
- A secure environment where patients can address their problems in safety and with dignity.
- Ongoing mental health assessment, which meets the needs of patients through their care pathway.
- Individualised evidence-based treatment packages, based upon assessment of need and risk.
- A multi-disciplinary approach to the provision of patient care and treatment resulting in the provision of an extensive range of therapeutic, educational and recreational opportunities, particularly:
  - Psychological therapies including family therapy and creative therapies.
  - Appropriate educational services within a DfE-registered provider which is subject to OFSTED inspection.
  - Activity programmes during periods where education is not provided.
  - Functional rehabilitation including via community leave.

- Development of young people's future care pathway, including planning of transition to adult mental health services when young people approach 18 years, to enable the effective, safe and timely community discharge or transfer to an alternative mental health setting.

Particular competencies required to deliver secure inpatient assessment and treatment to young people who present with a range of complex behaviours are:

- A comprehensive multi-disciplinary team (MDT) with a 'core team' of expert psychiatry, psychology (including clinical and forensic competencies), family therapy, social work, occupational therapy, education and nursing professionals.
- An ability to provide appropriate speech and language therapy and creative therapies.
- A therapeutic model based on the principles of child development and attachment that acknowledges the importance of relationships and the key role of primary caregivers as agents of change. The model informs the work of the multi-disciplinary team and is an underpinning principle of the nursing workforce in maintaining a safe, therapeutic and developmentally appropriate culture within the unit.
- A comprehensive multi-disciplinary assessment and formulation of a young person and their wider support network. A structured clinical judgement approach to clinical risk assessment and management, reviewed at regular intervals. The assessment will inform an individual formulation including risks and protective factors which will be clearly recorded and shared by the team, the young person and their wider system.
- A therapeutic regime able to effectively deliver a variety of psychological interventions at an individual and group level addressing interpersonal relationships, problem-solving, affect regulation and mental health in line with the clinical formulation. The interventions should be flexible and responsive to the needs of the young people.
- The ability to provide a spectrum of offender-related interventions commensurate with high-risk presentations.
- A therapeutic milieu comfortable with a psychological understanding of formulations.
- The capacity to effectively deliver interventions for protracted periods of time.
- A level of resilience capable of dealing effectively with chronic challenging young people with past significant adversity.
- Capability to operate within a robust safeguarding approach that is able to balance therapy delivery and safety of staff and patients.
- The provision of interventions drawing from the available evidence base, whilst recognising the limits of this evidence for a complex client group. When working outside the evidence base, innovative interventions should be theoretically sound and robustly evaluated and should evidence clinical outcomes and young person and carer satisfaction.

Clinical Characteristics across Adolescent Secure Inpatient Provision

Demand for secure adolescent inpatient treatment has increased considerably in recent years. As outlined above, this is despite enhanced community mental health provision and is due to the increasing complexity of some young people (particularly girls) who present with severe mental health difficulties. Of particular note is the increased recognition (and perhaps prevalence) of young people with psychopathology arising from difficult and often traumatic early life experiences, resulting in attachment problems. Resulting mental health presentations include significant risk of harm to self (and at times to others), in addition to the complex safeguarding needs of this patient group. Despite often similar risk behaviours, boys tend to be criminalised more than girls, whose care needs (mental health and social care) are more prominently recognised. Attachment difficulties are often complicated by co-morbid mental illnesses (including psychosis, depression and anxiety disorders, particularly post-traumatic stress disorder (PTSD)) and neurodevelopmental disorders (particularly autistic spectrum disorder and attention deficit hyperactivity disorder (ADHD)). Disordered eating resulting in food and fluid restriction (but separate from typical anorexia nervosa) is an increasingly common additional presentation. Young people who also have learning difficulties or a formal learning disability present with further complexity and additional needs.

The increased demand for secure (and non-secure) adolescent inpatient treatment is currently resulting in a significant strain on all levels of the care pathway. The PICU model of a short period of intensive psychiatric intensive care does not meet the need of many young people who require secure adolescent inpatient treatment; this is in contrast to within adult mental health where behavioural disturbance in the context of acute mental illness (often psychosis) is prevalent. Young people who present with risk behaviours in the context of attachment difficulties require a stable and consistent treatment approach via a carefully planned care pathway. However, many are admitted to General Adolescent Units and Adolescent PICUS at times of crisis, and are unable to progress within the Adolescent PICU timescales (six to eight weeks). This results in prolonged Adolescent PICU admissions and significant demand on Adolescent LSU beds. Adolescent LSU admissions are often lengthy (6–18 months) as treatment for this patient group is complex and primarily psychological in nature.

Admissions to Adolescent MSU have traditionally been for young people whose risk behaviours have resulted in (or presented at times of) contact with the criminal justice system, particularly secure custodial placements. However, the number of young people in custody has reduced significantly within the past 15 years, primarily due to changes in sentencing guidelines. This has resulted in a further increase in complexity within young people in the community and has changed the referral pattern to Adolescent MSUs. It is now increasingly common for young people in non-custodial settings to be referred; this includes girls in Adolescent LSU placements who also present with a significant risk of harm to others (often in the context of staff intervening to manage harm to self).

Case Study (1): Ben

Ben is a 16-year-old boy whose parents separated 10 years ago due to domestic violence. He has exhibited longstanding behavioural difficulties at school resulting in a number of temporary exclusions. He had contact with CAMHS from the age of ten years in the context of psychosomatic symptoms. Eight months ago he presented with an acute psychotic illness following taking multiple drugs. He was detained under the Mental Health Act and admitted to an Adolescent PICU due to his acute behavioural disturbance. He responded well to initial treatment for psychosis but continued to exhibit behavioural difficulties, including aggression to others, arising from inappropriate social interactions. He was transferred to Adolescent LSU for further assessment and specialist treatment; an autistic spectrum disorder was diagnosed, and interventions were provided via a Positive Behavioural Support (PBS) plan.

Case Study (2): Meera

Meera is a 15-year-old girl who has experienced early childhood neglect and sexual abuse. She was removed from the care of her family at the age of eight years and has been subject to a Full Care Order since, resulting in multiple social care placements. Since the age of 12 years she has exhibited increasing self-harm behaviours in the form of cutting, scratching and hair-pulling. She was found near a motorway bridge and admitted to a General Adolescent Unit one weekend at the age of 14 years. Her self-harm behaviour escalated following admission, and her attempts to leave the unit resulted in her being detained under the Mental Health Act and transferred to an Adolescent PICU where she began to tie ligatures. After two months she was referred to Adolescent LSU but was not transferred for a further three months due to lack of bed availability. She currently remains an inpatient on Adolescent LSU.

Case Study (3): Stephen

Stephen is a 17-year-old boy who lived with his family. He had no significant childhood adversity. He was doing well at school academically, but had no friends and was socially isolated. His longstanding interest in militaria developed into obsessional thoughts about weapons, and he had an extensive collection of knives, mainly obtained via the internet. One afternoon he hid in some undergrowth in a park near to his home and with two knives attacked an elderly man who was walking his dog; the man died at the scene. Stephen was arrested and remanded into custody, where his social interaction difficulties were pronounced. He was assessed and transferred to Adolescent MSU; a detailed multi-disciplinary team assessment concluded that he had an autistic spectrum disorder. He was deemed fit to plead and stand trial and convicted of manslaughter on the grounds of diminished responsibility. He was sentenced to a Hospital Order with a Restriction Order via sections 37 and 41 of the Mental Health Act. He remains in Adolescent MSU with a plan to be transferred to an adult forensic medium secure unit shortly following his 18th birthday.

Multiple-Choice Questions

See answers on page 674.

1. What is the expected length of admission in an Adolescent PICU?
    a. 3–4 weeks
    b. 6–8 weeks
    c. 3–6 months
    d. 6–12 months
2. What is the primary reason for the reduction in young people in custodial placements?
    a. Lack of funding
    b. Reducing crime
    c. Changes in sentencing guidelines
    d. Increased hospital placements
3. Which of the following is not a recognised care pathway to Adolescent LSU?
    a. Transfer from Tier 4 general adolescent inpatient services or (PICU or other Tier 4 low secure units).
    b. Stepping down from medium secure adolescent services.
    c. Admission from specialist education and welfare settings including welfare secure units.
    d. Acute out of hours admission via section 2 of the Mental Health Act.
4. Which of the following is not a secure adolescent inpatient service?
    a. General Adolescent Unit
    b. Adolescent PICU
    c. Adolescent LSU
    d. Adolescent MSU

Key References

Chitsabesan, P., Kroll, L., Bailey, S.U.E., Kenning, C., Sneider, S., MacDONALD, W.E.N.D.Y., Theodosiou, L., (2006). Mental health needs of young offenders in custody and in the community. *The British Journal of Psychiatry*, *188*(6): 534–540.

Department of Health, (2015). Future in mind: promoting, protecting and improving our children and young people's mental health and wellbeing. *NHS England Publication Gateway Ref. No 02939.*

NHS Mental Health Implementation Plan 2019/20–2023/4: https://www.longtermplan.nhs.uk/wp-content/uploads/2019/07/nhs-mental-health-implementation-plan-2019-20-2023-24.pdf.

In NHS England Service Specifications: https://www.england.nhs.uk/publication/?filter-publication=service-specification.

84 Specialist Services

Acute Inpatient

Hollie McGloughlin

KEY CONCEPTS

- Inpatient services provide a safe environment to assess and treat the most severely mentally ill children and young people.
- They can pose disadvantages such as institutionalising the child/young person, separating them from their support network and risking them picking up unhelpful behaviours.
- Inpatient services are under huge pressures, and there is a widespread lack of beds. Chronic under-resourcing in Tier 3 CAMHS compounds the problem.

Introduction

When a young person with severe mental illness has difficulties that cannot be managed by family or community services, they may require admission to an inpatient psychiatric unit. The usual reasons for an inpatient stay include:

- The severity of illness.
- The risk to self, usually suicide/self-harm, or to others.
- When there is uncertainty about diagnosis and a period of assessment is required.
- When treatment options in the community have been exhausted and it is felt that a more intensive approach may be of benefit.
- The need to try complex medication regimes such as Clozapine which is an atypical antipsychotic requiring close monitoring and weekly blood tests.

Inpatient services fall under Tier 4 child and adolescent mental health services and are commissioned by NHS England. Inpatient units vary across the country, with differing age ranges, criteria for admission, therapies on offer and average length of stay. They include general adolescent inpatient units (13–18 years), specialised units that deal with particular needs, e.g. children under 13 or those with eating disorders or learning disabilities, high-dependency and intensive care units, which provide care for young people with particularly complex needs and low and medium secure units for young people who need a higher level of security.

Summary of Inpatient Journey

Young people are usually referred to Tier 4 services via Tier 3, i.e. community CAMHS teams. Occasionally, they may be admitted via the acute hospitals in emergency scenarios, usually via the on-call psychiatric team. Young people can be admitted informally or under the Mental Health Act.

On admission all young people must have an initial assessment, including a risk assessment and physical examination, and care-plan completed within 24 hours. A comprehensive multi-disciplinary team (MDT) bio-psycho-social assessment and formulation of their needs and a care/treatment plan will be undertaken, in collaboration with the young person and their parents/carers. The aim of the formulation is to develop a shared understanding of the young person's difficulties and needs and to guide intervention. Risk management is an essential part of inpatient treatment.

Treatment will take place alongside assessments and, if appropriate, start at the point of admission. Treatment includes a range of pharmacological and psychological interventions. The young person will have input from occupational therapy, speech and language, social care and education. Psychological interventions include individual sessions and a structured programme of both recreational and therapeutic groups. Regular care programme approach (CPA) meetings will take place involving the young person, parents/carers, MDT, Tier 3 CAMHS and any other agencies involved. In general, local and weekend leave is built up for all young people during the process of the admission and extended, when approaching discharge.

For patients admitted for treatment of low-weight eating disorder the treatment plan will include regular monitoring of weight and other physical indices in accordance with current Junior Management of Really Sick Patients with Anorexia Nervosa (MARSIPAN) guidelines (Royal College of Psychiatrists) and a family programme.

There are risks and benefits to inpatient admission. Studies of general CAMHS inpatient units have shown positive health gain and sustained improvement in psychiatric symptoms. However, in randomised controlled trials based on patients with anorexia nervosa, inpatient care and community provision show similar results which has led to a debate about the value of inpatient treatment for this disorder. For young people with psychosis, intensive care in the community appears to be as effective as admission (Frith, 2017).

Advantages of Being Admitted to Hospital

When a young person is a risk to themselves, because of strong suicidal urges, or when a young person is a risk to others, because of the effect of severe mental illness on their behaviour, hospital admission can provide safety. Close supervision and modifications of their hospital environment will keep them safe and protect other people. This allows for a thorough psychiatric assessment and for intensive treatments to begin. In hospital the young person may benefit from contact with other young people in similar circumstances. The group process can be used for therapeutic purposes, as is the case of eating disorders, whereby the group effect is helpful in encouraging the individual to eat.

The young person often benefits from some separation from the family, who may require respite following the conflict and turmoil that accompanies mental illness in a family member. However, there can be disadvantages in this separation and the family should be included, wherever possible, in treatment planning and provision.

Hospital admission provides an opportunity to complete physical assessments and investigations, which may be very relevant to the cause of mental illness. It allows complex psychopharmacological treatment regimens to be introduced safely in a controlled environment with regular reviews of physical health parameters.

Disadvantages of Being Admitted to Hospital

Admission can be a frightening or disturbing experience. The nature of the inpatient environment can lead to high levels of disturbance, such as deliberate self-harm. There are the risks of stigma and labelling. Being with young people with similar difficulties can potentially reinforce difficulties. Young people may pick up other abnormal behaviours they witness on the unit (e.g. self-harm, avoidance and 'hearing voices'). The reasons for this vary but it is thought to be due to a desire to fit in with the peer group or an expression from the young person of how unwell they are and of their wish to remain in a therapeutic setting. Admission separates the child from their home environment and risks institutionalisation. Admission to hospital, where all their needs are taken care of, may interfere with the development of independence, which is particularly crucial at this stage in the young person's life. The child could be missing out on social, educational and occupational opportunities. It is always important to re-establish contact with the young person's family and community through leave, sharing the responsibility for protecting the young person well before discharge planning.

Admission potentially undermines the parents' ability to support the child and may cause disempowerment within the family system.

Disorders in Inpatient Settings

The National Inpatient Child and Adolescent Psychiatry Study (NICAPS, O'Herlihy et al., 2001) demonstrated that children and young people admitted to in-patient units have multiple co-morbid diagnoses and severe disorders. In male adolescents the most common diagnoses included psychotic illness (35%), mood disorders (22%), conduct disorders (22%) and eating disorders (6%). In female adolescents, the most common diagnoses were eating disorders (33%), mood disorders (19%) and psychotic illnesses (14%). In most units, the average length of stay is three months, but this does vary significantly on a case-by-case basis.

Challenges Facing Inpatient Services

Historically, the research evidence regarding inpatient care has been difficult to interpret, because of methodological problems in making comparisons between such different services. There have been a number of reviews of CAMHS Tier 4 inpatient provision over the past 15 years, often occurring in response to concerns about access and the level of provision. The NICAPS study undertaken in 2001 was a unique piece of research at the time, that described the state of inpatient CAMHS services across the UK and produced a set of standards against which all units could be assessed. Following this research, the Royal College of Psychiatrists developed the Quality Network for Inpatient CAMHS (QNIC) which assesses CAMHS inpatient services on a regular basis. QNIC demonstrates and improves the quality of child and adolescent psychiatric in-patient care through a system of reviews against standards.

The Royal College of Psychiatrists has proposed a proxy measure of appropriate bed numbers as between 2 and 4 beds per 100,000 population. The average ratio for England, 2.5, is at the low end of this scale. The consequences of too few inpatient beds include young people being inadequately supported in the community, admissions to paediatric wards, children being admitted to adult wards and children being admitted to inpatient hospitals far from home.

Following the Tier 4 review in 2014/15, the government provided £7 million additional funding for NHS England to provide over 50 additional CAMHS Tier 4 beds for young inpatients in the areas with the least provision and radically changed the referral system. In *Next Steps on the NHS Five Year Forward View* delivery plan, published in March 2017, the government have stated that there will be an additional increase of 150–180 beds.

Inpatient beds are only one aspect of the provision required. There is a need to consider other types of provision including crisis services, outreach and intensive home treatment services. There is a crucial relationship between Tier 4 and Tier 3 services in effectively meeting the needs of children and young people. There is widespread concern that, due to the lack of ability by CAMHS Tier 3 and other related community services in some areas to respond early to problems, there is often a deterioration in a child/young person's problems, that can lead to crisis, thereby increasing demand for inpatient services. Young people are frequently admitted to paediatric wards, following presentation in A&E departments. They may then remain on the ward beyond the time necessary to manage the medical aspects of the self-harm, waiting for the psychiatric assessment. If an inpatient admission is deemed appropriate, they may face an additional wait for an available bed. The paediatric wards are not equipped, and staff are not adequately trained, to deal with complex psychological problems The Royal College of Psychiatrists recommends that 'Intensive outreach services should be comprehensively commissioned by responsible commissioning groups and health boards to ensure an even distribution around the UK'. It is now government policy to increase access to intensive support within the community.

Case Study (1): Amira

Amira (14) presented with significant weight loss over a period of eight months. She currently weighs 39 kg with a weight for height of 75%. She is a high achiever hoping to study medicine in the future. She began to control her diet in an attempt to lose weight, as she was unhappy with her appearance. This coincided with end-of-year examinations and some friendship difficulties. She has been treated under the community eating disorders team. Amira had initially done well but recently has struggled to comply with the menu plan, lost weight and her parents can no longer cope. On admission, she was started on the refeeding meal plan which consists of eating a scheduled amount of calories per day, and placed on a supervised eating table with other young people. She had a physical health assessment, including a range of blood tests and a hormone profile and was commenced on multivitamins, thiamine and B12, due to the risk of refeeding.

She began group and individual therapy. Her family attended the family programme on the ward and came in for Amira's supervised meals and snacks. It became evident that Amira struggled with low self-esteem and anxiety. Although she made good progress on the ward she struggled to maintain her weight on leave. The team worked closely with the family and this started to improve. Over time, Amira's weight increased, she reached her target weight range, utilised more periods of extended leave and was discharged back into the community after a four-month admission, with ongoing care from the community eating disorders team to support her recovery.

Case Study (2): Connor

Connor (17) was admitted to hospital after a significant overdose of 30 paracetamol and 20 aspirin with intent to take his own life. There was a history of breakdown in living circumstances and recent relationship difficulties. On admission, he presented as low in mood. He did not regret his actions and was unable to give assurances that he could keep himself safe. Connor did not consent to admission and was placed under section 2 of the Mental Health Act.

It became clear that Connor was experiencing psychotic symptoms. He believed that people were 'out to get him' and trying to poison his food. Connor has a difficult background and is currently placed in foster care, due to previous neglect and violence within the family.

He was commenced on Fluoxetine treatment and subsequently Aripiprazole for his psychotic symptoms. Connor's mental state improved, and he was able to engage in therapy. He settled into the ward environment and formed some relationships with members of the team and other young people. The team worked with social services and found a new placement for Connor. Unfortunately, Connor started to self-harm on the ward by cutting when distressed and especially in the period preceding discharge. This reflected his apprehension about leaving hospital. He worked through this with the team and was discharged with the CAMHS home treatment service to help contain his feelings of rejection and manage the risk, with a plan for the community team to continue his on-going care.

Multiple-Choice Questions

See answers on page 674.

1. Which of the following is not a common reason why a child or young person may be admitted to a Tier 4 setting?
   a. The severity of mental health.
   b. The child's family no longer being able to cope at home.
   c. It is far more efficacious than treatment in the community for mental illness.
   d. There is significant risk to self and/or others posed by the young person.
   e. There is uncertainty about the diagnosis and an intensive period of assessment is required.
2. How many beds per 100,000 of the population do the Royal College of Psychiatrist recommend for adolescents?
   a. 1–3
   b. 2–4
   c. 3–6
   d. 9–12
   e. 12–15
3. Which of the following is not an advantage of being admitted to an inpatient unit?
   a. The group effect can be helpful in encouraging the individual to eat.
   b. The young person may benefit from having contact with people in similar circumstances.
   c. The young person often benefits from some separation from the family.
   d. The young person may pick up on behaviours they witness on the unit.
   e. Hospital admission can provide safety.
4. Which of the following is not provided in an inpatient setting?
   a. Input from occupational therapy, speech and language, social care and education.
   b. A comprehensive multi-disciplinary team (MDT) bio-psycho-social assessment and formulation of their needs and a care/treatment plan will be undertaken, in collaboration with the young person and their parents/carers.
   c. Intensive support on discharge with someone able to visit the young person at home on a daily basis.
   d. A programme of local and weekend leave.
   e. A structured programme of recreational as well as therapeutic groups.
5. Which of the following is not correct?
   a. A paediatric bed is an appropriate place for a young person to be admitted in a psychiatric crisis.
   b. There is a crucial relationship between Tier 4 and Tier 3 services in effectively meeting the needs of children and young people.
   c. There are widespread concerns due to the lack of ability by CAMHS Tier 3 and other related community services in some areas to respond early to problems.
   d. The average ratio for England is 2.5 inpatient CAMHS beds per 100,000 of the population.
   e. In-patient beds are only one aspect of the provision required and there is a need to consider other types of provision.

Key References

Faculty of Child and Adolescent Psychiatry, (2015). *Survey of Inpatient Admissions for Children and Young People with Mental Health Problems.* London: Royal College of Psychiatrists.

NHS England, (2017). *Five Year Forward View for Mental Health: One Year On.* London: NHS England.

O'Herlihy, A., et al., (2001). *National Inpatient Child and Adolescent Psychiatry Study.* London: College Research Unit of the Royal College of Psychiatrists and the Department of Health.

85 Specialist Services

An Inpatient Unit for Children with Complex Health Needs

Sally Wicks (updated by Margaret J.J. Thompson)

Introduction

Bursledon House is an example of a unit that meets the needs of children and young people with complex psychiatric/emotional/behavioural and or physical health problems. This unit is located in the grounds of the University Hospital Southampton. It is a 12-bedded residential unit for children and adolescents, with therapy/meeting rooms, kitchen and dining room, lounge, single and multiple bedrooms, a playground and with an integrated school, divided into junior- and senior-level classrooms. The unit is open from Monday to Friday. The children go home at weekends, with report forms to encourage their parents to feedback weekend progress to staff. Parents usually bring the child in on a Monday morning and take them home on Friday afternoons. Some children (up to five or six at a time) attend as day patients, usually at the end of an inpatient stay as part of a school reintegration plan.

KEY CONCEPTS

- Bursledon House is an example of a unit that meets the needs of children and young people with complex psychiatric/emotional/behavioural and or physical health problems.
- Due to the complexity of presenting children, it is staffed by a range of health and education specialists.
- Children and young people are commonly referred from CAMHS or community/inpatient paediatric services.
- Once admitted children, young people and their families are offered an individualised package of care including individual and family-based work.
- Close contact is maintained with the wider professional network around the child/young person, especially when reintegrating them into their own school.

Staffing

This unit lies within the Child Health Department, with all patients being admitted under the care either of a child psychiatry consultant or a paediatric consultant (either hospital or community based). There is daily medical input from an associate specialist in paediatrics and from the child psychiatry team including an ST3 and at times an ST4-6 as well as consultants. There is cover from nursing staff 24 hours a day Monday to Friday. In addition, there is a comprehensive multi-disciplinary team including psychologists, occupational therapists, physiotherapists, play specialists, a dietician, teaching staff and administrative staff.

Patient Group

Bursledon House is for children with psychiatric/emotional/behavioural problems and/or physical problems, which have impacted severely on day-to-day life and normal functioning, e.g. causing difficulties over school attendance or with family relationships. Common physical problems include constipation and soiling, wetting, feeding problems, chronic pain syndromes and children requiring neuro-rehabilitation. There is usually a mix of physical and emotional/behavioural difficulties in these children. Children who are too young for an adolescent psychiatric unit may be admitted with a range of mental health problems, including anorexia nervosa, obsessive-compulsive disorder, depression and anxiety. Patients can be admitted from infancy to age 16. Infants would be admitted with a parent/guardian, while school-age children do not have their parents resident.

Referral Process

Patients are referred to the team by clinicians, such as hospital consultants, community paediatricians or CAMHS consultant psychiatrists, by letter. The referral is discussed at the referral meeting. A decision is taken about which team members should carry out a pre-admission assessment with the family. This would be one member of the nursing staff with between one and four other members of the team including at least one doctor. The play specialist would usually also be involved.

At the pre-admission assessment, a decision is taken as to whether the child, or adolescent, is a suitable candidate for admission, i.e. whether the admission would help the family and whether they want to go ahead with it, or whether there may be other, more appropriate, management methods. Following this assessment, a detailed letter is sent to the referrer regarding the information gained, and if admission is felt to be appropriate, funding from commissioners in the patient's area is sought and then the patient is placed on the waiting list. If the child is to be admitted, the pre-admission assessment appointment is an opportunity for the family to familiarise themselves with the unit, so that when the admission day arrives, it is not as anxiety-provoking as it might otherwise have been. Sometimes a further visit might be arranged for this purpose.

The time spent on the waiting list may be several months. Urgent cases must take priority, and it is important to have the right inpatient mix at any time, to maintain a positive therapeutic environment.

Admission and Management

On admission, the family is seen for a 'catch-up' assessment of the on-going problems. These are then documented in the notes. The team will discuss the new patient at the ward round and a management plan will be agreed.

Management will consist of a combination of the following, as deemed appropriate to that particular case –

- **Individual work** with the child/adolescent, which may consist of supportive counselling, anger management, self-esteem work, cognitive behavioural therapy-based approaches, anxiety management provided by psychology or psychiatry.
- **Play sessions** particularly with younger children.
- **Sessions with the parents/family** to look at their concerns and at the issues which will need to be considered, and to enable the family to work collaboratively with the staff in helping their child/adolescent.
- **Physiotherapy** assessment and treatment.

- **Occupational therapy** assessment and treatment in daily living activities, fine and gross motor co-ordination, perceptual and sensory difficulties. Establishing the child's developmental level of functioning.
- **Dietary information and advice.**
- **Psychological assessment**, including cognitive and neuropsychological assessments and psychology-based individual work.
- **Assessment of ability in Bursledon House school.**
- **Observation and assessment of interaction** with other children and with staff, and of general behaviour.
- **Assessment of sleep** patterns, eating habits, self-care and mental state.
- **Re-integration** into the child's own school if appropriate.
- **Support and advice** to the parents/carers and own school staff.
- **Close liaison** with family/school/other professionals involved in the case.
- **Multi-disciplinary meetings** at appropriate intervals and pre-discharge meeting.
- **Full discharge summary** to referring clinician, parent and other professionals involved, including clear follow-up plan in the community.

Case Study (1): Stefan

Stefan, a 12-year-old boy, was admitted for rehabilitation following a head injury in a road traffic accident. Problems included:

- Right-sided limb weakness
- Behavioural difficulties
- Memory impairment
- Parents having difficulty accepting the severity of some of the changes

Rehabilitation Plan

- A structured weekly timetable including defined periods of time in the onsite school and periods of rest.
- Strategies to assist memory put in place including use of a memory book and signs on doors initially.
- Physiotherapy input twice daily with a particular focus on improving mobility.
- Occupational therapy directed at improving arm function and independence with activities of daily living.
- Regular liaison with paediatric neurology team.
- Behavioural management strategies devised between child psychiatrist, psychology and nursing staff.
- Ongoing psychological support for parents.
- Individual psychological support with child.
- Neuropsychology review with full assessment at six months post-head injury.
- ADHD assessment by child and adolescent psychiatrist.
- Liaison with own school leading to reintegration.

Progress

Stefan's behaviour improved after transfer from the paediatric wards, showing a good response to having a more structured timetable and nursing staff providing clear boundaries. The decision was made to carry out an ADHD assessment. History from parents did not suggest this diagnosis prior to the accident. It was felt that the poor concentration, over-activity and impulsiveness that had been present in the recovery period were becoming less prominent, so a policy of watch and wait was adopted. Eventually the decision was made that methylphenidate would not be required. With ongoing physiotherapy, Stefan became progressively steadier on his feet and in time was able to walk unaided. Less progress was made with the upper limb, but some functional use was regained. Stefan's parents initially found it difficult to accept that there were some cognitive/memory deficits and changes in temperament which were likely to be ongoing. They were supported in coming to terms with this. Multi-disciplinary team meetings were held to give professionals in the community a clear idea of Stefan's needs. An educational psychology assessment was initiated with plans for one-to-one support in school and follow-up arranged from local physiotherapists and occupational therapists. Stefan then had a reintegration to school and was discharged home.

Case Study (2): Holly

Holly, an eight-year-old girl, was admitted with concerns about her eating. Problems included:

- Longstanding narrow range of foods with poor intake and anxiety around food.
- Slow weight gain.
- Maternal stress due to poor eating and slow weight gain.

Management Plan

- Occupational therapy assessment for sensory and oral motor issues.
- Play programme including messy play and play with food to make food fun.
- Regular meetings with family to share progress and make plans for the weekend.
- Psychology input including anxiety management strategies and devising a hierarchy of new foods to try.
- Reward system involving stickers and prizes for trying new foods and for eating good amounts.
- Dietician's advice to staff and to family.

Progress

The occupational therapist's assessment did not show any significant sensory or oral motor issues. Holly made the decision alongside the psychologist working with her that she wanted to try new foods outside meal times, supported by one member of staff. At mealtimes, Holly was observed to be anxious, but this gradually improved with only familiar foods being offered initially and with gentle encouragement being given by staff. The distraction of social interaction with peers also appeared helpful. Holly soon began to earn stickers by eating greater quantities of familiar foods, and also, by eating very small amounts of new foods in individual sessions. With time it became possible for a couple of the 'new' foods to be incorporated at mealtimes. Parents were invited in to join some mealtimes and initially were observed to inadvertently be placing pressure on Holly to eat, but with advice from and modelling by nursing staff this improved. Eating at home at weekends improved, and Holly gained weight during the admission. At discharge parents were happy to know that Holly could eat reasonable amounts of food and had gained weight. They felt confident that the range of foods she would eat could gradually increase over time with a more relaxed approach to mealtimes.

Multiple-Choice Questions

See answers on page 674.

1. Which of the following physical complaints in children and young people would commonly be seen in a unit such as Bursledon House?
   a. Soiling and bed wetting
   b. Feeding problems
   c. Chronic fatigue problems
   d. Neurological problems
   e. All of the above
2. Which of the following professionals/services would *not* commonly refer directly into specialist units such as Bursledon house?
   a. Paediatric wards
   b. Community paediatricians
   c. Social services
   d. Community CAMHS
   e. All would commonly refer

Key References

Department of Health, (2003). *Every Child Matters*. London: HMSO.
Department of Health, (2004). *National Service Framework for Children, Young People and Maternity Services*. London: HMSO.

86 Specialist Services

Role of the Educational Psychologist

Helena Hoyos and Lucy Manger

Introduction

The role of the educational psychologist has developed and changed considerably since it was first established early in the 20th century. This has been particularly relevant during the last few years as a response to legislation set out in the Children and Families Act which became law on the 13 March 2014, and subsequent statutory guidance in the Special Educational Needs and Disability Code of Practice, published in July 2014. One key change was that the work of educational psychologists now focuses on children and young people from 0 to 25 years.

The process for how children and young people with special educational needs and disabilities are supported has also changed considerably through the introduction of Education Health and Care Plans (EHCPs) to replace the now defunct Statements of Special Educational Needs, with statutory guidance for all Statements to be transferred to EHCPs by 1 April 2018. Educational psychologists have a statutory role in the EHCP process and provide detailed advice to identify needs, necessary outcomes and the support required to achieve these. However, the majority of educational psychologists have a much wider role with children, schools and families, as well as contributing to educational research.

KEY CONCEPTS

- To apply psychological thinking and methodology to help children and young people develop and learn in all areas of their lives, including developing emotional wellbeing and resilience as well as more formal aspects of academic learning. This involves a range of methods, which may include direct assessment, observation, consultation, training and research.
- Educational psychologists work in a range of different contexts, and with different client groups. This includes work with children, parents and carers, schools and colleges, local authorities and other agencies concerned with education, social care and health.
- A key function is to provide psychological advice within the statutory framework for supporting children with Special Educational Needs (SEN), as set out in the Special Educational Needs and Disability Code of Practice: 0 to 25 years. This is the framework within which decisions are taken about the nature of a child or young person's need and the provision required to meet that need. An Educational Health and Care Plan (EHCP) may be issued as a result of this process.

The Main Roles of the Educational Psychologist

Assessment

Educational psychologists see assessment as a means of collecting information about a child or young person by a variety of means and, ideally, over time. It may involve gathering information from a wide range of sources, including the child/young person, parents/carers, teaching staff and other professionals. Educational psychologists are interested in the context in which the child/young person is developing, and assessment will usually encompass cognitive, emotional and social factors. Educational psychologists analyse what has been identified as the problem and form hypotheses about what underlying issues could be contributing to it. Assessment can be useful in testing out whether or not these hypotheses are valid and in helping to form alternatives, where appropriate. This may involve individual assessment work with the child/young person using a range of assessment tools including but not limited to standardised cognitive assessment, dynamic assessment, questionnaires, observation schedules, curriculum-based assessment and other approaches aimed at eliciting children's views.

Sometimes assessments carried out by educational psychologists are used to help inform local authority assessments of children and young people with special educational needs and disabilities to provide advice which may be incorporated into an EHCP. Educational psychology assessments are primarily used to help identify outcomes, plan future interventions to help the child/young person and review progress.

Consultation

Educational psychologists offer consultation to a variety of clients, including early years settings, schools (often liaising with the Special Educational Needs Coordinator – SENCo), colleges, parents, carers, partner agencies and local authority staff. Consultation can take place through meetings within the educational placement, at alternative venues within the community, in the home or on the telephone. The focus of consultation is on joint, collaborative problem-solving, informed by the understanding of psychological models and psycho-social processes which the educational psychologist brings. Sometimes specific techniques are used, such as solution circles, person-centred planning, rich pictures, PATHs, coaching, motivational interviewing and solution-focussed approaches.

Intervention

Educational psychologists draw on their professional knowledge and skills to develop and recommend carefully planned and evidence-based interventions, according to the needs of each individual with whom they work. This may include interventions which focus directly on an individual's particular skill set, but can also encompass group, whole-class, school-wide and parenting approaches. Interventions often address a range of different issues, including cognition and learning, communication and languages, social, emotional and mental health development, and approaches to behavioural management. At times educational psychologists may work directly with a child, young person or family to deliver an intervention, such as cognitive behavioural therapy or systemic work. They may also work directly with staff using an approach such as coaching.

Educational psychologists aim to help those living or working with the child/young person on a daily basis to develop their own capacity to support the child/young person. Interventions are usually developed in collaboration with these service users and may involve the educational psychologist delivering training and/or offering ongoing supervision. Educational psychologists collaborate with other professionals to help ensure that interventions are co-ordinated and do not overload the child/young person or compromise their inclusion within their peer group.

Training

Educational psychologists are trained to understand the psychological processes behind the learning, behaviour and development of children and young people and how these may be affected by the environment and social context in which the child/young person is growing up. Educational psychologists have some training in organisational and systemic psychology, which informs their understanding of the wider context within which children are developing. By offering training and support tailored to meet the needs of individual learners and groups, educational psychologists help others begin to link research and psychological theory with their everyday work with children and young people.

Educational psychologists are members of the Health and Care Professions Council, which carefully regulates practice and requires a rigorous level of ongoing training and other forms of continuing professional development. Educational psychologists need to remain aware of the local and national contexts within which they work in order to ensure that they are responding to developing priorities. Many educational psychologists also choose to extend their skills by undertaking further training. Typical examples include cognitive behavioural therapy, systemic family work, coaching and supervision.

Research

Educational psychologists are trained to carry out research in a range of settings. This may include reviewing the effectiveness of interventions at a local level or carrying out wider research to help design educational practice and policy. Since 2006 educational psychology training has been at doctoral level, with many previously qualified educational psychologists also completing doctoral research. As part of their roles many qualified and practising educational psychologists provide supervision for trainee educational psychologists who are completing research projects, as well as for practice placements.

Outcome Measures

Evidence-based practice is at the core of the work of an educational psychologist. Assessment of the impact of interventions is key in establishing their relevance and effectiveness, and will be central to the casework review process through progress data and test/re-test information. Qualitative information can also be gathered to add to this process through a variety of sources, which may often include the use of pre- and post-measures such as rating scales and questionnaires. The introduction of EHCPs has highlighted the importance of specific short- and long-term outcomes for young people and the particular provision required to help to achieve these.

Whilst acknowledging the importance of specific outcome measures, it is also important to recognise that there is a challenge in measuring a role which is primarily about empowering other people through the application of psychology. Therefore, to some extent, educational psychologists are reliant upon anecdotal accounts of impact, progress and increased wellbeing of those they support in order to gauge their effectiveness and the value of their contribution.

Case Study (1): Sanjay

Sanjay has Duchenne muscular dystrophy. Although he is independently mobile at present, he is likely to need a wheelchair within the next academic year. Due to his condition and its impact on his health and education, the county council carried out an assessment of Sanjay before he started school with a view to identifying what provision would be required to support him. As part of the assessment process, an educational psychologist visited Sanjay at home and in his pre-school. She talked to Sanjay's parents and his key worker and filled in a developmental chart with them. Through multi-agency meetings and by telephone, the educational psychologist liaised with Sanjay's paediatrician, physiotherapist, occupational therapist and specialist teacher. The educational psychologist observed Sanjay on two separate occasions in the different settings and played with him, using toys and some dynamic assessment tools. Sanjay was subsequently given an EHCP, which is ongoing and reviewed annually.

Sanjay is now in Year 2. With a view to his transition into junior school, the educational psychologist was asked to visit Sanjay again to update her advice in advance of the annual review. She carried out some more observations and repeated some of the dynamic assessments carried out previously, to gauge Sanjay's progress over time. The educational psychologist attended the annual review of Sanjay's EHCP, which was attended by his parents, class teacher, SENCo, physiotherapist and specialist teacher. Sanjay also attended the meeting for the last ten minutes to order to give his views about school. At the annual review meeting, all those involved with Sanjay considered together about how best to support Sanjay in his move to junior school and whether a change of placement or any adaptations to the current environment would be needed to accommodate his changing mobility needs. As a result, it was agreed that transfer to the mainstream junior school was appropriate, with additional hours of support and appropriate adaptations made to the physical environment. Sanjay was very keen to stay with his friends and this was taken into account when making the decision.

Case Study (2): Tessa

Tessa is in Year 4 at school. She is achieving age-related expectations in all her subjects, although her handwriting is causing some concern as she writes slowly and her letters are poorly formed. Her spelling in the context of her writing is weaker than it appears from her spelling test results. Tessa often appears angry or upset in the classroom and, at times, has been reluctant to go to school. She appears frustrated when asked to do her work, especially during written tasks. Her behaviour in response to this apparent frustration has escalated to the point where she often refuses to do the work or destroys the work she has attempted to do. She has not been aggressive to other children or to adults, but has occasionally kicked chairs and thrown things in the classroom. Her parents and teachers asked the educational psychologist to observe Tessa and work with her on some individual assessments to try and help them understand her behaviour better and to recommend ways of supporting her.

The observations led the educational psychologist to form the hypothesis that Tessa has some specific difficulties with aspects of learning. Her frustration seemed to be most noticeable during written tasks and when she had been listening to spoken lesson content and was then asked to complete a task independently. Subsequent individual assessment identified that Tessa has difficulties with auditory working memory and phonological processing speed. Her handwriting and spelling are also weaker than would be predicted based on her overall cognitive ability so she struggles to demonstrate her full knowledge and understanding on paper.

The educational psychologist met with Tessa's teacher and parents to discuss these results and plan how best to support her. As a result of this, adaptations were made in the classroom to help support Tessa's working memory and she was given extra time to complete tasks. She was also given the use of a laptop to record her work, and opportunities to learn touch typing. The educational psychologist also recommended that Tessa follow a 'Cued Spelling' intervention and provided training for staff on how to deliver this. The educational psychologist also recommended that Tessa have six support sessions with the school's emotional literacy support assistant (ELSA) to help her learn how to recognise and manage her emotions and develop her confidence and self-esteem in relation to learning. This work is supervised by the Educational Psychology Service, which also provided initial training for the ELSA.

Case Study (3): Tom

Tom was taken into care ten years ago at the age of five. He lives with his fourth foster family and has been with them for 18 months. He seems very unhappy at school and is struggling to learn, despite having been assessed by the educational psychologist as being of high average intelligence. Tom finds it very hard to settle to work, especially during structured, adult-led sessions, and appears to lack confidence in his ability. He can be very rude and aggressive to some of his teachers, although he has a strong relationship with his PE teacher. He has few consistent friendships, has been involved in several fights at lunchtimes and has been excluded from school for a total of 19 days this year. He is currently on a part-time timetable and spends part of each day in the school's inclusion unit. However, in spite of this provision the school is worried that they may have to exclude him permanently, if his behaviour does not improve and he is unable to attend mainstream lessons.

The educational psychologist has provided whole-school training on attachment theory and has met with Tom's teachers to increase staff empathy and explore how the training might be relevant to him. The educational psychologist also met with the SENCo to discuss specific strategies, for example increasing Tom's motivation by introducing an element of choice into tasks and increasing opportunities for positive reinforcement of his efforts. It was also recommended that a key adult be identified, with whom Tom could meet on a regular basis to share his concerns and strengthen his engagement with school. This could be facilitated through the inclusion unit, as staff in that context may be well placed to build a personal connection with Tom and help him work towards increasing his timetable. However, if Tom prefers, it may be possible to build on his existing relationship with his PE teacher. The sports department may also be able to help Tom develop more positive relationships with his peers, through including him in sports teams. Tom's progress is regularly monitored and is reviewed with the educational psychologist on a half termly basis to ensure that the risk of exclusion is reduced and that he is happier and more settled within school.

Key Reference

Department of Health, Department for Education, (2014). *Special Educational Needs and Disability Code of Practice: 0 to 25 years*. London: DH & DfE.

87 Specialist Services

Education for Children with Autism Spectrum Disorders and Social Stories for Parents of Autistic Children

Sandra Teale (updated by Margaret J.J. Thompson)

Introduction

Education is an area that has received much attention of late, with changes that are far-reaching in the realm of special needs. Special education is in flux. Funding implications impact on proposals for placements outside that of a named mainstream school. A growing number of local educational authorities are working to develop more inclusive policies and specialist 'in-county' provision to accommodate the growing number of children with an autistic spectrum condition diagnosis. For those children with a diagnosis, the support needs are variable and sometimes very complex.

However, any individual educational programme needs to be mindful of the variable abilities, intellectually and socially, that this population can exhibit. This will then influence the type of educational package needed.

KEY CONCEPTS

When identifying the most appropriate programme or placement, variables to consider include:

- The nature of the curriculum and how it is delivered.
- The experience of the staff.
- The child–staff ratio.
- The current peer groupings (re: ability and size).
- The involvement of parents.
- The opportunity for specialist advisory support, therapeutic input, e.g. speech and language therapy, occupational therapy, music therapy.
- Available resources.
- The opportunity to spend time with peers, with or without an autism diagnosis, should be taken into account.
- Meeting the individual's needs is paramount.

Many schools will attempt to identify and meet the needs of a child after initial 'in-school' assessment. The needs of children with disabilities in education are laid out in the Children and Families Act (2014) and subsequent statutory guidance in the Special Educational Needs and Disability Code of Practice (July 2014).

If a parent/carer or school feel that the needs of a child are not being addressed, they may apply to the local education authority for an Education Health and Care Plan (EHCP). This statement is a legal document issued by a local authority, setting out the educational and learning needs of the child and specifying how these should be addressed.

Local education authorities need to be creative in their placement of children on the autistic spectrum, focusing on the overall needs of the individual child.

Effective types of provision for ASD young people include:

- Mainstream schools with trained support staff and ASD-friendly ethos
- Mainstream schools with an ASD specialist unit attached
- Specialist day/residential provision for ASD/learning difficulties with possible links to a local mainstream school
- Home-based learning programme

Early intervention programmes vary from outreach support for families provided by local authorities linking them to specialist services, to home-based programmes that may receive funding from their local authority. An effective early-years programme would address the 'triad of impairments' and sensory needs and build positive relationships with those involved with the child.

The programme would focus on:

- Communication
- Social interaction
- Play, leisure and life skills

Access to a curriculum would include:

- Structure, visual learning and modelling
- Direct teaching of social skills
- Understanding the functions of behaviour and teaching acceptable behavioural responses

Mainstream School Case Study (1): Jim

Jim (nine) was a quiet boy with a diagnosis of Asperger syndrome and an extensive interest in airplanes. He was very compliant, eager to please and followed the school rules without question. The school staff were given training on ASD and were receptive to further professional support. Jim's teachers perceived him to be extremely polite and easy to manage. His peers were given training on ASD and others with different learning needs, developed a tolerance of Jim, seeing him as a bit of a 'geek', but non-threatening.

One other boy in the school described Jim as his best friend because they shared an interest in Pokémon. Jim found transitions challenging, and large groups of people made him anxious. The school worked with Jim using social stories and supported him in identifying the most stressful situations, allowing him the opportunity to avoid these settings until he could tolerate them and learn how to cope.

Jim had an experienced learning support assistant with an understanding of ASD and of Jim's specific sensory needs. Initially, she worked with Jim 1:1 and then expanded her time to support other students with ASD, running a social skills group and offering 1:1 sessions to Jim twice weekly.

Mainstream School with an ASD Specialist Unit Attached Case Study (2): Bob

Bob, a student with a diagnosis of high-functioning autism, became extremely anxious when he moved from a small primary school to a large comprehensive school. He was very worried by the thought of the many changes associated with his change of school. Bob was motivated to attend a mainstream school, wanting to participate in the variety of lessons on offer. It was decided that to support Bob with this transition, he would be best suited to attending a school where there was an ASD base that he could use as a place of refuge and support when his anxieties dictated. Bob began at the school using the base for his first lesson to help him organise his day, relax and talk through his anxieties, practising strategies he could use throughout the day. He had an agreed exit strategy that the teachers supported, allowing Bob to leave a classroom when his anxieties rose to an unmanageable level.

During his first two terms, Bob had a learning support assistant with him 1:1, with them fading their support during the latter part of the term. Bob is now in Year 10, receiving support from the ASD base through a social skills and life skills group, relaxation session and relationship/sex education lessons. He is on target to achieve his GCSEs at a high grade.

Specialist Day/Residential Provision for ASC/Learning Difficulties with Possible Links to a Local Mainstream School Case Study (3): Beth

Beth (16) had a diagnosis of ASD and attended a residential specialist school for learning difficulties with a high proportion of the student population with ASD. Beth had some provocative sexual behaviours around males and became challenging with intervention by staff. It was felt that her needs and vulnerabilities warranted that she be educated within a secure setting. Beth's 24-hour waking day programme followed the national curriculum in addition to life skills, social skills training, sensory integration, behavioural interventions and specialist relationship/sexuality education.

Beth had a special interest in food preparation and participated in a local college link provision for catering, supported by a learning support assistant. She secured a placement in further education in food preparation and is on course to begin in September.

Beth has been given the opportunity to develop a variety of activities, bringing her into contact with peers her own age. She is directly taught and coached on appropriate social skills 1:1, when in these situations. Although Beth's lack of understanding about relationships/sexuality makes her vulnerable, she is developing an awareness of her own feelings and emotions.

Home-Based Programme Case Study (4): Joe

Joe (14) had a diagnosis of ASD and found any educational provision so anxiety- producing that he became a school refuser. His parents felt that the educational provision would need to be home-based, if it was to support Joe.

The educational authority organised for Joe to have some of his programme delivered through a virtual school, accessing his computer with a tutor 1:1. He would progress onto joining a small group of three. Joe had the support of a specialist teacher in ASD, who visited him to teach him life and social skills, and an occupational therapist who identified his sensory needs, supporting him to develop coping strategies. During these sessions, Joe would be taught in a visual manner, helping him to explore social perspectives, social problem-solving and teaching him directly the skills needed in a variety of situations.

Joe had a support worker from social services who practiced these skills with him out in the community. Joe joined a weekly exercise class. He joined a local scout group with the encouragement of his support worker, helping him build peer relationships. Joe attended sessions with the local CAMHS specialist ASD team to help him understand his feelings of anxiety, benefiting from a sensory profile to understand the difficulties he had in regulating his sensory input. This information, coupled with CBT to address his anxiety, meant that Joe became aware of how to reduce his anxiety and practise coping strategies. Joe is currently investigating a small adult education class in computing and web design.

Educational provision for ASD children is varied and benefits from having the needs of the individual as the main focus to identify the most appropriate programme or placement.

Related Information

- **Autism Education Trust** (The Autism Education Trust (AET)) was launched in November 2007 with funding from the Department for Children, Schools and Families. It is dedicated to co-ordinating and improving education support for all children on the autism spectrum in England.
- **Inclusion Development Programme National Standards (IDP): Primary and Secondary: Teaching and supporting pupils on the autism spectrum** is an e-learning course that supports teachers in meeting the needs of pupils on the autism spectrum. The course is designed for teachers and teaching assistants, trainers and initial teacher training (ITT) providers, headteachers and leadership teams, support workers and student teachers in training
- **The National Autistic Society** (https://www.autism.org.uk/) is the leading UK charity for people with autism, including Asperger syndrome, and their families. They provide information, support and services for those needing to be signposted to appropriate help.
- **The National Autistic Society's Early Bird Programme**, a three-month programme for the parents/carers of pre-school children on the autism spectrum. It is delivered by licensed trainers who work with parents/carers on how to encourage the best from their child.
- **The Autism Good Practice Guidance (2009)** was developed by the Autism Working Group and gives practical advice to providers for children with autistic spectrum disorders, based on existing good practice, and helps them to reflect on their own practice and examples of good practice.
- **The National Autism Plan for Children (NAPC)** produced by the National Initiative for Autism: Screening and Assessment (NIASA). The plan covers the identification, assessment, diagnosis and access to early interventions for pre-school and primary school-aged children with autistic spectrum disorders. The guidelines are for parents and anyone who works with ASD children and were developed by a multi-disciplinary group of core professionals from health, education, social services and representatives of parents and the voluntary sector.
- Early Support Programme: the government programme to achieve better co-ordinated, family-focussed services for young disabled children and their families (https://www.rbkc.gov.uk/family-information-service/info-parents-and-carers/children-disabilities/early-support-programme).
- Early Years Foundation Stage is a government initiative setting the standards for learning, development and care for children from birth to five. It brings together Curriculum Guidance for the Foundation Stage (2000), the Birth to Three Matters (2002) framework and the National Standards for Under 8s Day Care and Childminding (2003), building

a coherent and flexible approach to care and learning. All providers are required to use the EYFS to ensure that whatever setting parents choose, they can be confident that their child will receive a quality experience that supports their development and learning. This has been updated: 2020 Early Years Foundation Stage: Assessment and Reporting Arrangements (ARA).

- National Portage Association: a charity offering support and information to parents and professionals involved in portage.
- Office for Advice, Assistance, Support and Information on Special Needs (OAASIS): a resource for parents and professionals caring for children and young people with autism/Asperger syndrome and other learning disabilities.

Social Stories for Parents of Autistic Children

KEY CONCEPTS

- Unique, tailor-made stories written in a specific format and from the perspective of the young person with ASD.
- To develop a better understanding of specific events, situations, skills or concepts, so that young people can work out how to respond or behave more appropriately.
- As the aim is to develop understanding rather than just learning a rote response, the focus should always be on describing rather than directing.
- Social stories can be used to help in any situation that is confusing, upsetting or that the young person is struggling in.
- Social stories are a specific technique designed to help improve the social understanding of young people with ASD.

Impairments in social understanding can mean that young people with autism spectrum disorder (ASD) are often unaware of the unwritten social rules and what is, or is not, expected in certain situations. Their difficulties with understanding and making sense of others can mean that they struggle to work out what other people might be thinking and feeling or why they are doing what they are doing. Social stories, originally developed by Carol Gray in 1991, are designed to help improve the social understanding of young people with ASD.

What Are Social Stories?

Social stories are short, unique, tailor-made stories written in a specified style and format. Each story focusses on a specific event, situation, skill or concept and aims to help the young person understand this better. Stories may draw attention to unwritten social rules or taboos, relevant social cues, others' perspectives or the consequences of certain actions.

How Do Social Stories Work?

Increasing the social understanding of young people with ASD can decrease the frustration and anxiety that they experience in certain situations. It may reduce the inappropriate or challenging behaviour that not understanding a social situation, and/or experiencing high levels of distress, can result in. Increased understanding allows young people to adapt and modify their behaviour. Social stories can help other people see things from the point of view of the young person with ASD, thereby increasing their understanding of the young person.

The evidence base for the efficacy of social stories with young people with ASD is growing. Due to their highly specific, individual nature, most research comprises very small numbers of subjects, case studies or single-case experimental designs.

What Do Social Stories Look Like?

Social stories are written in the first person, as though the young people with ASD are describing the event themselves. They describe situations in a series of logical steps.

Four types of sentences are used:

- **Descriptive** – relevant factual information.
- **Perspective** – information about others' thoughts, feelings, reasons and motives.
- **Directive** – appropriate responses the young person could try.
- **Affirmative** – reassurance and motivation for the young person.

The basic ratio of zero to one directive sentence for every two to five descriptive or perspective sentences ensures that the focus of the story is to help develop young people's social understanding, rather than teaching them a rote response. The length, vocabulary and style of writing are tailored to the young person's age and level of understanding. Illustrations, photos or symbols can be used for younger children, and more creative adaptations, e.g. presenting them as a short film or in a multimedia format, are possible.

Once written, social stories need to be read and re-read with the young person. Frequent repetition facilitates the learning. Re-reading stories before a young person enters a specific situation is particularly helpful, as the information about that situation will be fresh in the mind and can be applied straight away.

When Can Social Stories Be Used?

Social stories can be used in any situation that is confusing or upsetting for a young person. These could include introducing changes to routine, preparing for trips or visits and any other new situations that the young person needs help to understand. They can be used to describe social situations, e.g. clubs, break times and expectations and appropriate behaviour for those or to help young people understand when and why to use specific social skills. Emotions, such as fear and anger, can be the topic of a social story, focussing on increasing the young person's ability to recognise, label and manage these emotions.

Multiple-Choice Questions

See answers on page 674.

1. What considerations should be considered when identifying an appropriate placement for a child with ASC?
    a. The special advisory support
    b. Peer group sizes and abilities
    c. The opportunity to mix with ASC and non-ASC children
    d. The expertise of staff
    e. All of the above

2. What are the characteristics of an effective early-years programme?
   a. Communication, social interaction, play, leisure and life skills.
   b. Access to a curriculum would include structure, visual learning and modelling and direct teaching of social skills.
   c. Understanding the functions of behaviour and teaching acceptable behavioural responses.
   d. A, B and C.
   e. Role modelling from peers that have no ASC diagnosis.
3. Which of these statements about social stories is not true?
   a. Social stories aim to increase a young person's social understanding.
   b. Social stories tell young people what they should do in certain situations.
   c. Social stories are written from the point of view of the young person.
   d. Social stories can be presented in a range of mediums.
   e. Social stories can help others to understand young people with ASD better.

Key References

Attwood, T., (1998). *Asperger's Syndrome: A Guide for Parents and Professionals.* London: Jessica Kingsley Publishers.

Jordan, R.R., (2003). *Educational Provision: Making Mainstream Schools Autism-Friendly & Inclusion.* School of Education, University of Birmingham.

Wing, L., (1993). The definition and prevalence of autism: a review. *European Child and Adolescent Psychiatry*, 2(2): 61–74.

88 Specialist Services

Working with Children in Care and Residential Schools (a Whole Service/Systems Approach to Emotion-Regulation)

Cathie O'Brien

This chapter looks at the organisational system that children and young people (CYP) who live away from home live in, and proposes a sustainable therapeutic model, at a whole service level, that can be used at every level of the service/system from professionals through to children and families. This model builds resilience via a good understanding of a relational approach, through an attachment theory and gestalt therapy lens.

Attachment Theory through a Gestalt Therapy Lens

Gestalt therapy works in the here and now with the whole individual or group, working with their thoughts, feelings and nervous system in the present situation and is interested in 'how' relationships are co-created. For instance, when a professional is teaching children or putting in place a therapeutic intervention, they and the environment are part of the relationship that is created, they are part of the resulting action. These are the implicit, non-verbal and often unaware and unacknowledged aspects of being human, and gestalt pays particular attention to this. It uses the four stages of contact and withdrawal, shown in Figure 88.1 on the outside of the circle, as a framework to explore this co-creation, which I have integrated with attachment theory, shown in the inner circle (O'Brien, 2011). I integrated the two because both are regulatory theories and recognise how the personality develops through a process of interactions with the environment. Also, attachment theory and the terms self-/emotion-regulation have become a common language in services but with little understanding of 'how' this occurs. Individuals can either focus on immediate attachment or high avoidance of attachment with little understanding of the process of attachment. This lack of understanding can unintentionally lead to CYP losing their placements or gaining a criminal record due to professionals activating their attachment behaviour system through conventional ways of relating, not understanding their invisible trauma. Once the attachment system is activated in a way CYP cannot manage, this can lead to the child self-harming or harming others. Professionals need to learn how to adapt to this invisible trauma, developing disciplined awareness of the relationship – which can sometimes feel counter-intuitive.

Figure 88.1 shows the first stage of contact which is sensation, and in attachment theory this is the activation of the attachment system; this is a sensory experience which could be triggered by thoughts, feelings or other/environment. This is followed by attachment behaviour and how we creatively adjust to internal sensations in relation to other/environment. For example, a child in school may need to go to the toilet, an internal sensation, but the child's external experience may be that others will shame them so they may adapt to the situation by becoming disruptive in order to leave the classroom. When this process is healthy, contact and

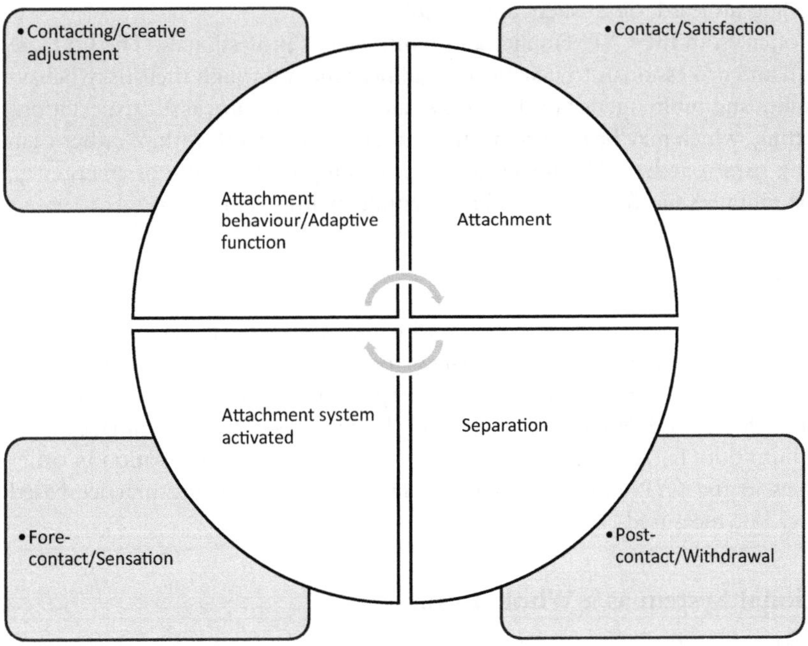

Figure 88.1 The four stages of contact in gestalt therapy integrated with the process of attachment and separation in attachment theory. (Source: Cathie O'Brien © 2011.)

withdrawal/attachment and separation are achieved spontaneously and with little effort, but when people have suffered interpersonal trauma they can get stuck at different stages along the cycle.

The Child That Enters into the System

An example of a child that may enter into such a system is 14-year-old Sarah, who has injured another member of staff in the residential setting, and this behaviour has become increasingly unpredictable. She self-harms, uses drugs and alcohol, has unsafe sex and absconds for long periods of time with no one knowing where she is or who she is with. Her presentation is chaotic, and she finds both closeness and distance in relation to professionals and family difficult to manage. She has a complex understanding of her family, and she has an innate need to return home while simultaneously wanting to withdraw. She has also gained, over time, a variety of working diagnoses from ADHD and autism to attachment disorder and is starting to develop a criminal record.

The System

The systems are dealing with many forces and constraints. The constraints are often outside of the system such as Ofsted, CQC, commissioners and government initiatives and are outcome-driven. These constraints lead many organisations into left-brain levels of communication, using paperwork trails and statistics only to measure outcomes or analyse a situation. This can often leave staff feeling unheard, dissatisfied, and fearful.

The forces are often from the CYP, families and multi-agency professionals. The CYP are literally forcing staff and professionals to take notice and hear them through their risky behaviours, and the families and multi-agency professionals can try to place unrealistic expectations on a residential setting, which may be counter to the legislation they work within, rather than holding and sharing risks together. The forces are often coming from a sense of emergency, defence, protection, impulse and frightened and frightening environments.

Organisational Symptoms

These organisations are often in a parallel process with the wider system, families and the young people and often express feelings of helplessness, powerlessness, anxiety, anger, taking control or no control, overwhelming amounts of time spent on political and organisational dynamics and feeling blamed and deskilled, all potentially leading to secondary trauma, exhaustion, sickness and burn out. These symptoms need to be reduced in the organisation in order to reduce symptoms in the CYP and wider systems, and through collecting practice-based evidence progress can be measured.

The Organisational System as a Whole Brain

The wave analogy shown in Figure 88.2 (Chidiac, 2018) can be a useful assessment tool to help organisations gain insight into their organisational relational style. I added in the forces and constraints so organisations can gain a clear sense of what may drive their culture, and attachment styles so they can see their organisation from a whole brain perspective, gain a sense of their relational style, what style the workforce may favour and how they may influence the CYP's relational style. For instance, an over-emphasis on ego function involving processes and systems with no time for interactions between colleagues could lead to isolation and high

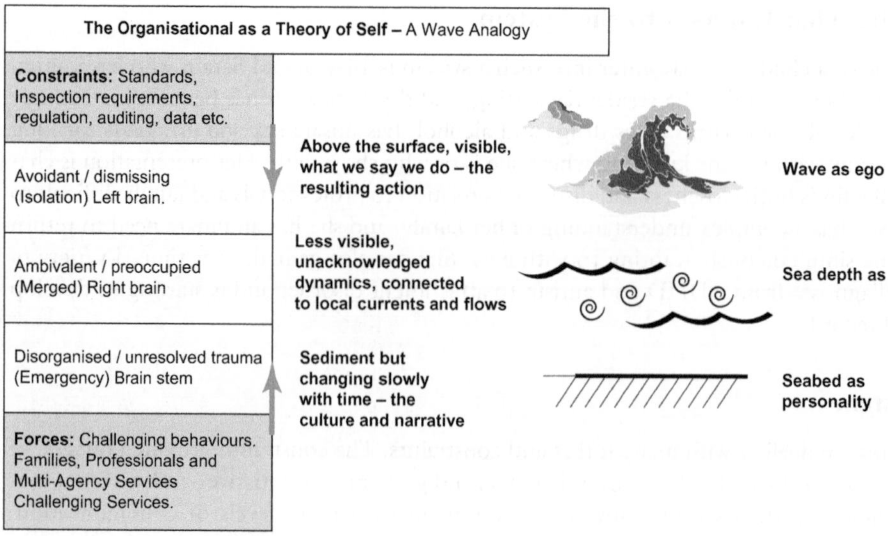

Figure 88.2 The organisational system as a whole brain.

avoidance; this in turn could lead to ambivalence in relationships, the id function, with emphasis on seeking relationships for reassurance, gossip and splitting off, a more destructive relational style, and this in turn can also be the cause of the aforementioned avoidance. Altogether, they can create a trauma environment and a culture of emergency, often seen in disorganised patterns of attachment.

Creating a Safe Emergency: A Bottom Approach

The child that enters into this system is already in a state of emergency due to interpersonal trauma as well as the trauma of being removed from their home and the area they live in or after experiencing many placement breakdowns; therefore the organisation needs to create the safe conditions for CYP to be able to manage their sense of emergency which is often triggered through relationships. This involves the organisation feeling safe first and foremost, not just for the CYP but also for the professionals in it.

A bottom-up approach attends to the emergency, the brain stem/nervous system of the organisation, which in residential environments can become the overall culture of the organisation. This mirrors the order of brain development in new-borns and is essential in trauma work involving a real understanding of emotion-regulation.

This is achieved firstly through training, followed by reflective practice. The focussed and direct work in training can act as a safe container, creating the conditions for teams to develop relationships with themselves and each other and is the starting point for developing tolerance for reflective practice which has more emphasis on how individuals feel in relation to young people, each other and the whole system, drawing upon the training elements to consolidate learning. (See Figure 88.3.)

Training

The training involves fun, non-threatening, experiential learning in attachment and trauma and the recognition that the relationship is the main cause for alarm. The aim is to help staff become aware of their own sensations and how they adapt in relation to others and the situation. This awareness can help them to understand the CYP they work with as well as developing disciplined awareness and ethical presence when working relationally with interpersonal trauma.

Sensation

An example of this would be to ask staff to work in pairs with one of them blindfolded while the other talks them through different sensory objects. This is graded, with importance placed on noticing 'how' they feel before starting the exercise rather than on the outcome of the exercise. If staff notice they don't want to be blindfolded, then this is key over and above anything else, and I help staff understand why this awareness would be empowering to young people who struggle to manage their sensory motor system. Sensory work with CYP, done in a fun, non-threatening environment, is a precursor to naming emotion. Teams also notice how the sensory objects can trigger happy or sad memories, and this helps them to further understand trauma and how behaviours can be triggered by the senses, which can activate the nervous/attachment system and that CYP may have no control or understanding over their resulting behaviour.

The Adaptive Function

Another exercise is to ask staff to stand opposite each other in pairs and then walk towards each other, noticing when they feel the need to stop, and then to experiment with closeness and

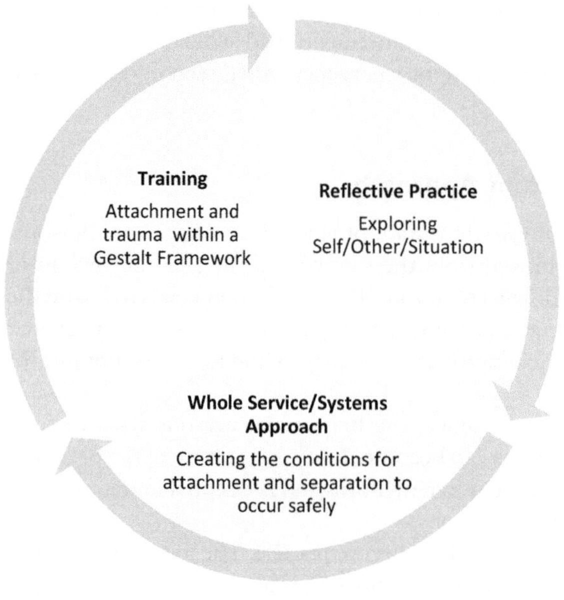

Figure 88.3 A whole service/systems approach to emotion-regulation – a model of work.

distance between each other. When do they feel most comfortable: face to face, side to side or back to back? What are the sensations and resulting actions?

Through this exercise staff become very aware of the different ways they adapt, and this helps them to understand children's behaviours and the adaptive function, as many staff will adapt to the situation by laughing, high energy, excessive noise and they could be considered as 'naughty children' who won't sit still or do as they are told. This helps them to become aware of how risky it feels for children in a learning or group environment and why they may adapt in the way they do.

The Contact Boundary

These exercises set the scene and underpin the theory around working with interpersonal trauma, teaching staff through experience, the process of contact and withdrawal/attachment and separation, and that it is the adaptive function, called the contact boundary in gestalt, the relationship 'between', that has suffered and never truly developed in vulnerable CYP.

In order to help teams work at the contact boundary, the relationship between, I ask them to pretend they have a hula hoop around their waist. The hula hoop analogy acts as a contact boundary and helps staff to remain aware of working 'between' self and other, noticing the others' tolerance for relationships – developing disciplined awareness rather than becoming merged or rejecting. This process gently stimulates and simultaneously contains the adaptive function/attachment behaviour system, allowing CYP to remain aware and develop psychologically while being in a relationship.

Teamwork

Lastly I talk about teamwork. For instance, when a professional's needs are placed over the good of the whole and the child in their care, for example an individual needing to be liked, this can create splits within the organisation and therefore the child's psychological state. When the team work as one, which I call 'the we', this can calm the child, the whole organisation and the systems around the child.

For instance, 'We have agreed that this maybe the best way forward', or 'we have taken what you have said very seriously and we will discuss this as a team at the next hand over', rather than 'I don't know go and ask…', or 'so and so made the decision and I don't agree with it'. Staff have been badly hurt under the latter when left on their own to make a difficult decision. This way of working can involve parents, carers and multi-agency professionals jointly making difficult decisions and holding risks, and I explain how they have become a healthy other in relation to the child rather than a fragmented other.

The Voice of the Child

It is really important to note that the voice of the child is paramount. 'The we' should not be used as an oppressive controlling behaviour strategy. Its intention is to decrease anxiety in organisations and systems so staff do not feel isolated and as a result become frightened or frightening. When teams develop a compassionate and reflective culture and as a result work well together, this way of working can be freeing for both staff and CYP, allowing both to regulate in a healthy manner (O'Brien, 2011/2017).

Reflective Practice

The training underpins reflective practice, and the cycle of contact and withdrawal (Figure 88.1) is drawn upon when considering the young people and the organisation, as well as the families and multi-agency systems. In gestalt this is a constant process of self, other, situation (Denham-Vaughan and Chidiac, 2013). For those interested in further theoretical understanding, the layers of skill that sit behind these processes are phenomenology, dialogue and field theory as shown in Figure 88.4.

Reflective practice can offer and role model the safe conditions needed to explore emergencies and feelings in relation to working with extremely distressed CYP and a place to reflect on practice. In the early stages it is important that teams are helped to learn how to communicate with each other from a place of self-responsibility and ownership of feelings, sensitivity towards the other and taking account of the whole situation. Reflective practice needs to become a safe space where staff can explore different perceptions of the same situation and the many different ways in which individuals manage this, as well as becoming aware of their differences in terms of experience, age, gender and culture and how the young people may treat them all differently.

Self	**Phenomenology:** Tracking thoughts, feelings, and sensations in the here and now.
Other	**Dialogical:** An interpersonal approach working between self and other.
Situation	**Field Theory:** Isolated elements are considered as part of the whole situation and consideration is given to how they impact each other.

Figure 88.4 Phenomenology, dialogue and field theory.

Teamwork is also important to explore, especially unhealthy competition where staff who are struggling with a young person are told 'they are alright with me!' This can leave the young person and both staff members vulnerable, and it is useful to explore these dynamics from a self/other/situation perspective. Once teams feel safe, then courageous conversations can be encouraged and difference/different opinions can be better tolerated, developing connection through difference and as a result safety. Reflective practice helps teams to feel the process of contact and withdrawal, in the here and now, putting theory into practice, developing skills and good teamwork. This felt sense and way of working are then naturally disseminated through the organisation down to the young people.

This is not the same as supervision, which is usually delivered from professional to professional within the same field, with emphasis on strategies and outcomes. This approach gives teams more flexibility and fluidity to assess individual situations, using the skills developed around teamwork, and working at the contact boundary. This flexibility as a team is key with vulnerable young people who regularly change the goal posts when a fixed strategy is put in place, leaving both staff and children vulnerable.

Contact: Bringing the Whole Together

This process is the integration of the whole individual and organisation, and as teams experience this then it becomes part of them; similar to a sports team who want to achieve a particular technical set piece, they will spend hours practicing parts of the technique, stretching their minds and body, adapting to each other's strengths and weaknesses, until it suddenly comes together – they make contact. It is effortless when it occurs and is integrated at an explicit and implicit level and therefore has long-lasting results. As a result this natural integration of the whole brain organisation can lead to a natural integration of the whole child.

Outcomes

A relational approach should show a decrease in the organisational symptoms described previously which should decrease the young people's symptoms shown through behaviours. Please see Figure 88.5.

Staff

Reduction in:

- Anxiety amongst the team which decreases anxiety in the young people.
- Time spent on organizational and political dynamics.
- Sickness.

Increase in:

- Job satisfaction.
- Staff development and increased team work.
- A team that feels grounded and valued.
- A relational approach.
- A greater respect for difference.

Children and young people

Reduction in:

- Staff being physically hurt.
- The young people gaining a criminal record.
- Incidents.
- Safeguarding – i.e. cause for concern.
- Self-harm.
- Absconding.

Increase in:

- A more grounded young person.
- An increased ability to contain and regulate emotion.
- Development of mutual trust in relationships.
- Ability to engage in other activities.

Figure 88.5 Benefits of the relational approach.

Conclusion

This chapter is a brief overview of this complex work and shows a model of work that can assess the health of the organisation from an attachment and trauma perspective and its impact on both staff and the developing brains of the young people in their care. It shows the importance of attending to the environment, developing a safe emergency and how the whole service and systems around CYP can work therapeutically with interpersonal trauma. There is particular emphasis on a relational approach and creating the conditions for safe contact and withdrawal/attachment and separation, with the potential to reduce risk and help towards the integration of the whole brain child. Therapy alone, in my opinion, will not bring about change when the environment is in a state of emergency.

Multiple-Choice Questions

See answers on page 674.

1. What is the focus of gestalt therapy?
   a. The past
   b. The here and now
   c. The future
2. What is the adaptive function?
   a. Attachment
   b. Attachment system
   c. Attachment behaviour
3. How could you assess the relational health of the organisation?
   a. Using the wave analogy
   b. Using the process of contact and withdrawal
   c. Using the process of self/other/situation
4. What tool could you use to help professionals in residential environments work at the contact boundary?
   a. Sensory work
   b. The hula hoop analogy
   c. The we analogy
5. Why is it important to create safe conditions for CYP to practice contact and withdrawal?
   a. So they can talk about the process of contact and withdrawal.
   b. To contain them.
   c. To enable CYP to develop psychologically and reduce risks.

Key References

Chidiac, M.A., (2018). *Relational Organisational Gestalt—An Emergent Approach to Organisational Development.* London: Routledge.

Denham-Vaughan, S., Chidiac, M.A., (2013). SOS: A relational orientation towards social inclusion. *Mental Health and Social Inclusion*, 17(2): 100–107.

O'Brien, C., (2011). Disorganised and in care. British Association of Counselling and Psychotherapy. *Children Young People and Families Journal.*

O'Brien, C., (2017). Self, other and the we. British Association of Counselling and Psychotherapy. *Children Young People and Families Journal.*

89 Social Care Provision for Children and Families in CAMHS

The Importance of the Role of a Social Worker within CAMHS Teams … without Becoming a Therapist

Gabrielle Loades

KEY CONCEPTS

- Socio-economic environment, poverty, neglect and abuse have adverse effects on people's mental health and overall functioning.
- Such factors affect a child's global, i.e. cognitive and behavioural, development in addition to their wellbeing.
- Social workers aim to intervene in those situations by protecting vulnerable adults or children from abuse and by empowering and supporting individuals and families in making safe and informed decisions.

A brief history of social work within our society helps us to understand how the profession came about. We began to recognise our innate responsibility to support others in need during the Elizabethan era. The Poor Law Act (1601) ensured that poor people received reasonably good support through their parishes (Payne, 2005). The changes made to the Poor Law Act in 1834 were sadly less favourable. It was then that the state started to differentiate between the 'deserving' and the 'undeserving' poor, i.e. those that were disabled and those that were 'just' unemployed.

It was then that the workhouses were created, intended as deterrents to unemployment. In 1869, the Charity Organisation Society (COS) and in 1884, The Settlement Movement (TSM) were established. It could be argued that these organisations paved the way for social work as we know it today. The COS developed casework and laid the foundation for making judgements that were 'based on detailed assessments of the applicant's circumstances, requiring home visits'. The TSM's aim was to 'establish settlements in deprived parts of cities' where people that were better-off could educate those that were poor, uneducated and in need of help (Wilson et al., 2011). The first social work training began in the mid-1950s, and in 1999, it was recommended by the Department of Health, Social Services and Public Safety that social work education was to be extended to degree level to ensure that all potential social workers receive comprehensive training that would enable them to support individuals and communities. The 'social work' title has itself been protected since 1 April 2005, and all practising social workers are required to be registered with a regulatory body.

The British Association of Social Workers (BASW) is the professional association for social workers in the United Kingdom. Social workers can register with BASW for a monthly fee. BASW offers services that protect, support and develop social work careers. They initiated the Code of Ethics for Social Workers that states the values and ethical principles on which the profession is based. These are: human rights, social justice and professional integrity. There are a further 17 Ethical Practice Principles (Figure 89.1).

What Do Social Workers Actually Do and Why Is Their Role So Important in CAMHS?

In simple terms, social workers are committed to social justice, protection, safeguarding, empowerment and welfare of people in need. To achieve this, social workers need to have a variety of skills.

- Transferrable skills
- Assessment skills
- Safeguarding

Promote Partnership Working

Partnership is one of those words that is used over and over without professionals, at times, really paying attention to its true value. Serious case reviews very often point to the lack of it. Why do professionals struggle with it? What initiatives are there to support partnership working?

Section 11 of the Children Act 2004 places duties on a range of organisations, including the NHS, other agencies and individuals, to ensure that their functions, and any services that they contract out to others, are discharged with regard to the need to 'safeguard and promote

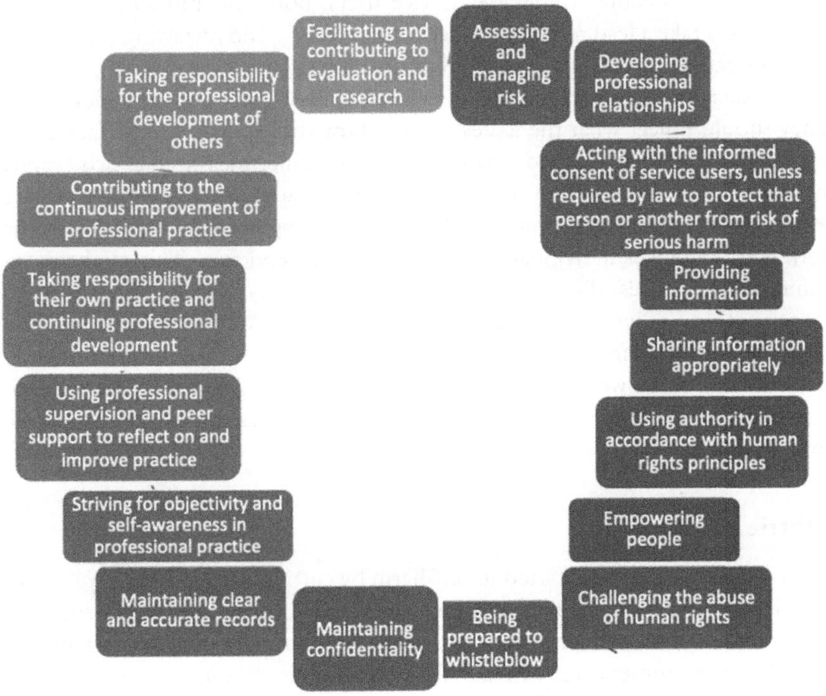

Figure 89.1 Ethical Practice Principles.

the welfare of children' (*Working Together to Safeguard Children*, 2018). This means that children's services, police and the NHS must work together and must have comprehensive safeguarding policies in place. Whilst nowadays we have many integrated teams thanks to the Health Act 1999, meaning that health and social care professionals work, e.g. from the same base, use the same processes and access the same training and pool budgets, it does not always mean that these teams work more effectively.

A review of multiple studies around joint working (Cameron et al., 2015) shows that sometimes bringing in professionals from differing disciplines can hinder joint working. One of the studies cited showed that 'social work values and, in particular, the social models, were not respected by health professionals and this led to a lack of appreciation of their contribution within multi-professional teams'. This happens perhaps because of the use of non-medical models in social work practice and misconceptions that mental health disorders can be socially driven. Social workers in mental health teams often struggle to maintain their identity for this reason. Often, the role of the social worker is overtaken by the role of a therapist, and eventually the value of the social work role within CAMHS is lost. Being aware of this possibility is vital in being able to maintain own's identity in addition to effectively safeguarding children. Assimilation is not an effective mode of partnership.

Care Planning and Care Management

These terms are used within all types of social work, be it social work with children and families, disabled adults or elderly people. Originally, care management came about in 1991 (DOH) as the response to providing more individualised care to adult service users. It is now applied within children and family services. Social workers bring a wealth of **transferrable skills** to mental health teams. Care planning and management is one of them. The social worker's role is about empowering and protecting vulnerable service users, both children and adults. To achieve this, social workers take a lead role in organising, monitoring and reviewing services for adults and children. Effective care planning leads to positive outcomes for children.

Care plans need to be reviewed on a regular basis with the involvement of the children and their families. They should reflect what the issues are and how those issues will be tackled to ensure that a positive outcome is achieved. Plans must be specific, measurable, achievable, realistic and time bound (SMART), so that they can be managed appropriately. Care plans are fluid, in that they can be changed at any time to reflect the changing needs of individuals. The aim of social work is to empower individuals and to foster independence. This might mean that at the beginning of the process direct support would be necessary, but the aim is that, by the end of the intervention, individuals/children will be able to tackle issues independently through learned management techniques.

Now that we know what social work is and what the profession brings into supporting people in need, we can consider the value of social workers in CAMHS teams. This case study will demonstrate some of its value.

Case Study: Nittie

Nittie (16) is originally from India. She started to self-harm by cutting herself about a year ago. The referral to CAMHS came from the family GP, who described the family as very supportive of their daughter. Nittie attended a routine assessment appointment at CAMHS with her father, Mr Sharma. The appointment was with a male social worker, Adam.

At the beginning of the assessment Adam told both Nittie and her father that he would need to see Nittie alone as part of the assessment. Her father was not happy about that and said that in their culture, it would not be appropriate for Nittie to be alone with another male. All the family wanted was for CAMHS to sort out their daughter's self-harming behaviour. Adam agreed to continue with the assessment nevertheless, as he was aware that Nittie had been waiting for assessment for over four months. Throughout the assessment, Adam noticed that it was Mr Sharma who answered all the questions, despite the fact that Nittie was 16 years old.

He showed little warmth towards Nittie and was very critical of her self-harming behaviour, calling her an 'attention seeker' and saying that she was bringing shame on their family. Nittie showed little eye contact and seemed very uncomfortable. She shared very little with Adam and would respond only to closed questions.

Q. Are there serious enough concerns in respect of Nittie to make a referral to children's services?

A. Not yet at this stage. Adam will need to carry out further investigation that would involve contacting other agencies, e.g. Nittie's school. He will need to be creative in finding out further information about Nittie to be able to make an informed decision.

Q. How could Adam find more information directly from Nittie whilst at the same time respecting her culture?

A. Adam could try to involve his female colleagues in asking Nittie questions in private, without her father being present. Sometimes, children do not want to disclose information in front of their parents because of perceived shame or because they might be scared of the consequences. Whilst we must respect other cultures, we have a duty to safeguard children. Children's rights and needs are always paramount.

Q. What should Adam be guided by when working with children and families?

A. Adam should always strive to keep in mind BASW Codes of Ethics. Social workers do not have to actually subscribe to BASW Codes of Ethics, but they should abide and practice within them at all times.

Key References

Cameron, A., Lart, R., Bostock, L., Coomber, C., (2015). Factors that promote and hinder joint and integrated working between health and social care services. Online: Social care institute for excellence.

Cree, V., Mayers, S., (2008). *Social Work, Making a Difference.* Bristol: Policy Press.

Payne, M., (2005). *The origins of Social Work, Continuity and Change.* Basingstoke: Palgrave Macmillan.

Wilson, K., Ruch, G., Lymbery, M., Cooper, A., (2011), *Social Work, An Introduction to Contemporary Practice.* London: Pearsons Education Limited.

References

Abdulkadir, M., Londono, D., Gordon, D., Fernandez, T. V., Brown, L. W., Cheon, K. A., ... Dietrich, A. (2018). Investigation of previously implicated genetic variants in chronic tic disorders: a transmission disequilibrium test approach. *European Archives of Psychiatry and Clinical Neuroscience*, 268(3), 301–316. doi: 10.1007/s00406-017-0808-8

Abrahamson, A. C., Baker, L. A., & Caspi, A. (2002). Rebellious teens? Genetic and environmental influences on the social attitudes of adolescents. *Journal of Personality and Social Psychology*, 83(6), 1392.

Achenbach, T. M. (1991). *Integrative Guide to the 1991 CBCL/4-18, YSR, and TRF Profiles*. Burlington, USA: University of Vermont, Department of Psychology.

Achenbach, T. M. (2001). Achenbach system of empirically based assessment: school age forms and profiles, child behavior checklist for ages. *Aseba*, 6–18.

Aepli, A., Kurth, S., Tesler, N., Jenni, O. G., & Huber, R. (2015). Caffeine consuming children and adolescents show altered sleep behavior and deep sleep. *Brain Sciences*, 5(4), 441–455.

Ainsworth, M. D. S. (1967). *Infancy in Uganda: Infant Care and the Growth of Love*. Baltimore: Johns Hopkins University Press.

Ainsworth, M. D. S., Blehar, M. C., Waters, E., & Wall, S. (1978). *Patterns of Attachment: A Psychological Study of the Strange Situation*. Hillsdale, NJ: Erlbaum.

Al-Adawi, S., Bax, B., Bryant-Waugh, R., Claudino, A. M., Hay, P., Monteleone, P., ... Uher, R. (2013). Revision of ICD–status update on feeding and eating disorders. *Advances in Eating Disorders*, 1(1), 10–20.

Alam, N., Wojtyniak, B., & Rahaman, M. M. (1989). Anthropometric indicators and risk of death. *The American Journal of Clinical Nutrition*, 49(5), 884–888.

Al-Diwani, A. A., Pollak, T. A., Irani, S. R., & Lennox, B. R. (2017). Psychosis: an autoimmune disease? *Immunology*, 152(3), 388–401.

Alexander-Bloch, A. F., Vértes, P. E., Stidd, R., Lalonde, F., Clasen, L., Rapoport, J., ... Gogtay, N. (2013). The anatomical distance of functional connections predicts brain network topology in health and schizophrenia. *Cerebral cortex*, 23(1), 127–138.

Alison, Chown (2014). *Play Therapy in the Outdoors: Taking Play Therapy out of the Playroom and into Natural Environment*. JKP.

Allen, L. R., Watson, L. B., Egan, A. M., & Moser, C. N. (2019). Well-being and suicidality among transgender youth after gender-affirming hormones. *Clinical Practice in Pediatric Psychology*, 7(3), 302–311.

American Psychiatric Association (2013). *Diagnostic and Statistical Manual of Mental Disorders (DSM-5®)*. American Psychiatric Pub.

Angst, J. (2013). Bipolar disorders in DSM-5: strengths, problems and perspectives. *International Journal of Bipolar Disorders*, 1, 12. https://doi.org/10.1186/2194-7511-1-12

APA (2013). *Diagnostic and Statistical Manual of Mental Disorders* (5th edition). Washington, DC: American Psychiatric Association.

Appleby, L., Cooper, J., Amos, T., & Faragher, B. (1999). Psychological autopsy study of suicides by people aged under 35. *British Journal of Psychiatry*, 175, 168–174.

Arcelus, J., Bouman, W. P., Van Den Noortgate, W., Claes, L., Witcomb, G., & Fernandez-Aranda, F. (2015). Systematic review and meta-analysis of prevalence studies in transsexualism. *European Psychiatry*, 30(6), 807–815.

Arcelus, J., Haslam, M., Farrow, C., & Meyer, C. (2013). The role of interpersonal functioning in the maintenance of eating psychopathology: a systematic review and testable model. *Clinical Psychology Review*, 33(1), 156–167.

Arthur, G. K., & Monnell, K. (2005). *Body Dysmorphic Disorder*. Emedicine–com. com–2004.

Astill, R. G., Van der Heijden, K. B., Van Ijzendoorn, M. H., & Van Someren, E. J. (2012). Sleep, cognition, and behavioral problems in school-age children: a century of research meta-analyzed. *Psychological Bulletin*, 138(6), 1109–1138.

Axline, V. (1989). *Play Therapy*. London: Churchill Livingstone.

Baker, M., & Bishop, F. L. (2015). Out of school: a phenomenological exploration of extended non-attendance. *Educational Psychology in Practice*, 31(4), 354–368.

Balázs, J., Miklósi, M., Keresztény, A., Hoven, C. W., Carli, V., Wasserman, C., Apter, A., Bobes, J., Brunner, R., Cosman, D., Cotter, P., Haring, C., Iosue, M., Kaess, M., Kahn, J. P., Keeley, H., Marusic, D., Postuvan, V., Resch, F., Saiz, P. A., Sisask, M., Snir, A., Tubiana, A., Varnik, A., Sarchiapone, M., & Wasserman, D. (2013). Adolescent subthreshold-depression and anxiety: psychopathology, functional impairment and increased suicide risk. *Journal of Child Psychology and Psychiatry*, 54(6), 670–677. doi: 10.1111/jcpp.12016. Epub 2013 Jan 18. Erratum in: *J Child Psychol Psychiatry*. 2017 Sep;58(9), E1. PMID: 23330982.

Baldwin, J. R., Reuben, A., Newbury, J. B., & Danese, A. (2019). Agreement between prospective and retrospective measures of childhood maltreatment: a systematic review and meta-analysis. *JAMA Psychiatry*, 76(6), 584–593. doi: 10.1001/jamapsychiatry.2019.0097. PMID: 30892562; PMCID: PMC6551848.

Bandelow, B., & Michaelis, S. (2015). Epidemiology of anxiety disorders in the 21st century. *Dialogues Clinical Neuroscience*, 17(3), 327–335. doi: 10.31887/DCNS.2015.17.3/bbandelow. PMID: 26487813; PMCID: PMC4610617.

Bandura, A. (1997). Self-efficacy and health behaviour. In A. Baum, S. Newman, J. Wienman, R. West, & C. McManus (Eds.), *Cambridge Handbook of Psychology, Health and Medicine* (pp. 160–162). Cambridge: Cambridge University Press.

Barbano, A. C., van der Mei, W. F., Bryant, R. A., et al. (2019). Clinical implications of the proposed ICD-11 PTSD diagnostic criteria. *Psychological Medicine*, 49(3), 483–490. https://doi.org/10.1017/S0033291718001101.

Baroni, A., Lunsford, J. R., Luckenbaugh, D. A., Towbin, K. E., & Leibenluft, E. (2009). Practitioner review: the assessment of bipolar disorder in children and adolescents. *Journal of Child Psychology and Psychiatry*, 50(3), 203–215. doi: 10.1111/j.1469-7610.2008.01953.x

Barkley, R. A. (2002). Major life activity and health outcomes associated with attention-deficit/hyperactivity disorder. *The Journal of Clinical Psychiatry*.

Barkley, R. A. (2013). *Defiant Children: A Clinician's Manual for Assessment and Parent Training*. Guilford Press.

Barkley, R. A., DuPaul, G. J., & McMurray, M. B. (1990). Comprehensive evaluation of attention deficit disorder with and without hyperactivity as defined by research criteria. *Journal of Consulting and Clinical Psychology*, 58(6), 775–789.

Barkley, R. A., Murphy, K. R., Dupaul, G. J., & Bush, T. (2002). Driving in young adults with attention deficit hyperactivity disorder: knowledge, performance, adverse outcomes, and the role of executive functioning; Driving and ADHD; RA Barkley et al. *Journal of the International Neuropsychological Society: JINS*, 8(5), 655.

Barkley, R. A., Murphy, K., & Kwasnik, D. (1996). Psychological adjustment and adaptive impairments in young adults with ADHD. *Journal of Attention Disorders*, 1(1), 41–54.

Baron-Cohen, S. (1999). The evolution of a theory of mind. In Corballis M. C., & Lea S. E. G. (Eds.), *The Descent of Mind: Psychological Perspectives on Hominid Evolution* (pp. 261–277). Oxford University Press.

Bass, N., & Skuse, D. (2018). Genetic testing in children and adolescents with intellectual disability. *Current Opinion in Psychiatry*, 31(6), 490–495.

Bateson, G. (1962). A note on the double bind. In C. Sluzki, & D. Ransom (Eds.), *Double Bind: The Foundation of the Communicational Approach to the Family* (pp. 39–42). New York: Grune & Stratton.

Battaglia, M., Garon-Carrier, G., Côté S. M., Dionne, G., Touchette, E., Vitaro, F., Tremblay, R. E., & Boivin, M. (2017). Early childhood trajectories of separation anxiety: bearing on mental health, academic achievement, and physical health from mid-childhood to preadolescence. *Depress Anxiety*, 34(10), 918–927. doi: 10.1002/da.22674. Epub 2017 Aug 18. PMID: 28833904.

Baune, B. T., & Malhi, G. S. (2015). A review on the impact of cognitive dysfunction on social, occupational, and general functional outcomes in bipolar disorder. *Bipolar Disorders*, 17(Suppl 2), 41–55. doi: 10.1111/bdi.12341. PMID: 26688289.

Baxter, A. J., Brugha, T. S., Erskine, H. E., Scheurer, R. W., Vos, T., & Scott, J. G. (2015). The epidemiology and global burden of autism spectrum disorders. *Psychological Medicine*, 45(3), 601–613. https://doi.org/10.1017/S003329171400172X.

Becerra-Culqui, T. A., Liu, Y., Nash, R., et al. (2018). Mental health of transgender and gender nonconforming youth compared With their peers. *Pediatrics*, 141(5), e20173845.

Ben-Shlomo, Y., Scharf, J. M., Miller, L. L., & Mathews, C. A. (2016). Parental mood during pregnancy and post-natally is associated with offspring risk of Tourette syndrome or chronic tics: prospective data from the Avon Longitudinal Study of Parents and Children (ALSPAC). *European Child and Adolescent Psychiatry*, 25(4), 373–381. doi: 10.1007/s00787-015-0742-0

Berens, A. E., Jensen, S. K. G., & Nelson, C. A. 3rd. (2017). Biological embedding of childhood adversity: from physiological mechanisms to clinical implications. *BMC Medicine*, 15(1), 135. doi: 10.1186/s12916-017-0895-4. PMID: 28724431; PMCID: PMC5518144.

Berg, Lewis M. (1996). School avoidance, school phobia, and truancy. In M. Lewis (Ed.), *Child and Adolescent Psychiatry: A Comprehensive Textbook* (pp. 1104–1110). Sydney: Williams & Wilkins.

Biby, E. L. (1998). The relationship between body dysmorphic disorder and depression, self-esteem, somatization, and obsessive–compulsive disorder. *Journal of Clinical Psychology*, 54(4), 489–499.

Bierman, K. L., Nix, R. L., Heinrichs, B. S., et al. (2014). Effects of Head Start REDI on children's outcomes 1 year later in different kindergarten contexts. *Child Development*, 85(1), 140–159. doi: 10.1111/cdev.12117

Bisson, J. I., Roberts, N. P., Andrew, M., Cooper, R., & Lewis, C. (2013). Psychological therapies for chronic post-traumatic stress disorder (PTSD) in adults. *Cochrane Database of Systematic Reviews*, 12(12). Https://doi.org/10.1002/14651858.CD003388.pub4.

Black, K. J., Black, E. R., Greene, D. J., & Schlaggar, B. L. (2016). Provisional tic disorder: what to tell parents when their child first starts ticcing. *F1000Res*, 5, 696. doi: 10.12688/f1000research.8428.1

Blacker, C. P. (1946). PEP Web - Neurosis and the Mental Health Services. (Oxford University Press, 1946. Pp. 218. Price, 21s.) Pep-web.org. http://www.pep-web.org/document.php?id=ijp.027.0065d

Blair, R. J., Finger, E., & Marsh, A. (2009). The development and neural bases of psychopathy. In De Haan M., & Gunnar, M.R (Eds.), *Handbook of Developmental Social Neuroscience* (pp. 419–434). Guildford Press.

Bliss, J. (1980). Sensory experiences of Gilles de la Tourette syndrome. *Archives of General Psychiatry*, 37(12), 1343–1347.

Boivin, L., Notredame, C.-E., Jardri, R., & Medjkane, F. (2020). Supporting parents of transgender adolescents: yes, but how? *Archives of Sexual Behavior*, 49(1), 1–3.

Bos, K., Zeanah, C. H., Fox, N. A., Drury, S. S., McLaughlin, K. A., & Nelson, C. A. (2011). Psychiatric outcomes in young children with a history of institutionalization. *Harvard Review of Psychiatry*, 19(1), 15–24. https://doi.org/10.3109/10673229.2011.549773.

Bor, W., Sanders, M. R., & Markie-Dadds, C. (2002). The effects of the Triple P-Positive Parenting Program on preschool children with co-occurring disruptive behaviour and attentional/hyperactive difficulties. *Journal of Abnormal Child Psychology*, 30, 571–587.

Bould, H., De Stavola, B., Lewis, G., & Micali, N. (2018). Do disordered eating behaviours in girls vary by school characteristics? A UK cohort study. *European Child & Adolescent Psychiatry*, 27(11), 1473–1481.

Bowlby, J. (1973). *Attachment and Loss Volumes 2 and 3.* New York: Basic Books.
Bowman, M. L., & Yehuda, R. (2004). Risk factors and the adversity-stress model. In: G. M. Rosen (Ed.), *Posttraumatic Stress Disorder: Issues and Controversies*, 15–38. John Wiley & Sons Ltd.
Brabson, L. A., Brown, J. L., Capriotti, M. R., Ramanujam, K., Himle, M. B., Nicotra, C. M., ... Specht, M. W. (2016). Patterned changes in urge ratings with tic suppression in youth with chronic tic disorders. *Journal of Behavior Therapy and Experimental Psychiatry*, 50, 162–170. doi: 10.1016/j.jbtep.2015.07.004
Brand, S., Gerber, M., Beck, J., Hatzinger, M., Pühse, U., & Holsboer-Trachsler, E. (2010). Exercising, sleep-EEG patterns, and psychological functioning are related among adolescents. *World Journal of Biological Psychiatry*, 11(2), 129–140.
Brandt, V. C., Beck, C., Sajin, V., Baaske, M. K., Baumer, T., Beste, C., ... Munchau, A. (2016). Temporal relationship between premonitory urges and tics in Gilles de la Tourette syndrome. *Cortex*, 77, 24–37. doi: 10.1016/j.cortex.2016.01.008
Bratton, S. C., Ray, D., Rhine, T., & Jones, L. (2005). The efficacy of play therapy with children: a meta-analytic review of treatment outcomes. *Professional Psychology: Research and Practice*, 36(4), 376–390. https://doi.org/10.1037/0735-7028.36.4.376
Breeden, A. L., Cardinale, E. M., Lozier, L. M., VanMeter, J. W., & Marsh, A. A. (2015). Callous-unemotional traits drive reduced white-matter integrity in youths with conduct problems. *Psychological Medicine*, 45(14), 3033.
Brennan, P. A., Grekin, E. R., & Mednick, S. A. (2003). Prenatal and perinatal influences on conduct disorder and serious delinquency.
Bretherton, I. (1985). Attachment theory: retrospect and prospect. *Monographs of the Society for Research in Child Development*, 50(1 & 2), 3–35.
Brewin, C. R., Andrews, B., & Valentine, J. D. J. J. o. (2000). Meta-analysis of risk factors for posttraumatic stress disorder in trauma-exposed adults. *Journal of Consulting and Clinical Psychology*, 68(5), 748.
Brisch, K. H. (2002). *Treating Attachment Disorders: From Theory to Therapy.* New York, London: Guilford Press.
Brouwer-Borghuis, M. L., Heyne, D., Sauter, F. M., & Scholte, R. H. (2019). The link: an alternative educational program in the Netherlands to reengage school-refusing adolescents with schooling. *Cognitive and Behavioral Practice*, 26(1), 75–91.
Buse, J., Schoenefeld, K., Munchau, A., & Roessner, V. (2012). Neuromodulation in tourette syndrome: dopamine and beyond. *Neuroscience and Biobehavioral Reviews*, doi: S0149-7634(12)00171-6 [pii] 10.1016/j.neubiorev.2012.10.004
Burke, J. D., Loeber, R., Lahey, B. B., & Rathouz, P. J. (2005). Developmental transitions among affective and behavioral disorders in adolescent boys. *Journal of Child Psychology and Psychiatry*, 46(11), 1200–1210.
Butler, G., De Graaf, N., Wren, B., & Carmichael, P. (2018). Assessment and support of children and adolescents with gender dysphoria. *Archives of Disease in Childhood*, 103(7), 631–636.
Byng-Hall, J. (1995). *Rewriting Family Scripts: Improvisation and Systems Change.* New York: Guilford Publications.
Calhoun, S. L., Fernandez-Mendoza, J., Vgontzas, A. N., Liao, D., & Bixler, E. O. (2014). Prevalence of insomnia symptoms in a general population sample of young children and preadolescents: gender effects. *Sleep Medicine*, 15(1), 91–95.
Cameron, A., Lart, R., Bostock, L., & Coomber, C. (2015). Factors that promote and hinder joint and integrated working between health and social care services. *Health and Social Care in the Community*, 22(3), 225–233.
Cannon, Walter B., & Rosenberg, Charles E. (1932). *The Wisdom of the Body.* New York: W.W Norton & Company inc.
Capriotti, M. R., Brandt, B. C., Turkel, J. E., Lee, H. J., & Woods, D. W. (2014). Negative reinforcement and premonitory urges in youth with tourette syndrome: an experimental evaluation. *Behavior Modification*, 38(2), 276–296. doi: 10.1177/0145445514531015
Care Quality Commission. 2019. *Are We Listening? A Review of Children and Young People's Mental Health Services.* London: CQC.

Carter, B., Rees, P., Hale, L., Bhattacharjee, D., & Paradkar, M. S. (2016). Association Between portable screen-based media device access or use and sleep outcomes: a systematic review and meta-analysis. *JAMA Pediatrics*, 170(12), 1202–1208.

Carter, M. R., & Barrett, C. B. (2006). The economics of poverty traps and persistent poverty: an asset-based approach. *Journal of Development Studies*, 42(2), 178–199. doi: 10.1080/00220380500405261

Carter, A. S., Briggs-Gowan, M. J., & Davis, N. O. (2004). Assessment of young children's social-emotional development and psychopathology: recent advances and recommendations for practice. *Journal of Child Psychology and Psychiatry*, 45(1), 109–134.

Caspi, A., et al. (2016). Childhood forecasting of a small segment of the population with large economic burden. *Nature Human Behaviour*, 1. doi: 10.1038/s41562-016-0005

Cattanach, A. (2008a). *Narrative Approaches in Play Therapy with Children* 2nd Edition. London: Jessica Kingsley.

Cavill, S. (2000). Psychology in practice: welfare of refugees. *The Psychologist*, 13(11), 552–554.

Chao, T. K., Hu, J., & Pringsheim, T. (2014). Prenatal risk factors for Tourette Syndrome: a systematic review. *BMC Pregnancy and Childbirth*, 14(1), 53. doi: 10.1186/1471-2393-14-53

Charney, A. W., Stahl, E. A., Green, E. K., et al. (2019). Contribution of rare copy number variants to bipolar disorder risk is limited to schizoaffective cases. *Biological Psychiatry*. https://doi.org/10.1016/j.biopsych.2018.12.009.

Chen, W., & Taylor, E. (2006). Parental account of children's symptoms (PACS), ADHD phenotypes and its application to molecular genetic studies. *Attention-deficit/hyperactivity Disorder and the Hyperkinetic Syndrome: Current ideas and Ways Forward, 11788*, 3–20.

Cherry, K. (2019). http://psychology.about.com/od/psychosocialtheories/a/psychosocial_3.htm [updated 2019] (Accessed 16.0.2020).

Children and young people in mind: the final report of the National CAMHS review (2008). Doh.

Chiniara, L. N., Viner, C., Palmert, M., & Bonifacio, H. (2019).Perspectives on fertility preservation and parenthood among transgender youth and their parents. *Archives of Disease in Childhood*, 104(8), 739–744.

Chronaki, G. (2016). Event-related potentials and emotion processing in child psychopathology. *Frontiers in Psychology*, 7, Article 564. https://doi.org/10.3389/fpsyg.2016.00564

Chu, B. C., Rizvi, S. L., Zendegui, E. A., & Bonavitacola, L. (2015). Dialectical behavior therapy for school refusal: treatment development and incorporation of web-based coaching. *Cognitive and Behavioral Practice*, 22(3), 317–330.

Clark, T. C., Lucassen, M. F., Bullen, P., Denny, S. J., Fleming, T. M., Robinson, E. M., & Rossen, F. V. (2014). The health and well-being of transgender high school students: results from the New Zealand adolescent health survey (Youth'12). *Journal of Adolescent Health* , 55(1), 93–99.

Clarke, T. K., Weiss, A. R. D., & Berrettini, W. H. (2012). The genetics of anorexia nervosa. *Clinical Pharmacology & Therapeutics*, 91(2), 181–188.

Clegg, J., Hollis, C., & Rutter, M. (1999). Life Sentence – What Happens to Children with Developmental Language Disorders in Later Life? Royal College of Speech and Language Therapists Bulletin November

Cline,T., Gulliford, A., & Birch, S. (2015). *Educational Psychology*. Routledge.

Coghill, D. (2019). Debate: are stimulant medications for attention-deficit/hyperactivity disorder effective in the long term? (For). *Journal of the American Academy of Child and Adolescent Psychiatry*, 58(10), 938–939.

Cohen-Kettenis, P. T., & van Goozen, S. H. M. (1998). Pubertal delay as an aid in diagnosis and treatment of a transsexual adolescent. *European Child and Adolescent Psychiatry*, 7(4), 246–248.

Cole, J., Ball, H. A., Martin, N. C., Scourfield, J., & Mcguffin, P. (2009). Genetic overlap Between measures of hyperactivity/inattention and mood in children and adolescents. *Journal of the American Academy of Child and Adolescent Psychiatry*, 48(11), 1094–1101.

Cole, T. J., Flegal, K. M., Nicholls, D., & Jackson, A. A. (2007). Body mass index cut offs to define thinness in children and adolescents: international survey. *BMJ*, 335(7612), 194.

Coleman, E., Bockting, W., Botzer, M., et al. (2012). Standards of care for the health of transsexual, transgender, and gender-nonconforming people. *International Journal of Transgenderism*, 13(4), 165–232.

Collier, K. L., Van Beusekom, G., Bos, H. M., & Sandfort, T. G. (2013). Sexual orientation and gender identity/expression related peer victimization in adolescence: a systematic review of associated psychosocial and health outcomes. *Journal of Sex Research*, 50(3–4), 299–317. https://doi.org/10.1080/00224499.2012.750639.

Conelea, C. A., Woods, D. W., Zinner, S. H., Budman, C. L., Murphy, T. K., Scahill, L. D., … Walkup, J. T. (2013). The impact of Tourette Syndrome in adults: results from the Tourette Syndrome impact survey. *Community Mental Health Journal*, 49(1), 110–120. doi: 10.1007/s10597-011-9465-y

Cooper, et al. (2009, 2013, 2015). *Counselling & Psychotherapy Research*. https://www.tandfonline.com/toc/rcpr20/current

Cortese, S. (2019). The Association between ADHD and Obesity: intriguing, progressively more investigated, but still puzzling. *Brain Sciences*, 9(10), 256.

Cortese, S., Adamo, N., Del Giovane, C., Mohr-Jensen, C., Hayes, A. J., Carucci, S., … Hollis, C. (2018). Comparative efficacy and tolerability of medications for attention-deficit hyperactivity disorder in children, adolescents, and adults: a systematic review and network meta-analysis. *The Lancet Psychiatry*, 5(9), 727–738.

Cortese, S., Ferrin, M., Brandeis, D., Buitelaar, J., Daley, D., Dittmann, R. W., Holtmann, M., Santosh, P., Stevenson, J., Stringaris, A., Zuddas, A., Sonuga-Barke, E. J.; & European ADHD Guidelines Group (EAGG) (2015). Cognitive training for attention-deficit/hyperactivity disorder: meta-analysis of clinical and neuropsychological outcomes from randomized controlled trials. *Journal of the American Academy of Child and Adolescent Psychiatry*, 54(3), 164–174.

Cortese, S., Ferrin, M., Brandeis, D., Holtmann, M., Aggensteiner, P., Daley, D., Santosh, P., Simonoff, E., Stevenson, J., Stringaris, A., Sonuga-Barke, E. J.; & European ADHD Guidelines Group (EAGG) (2016). Neurofeedback for attention-deficit/hyperactivity disorder: meta-analysis of clinical and neuropsychological outcomes from randomized controlled trials. *Journal of the American Academy of Child and Adolescent Psychiatry*, 55(6), 444–455.

Cortese, S., Holtmann, M., Banaschewski, T., Buitelaar, J., Coghill, D., Danckaerts, M., Dittmann, R. W., Graham, J., Taylor, E., Sergeant, J.; & European ADHD Guidelines Group (2013). Practitioner review: current best practice in the management of adverse events during treatment with ADHD medications in children and adolescents. *Journal of Child Psychology and Psychiatry*, 54(3), 227–246.

Cortese, S., & Rohde, L. A. (2019). ADHD diagnoses: are 116 200 permutations enough? *The Lancet. Child & Adolescent Health*, 3(12), 844.

Cortese, S., Tomlinson, A., & Cipriani, A. (2019). Meta-review: network meta-analyses in child and adolescent psychiatry. *Journal of the American Academy of Child and Adolescent Psychiatry*, 58(2), 167–179.

Costello, E. J., Egger, H., & Angold, A. (2005). 10-year research update review: the epidemiology of child and adolescent psychiatric disorders: in methods and public health burden. *Journal of the American Academy of Child and Adolescent Psychiatry*, 44(10), 972–986. https://doi.org/10.1097/01.chi.0000172552.41596.6f.

CQC. (2016). *Not Seen, Not Heard*. https://www.cqc.org.uk/sites/default/files/20160707_not_seen_not_heard_report.pdf

Crawley, E. (2014). The epidemiology of chronic fatigue syndrome/myalgic encephalitis in children. *Archives of Disease in Childhood*, 99(2), 171–174.

Cree,V., & Mayers, S. (2008). *Social Work, Making a Difference*. Bristol : The Policy Press.

Cross-Disorder Group of the Psychiatric Genomics Consortium, C.-D. G. of the P. G. (2013). Identification of risk loci with shared effects on five major psychiatric disorders: a genome-wide analysis. *Lancet (London, England)*, 381(9875), 1371–1379. https://doi.org/10.1016/S0140-6736(12)62129-1.

Cummings, C. M., Caporino, N. E., & Kendall, P. C. (2014). Comorbidity of anxiety and depression in children and adolescents: 20 years after. *Psychological Bulletin*, 140(3), 816–845. doi: 10.1037/a0034733. Epub 2013 Nov 11. PMID: 24219155; PMCID: PMC4006306.

Curtis, D., Adlington, K., & Bhui, K. S. (2019). Pursuing parity: genetic tests for psychiatric conditions in the UK National Health Service. *The British Journal of Psychiatry* , 214(5), 248–250. https://doi.org/10.1192/bjp.2019.48.

Daley, D., van der Oord, S., Ferrin, M., Danckaerts, M., Doepfner, M., Cortese, S., Sonuga-Barke, E. J.; & European ADHD Guidelines Group. (2014). Behavioral interventions in attention-deficit/hyperactivity disorder: a meta-analysis of randomized controlled trials across multiple outcome domains. *Journal of the American Academy of Child and Adolescent Psychiatry*, 53(8), 835–847.

Davison, F., & Howlin, P. (1997). A follow-up study of children attending a primary age language unit. *European Journal of Disorders of Communication* , 32(1), 19–36.

Dawson, G., Webb, S. J., Carver, L., Panagiotides, H., & McPartland, J. (2004). Young children with autism show atypical brain responses to fearful versus neutral facial expressions of emotion. *Developmental Science*, 7(3), 340–359.

de Graaf, N. M., & Carmichael, P. (2019). Reflections on emerging trends in clinical work with gender diverse children and adolescents. *Clinical Child Psychology and Psychiatry*, 24(2), 353–364.

de Graaf, N. M., Manjra, I. I., Hames, A., & Zitz, C. (2019). Thinking about ethnicity and gender diversity in children and young people. *Clinical Child Psychology and Psychiatry*, 24(2), 291–303.

Demkow, U., & czyk, T. (2017). Genetic tests in major psychiatric disorders—Integrating molecular medicine with clinical psychiatry—Why is it so difficult? *Translational Psychiatry*, 7(6), e1151. https://doi.org/10.1038/tp.2017.106.

Demmler, J. C., Brophy, S. T., Marchant, A., John, A., & Tan, J. O. (2020). Shining the light on eating disorders, incidence, prognosis and profiling of patients in primary and secondary care: national data linkage study. *The British Journal of Psychiatry*, 216(2), 105–112.

Demontis, D., Walters, R. K., Martin, J., et al. (2019). Discovery of the first genome-wide significant risk loci for attention deficit/hyperactivity disorder. *Nature Genetics*, 51(1), 63–75. https://doi.org/10.1038/s41588-018-0269-7.

Denham, S. A. (1986). Social cognition, prosocial behavior, and emotion in preschoolers: contextual validation. *Child Development*, 57(1), 194–201. https://doi.org/10.2307/1130651

Department for Children, Schools and Families/Office of National Statistics. (2009). Children looked after in England (including adoption and care) year ending 31 March 2009. London: Department for Children, Schools and Families.

Department of Health JSNA Guidance. (2007, p. 7). http://www.publichealth.southampton.gov.uk/healthintelligence/jsna/background.aspx

Department of Health & NHS England. (2015). *Future in Mind Promoting, Protecting and Improving Our Children and Young People's Mental Health and Wellbeing*. London: Department of Health.

de Vries, A. L., & Cohen-Kettenis, P. T. (2012). Clinical management of gender dysphoria in children and adolescents: the Dutch approach. *Journal of Homosexuality*, 59(3), 301–320.

De Vries, A. L., McGuire, J. K., Steensma, T. D., Wagenaar, E. C., Doreleijers, T. A., & Cohen-Kettenis, P. T. (2014). Young adult psychological outcome after puberty suppression and gender reassignment. *Pediatrics*, 134(4), 696–704.

de Vries, A. L., Noens, I. L., Cohen-Kettenis, P. T., van Berckelaer-Onnes, I. A., & Doreleijers, T. A. (2010). Autism spectrum disorders in gender dysphoric children and adolescents. *Journal of Autism and Developmental Disorders*, 40(8), 930–936.

De Vries, A. L., Steensma, T. D., Doreleijers, T. A., & Cohen-Kettenis, P. T. (2011). Puberty suppression in adolescents with gender identity disorder: a prospective follow-up study. *Journal of Sexual Medicine*, 8(8), 2276–2283.

Dewald, J. F., Meijer, A. M., Oort, F. J., Kerkhof, G. A., & Bögels, S. M. (2010). The influence of sleep quality, sleep duration and sleepiness on school performance in children and adolescents: a meta-analytic review. *Sleep Medicine Reviews*, 14(3), 179–189.

DfE (Department for Education). (2017). Available from: https://www.gov.uk/government/uploads/system

DH. (2004). *National Service Framework for Children, Young People and Maternity Services.* London: HMSO.

DH & DfES. 2017. *Transforming Children and Young People's Mental Health Provision: A Green Paper*. London: HMSO.
DiMaio, S., Grizenko, N., & Joober, R. (2003). Dopamine genes and attention-deficit hyperactivity disorder: a review. *Journal of Psychiatry and Neuroscience.*
Dobrescu, S. R., Dinkler, L., Gillberg, C., Råstam, M., Gillberg, C., & Wentz, E. (2020). Anorexia nervosa: 30-year outcome. *The British Journal of Psychiatry*, 216(2), 97–104.
Doherty, J. L., & Owen, M. J. (2014). Genomic insights into the overlap between psychiatric disorders: implications for research and clinical practice. *Genome Medicine*, 6(4), 29.
Domènech-Llaberia, E., Viñas, F., Pla, E., Jané, M. C., Mitjavila, M., Corbella, T., & Canals, J. (2009). Prevalence of major depression in preschool children. *European Child and Adolescent Psychiatry*, 18(10), 597–604.
Doyle. (2012). Chapter 23. In Sue Pattison, Maggie Robson, Ann Beynon (Eds.), *The Handbook of Counselling Children & Young People* (p. 238).
Dramaix, M., Brasseur, D., Donnen, P., Bawhere, P., Porignon, D., Tonglet, R., & Hennart, P. (1996). Prognostic indicates for mortality of hospitalized children in Central Africa. *American Journal of Epidemiology*, 143(12), 1235–1243.
Draper, A., Jackson, G. M., Morgan, P. S., & Jackson, S. R. (2015). Premonitory urges are associated with decreased grey matter thickness within the insula and sensorimotor cortex in young people with Tourette syndrome. *Journal of Neuropsychology*, doi: 10.1111/jnp.12089
Drescher, J. (2015). Out of DSM: depathologizing homosexuality. *Behavioral Sciences*, 5(4), 565–575.
Drescher, J., & Byne, W. (2012). Gender dysphoric/gender variant (GD/GV) children and adolescents: summarizing what we know and what we have yet to learn. *Journal of Homosexuality*, 59(3), 501–510.
Drescher, J., & Byne, W. (2014). *Treating Transgender Children and Adolescents: An Interdisciplinary Discussion*. Routledge.
Driver, D. I., Gogtay, N., & Rapoport, J. L. (2013). Childhood onset schizophrenia and early onset schizophrenia spectrum disorders. *Child and Adolescent Psychiatric Clinics of North America*, 22(4), 539–555. https://doi.org/10.1016/j.chc.2013.04.001.
Drossman, D. A. (2006). Rome III: the new criteria. *Chinese Journal of Digestive Diseases*, 7, 181–185. https://doi.org/10.1111/j.1443-9573.2006.00265.x
Drummond, K. D., Bradley, S. J., Peterson-Badali, M., & Zucker, K. J. (2008). A follow-up study of girls with gender identity disorder. *Developmental Psychology*, 44(1), 34–45.
Duffy, A., Horrocks, J., Doucette, S., Keown-Stoneman, C., McCloskey, S., & Grof, P. (2014). The developmental trajectory of bipolar disorder. *British Journal of Psychiatry*, 204(2), 122–128. doi: 10.1192/bjp.bp.113.126706
Durwood, L., McLaughlin, K. A., & Olson, K. R. (2017). Mental health and self-worth in socially transitioned transgender youth. *Journal of the American Academy of Child and Adolescent Psychiatry*, 56(2), 116–123.
Eddy, C. M., & Cavanna, A. E. (2013). 'It's a curse!': coprolalia in Tourette syndrome. *European Journal of Neurology*, 20(11), 1467–1470. doi: 10.1111/ene.12207
Eddy, K. T., Dorer, D. J., Franko, D. L., Tahilani, K., Thompson-Brenner, H., & Herzog, D. B. (2008). Diagnostic crossover in anorexia nervosa and bulimia nervosa: implications for DSM-V. *American Journal of Psychiatry*, 165(2), 245–250.
Education Policy Institute (2017).
Edwards-Leeper, L., Leibowitz, S., & Sangganjanavanich, V. F. (2016). Affirmative practice with transgender and gender nonconforming youth: expanding the model. *Psychology of Sexual Orientation and Gender Diversity*, 3(2), 165.
Ehrenreich-May, J., Rosenfield, D., Queen, A. H., Kennedy, S. M., Remmes, C. S., & Barlow, D. H. (2017). An initial waitlist-controlled trial of the unified protocol for the treatment of emotional disorders in adolescents. *Journal of Anxiety Disorders*, 46, 46–55. doi: 10.1016/j.janxdis.2016.10.006. Epub 2016 Oct 17. PMID: 27771133.
Ehrensaft, D. (2011). *Gender Born, Gender Made: Raising Healthy Gender-Nonconforming Children*. New York: Workman Publishing.

Ehrensaft, M. K., Cohen, P., & Johnson, J. G. (2006). Development of personality disorder symptoms and the risk for partner violence. *Journal of Abnormal Psychology*, 115(3), 474.

Ehrensaft, M. K., Moffitt, T. E., & Caspi, A. (2004). Clinically abusive relationships in an unselected birth cohort: men's and women's participation and developmental antecedents. *Journal of Abnormal Psychology*, 113(2), 258.

Ein-Dor, T., & Hirschberger, G. (2016). Rethinking attachment theory. *Current Directions in Psychological Science*, 25(4), 223–227.

Eisenberg, M. E., Gower, A. L., McMorris, B. J., Rider, G. N., Shea, G., & Coleman, E. (2017). Risk and protective factors in the lives of transgender/gender nonconforming adolescents. *Journal of Adolescent Health*, 61(4), 521–526.

Eley, T. C., Deater-Deckard, K., Fombonne, E., Fulker, D. W., & Plomin, R. (1998). An adoption study of depressive symptoms in middle childhood. *Journal of Child Psychology and Psychiatry, and Allied Disciplines*, 39(3), 337–345.

Eley, T. C., Napolitano, M., Lau, J. Y., & Gregory, A. M. (2010). Does childhood anxiety evoke maternal control? A genetically informed study. *Journal of Child Psychology and Psychiatry*, 51(7), 772–779. doi: 10.1111/j.1469-7610.2010.02227.x. Epub 2010 Feb 24. PMID: 20202040.

Elia, J., Glessner, J. T., Wang, K., et al. (2011). Genome-wide copy number variation study associates metabotropic glutamate receptor gene networks with attention deficit hyperactivity disorder. *Nature Genetics*, 44(1), 78–84. https://doi.org/10.1038/ng.1013.

Emerson, E. (1995). *Challenging Behaviour: Analysis and Intervention in People with Learning Disabilities*. Cambridge: Cambridge University Press.

Emerson, E. (2003). Prevalence of psychiatric disorders in children and adolescents with and without intellectual disability. *Journal of Intellectual Disability Research*, 47(1), 51–58.

Emerson, E., & Hatton, C. (2007). *The Mental Health of Children and Adolescents with Learning Disabilities in Britain*. Foundation for People with Learning Disabilities. Lancaster, UK: Lancaster University.

Emerson, E., Moss, S., & Kiernan, C. (1999). The relationship between challenging behaviour and psychiatric disorders in people with severe developmental disabilities. In N. Bouras (Ed.), *Psychiatric and Behavioural Disorders in Developmental Disabilities and Mental Retardation*, 38–48. Cambridge: Cambridge University Press.

Emerson, E., Robertson, J., Gregory, N., Hatton, C., Kessissoglou, S., Hallam, A., & Hillery, J. (2000). Treatment and management of challenging behaviours in residential settings. *Journal of Applied Research in Intellectual Disabilities*, 13(4), 197–215.

Eminson, M., Benjamin, S., Shortall, A., Woods, T., & Faragher, B. (1996). Physical symptoms and illness attitudes in adolescents: an epidemiological study. *Journal of Child Psychology and Psychiatry*, 37(5), 519–528.

English, D. J., & the LONGSCAN Investigators (1997). Modified Maltreatment Classification System. https://www.unc.edu/depts/sph/longscan/pages/maltx/index.htm

Esbjørn, B. H., Normann, N., Christiansen, B. M., & Reinholdt-Dunne, M. L., 2018). The efficacy of group metacognitive therapy for children (MCT-c) with generalized anxiety disorder: an open trial. *Journal of Anxiety Disorders*, 53, 16–21. doi: 10.1016/j.janxdis.2017.11.002. Epub 2017 Nov 10. PMID: 29145078.

Evers, R. A., & van de Wetering, B. J. (1994). A treatment model for motor tics based on a specific tension-reduction technique. *Journal of Behavior Therapy and Experimental Psychiatry*, 25(3), 255–260.

Fairchild, G., Van Goozen, S. H., Calder, A. J., & Goodyer, I. M. (2013). Research review: evaluating and reformulating the developmental taxonomic theory of antisocial behaviour. *Journal of Child Psychology and Psychiatry*, 54(9), 924–940.

Fairchild, G., Van Goozen, S. H., Calder, A. J., Stollery, S. J., & Goodyer, I. M. (2009a). Deficits in facial expression recognition in male adolescents with early-onset or adolescence-onset conduct disorder. *Journal of Child Psychology and Psychiatry*, 50(5), 627–636.

Fairchild, G., van Goozen, S. H., Stollery, S. J., Aitken, M. R., Savage, J., Moore, S. C., & Goodyer, I. M. (2009b). Decision making and executive function in male adolescents with early-onset or adolescence-onset conduct disorder and control subjects. *Biological Psychiatry*, 66(2), 162–168.

Fani, T., & Ghaemi, F. (2011). Implications of Vygotsky's zone of proximal development (ZPD) in teacher education: ZPTD and self-scaffolding. *Procedia-Social and Behavioral Sciences*, 29, 1549–1554.

Faraone, S. V., Asherson, P., Banaschewski, T., et al. (2015). Attention-deficit/hyperactivity disorder. *Nature Reviews. Disease Primers*, 1(1), 15020. https://doi.org/10.1038/nrdp.2015.20.

Faraone, S. V., Biederman, J., & Monuteaux, M. C. (2000). Attention-deficit disorder and conduct disorder in girls: evidence for a familial subtype. *Biological Psychiatry*, 48(1), 21–29.

Faraone, S. V., Biederman, J., & Mick, E. (2006). The age-dependent decline of attention deficit hyperactivity disorder: a meta-analysis of follow-up studies. *Psychological Medicine*, 36(2), 159–165.

Faraone, S. V., Biederman, J., & Wozniak, J. (2012). Examining the comorbidity Between attention deficit hyperactivity disorder and bipolar I disorder: a meta-analysis of family genetic studies. *American Journal of Psychiatry*, 169(12), 1256–1266. https://doi.org/10.1176/appi.ajp.2012.12010087.

Faraone, S. V., & Doyle, A. E. (2000). Genetic influences on attention deficit hyperactivity disorder. *Current Psychiatry Reports*, 2(2), 143–146.

Faraone, S. V., Ghirardi, L., Kuja-Halkola, R., Lichtenstein, P., & Larsson, H. (2017). The familial co-aggregation of attention-deficit/hyperactivity disorder and intellectual disability: a register-based family study. *Journal of the American Academy of Child and Adolescent Psychiatry*, 56(2), 167–174.e1. https://doi.org/10.1016/j.jaac.2016.11.011.

Faraone, S. V., & Larsson, H. (2019). Genetics of attention deficit hyperactivity disorder. *Molecular Psychiatry*, 24(4), 562–575. https://doi.org/10.1038/s41380-018-0070-0.

Farrell, L. J., Kershaw, H., & Ollendick, T. (2018). Play-modified one-session treatment for young children with a specific phobia of dogs: a multiple baseline case series. *Child Psychiatry & Human Development*, 49(2), 317–329. doi: 10.1007/s10578-017-0752-x. PMID: 28766176.

Fast, A. A., & Olson, K. R. (2018). Gender development in transgender preschool children. *Child Development*, 89(2), 620–637.

Felitti, V. J., Anda, R. F., Nordenberg, D., Williamson, D. F., Spitz, A. M., Edwards, V., Koss, M. P., & Marks, J. S. (1998). Relationship of childhood abuse and household dysfunction to many of the leading causes of death in adults. The Adverse Childhood Experiences (ACE) Study. *American Journal of Preventive Medicine*, 14(4), 245–258. doi: 10.1016/s0749-3797(98)00017-8. PMID: 9635069.

Ferber, R. (1985). Sleep, sleeplessness, and sleep disruptions in infants and young children. *Annals of Clinical Research*, 17(5), 227–234.

Fernandez, T. V., State, M. W., & Pittenger, C. (2018). Tourette disorder and other tic disorders. In D. H. Geschwind, H. L. Paulson and C. Klein (Eds.), *Handbook of Clinical Neurology* (Vol. 147, pp. 343–354). Elsevier B.V.

Ferrari, A. J., Stockings, E., Khoo, J.-P., Erskine, H. E., Degenhardt, L., Vos, T., & Whiteford, H. A. (2016). The prevalence and burden of bipolar disorder: findings from the global burden of disease study 2013. *Bipolar Disorders*, 18(5), 440–450. https://doi.org/10.1111/bdi.12423.

Ferro, M. A. (2016). Major depressive disorder, suicidal behaviour, bipolar disorder, and generalised anxiety disorder among emerging adults with and without chronic health conditions. *Epidemiology and Psychiatric Sciences*, 25(5), 462–474.

Fielding, J., & Bass, C. (2018). Individuals seeking gender reassignment: marked increase in demand for services. *BJPsych Bulletin*, 42(5), 206–210.

Van Fleet, R., & Guerney, L. (2003). *Casebook of Filial Therapy*. Play Therapy Press.

Flint, J., & Yule, W. (1993). Behavioural phenotypes. In M. Rutter and L. Hersov (Eds.), *Recent Advances in Child and Adolescent Psychiatry*, 3rd Edition. Oxford: Blackwell Scientific.

Flint, J., & Yule, W. (1994). Behavioural phenotypes. In M. Rutter, E. Taylor, & L. Hersov (Eds.), *Child and Adolescent Psychiatry: Modern Approaches* (3rd ed., pp. 666–687). London: Blackwell Scientific.

Ford, T., Goodman, R., & Meltzer, H. (2003). The British child and adolescent mental health survey 1999: the prevalence of DSM-IV disorders. *Journal of the American Academy of Child & Adolescent Psychiatry*, 42(10), 1203–1211.

Formby, E. (2015). Limitations of focussing on homophobic, biphobic and transphobic 'bullying' to understand and address LGBT young people's experiences within and beyond school. *Sex Education*, 15(6), 626–640.

Fox, C., & Hawton, K. (2004). *Deliberate Self-Harm in Adolescence*. London: Jessica Kingsley.

Frare, F., Perugi, G., Ruffolo, G., & Toni, C. (2004). Obsessive–compulsive disorder and body dysmorphic disorder: a comparison of clinical features. *European Psychiatry*, 19(5), 292–298.

Freeman, D., Lister, R., Waite, F., Yu, L. M., Slater, M., Dunn, G., & Clark, D. (2019). Automated psychological therapy using virtual reality (VR) for patients with persecutory delusions: study protocol for a single-blind parallel-group randomised controlled trial (THRIVE). *Trials*, 20(1), 87.

Frías, Á., Palma, C., & Farriols, N. (2015). Comorbidity in pediatric bipolar disorder: prevalence, clinical impact, etiology and treatment. *Journal of Affective Disorders*, 174, 378–389. doi: 10.1016/j.jad.2014.12.008. Epub 2014 Dec 12. PMID: 25545605.

Frith, E. *Inpatient Provision for Children and Young People with Mental Health Problems.*

Gardner, H., 1983. *Frames of Mind*. New York: Basic Books.

Gaskill, R. L., & Perry, B. D. (2017). A neurosequential therapeutics approach to guided play, play therapy, and activities for children who won't talk. In C. A. Malchiodi, D. A. Crenshaw (Eds.), *What to Do When Children Clam Up in Psychotherapy: Interventions to Facilitate Communication* (pp. 38–66). Guilford Press.

Gaugler, T., Klei, L., Sanders, S. J., et al. (2014). Most genetic risk for autism resides with common variation. *Nature Genetics*, 46(8), 881–885. https://doi.org/10.1038/ng.3039.

Geller, B., Zimerman, B., Williams, M., Delbello, M. P., Frazier, J., & Beringer, L. (2002). Phenomenology of prepubertal and early adolescent bipolar disorder: examples of elated mood, grandiose behaviors, decreased need for sleep, racing thoughts and hypersexuality. *Journal of Child and Adolescent Psychopharmacology*, 12(1), 3–9. doi: 10.1089/10445460252943524. PMID: 12014593.

Gejman, P. V., Sanders, A. R., & Kendler, K S. (2011). Genetics of schizophrenia: new findings and challenges. *Annual Review of Genomics and Human Genetics*, 12, 121–144.

Gerhardt, S. (2004). *Why Love Matters: How Affection Shapes a Baby's Brain*. London & New York: Routledge.

Geschwind, D. H., & State, M. W. (2015). Gene hunting in autism spectrum disorder: on the path to precision medicine. *The Lancet. Neurology*, 14(11), 1109–1120. https://doi.org/10.1016/S1474-4422(15)00044-7.

Ghirardi, L., Brikell, I., Kuja-Halkola, R., et al. (2018). The familial co-aggregation of ASD and ADHD: a register-based cohort study. *Molecular Psychiatry*, 23(2), 257–262. https://doi.org/10.1038/mp.2017.17.

Giddan, J. J., Milling, L., & Campbell, N. B. (1996). Unrecognised language and speech deficits in pre-adolescent psychiatric inpatients. *American Journal of Orthopsychiatry*, 66(1), 85–92.

GIDS (2020). Gender Identity Development Service (GIDS). https://gids.nhs.uk/.

Gilles de la Tourette, G. (1885). Etude sur une affection nerveuse caracterisee par le l'incoordination motrice accompagnee d'echolalie et de coprolalie. *Archives de Neurologie*, 9(19–42), 158–200.

Gilmour, J., Hill, B., Place, M., & Skuse, D. H. (2004). Social communication deficits in conduct disorder: a clinical and community survey. *Journal of Child Psychology and Psychiatry*, 45(5), 967–978.

Giovanardi, G. (2017). Buying time or arresting development? The dilemma of administering hormone blockers in trans children and adolescents. *Porto Biomedical Journal*, 2(5), 153–156.

Gledhill, J., Rangel, L., & Garralda, E. (2000). Surviving chronic physical illness: psychosocial outcome in adult life. *Archives of Disease in Childhood*, 83(2), 104–110.

Glidden, D., Bouman, W. P., Jones, B. A., & Arcelus, J. (2016). Gender dysphoria and autism spectrum disorder: a systematic review of the literature. *Sexual Medicine Reviews*, 4(1), 3–14.

Glowinski, A. L., Madden, P. A. F., Bucholz, K. K., Lynskey, M. T., & Heath, A. C. (2003). Genetic epidemiology of self-reported lifetime DSM-IV major depressive disorder in a population-based twin sample of female adolescents. *Journal of Child Psychology and Psychiatry, and Allied Disciplines*, 44(7), 988–996.

Golan, O., Baron-Cohen, S., Hill, J. J., & Golan, Y. (2006). The "reading the mind in films" task: complex emotion recognition in adults with and without autism spectrum conditions. *Social Neuroscience*, 1(2), 111–123. doi: 10.1080/17470910600980986. PMID: 18633780.

Goldsmith, T., Shapira, N. A., Phillips, K. A., & McElroy, S. L. (1998). Conceptual foundations of obsessive-compulsive spectrum disorders. *Obsessive-Compulsive Disorder: Theory, Research, and Treatment.* New York: Guilford, 397–425.

Goldstein, B. I., Birmaher, B., Carlson, G. A., DelBello, M. P., Findling, R. L., Fristad, M., Kowatch, R. A., Miklowitz, D. J., Nery, F. G., Perez-Algorta, G., Van Meter, A., Zeni, C. P., Correll, C. U., Kim, H. W., Wozniak, J., Chang, K. D., Hillegers, M., & Youngstrom, E. A. (2017). *The International Society for Bipolar Disorders* Task Force report on pediatric bipolar disorder: knowledge to date and directions for future research. *Bipolar Disorders*, 19(7), 524–543. doi: 10.1111/bdi.12556. Epub 2017 Sep 25. PMID: 28944987; PMCID: PMC5716873.

Goodlin-Jones, B., Tang, K., Liu, J., & Anders, T. F. (2009). Sleep problems, sleepiness and daytime behavior in preschool-age children. *Journal of Child Psychology and Psychiatry, and Allied Disciplines*, 50(12), 1532–1540.

Goodman, R. (1997). The strength and difficulties questionnaire: a research note. *Journal of Child Psychology and Psychiatry*, 38, 581–586.

Goodman, W. K., Price, L. H., Rasmussen, S. A., Riddle, M. A., & Rapoport, J. L. (1991). *Children's Yale-Brown Obsessive Compulsive Scale (CY-BOCS).* New Haven: Department of Psychiatry, Yale University School of Medicine.

Government equalities office (2018). *LGBT Action Plan: Improving the Lives of Lesbian, Gay, Bisexual and Transgendered People.* London: HM Government.

Gradisar, M., Jackson, K., Spurrier, N. J., et al. (2016). Behavioral interventions for infant sleep problems: a randomized controlled trial. *Pediatrics*, 137(6). https://carolgraysocialstories.com.

Gray, C. (2015). The *New Social Story Book: Illustrated Edition.* Arlington: Future Horizons Inc.

Gray, C., & Garand, J. (1993). Social stories: improving responses of students with autism with accurate social information. Research Article. https://doi.org/10.1177/108835769300800101

Gray, C., & White, W. L. (2000). *My Social Stories Book.* London: Jessica Kingsley Publishers.

Green, E. K., Rees, E., Walters, J. T. R., et al. (2016). Copy number variation in bipolar disorder. *Molecular Psychiatry*, 21(1), 89–93. https://doi.org/10.1038/mp.2014.174.

Green, J. (2006). Annotation: the therapeutic alliance – a significant but neglected variable in child mental health treatment studies. *Journal of Child Psychology and Psychiatry*, 47(5), 425–435.

Gregory, A. M., Van der Ende, J., Willis, T. A., & Verhulst, F. C. (2008). Parent-reported sleep problems during development and self-reported anxiety/depression, attention problems, and aggressive behavior later in life. *Archives of Pediatrics and Adolescent Medicine*, 162(4), 330–335.

Gringras, P. (2008). When to use drugs to help sleep. *Archives of Disease in Childhood*, 93(11), 976–981.

Grossman, A. H., D'augelli, A. R., & Frank, J. A. (2011). Aspects of psychological resilience among transgender youth. *Journal of LGBT Youth*, 8(2), 103–115.

Grove, J., Ripke, S., Als, T. D., et al. (2019b). Identification of common genetic risk variants for autism spectrum disorder. *Nature Genetics*, 51(3), 431–444. https://doi.org/10.1038/s41588-019-0344-8.

Groves, S., Backer, Hilmar S., Van den Bosch, Wies, & Miller, A. (2011). Dialetical behaviour therapy with adolescents. *Child and Adolescent Mental Health*, 17(12).

Gunderson, J. G. (2011). Borderline personality disorder. *New England Journal of Medicine*, 364(21), 2037–2042.

Grych, J. H., & Cardoza-Fernandes, S. (2001). Understanding the Impact of Interparental Conflict on Children: The Role of Social Cognitive Processes.

Hall, D., & Williams, J. (2008). Safeguarding, child protection and mental health. *Archives of Disease in Childhood*, 93, 11–13.

Hall, J., Trent, S., Thomas, K. L., O'Donovan, M. C., & Owen, M. J. (2015). Genetic risk for schizophrenia: convergence on synaptic pathways involved in plasticity. *Biological Psychiatry*, 77(1), 52–58. https://doi.org/10.1016/j.biopsych.2014.07.011.

Harlow, H. F., & Zimmermann, R. R. (1959). Affectional responses in the infant monkey. *Science*, 130, 421–432.

Hassan, N., & Cavanna, A. E. (2012). The prognosis of Tourette syndrome: implications for clinical practice. *Functional Neurology*, 27(1), 23–27.

Hastings, R. P., & Brown, T. (2000). Functional assessment and challenging behaviors: some future directions. *Journal of the Association for Persons with Severe Handicaps*, 25(4), 229–240.

Hart & Risley. (1995). Meaningful Differences National Strategies Every Child a Talker Project 2008-2011.

Hartshorne, M., Freeman, K., & Parrott, J. (2006). The cost to the nation of children's poor communication. I CAN Talk Communication Disability and Literacy Difficulties Issue 1.

Hellerstedt, W. L., Madsen, N. J., Gunnar, M. R., Grotevant, H. D., Lee, R. M., & Johnson, D. E. (2008). The international adoption project: population-based surveillance of Minnesota parents who adopted children internationally. *Maternal and Child Health Journal*, 12(2), 162–171. doi: 10.1007/s10995-007-0237-9

Hembree, W. C., Cohen-Kettenis, P. T., Gooren, L., et al. (2017). Endocrine treatment of gender-dysphoric/gender-incongruent persons: an Endocrine Society* clinical practice guideline. *The Journal of Clinical Endocrinology and Metabolism*, 102(11), 3869–3903.

Herle, M., De Stavola, B., Hübel, C., Abdulkadir, M., Ferreira, D. S., Loos, R. J., ... Micali, N. (2020). A longitudinal study of eating behaviours in childhood and later eating disorder behaviours and diagnoses. *The British Journal of Psychiatry*, 216(2), 113–119.

Heron-Delaney, M., Kenardy, J., Charlton, E., & Matsuoka, Y. (2013). A systematic review of predictors of posttraumatic stress disorder (PTSD) for adult road traffic crash survivors. *Injury*, 44(11), 1413–1422. https://doi.org/10.1016/j.injury.2013.07.011.

Herrenkohl, R. C., & Herrenkohl, T. I. (2009). Assessing a child's experience of multiple maltreatment types: some unfinished business. *Journal of Family Violence*, 24(7), 485–496. https://doi.org/10.1007/s10896-009-9247-2

Hienert, M., Gryglewski, G., Stamenkovic, M., Kasper, S., & Lanzenberger, R. (2018). Striatal dopaminergic alterations in Tourette's syndrome: a meta-analysis based on 16 PET and SPECT neuroimaging studies. *Transl Psychiatry*, 8(1), 143. doi: 10.1038/s41398-018-0202-y

Hilker, R., Helenius, D., Fagerlund, B., et al. (2018). Heritability of schizophrenia and schizophrenia spectrum based on the nationwide Danish twin register. *Biological Psychiatry*, 83(6), 492–498. https://doi.org/10.1016/j.biopsych.2017.08.017.

Hill, J. (2002). Biological, psychological and social processes in the conduct disorders. *Journal of Child Psychology and Psychiatry*, 43(1), 133–164.

Hisle-Gorman, E., Landis, C. A., Susi, A., Schvey, N. A., Gorman, G. H., Nylund, C. M., & Klein, D. A. (2019). Gender dysphoria in children with autism spectrum disorder. *LGBT Health*, 6(3), 95–100.

HM Government (2014). *Children and Families Act*. London: HM Govt.

HM Government. (2018). *Working Together to Safeguard Children A Guide to Inter-Agency Working to Safeguard and Promote the Welfare of Children*. London: HMSO.

Hoek, H. W., & Van Hoeken, D. (2003). Review of the prevalence and incidence of eating disorders. *International Journal of Eating Disorders*, 34(4), 383–396.

Hoffman, M. (1991). *Empathy, Social Cognition and Moral Action*. Lawrence, Erlbaum.

Holley, S., Hill, C. M., & Stevenson, J. (2011). An hour less sleep is a risk factor for childhood conduct problems. *Child: Care, Health and Development*, 37(4), 563–570.

Hong, M. P., & Erickson, C. A. (2019). Investigational drugs in early-stage clinical trials for autism spectrum disorder. *Expert Opinion on Investigational Drugs*, 28(8), 709–718. doi: 10.1080/13543784.2019.1649656. Epub 2019 Aug 12.

Howard, D. M., Adams, M. J., Clarke, T.-K., et al. (2019). Genome-wide meta-analysis of depression identifies 102 independent variants and highlights the importance of the prefrontal brain regions. *Nature Neuroscience*, 22(3), 343–352. https://doi.org/10.1038/s41593-018-0326-7.

Howes, O., McCutcheon, R., & Stone, J. (2015). Glutamate and dopamine in schizophrenia: an update for the 21st century. *Journal of Psychopharmacology*, 29(2), 97–115.

Howes, O. D., Bose, S. K., Turkheimer, F., Valli, I., Egerton, A., Valmaggia, L. R., ... McGuire, P. (2011). Dopamine synthesis capacity before onset of psychosis: a prospective [18F]-DOPA PET imaging study. *American Journal of Psychiatry*, 168(12), 1311–1317.

Huebner, T., Vloet, T. D., Marx, I., Konrad, K., Fink, G. R., Herpertz, S. C., & Herpertz-Dahlmann, B. (2008). Morphometric brain abnormalities in boys with conduct disorder. *Journal of the American Academy of Child & Adolescent Psychiatry*, 47(5), 540–547.

Hutchinson, A., Midgen, M., & Spiliadis, A. (2020). In support of research Into rapid-onset gender dysphoria. *Archives of Sexual Behavior*, 1–2.

Hyde, T. M., Aaronson, B. A., Randolph, C., Rickler, K. C., & Weinberger, D. R. (1992). Relationship of birth weight to the phenotypic expression of Gilles de la Tourette's syndrome in monozygotic twins. *Neurology*, 42(3 Pt 1), 652–658.

IACAPAP. (2019). https://iacapap.org/content/uploads/A.7-Psychopharmacology-2019.1.pdf

Iossifov, I., O'Roak, B. J., Sanders, S. J., et al. (2014). The contribution of de novo coding mutations to autism spectrum disorder. *Nature*, 515(7526), 216. https://doi.org/10.1038/NATURE13908.

Isaacs, J. B. (2007). Impacts of Early Childhood Programs First Focus Making Children and Families the Priority. tomorrowsyouth.org

James, A. C., James, G., Cowdrey, F. A., Soler, A., & Choke, A. (2013). Cognitive behavioural therapy for anxiety disorders in children and adolescents. *Cochrane Database Systematic Review*, 3(6), CD004690. doi: 10.1002/14651858.CD004690.pub3. Update in: Cochrane Database Syst Rev. 2015;(2):CD004690. PMID: 23733328.

Janssen, X. MA, Hughes, A. R., Hill, C. M., Kotronoulas, G., Kipping, R., & Kesketh, K. (2019). Are screen-exposure time and daytime physical activity associated with sleep in under 5s: a systematic review. *Sleep Medicine Reviews*.

Jarrett, M. A., & Ollendick, T. H. (2008). A conceptual review of the comorbidity of attention-deficit/hyperactivity disorder and anxiety: implications for future research and practice. *Clinical Psychology Review*, 28(7), 1266–1280. doi: 10.1016/j.cpr.2008.05.004. Epub 2008 May 17. PMID: 18571820.

Jennings, S. (2011). *Healthy Attachments and Neuro-Dramatic-Play (Arts Therapies)*. Jessica Kingsley.

Johnson, E. K., & Finlayson, C. (2016). Preservation of fertility potential for gender and sex diverse individuals. *Transgender Health*, 1(1), 41–44.

Joint Formulary Committee. (2010). British National Formulary for Children. 2010–2011. London: BMJ Group and Pharmaceutical Press.

Jones, H. J., Stergiakouli, E., Tansey, K. E., et al. (2016). Phenotypic manifestation of genetic risk for schizophrenia During adolescence in the general population. *JAMA Psychiatry*, 73(3), 221–228. https://doi.org/10.1001/jamapsychiatry.2015.3058.

Jones, A. P., Laurens, K. R., Herba, C. M., Barker, G. J., & Viding, E. (2009). Amygdala hypoactivity to fearful faces in boys with conduct problems and callous-unemotional traits. *American Journal of Psychiatry*, 166(1), 95–102.

Jones, K., Daley, D., Hutchings, J., et al. (2007). Efficacy of the incredible years basic parenting programas an early intervention for conduct problems and ADHD child care. *Health and Development*, 33, 749–756.

Joslyn, C., Hawes, D. J., Hunt, C., & Mitchell, P. B. (2016), Is age of onset associated with severity, prognosis, and clinical features in bipolar disorder? A meta-analytic review. *Bipolar Disorders*, 18, 389–403. doi: 10.1111/bdi.12419

Joyce, K., Thompson, A., & Marwaha, S. (2016). Is treatment for bipolar disorder more effective earlier in illness course? A comprehensive literature review. *International Journal of Bipolar Disorders*, 4, 19. https://doi.org/10.1186/s40345-016-0060-6

Kahn, R. S., van Rossum, I. W., Leucht, S., McGuire, P., Lewis, S. W., Leboyer, M., ... Díaz-Caneja, C. M. (2018). Amisulpride and olanzapine followed by open-label treatment with clozapine in first-episode schizophrenia and schizophreniform disorder (OPTiMiSE): a three-phase switching study. *The Lancet Psychiatry*, 5(10), 797–807.

Kalanithi, P. S., Zheng, W., Kataoka, Y., DiFiglia, M., Grantz, H., Saper, C. B., ... Vaccarino, F. M. (2005). Altered parvalbumin-positive neuron distribution in basal ganglia of individuals with Tourette syndrome. *Proceedings of the National Academy of Sciences of the United States of America*, 102(37), 13307–13312. doi: 10.1073/pnas.0502624102

Kaltiala, R., Bergman, H., Carmichael, P., et al. (2020). Time trends in referrals to child and adolescent gender identity services: a study in four Nordic countries and in the UK. *Nordic Journal of Psychiatry*, 74(1), 40–44.

Kaltiala-Heino, R., Sumia, M., Työläjärvi, M., & Lindberg, N. (2015). Two years of gender identity service for minors: overrepresentation of natal girls with severe problems in adolescent development. *Child and Adolescent Psychiatry and Mental Health*, 9(1), 9.

Kaminski, J. W., Valle, L. A., Filene, J. H., & Boyle, C. L. (2008). A meta-analytic review of components associated with parent training program effectiveness. *Journal of Abnormal Child Psychology*, 36(4), 567–589.

Kataoka, Y., Kalanithi, P. S., Grantz, H., Schwartz, M. L., Saper, C., Leckman, J. F., & Vaccarino, F. M. (2010). Decreased number of parvalbumin and cholinergic interneurons in the striatum of individuals with Tourette syndrome. *Journal of Comparative Neurology*, 518(3), 277–291. doi: 10.1002/cne.22206

Kazdin, A. E. (1997). Practitioner review: psychosocial treatments for conduct disorder in children. *Journal of Child Psychology and Psychiatry*, 38(2), 161–178.

Keane, T., Marshall, A., & Taft, C. (2006). Posttraumatic stress disorder: etiology, epidemiology, and treatment outcome. *Annual Review of Clinical Psychology*, 2(1), 161–197.

Keane, T. M., Marshall, A. D., & Taft, C. T. (2006). Posttraumatic stress disorder: etiology, epidemiology, and treatment outcome, *Annual Review of Clinical Psychology*, 2(1), 161–197. https://doi.org/10.1146/annurev.clinpsy.2.022305.095305.

Kearney, C. A. (2002). Identifying the function of school refusal behavior: a revision of the School Refusal Assessment Scale. *Journal of Psychopathology and Behavioral Assessment*, 24(4), 235–245.

Kearney, C. A. (2007). Forms and functions of school refusal behavior in youth: an empirical analysis of absenteeism severity. *Journal of Child Psychology and Psychiatry*, 48(1), 53–61.

Kearney, C. A., & Silverman, W. K. (1999). Functionally based prescriptive and nonprescriptive treatment for children and adolescents with school refusal behaviour. *Behaviour Therapy*, 30, 673–695.

Keel, P. K., Brown, T. A., Holm-Denoma, J., & Bodell, L. P. (2011). Comparison of DSM-IV versus proposed DSM-5 diagnostic criteria for eating disorders: reduction of eating disorder not otherwise specified and validity. *International Journal of Eating Disorders*, 44(6), 553–560.

Kendall, K. M., Rees, E., Bracher-Smith, M., et al. (2019). Association of rare copy number variants With risk of depression. *JAMA Psychiatry*. https://doi.org/10.1001/jamapsychiatry.2019.0566.

Kendler, K. S., Prescott, C. A., Myers, J., & Neale, M. C. (2003). The structure of genetic and environmental risk factors for common psychiatric and substance use disorders in men and women. *Archives of General Psychiatry*, 60(9), 929–937. doi: 10.1001/archpsyc.60.9.929. PMID: 12963675.

Kernot, C., Tomlinson, A., Chevance, A., & Cipriani, A. (2019). One step closer to personalised prescribing of antidepressants: using real-world data together with patients and clinicians' preferences. *Evidence-Based Mental Health*, 22(3), 91–92.

Kessler, R. C. (1995). *The National Comorbidity Survey: Preliminary Results and Future Directions.*

Kessler, R. C., Avenevoli, S., & Ries Merikangas, K. (2001). Mood disorders in children and adolescents: an epidemiologic perspective. *Biological Psychiatry*, 49(12), 1002–1014.

Kessler, R. C., Berglund, P., Demler, O., Jin, R., Merikangas, K. R., & Walters, E. E. (2005). Lifetime prevalence and age-of-onset distributions of DSM-IV disorders in the national comorbidity survey replication. *Archives of General Psychiatry*, 62(6), 593–602. https://doi.org /10.1001/archpsyc.62.6.593.

Kirov, G. (2015). CNVs in neuropsychiatric disorders. *Human Molecular Genetics*, 24(R1), R45–R49. https://doi.org/10.1093/hmg/ddv253.

Kim, S., Greene, D. J., Bihun, E. C., Koller, J. M., Hampton, J. M., Acevedo, H., ... Black, K. J. (2019). Provisional tic disorder is not so transient. *Scientific Reports*, 9(1), 3951. doi: 10.1038/ s41598-019-40133-4

Knefel, M., Lueger-Schuster, B., Bisson, J., Karatzias, T., Kazlauskas, E., & Roberts, N. P. (2019). A cross-cultural comparison of ICD-11 complex posttraumatic stress disorder symptom networks in Austria, the United Kingdom, and Lithuania. *Journal of Traumatic Stress*, 33(1), 41–51. https://doi.org/10.1002/jts.22361.

Knollmann, M., Reissner, V., & Hebebrand, J. (2019). Towards a comprehensive assessment of school absenteeism: development and initial validation of the inventory of school attendance problems. *European Child & Adolescent Psychiatry*, 28(3), 399–414.

Knudsen, E. I. (2004). Sensitive periods in the development of the brain and behavior. *Journal of Cognitive Neuroscience*, 16(8), 1412–1425. doi: 10.1162/0898929042304796. PMID: 15509387.

Kosciw, J. G., Greytak, E. A., & Diaz, E. M. (2009). Who, what, where, when, and why: demographic and ecological factors contributing to hostile school climate for lesbian, gay, bisexual, and transgender youth. *Journal of Youth and Adolescence*, 38(7), 976–988.

Kossowsky, J., Pfaltz, M. C., Schneider, S., Taeymans, J., Locher, C., & Gaab, J. (2013). The separation anxiety hypothesis of panic disorder revisited: a meta-analysis. *American Journal of Psychiatry*, 170(7), 768–781. doi: 10.1176/appi.ajp.2012.12070893. PMID: 23680783.

Kotimaa, A. J., Moilanen, I., Taanila, A., Ebeling, H., Smalley, S. L., Mcgough, J. J., ... Järvelin, M. R. (2003). Maternal smoking and hyperactivity in 8-year-old children. *Journal of the American Academy of Child & Adolescent Psychiatry*, 42(7), 826–833.

Kovshoff, H., Vrijens, M., Thompson, M., Yardley, L., Hodgkins, P., Sonuga-Barke, E. J., & Danckaerts, M. (2013). What influences clinicians' decisions about ADHD medication? Initial data from the Influences on Prescribing for ADHD Questionnaire (IPAQ). *European Child & Adolescent Psychiatry*, 22(9), 533–542.

Kroon, J. S., Wohlfarth, T. D., Dieleman, J., et al. (2013). Incidence rates and risk factors of bipolar disorder in the general population: a population-based cohort study. *Bipolar Disorders*, 15(3), 306–313. https://doi.org/10.1111/bdi.12058.

Kumsta, R., Kreppner, J., Kennedy, M., Knights, N., Rutter, M., & Sonuga-Barke, E. (2015). Psychological consequences of early global deprivation. *European Psychologist*, 20(2), 138–151.

Kutcher, S., et al. (2004). International consensus statement on attention-deficit/hyperactivity disorder (ADHD) and disruptive behaviour disorders (DBDs): clinical implications and treatment practice suggestions. *European Neuropsychopharmacology*, 14(1), 11–28.

Kuvalanka, K. A., Weiner, J. L., Munroe, C., Goldberg, A. E., & Gardner, M. (2017). Trans and gender-nonconforming children and their caregivers: gender presentations, peer relations, and well-being at baseline. *Journal of Family Psychology* , 31(7), 889.

Kwak, C., Dat Vuong, K., & Jankovic, J. (2003). Premonitory sensory phenomenon in Tourette's syndrome. *Movement Disorders*, 18(12), 1530–1533. doi: 10.1002/mds.10618

Labuschagne, I., Phan, K. L., Wood, A., Angstadt, M., Chua, P., Heinrichs, M., ... Nathan, P. J. (2010). Oxytocin attenuates amygdala reactivity to fear in generalized social anxiety disorder. *Neuropsychopharmacology*, 35(12), 2403–2413.

Lahey, B. B., Van Hulle, C. A., Singh, A. L., Waldman, I. D., & Rathouz, P. J. (2011). Higher-order genetic and environmental structure of prevalent forms of child and adolescent psychopathology. *Archives of General Psychiatry*, 68(2), 181–189. doi: 10.1001/archgenpsychiatry.2010.192. Erratum in: JAMA Psychiatry. 2015 Aug; 72(8), 851. PMID: 21300945; PMCID: PMC3322461.

Landreth, G. (2002). *Play Therapy, The Art of the Relationship*. New York: Brunner Routledge.

Lapidus, N., Minetti, A., Djibo, A., Guerin, P. J., Hustache, S., Gaboulaud, V., & Grais, R. F. (2009). Mortality risk among children admitted in a large-scale nutritional program in Niger, 2006. *PLoS One*, 4(1), e4313.

Larsson, H., Anckarsater, H., Råstam, M., Chang, Z., & Lichtenstein, P. (2012). Childhood attention-deficit hyperactivity disorder as an extreme of a continuous trait: a quantitative genetic study of 8,500 twin pairs. *Journal of Child Psychology and Psychiatry*, 53(1), 73–80. doi: 10.1111/j.1469-7610.2011.02467.x. Epub 2011 Sep 16. PMID: 21923806.

Larsson, H., Chang, Z., D'Onofrio, B., & Lichtenstein, P. (2013). The heritability of clinically diagnosed attention deficit hyperactivity disorder across the lifespan. *Psychological Medicine*, 44(10), 2223–2229.

Lask, B., Gordon, I., Christie, D., Frampton, I., Chowdhury, U., & Watkins, B. (2005). Functional neuroimaging in early-onset anorexia nervosa. *International Journal of Eating Disorders*, 37(S1), S49–S51.

Leve, L. D., & Chamberlain, P. (2007). A randomized evaluation of Multidimensional Treatment Foster Care: effects on school attendance and homework completion in juvenile justice girls. *Research on Social Work Practice*, 17(6), 657–663.

Lateef, T. M., Merikangas, K. R., He, J., Kalaydjian, A., Khoromi, S., Knight, E., & Nelson, K. B. (2009). Headache in a national sample of American children: prevalence and comorbidity. *Journal of Child Neurology*, 24(5), 536–543.

Leckman, J. F., Walker, D. E., & Cohen, D. J. (1993). Premonitory urges in Tourette's syndrome. *American Journal of Psychiatry*, 150(1), 98–102. doi: doi.org/10.1176/ajp.150.1.98

Leeb, Rebecca, Paulozzi, Leonard, Melanson, Cindi, Simon, Thomas, & Arias, Ileana (2008). Child maltreatment surveillance: uniform definitions for public health and recommended data elements. Division of Violence Prevention, program of the Centers for Disease Control and Prevention, 3 pgs.

Leigh, E., & Clark, D. M. (2018). Understanding social anxiety disorder in adolescents and improving treatment outcomes: applying the cognitive model of clark and wells (1995). *Clinical Child and Family Psychology Review*, 21(3), 388–414. doi: 10.1007/s10567-018-0258-5. PMID: 29654442; PMCID: PMC6447508.

Lenzi, F., Cortese, S., Harris, J., & Masi, G. (2018). Pharmacotherapy of emotional dysregulation in adults with ADHD: a systematic review and meta-analysis. *Neuroscience & Biobehavioral Reviews*, 84, 359–367.

Leve, L. D., & Chamberlain, P. (2007). A randomized evaluation of Multidimensional Treatment Foster Care: effects on school attendance and homework completion in juvenile justice girls. *Research on Social Work Practice*, 17(6), 657–663.

Leverich, G. S., Post, R. M., Keck, P. E. Jr., Altshuler, L. L., Frye, M. A., Kupka, R. W., Nolen, W. A., Suppes, T., McElroy, S. L., Grunze, H., Denicoff, K., Moravec, M. K., & Luckenbaugh, D. (2007). The poor prognosis of childhood-onset bipolar disorder. *Journal of Pediatrics*, 150(5), 485–490. doi: 10.1016/j.jpeds.2006.10.070. PMID: 17452221.

Levine, M. P., & Smolak, L. (2002). Body image development in adolescence. *Body Image: A Handbook of Theory, Research, and Clinical Practice*, 74–82.

Lichtenstein, P., Carlström, E., Råstam, M., Gillberg, C., & Anckarsäter, H. (2010). The genetics of autism spectrum disorders and related neuropsychiatric disorders in childhood. *American Journal of Psychiatry*, 167(11), 1357–1363. doi: 10.1176/appi.ajp.2010.10020223. Epub 2010 Aug 4. PMID: 20686188.

de Lijster, J. M., Dieleman, G. C., Utens, E. M. W. J., Dierckx, B., Wierenga, M., Verhulst, F. C., & Legerstee, J. S. (2018). Social and academic functioning in adolescents with anxiety disorders: a systematic review. *Journal of Affective Disorders*, 230, 108–117. doi: 10.1016/j.jad.2018.01.008. Epub 2018 Jan 31. PMID: 29407534.

Lewis, G., Rice, F., Harold, G. T., Collishaw, S., & Thapar, A. (2011). Investigating environmental links between parent depression and child depressive/anxiety symptoms using an assisted conception design. *Journal of the American Academy of Child & Adolescent Psychiatry*, 50(5), 451–459.

Lim, L., Hart, H., Mehta, M. A., Simmons, A., Mirza, K., & Rubia, K. (2015). Neural correlates of error processing in young people With a history of severe childhood abuse: an fMRI study. *American Journal of Psychiatry*, 172(9), 892–900. https://doi.org/10.1176/appi.ajp.2015.14081042.

Lim, L., Radua, J., & Rubia, K. (2014). Gray matter abnormalities in childhood maltreatment: a voxel-wise meta-analysis. *American Journal of Psychiatry*, 171(8), 854–863. https://doi.org/10.1176/appi.ajp.2014.13101427.

Lin, H., Katsovich, L., Ghebremichael, M., et al. (2007). Psychosocial stress predicts future symptom severities in children and adolescents with Tourette syndrome and/or obsessive-compulsive disorder. *Journal of Child Psychology and Psychiatry*, 48(2), 157–166. https://doi.org/10.1111/j.1469-7610.2006.01687.x.

Linehan, Marsha M. (1993). *Skills training manual for treating borderline personality disorder*. New York: The Guildford Press.

Littman, L. (2018). Rapid-onset gender dysphoria in adolescents and young adults: a study of parental reports. *PLOS ONE*, 13(8), e0202330.

Lloyd, S. (2016). *Improving Sensory Processing in Traumatized Children: Practical Ideas to Help Your Child's Movement, Coordination and Body Awareness.* London: Jessica Kingsley.

LoBue, V., Pérez-Edgar, K., & Buss, K. (2019). *Handbook of Emotional Development.* Springer.

Loeber, R., Burke, J. D., Lahey, B. B., Winters, A., & Zera, M. (2000). Oppositional defiant and conduct disorder: a review of the past 10 years, Part I. *Journal of the American Academy of Child and Adolescent Psychiatry*, 39(12), 1468–1484.

Long, P., Forehand, R., Wierson, M., & Morgan, A. (1994). Does parent training with young noncompliant children have long-term effects? *Behaviour Research and Therapy*, 32(1), 101–107.

Lonigan, C. J., Phillips, B. M., Wilson, S. B., & Allan, N. P. (2011). Temperament and anxiety in children and adolescents. In: W. K. Silverman and A. P. Field (Eds.), *Anxiety Disorders in Children and Adolescents*, 198–224. Cambridge: Cambridge University Press.

Lorenz, K. (1979). *The Year of the Greylag Goose.* New York: Harcourt Brace Janovich.

Lougher, L. (2000). *Occupational Therapy for Child and Adolescent Mental Health* (1st edition). College of Occupational Therapists. www.cot.co.uk.

Luby, J., Lenze, S., & Tillman, R. (2012). A novel early intervention for preschool depression: findings from a pilot randomized controlled trial. *Journal of Child Psychology and Psychiatry, and Allied Disciplines*, 53(3), 313–322.

Luman, M., Sergeant, J. A., Knol, D. L., & Oosterlaan, J. (2010). Impaired decision making in oppositional defiant disorder related to altered psychophysiological responses to reinforcement. *Biological Psychiatry*, 68(4), 337–344.

Lynam, D. R., & Gudonis, L. (2005). The development of psychopathy. *Annual Review of Clinical Psychology*, 1, 381–407.

MacDonald, D. E., McFarlane, T. L., & Olmsted, M. P. (2014). "Diagnostic shift " from eating disorder not otherwise specified to bulimia nervosa using DSM-5 criteria: a clinical comparison with DSM-IV bulimia. *Eating Behaviors*, 15(1), 60–62.

Magee, W. J., Eaton, W. W., Wittchen, H. U., McGonagle, K. A., & Kessler, R. C. (1996). Agoraphobia, simple phobia, and social phobia in the National Comorbidity Survey. *Archives of General Psychiatry*, 53(2), 159–168. doi: 10.1001/archpsyc.1996.01830020077009. PMID: 8629891.

Main, M., Goldwyn, R., & Hesse, E. (2002). *Adult Attachment Scoring and Classification Systems*, Version 7.0. University of California at Berkeley: Unpublished manuscript.

Malchiodi, C., & Crenshaw, D. (2014). *Creative Arts and Play Therapy.* Guildford.

Malhi, G. S., Morris, G., Hamilton, A., Outhred, T., & Mannie, Z. (2017). Is "early intervention" in bipolar disorder what it claims to be? *Bipolar Disorders*, 19, 627–636. https://doi.org/10.1111/bdi.12576

Mannuzza, S., Klein, R. G., Bessler, A., Malloy, P., & LaPadula, M. (1993). Adult outcome of hyperactive boys: educational achievement, occupational rank, and psychiatric status. *Archives of General Psychiatry*, 50(7), 565–576.

March, J. S., & Mulle, K. (1998). *OCD in Children and Adolescents: A Cognitive-Behavioral Treatment Manual.* Guilford Press.

Marco, R., Miranda, A., Schlotz, W., Melia, A., Mulligan, A., Müller, U., ... Medad, S. (2009). Delay and reward choice in ADHD: an experimental test of the role of delay aversion. *Neuropsychology*, 23(3), 367.

Marsh, A. A., et al. (2008). Reduced amygdala response to fearful expressions in children and adolescents with callous-unemotional traits and disruptive behavior disorders. *American Journal of Psychiatry*, 165(6), 712–720.

Mataix-Cols, D., Isomura, K., Perez-Vigil, A., Chang, Z., Ruck, C., Larsson, K. J., ... Lichtenstein, P. (2015). Familial risks of Tourette syndrome and chronic tic disorders a population-based cohort study. *Jama Psychiatry*, 72(8), 787–793. doi: 10.1001/jamapsychiatry.2015.0627

Matthijssen, A. M., Dietrich, A., Bierens, M., Kleine, Deters R., van de Loo-Neus, G. H. H., van den Hoofdakker, B. J., Buitelaar, J. K., & Hoekstra, P. J. (2019). Continued benefits of methylphenidate in ADHD after 2 years in clinical practice: a randomized placebo-controlled discontinuation study. *American Journal of Psychiatry*, 176(9), 754–762.

Mauriac, F. (1952). *The Desert of Love*. New York: Bantam.

Mayville, S., Katz, R. C., Gipson, M. T., & Cabral, K. (1999). Assessing the prevalence of body dysmorphic disorder in an ethnically diverse group of adolescents. *Journal of Child and Family Studies*, 8(3), 357–362.

McAdams, T. A., Rijsdijk, F. V., Neiderhiser, J. M., Narusyte, J., Shaw, D. S., Natsuaki, M. N., Spotts, E. L., Ganiban, J. M., Reiss, D., Leve, L. D., Lichtenstein, P., & Eley, T. C. (2015). The relationship between parental depressive symptoms and offspring psychopathology: evidence from a children-of-twins study and an adoption study. *Psychological Medicine*, 45(12), 2583–2594. doi: 10.1017/S0033291715000501. Epub 2015 May 21. PMID: 25994116; PMCID: PMC4523449.

McClellan, J., Stock, S.; & American Academy of Child and Adolescent Psychiatry (AACAP) Committee on Quality Issues (CQI) (2013). Practice parameter for the assessment and treatment of children and adolescents with schizophrenia. *Journal of the American Academy of Child and Adolescent Psychiatry*, 52(9), 976–990.

McDougall, T. (2006). *Nursing Children and Young People with Learning Disabilities and Mental Health Problems in T. McDougall Child and Adolescent Mental Health Nursing*. Oxford: Blackwell Publishing.

McGee, R., Makinson, T., Williams, S., Simpson, A., & Silva, P. A. (1984). A longitudinal study of enuresis from five to nine years. *Journal of Paediatrics and Child Health*, 20, 39–42. https://doi.org/10.1111/j.1440-1754.1984.tb00034.x

McGuffin, P., Rijsdijk, F., Andrew, M., Sham, P., Katz, R., & Cardno, A. (2003). The heritability of bipolar affective disorder and the genetic relationship to unipolar depression. *Archives of General Psychiatry*, 60(5), 497. https://doi.org/10.1001/archpsyc.60.5.497.

McGuire, J. F., Piacentini, J., Brennan, E. A., Lewin, A. B., Murphy, T. K., Small, B. J., & Storch, E. A. (2014). A meta-analysis of behavior therapy for Tourette syndrome. *Journal of Psychiatric Research*, 50, 106–112. https://doi.org/10.1016/j.jpsychires.2013.12.009.

McKay, Matthew, Wood, Jeffrey C., & Brantley, J. (2007). *The Dialetical Behavior Therapy Skills Workbook*. Oakland: New Harbinger Publications, Inc.

McKay-Brown, L., McGrath, R., Dalton, L., Graham, L., Smith, A., Ring, J., & Eyre, K. (2019). Reengagement with education: a multidisciplinary home school clinic approach developed in Australia for school refusing youth. *Cognitive and Behavioral Practice*, 26(1), 92–106.

McLaughlin, K. A. (2016). Future directions in childhood adversity and youth psychopathology. *Journal of Clinical Child and Adolescent Psychology* , 45(3), 361–382.

McLaughlin, K. A., Greif, Green J., Gruber, M. J., Sampson, N. A., Zaslavsky, A. M., & Kessler, R. C. (2012). Childhood adversities and first onset of psychiatric disorders in a national sample of US adolescents. *Archives of General Psychiatry*, 69(11), 1151–1160. doi: 10.1001/archgenpsychiatry.2011.2277. PMID: 23117636; PMCID: PMC3490224.

McLaughlin, K. A., Sheridan, M. A., Winter, W., Fox, N. A., Zeanah, C. H., & Nelson, C. A. (2014). Widespread reductions in cortical thickness following severe early-life deprivation: a neurodevelopmental pathway to attention-deficit/hyperactivity disorder. *Biological Psychiatry*, 76(8), 629–638. https://doi.org/10.1016/j.biopsych.2013.08.016.

McLeod, S. (2015). *Skinner-Operant Conditioning*. Retrieved from. Retrieved April 2020 - academia.edu

McNicholas, F., Adamson, M., McNamara, N., et al. (2015). Who is in the transition gap? Transition from CAMHS to AMHS in the Republic of Ireland. *Irish Journal of Psychological Medicine*, 32, 61–69.

Meadows, S. (1992). *Understanding Child Development*. Hove: Routledge.

Medical Act. (1983). http://www.legislation.gov.uk/ukpga/1983/54/contents

Medicine AAoS. (2014). *International Classification of Sleep Disorders* (3rd edition). American Academy of Sleep Medicine.

Mehta, M. A., Gore-Langton, E., Golembo, N., Colvert, E., Williams, S. C. R., & Sonuga-Barke, E. J. S. (2010). Hyporesponsive reward anticipation in the Basal Ganglia following severe institutional deprivation early in life. *Journal of Cognitive Neuroscience*, 22(10), 2316–2325. https://doi.org/10.1162/jocn.2009.21394.

Meltzer, H., Gatward, R., Goodman, R., & Ford, T. (2003). Mental health of children and adolescents in Great Britain. *International Review of Psychiatry*, 15(1–2), 185–187. doi: 10.1080/0954026021000046155. PMID: 12745331.

Meltzer, L. J., & Mindell, J. A. (2014). Systematic review and meta-analysis of behavioral interventions for pediatric insomnia. *Journal of Pediatric Psychology*, 39(8), 932–948. Meltzer, L. J., & Mindell, J. A. (2007). Relationship between child sleep disturbances and maternal sleep, mood, and parenting stress: a pilot study. *Journal of Family Psychology* , 21(1), 67–73.

Mennin, D., Biederman, J., Mick, E., & Faraone, S. V. (2000). Towards defining a meaningful anxiety phenotype for research in ADHD children. *Journal of Attention Disorders*, 3(4), 192–199.

Mental Health Foundation (2006). *Truth Hurts: Report of the National Inquiry into Self-Harm among Young People*. London: Mental Health Foundation. https://doi.org/10.1017/S0033291715000501.

Mental health of children and young people in England (2017). Emotional Disorders.

Merikangas, K. R., He, J. P., Burstein, M., et al. (2010). Lifetime prevalence of mental disorders in US adolescents: results from the National Comorbidity Survey Replication-Adolescent Supplement (NCS-A). *Journal of the American Academy of Child and Adolescent Psychiatry*, 49(10), 980–989.

Van Meter, A. R., Burke, C., Youngstrom, E. A., Faedda, G. L., & Correll, C. U. (2016). The bipolar prodrome: meta-analysis of symptom prevalence prior to initial or recurrent mood episodes. *Journal of the American Academy of Child and Adolescent Psychiatry*, 55(7), 543–555. doi: 10.1016/j.jaac.2016.04.017. Epub 2016 May 11. PMID: 27343882.

Mick, E., Santangelo, S. L., Wypij, D., & Biederman, J. (2000). Impact of maternal depression on ratings of comorbid depression in adolescents with attention-deficit/hyperactivity disorder. *Journal of the American Academy of Child and Adolescent Psychiatry*, 39(3), 314–319.

Mill, J., & Petronis, A. (2008). Pre-and peri-natal environmental risks for attention-deficit hyperactivity disorder (ADHD): the potential role of epigenetic processes in mediating susceptibility. *Journal of Child Psychology and Psychiatry, and Allied Disciplines*, 49(10), 1020–1030.

Miller, M., Musser, E. D., Young, G. S., Olson, B., Steiner, R. D., & Nigg, J. T. (2019). Sibling recurrence risk and cross-aggregation of attention-deficit/hyperactivity disorder and autism spectrum disorder. *JAMA Pediatrics*, 173(2), 147. https://doi.org/10.1001/jamapediatrics.2018.4076.

Miller-Lewis, L. R., Baghurst, P. A., Sawyer, M. G., Prior, M. R., Clark, J. J., Arney, F. M., & Carbone, J. A. (2006). Early childhood externalising behaviour problems: child, parenting, and family-related predictors over time. *Journal of Abnormal Child Psychology*, 34(6), 886–901.

Milrod, C. (2014). How young is too young: ethical concerns in Genital surgery of the transgender MTF adolescent. *Journal of Sexual Medicine*, 11(2), 338–346.

MindEd www.minded.org.uk.

Mindell, J. A., Bartle, A., Wahab, N. A., et al. (2011). Sleep education in medical school curriculum: a glimpse across countries. *Sleep Medicine*, 12(9), 928–931.

Mindell, J. A., Meltzer, L. J., Carskadon, M. A., & Chervin, R. D. (2009). Developmental aspects of sleep hygiene: findings from the 2004 National Sleep Foundation Sleep in America Poll. *Sleep Medicine*, 10(7), 771–779.

Mindell, J. A., & Owens, J. A. (2015). *Sleep in the Pediatric Practice in A Clinical Guide to Pediatric Sleep*. South Holland, Netherlands: Wolters Kluwer.

Mitchell, A. J., Chan, M., Bhatti, H., Halton, M., Grassi, L., Johansen, C., & Meader, N. (2011). Prevalence of depression, anxiety, and adjustment disorder in oncological, haematological, and palliative-care settings: a meta-analysis of 94 interview-based studies. *The Lancet Oncology*, 12(2), 160–174.

Moffitt, T. E., Caspi, A., Dickson, N., Silva, P., & Stanton, W. (1996). Childhood-onset versus adolescent-onset antisocial conduct problems in males: natural history from ages 3 to 18 years. *Development and Psychopathology*, 8(2), 399–424.

Moffitt, T. E., Harrington, H., Caspi, A., Kim-Cohen, J., Goldberg, D., Gregory, A. M., & Poulton, R. (2007). Depression and generalized anxiety disorder: cumulative and sequential comorbidity in a birth cohort followed prospectively to age 32 years. *Archives of General Psychiatry*, 64(6), 651–660.

Moffitt, T. E., & Scott, S. (2008). Conduct disorders of childhood and adolescence. *Rutter's Child and Adolescent Psychiatry*, 5, 543–564.

Mohr, C., & Schneider, S. (2013). Anxiety disorders. *European Child and Adolescent Psychiatry*, 22(Supplement 1), S17–S22. https://doi.org/10.1007/s00787-012-0356-8.

Molina, B. S., Hinshaw, S. P., Swanson, J. M., et al. (2009).The MTA at 8 years: prospective follow-up of children treated for combined-type ADHD in a multisite study. *Journal of the American Academy of Child and Adolescent Psychiatry*, 48(5), 484–500.

Möller, E. L., Nikolić, M., Majdandžić, M., & Bögels, S. M. (2016). Associations between maternal and paternal parenting behaviours, anxiety and its precursors in early childhood: a meta-analysis. *Clinical Psychology Review*, 45, 17–33. https://doi.org/10.1016/j.cpr.2016.03.002.

Moncrieff, J., & Timimi, S. (2013). The social and cultural construction of psychiatric knowledge: an analysis of NICE guidelines on depression and ADHD. *Anthropology and Medicine*, 20(1), 59–71.

Montano, C. B., & Young, J. (2012). Discontinuity in the transition from pediatric to adult health care for patients with attention-deficit/hyperactivity disorder. *Postgraduate Medical*, 124, 23–32.

Moreno, C., Sánchez-Queija, I., Muñoz-Tinoco, V., et al. (2009). Cross-national associations between parent and peer communication and psychological complaints. *International Journal of Public Health*, 54(2)(Supplement 2), 235–242.

Moreno-Alcázar, A., Treen, D., Valiente-Gómez, A., Sio-Eroles, A., Pérez, V., Amann, B. L., & Radua, J. (2017). Efficacy of eye movement desensitization and reprocessing in children and adolescent with post-traumatic stress disorder: a meta-analysis of randomized controlled trials. *Frontiers in Psychology*, 8, 1750. https://doi.org/10.3389/fpsyg.2017.01750.

Morrell, J., & Murray, L. (2003). Parenting and the development of conduct disorder and hyperactive symptoms in childhood: a prospective longitudinal study from 2 months to 8 years. *Journal of Child Psychology and Psychiatry, and Allied Disciplines*, 44(4), 489–508.

Mul, D., & Hughes, I. (2008). The use of GnRH agonists in precocious puberty. *European Journal of Endocrinology*, 159(Supplement 1), S3–S8.

Müller-Vahl, K. R., Loeber, G., Kotsiari, A., Müller-Engling, L., & Frieling, H. (2017). Gilles de la Tourette syndrome is associated with hypermethylation of the dopamine D2 receptor gene. *Journal of Psychiatric Research*, 86, 1–8. https://doi.org/10.1016/j.jpsychires.2016.11.004.

Munro, E. (2011). *The Munro Review of Child Protection: Final Report. A Child-Centred System.* London: Department for Education.

Muris, P., & Ollendick, T. H. (2015). Children who are anxious in silence: a review on selective mutism, the new anxiety disorder in DSM-5. *Clinical Child and Family Psychology Review*, 18(2), 151–169. https://doi.org/10.1007/s10567-015-0181-y.

Muris, P. L., Merckelbach, H., Gadet, B., & Moulaert, V. (2000). Fears, worries, and scary dreams in 4-to 12-year-old children: their content, developmental pattern, and origins. *Journal of Clinical Child Psychology*, 29(1), 43–52. Https://doi.org/10.1207/S15374424jccp2901_5.

Murphy, T. K., Lewin, A. B., Storch, E. A., Stock, S., & American Academy of, C., & Adolescent Psychiatry Committee on Quality, I. (2013). Practice parameter for the assessment and treatment of children and adolescents with tic disorders. *Journal of the American Academy of Child & Adolescent Psychiatry*, 52(12), 1341–1359. https://doi.org/10.1016/j.jaac.2013.09.015.

Music, G. (2011). *Nurturing Natures—Attachment and Children.' Rturing Natures—Attachment and Childrenescent.* East Sussex: Psychology Press.

My Asperger Child. www.MyAspergerChild.com/Help for parents with Asperger children developing social skills at home and school (Accessed March 28 2011).

Nahata, L., Tishelman, A. C., Caltabellotta, N. M., & Quinn, G. P. (2017). Low fertility preservation utilization among transgender youth. *Journal of Adolescent Health* , 61(1), 40–44.
Nakao, T., Radua, J., Rubia, K., & Mataix-Cols, D. (2011). Gray matter volume abnormalities in ADHD: voxel-based meta-analysis exploring the effects of age and stimulant medication. *American Journal of Psychiatry*, 168(11), 1154–1163.
National Audit Office (2018). *Improving Children's' and Young Peoples' Mental Health Services.* London.
National Confidential Inquiry into Suicide and Safety in Mental Health Access (February 2020).
National Institute for Clinical Excellence (2004). Self-harm: the short-term physical and psychological management and secondary prevention of self-harm in primary and secondary care.
Nelson, C., Fox, N., & Zeanah, C. (2014). *Romania's Abandoned Children.* Cambridge, MA: Harvard University Press.
Nelson, R. J., & Trainor, B. C. (2007). Neural mechanisms of aggression. *Nature Reviews. Neuroscience*, 8(7), 536–546.
Neuropsychiatric Genetics: the Official Publication of the International Society of Psychiatric Genetics, 168(8), 730–738. https://doi.org/10.1002/ajmg.b.32378.
Newman, M. G., Llera, S. J., Erickson, T. M., Przeworski, A., & Castonguay, L. G. (2013). Worry and generalized anxiety disorder: a review and theoretical synthesis of evidence on nature, etiology, mechanisms, and treatment. *Annual Review of Clinical Psychology*, 9 275–297. doi: 10.1146/annurev-clinpsy-050212-185544. PMID: 23537486; PMCID: PMC4964851.
NHS Advisory Service. (1986). *Bridges Over Troubled Waters: A Report from the NHS Health Advisory Service on Services for Disturbed Adolescents.* NHS Advisory Service.
NHS Digital (2018) National study of Health and Wellbeing: children and Young People. London. NHS England (2019) NHS Long-term Plan. London. National CAMHS Review 2008.
NHS Digital. 2019. *Psychological Therapies, Annual Report on the Use of IAPT Services 2018-19.* London: NHS Digital.
NHS England (2014). Child and adolescent mental health services tier 4 report.
NHS England (2016). Five Year Forward View for Mental Health. London.
NHS England (2017). Five Year Forward View for Mental Health: One Year on.
NHS England (2019). NHS Long-Term Plan. London.
NHS Mental Health Implementation Plan 2019/20–2023/24: https://www.longtermplan.nhs.uk/wp-content/uploads/2019/07/nhs-mental-health-implementation-plan-2019-20-2023-24.pdf
Niarchou, M., Martin, J., Thapar, A., Owen, M. J., & van den Bree, M. B. M. (2015). The clinical presentation of attention deficit-hyperactivity disorder (ADHD) in children with 22q11.2 deletion syndrome. *American Journal of Medical Genetics,. Part B.*
NICE. https://www.nice.org.uk/guidance/ng134
NICE. (2011). Guidelines on longer management of Self-harm Self Harm.
NICE (2016). Transition from Children's to Adults' Services for Young People Using Health or Social Care Services.
NICE 2018 guidelines for ADHD. Available at nice.org.uk/guidance/ng87 (New Forest Parent Programme cited on page 107 and 123).
NICE guidelines for treatment of Nocturnal Enuresis May 2010.
NICE (2010). *Guidelines Constipation in Children and Young People May 2010.* London: NICE.
NICE. (2010). *NICE Guidelines for Treatment of Nocturnal Enuresis May 2010.* London: NICE.
NICE. Psychosis and schizophrenia in children and young people: recognition and management. Vol. NICE guideline CG155 2013, www.nice.org.uk/CG155.
NICE. (2019). *Depression in Children and Young People: Identification and Management.* London.
Nicholls, D., & Becker, A. (2020). Food for thought: bringing eating disorders out of the shadows. *The British Journal of Psychiatry* , 216(2), 67–68.
Nicole Petrowski, Claudia Cappa, & Peter Gross (2017). Estimating the number of children in formal alternative care: challenges and results. *Child Abuse & Neglect*, 70, 388–398, ISSN 0145-2134.

Nixon, G. M., Thompson, J. M., Han, D. Y., et al. (2009). Falling asleep: the determinants of sleep latency. *Archives of Disease in Childhood*, 94(9), 686–689.

Nock, M. K., & Kazdin, A. E. (2001). Parent expectancies for child therapy: assessment and relation to participation in treatment. *Journal of Child and Family Studies*, 10(2), 155–180.

Nock, M. K., Kazdin, A. E., Hiripi, E., & Kessler, R. C. (2007). Lifetime prevalence, correlates, and persistence of oppositional defiant disorder: results from the National Comorbidity Survey Replication. *Journal of Child Psychology and Psychiatry*, 48(7) 703–713.

Norman, R. E., Byambaa, M., De, R., Butchart, A., Scott, J., & Vos, T. (2012). The long-term health consequences of child physical abuse, emotional abuse, and neglect: a systematic review and meta-analysis. *PLoS Medicine*, 9(11), e1001349. doi: 10.1371/journal.pmed.1001349. Epub 2012 Nov 27. PMID: 23209385; PMCID: PMC3507962.

Norton, P. J., & Paulus, D. J. (2017). Transdiagnostic models of anxiety disorder: theoretical and empirical underpinnings. *Clinical Psychology Review*, 56, 122–137. doi: 10.1016/j.cpr.2017.03.004. Epub 2017 Mar 27. PMID: 28450042.

Nottingham City Council (2019). Nottingham Youth Justice Service Youth Justice Plan 2017-20: 2019-20 Update, pp.3.

Nottingham Insight. (2019). Indices of Deprivation [online] Available at https://www.nottinghaminsight.org.uk/themes/deprivation-and-poverty/indices-of-deprivation-2019/ [Accessed February 19th, 2020]

Nowicki, S., & Carton, J. (1993). The measurement of emotional intensity from facial expressions. *Journal of Social Psychology*, 133(5), 749–750. doi: 10.1080/00224545.1993.9713934

Nyhan, W. L. (1972). Behavioural Phenotypes in Organic Brain Disease. Presidential address to the Society for Pediatric Research, May 1, 1971. Paediatric Research 6. In G. O'Brien and W. Yule (Eds.), *Behavioural Phenotypes (Clinics in Developmental Medicine No. 138)*, 1–9. London: Cambridge University Press.

Nyhan, W. L. (1976). Behavior in the Lesch-Nyhan syndrome. *Journal of Autism and Childhood Schizophrenia*, 6(3), 235–252.

Oar, E. L., Farrell, L. J., & Ollendick, T. H. (2015). One session treatment for specific phobias: an adaptation for paediatric blood-injection-injury phobia in youth. *Clinical Child and Family Psychology Review*, 18(4), 370–394. https://doi.org/10.1007/s10567-015-0189-3. PMID: 26374227.

O'Brien, C. (2011). Disorganised and in Care. British Association of Counselling and Psychotherapy—Children young people and families Journal.

O'Brien, C. (2017). Self, Other and the We. British Association of Counselling and Psychotherapy—Children young people and families Journal.

O'Donovan, M. C., & Owen, M. J. (2016). The implications of the shared genetics of psychiatric disorders. *Nature Medicine*, 22(11), 1214–1219. https://doi.org/10.1038/nm.4196.

O'Flynn, N. (2011). Nocturnal enuresis in children and young people: NICE clinical guideline. *British Journal of General Practice* , 61(586), 360–362.

Ogden, T., & Hagen, K. A. (2018). *Adolescent Mental Health: Prevention and Intervention.* Routledge.

Ogundele, M., & Omenaka, I. (2012). An audit of transitional care for adolescents with ADHD in a North West England district. *Archives of Disease in Childhood*, 97(Suppl. 1), A129.

O'Herlihy, A., et al. (2001). *National Inpatient Child and Adolescent Psychiatry Study London: College Research Unit of the Royal College of Psychiatrists and the Department of Health.*

Ohman, A. (2005). The role of the amygdala in human fear: automatic detection of threat. *Psychoneuroendocrinology*, 30(10), 953–958. https://doi.org/10.1016/j.psyneuen.2005.03.019.

Ollendick, T. H., Öst, L. G., Ryan, S. M., Capriola, N. N., & Reuterskiöld, L. (2017). Harm beliefs and coping expectancies in youth with specific phobias. *Behaviour Research and Therapy*, 91, 51–57. https://doi.org/10.1016/j.brat.2017.01.007.

Olsen, D. (2000). Cicumplex model of marital and family systems. *Journal of Family Therapy* 22, 144–167.

Olson-Kennedy, J., Chan, Y.-M., Garofalo, R., et al. (2019). Impact of early medical treatment for transgender youth: protocol for the longitudinal, observational Trans Youth Care Study. *JMIR Research Protocols*, 8(7), e14434.

Olweus, D. (1997). Bully/victim problems in school: facts and intervention. *European Journal of Psychology of Education*, 12(4), 495.

Osborne, C., & Burton, S. (2014). Emotional Literacy Support Assistants' views on supervision provided by educational psychologists: what EPs can learn from group supervision. *Educational Psychology in Practice*, 30(2), 139–155.

Osland, S. T., Steeves, T. D., & Pringsheim, T. (2018). Pharmacological treatment for attention deficit hyperactivity disorder (ADHD) in children with comorbid tic disorders. *Cochrane Database of Systematic Reviews*, 6, CD007990. Https://doi.org/10.1002/14651858.CD007990.pub3.

Otowa, T., Hek, K., Lee, M., et al. (2016). Meta-analysis of genome-wide association studies of anxiety disorders [published correction appears in Mol Psychiatry. 2016 Oct;21(10):1485]. *Molecular Psychiatry*, 21(10), 1391–1399. doi: 10.1038/mp.2015.197

Ougrin, D., Zundel, T., Kyriakopoulos, M., Banarsee, R., Stahl, D., & Taylor, E. (2012). Adolescents with suicidal and nonsuicidal self-harm: clinical characteristics and response to therapeutic assessment. *Psychological Assessment*, 24(1), 11.

Owen, M. J., Sawa, A., & Mortensen, P. B. (2016). Schizophrenia. *The Lancet*, 388(10039), 86–97. https://doi.org/10.1016/S0140-6736(15)01121-6.

Owens, J. A., & Witmans, M. (2004). Sleep problems. *Current Problems in Pediatric and Adolescent Health Care*, 34(4), 154–179.

Ozer, E. J., Best, S. R., Lipsey, T. L., & Weiss, D. S. J. P. b. (2003). Predictors of posttraumatic stress disorder and symptoms in adults: a meta-analysis, 129(1), 52.

Paavonen, E. J., Porkka-Heiskanen, T., & Lahikainen, A. R. (2009). Sleep quality, duration and behavioral symptoms among 5–6-year-old children. *European Child and Adolescent Psychiatry*, 18(12), 747–754.

Pakman, M. (2000). Disciplinary knowledge: postmodernism and globalization: a call for Donald Schoen's 'reflective turn' for the mental health professions. *Cybernetics and Human Knowing*, 7, 105–126.

Panksepp, J. (2004). *Affective Neuroscience: The Foundations of Humane and Animal Emotions.* Oxford: Oxford University Press.

Papadopoulos, I. (2006). The Papadopoulos, Tilki and Taylor model of developing Cultural Competence. In: I. Papadopoulos (Ed.), *Transcultural Health and Social Care: Developing Culturally Competent Practitioners.* Oxford: Elsevier.

Pappert, E. J., Goetz, C. G., Louis, E. D., Blasucci, L., & Leurgans, S. (2003). Objective assessments of longitudinal outcome in Gilles de la Tourette's syndrome. *Neurology*, 61(7), 936–940. doi: http://dx.doi.org/10.1212/01.WNL.0000086370.10186.7C

Pardiñas, A. F., Holmans, P., Pocklington, A. J., et al. (2018). Common schizophrenia alleles are enriched in mutation-intolerant genes and in regions under strong background selection. *Nature Genetics*, 50(3), 381–389. https://doi.org/10.1038/s41588-018-0059-2.

Passamonti, L., Fairchild, G., Goodyer, I. M., Hurford, G., Hagan, C. C., Rowe, J. B., & Calder, A. J. (2010). Neural abnormalities in early-onset and adolescence-onset conduct disorder. *Archives of General Psychiatry*, 67(7), 729–738.

Patel, D. R., Feucht, C., Brown, K., & Ramsay, J. (2018). Pharmacological treatment of anxiety disorders in children and adolescents: a review for practitioners. *Translational Pediatrics*, 7(1), 23–35. doi: 10.21037/tp.2017.08.05

Patterson, G. R. (1982). *Coercive Family Process.* Eugene, OR: Castalia.

Payne, M. (2005). *The Origins of Social Work, Continuity and Change.* Basingstoke: Palgrave Macmillan.

Pentecost, D. (2000). *Parenting the ADD Child.* London: Jessica Kingsley Publishers.

Percy, R., Creswell, C., Garner, M., O'Brien, D., & Murray, L. (2016). Parents' verbal communication and childhood anxiety: a systematic review. *Clinical Child and Family Psychology Review*, 19(1),

55–75. ISSN 1573 2827 doi: https://doi.org/10.1007/s1056701501982 Available at http://centaur.reading.ac.uk/46745/

Perry. (2016). *Early Childhood Development: Concepts, Methodologies, Tools, and Applications.* Management Association, Information Resources.

Peterson, R. L., Boada, R., McGrath, L. M., Willcutt, E. G., Olson, R. K., & Pennington, B. F. (2016). Cognitive prediction of reading, math, and attention shared and unique influences. *Journal of Learning Disabilities*, 0022219415618500.

Pettersson, E., Sjölander, A., Almqvist, C., Anckarsäter, H., D'Onofrio, B. M., Lichtenstein, P., & Larsson, H. (2015). Birth weight as an independent predictor of ADHD symptoms: a within-twin pair analysis. *Journal of Child Psychology and Psychiatry*, 56(4), 453–459.

Phillips, K. A., Atala, K. D., & Albertini, R. S. (1995). Case study: body dysmorphic disorder in adolescents. *Journal of the American Academy of Child & Adolescent Psychiatry*, 34(9), 1216–1220.

Pickering, L., Hadwin, J. A., & Kovshoff, H. (2020). The role of peers in the development of social anxiety in adolescent girls: a systematic review. *Adolescent Research Review*, 5, 341–362. https://doi.org/10.1007/s40894-019-00117-x

Pine, D. S., & Monk, C. S. (2009). The development and cognitive neuroscience of anxiety. In C. A. Nelson, & M. Luciana (Eds.), (2008). *Handbook of Developmental Cognitive Neuroscience* (pp. 755–770). MIT Press.

Pingault, J.-B., Viding, E., Galéra, C., Greven, C. U., Zheng, Y., Plomin, R., & Rijsdijk, F. (2015). Genetic and environmental influences on the developmental course of attention-deficit/hyperactivity disorder symptoms From childhood to adolescence. *JAMA Psychiatry*, 72(7), 651. https://doi.org/10.1001/jamapsychiatry.2015.0469.

Pinquart, M., & Kauser, R. (2018). Do the associations of parenting styles with behavior problems and academic achievement vary by culture? Results from a meta-analysis. *Cultural Diversity and Ethnic Minority Psychology*, 24(1), 75–100. https://doi.org/10.1037/cdp0000149

Piotrowski, A. (2015). Conduct disorder: a result of the environment. *Debating Diagnosis*, 111.

Plomin, R. (1994). *Genetics and Experience: The Interplay between Nature and Nurture.* Sage Publications, Inc.

Plomin, R. (1994). *Genetics and Experience: The Interplay between Nature and Nurture.* Sage Publications, Inc.

Polanczyk, G. V., Willcutt, E. G., Salum, G. A., Kieling, C., & Rohde, L. A. (2014). ADHD prevalence estimates across three decades: an updated systematic review and meta-regression analysis. *International Journal of Epidemiology*, 43(2), 434–442.

Polderman, T. J., Benyamin, B., de Leeuw, C. A., Sullivan, P. F., van Bochoven, A., Visscher, P. M., & Posthuma, D. (2015). Meta-analysis of the heritability of human traits based on fifty years of twin studies. *Nature Genetics*, 47(7), 702–709. doi: 10.1038/ng.3285

Posada, G., & Jacobs, A. (2001). Child-mother attachment relationships and culture. *American Psychologist*, 56(10), 821–822.

Posner, J. (2020). Burden of ADHD. *Epidemiology.*

Poteat, V. P., Scheer, J. R., & Mereish, E. H. (2014). Factors affecting academic achievement among sexual minority and gender-variant youth. *Advances in Child Development and Behavior*, 47, 261–300.

Pottick, K. J., Bilder, S., Vander Stoep, A., et al. (2008). US patterns of mental health service utilization for transition-age youth and young adults. *Journal of Behavioral Health Services & Research*, 35, 373–389.

Power, R. A., Tansey, K. E., Buttenschøn, H. N., et al. (2017). genome-wide association for major depression through age at onset stratification: major depressive disorder working group of the psychiatric genomics consortium. *Biological Psychiatry*, 81(4), 325–335. https://doi.org/10.1016/j.biopsych.2016.05.010.

Preamble to the Constitution of WHO as adopted by the International Health Conference, New York, 19 June–22 July 1946; signed on 22 July 1946 by the representatives of 61 States (Official Records of WHO, no. 2, p. 100) and entered into force on 7 April 1948.

Prentice, P., & Viner, R. M. (2013). Pubertal timing and adult obesity and cardiometabolic risk in women and men: a systematic review and meta-analysis. *International Journal of Obesity*, 37(8), 1036–1043.

Price, A. M., Wake, M., Ukoumunne, O. C., & Hiscock, H. (2012). Five-year follow-up of harms and benefits of behavioral infant sleep intervention: randomized trial. *Pediatrics*, 130(4), 643–651.

Price, R. A., Kidd, K. K., Cohen, D. J., Pauls, D. L., & Leckman, J. F. (1985). A twin study of Tourette syndrome. *Archives of General Psychiatry*, 42(8), 815–820.

Puckering, C. (2004). Mellow parenting, an intensive intervention to change relationships. *Signal (Bulletin of the World Association for Infant Mental Health)*, 12, 1–5.

Purnell, L. (2005). The Purnell model for cultural competence. *The Journal of Multicultural Nursing & Health*, 11(2), 7–15.

Putwain, D. (2007). Researching academic stress and anxiety in students: some methodological considerations. *British Educational Research Journal*, 33(2), 207–219. https://doi.org/10.1080/01411920701208258

Quach, J., Hiscock, H., Canterford, L., & Wake, M. (2009). Outcomes of child sleep problems over the school-transition period: australian population longitudinal study. *Pediatrics*, 123(5), 1287–1292.

Rangel, L., Garralda, M. E., Levin, M., & Roberts, H. (2000). The course of severe chronic fatigue syndrome in childhood. *Journal of the Royal Society of Medicine*, 93(3), 129–134.

Rapoport, J. L., & Gogtay, N. (2011). Childhood onset schizophrenia: support for a progressive neurodevelopmental disorder. *International Journal of Developmental Neuroscience* , 29(3), 251–258. https://doi.org/10.1016/j.ijdevneu.2010.10.003.

Rasquin, A., Di Lorenzo, C., Forbes, D., Guiraldes, E., Hyams, J. S., Staiano, A., & Walker, L. S. (2006). Childhood functional gastrointestinal disorders: child/adolescent. *Gastroenterology*, 130(5), 1527–1537. doi: 10.1053/j.gastro.2005.08.063. PMID: 16678566; PMCID: PMC7104693.

Reed, P. (2016). Researching taboos: research in play therapy. In Le Vay, E. Cuschieri (Eds.), *Challenges in the Theory and Practice of Play Therapy*. Routledge.

Reid, J. B., & Patterson, G. R. (1989). The development of antisocial behaviour patterns in childhood and adolescence. *European Journal of Personality*, 3(2), 107–119.

Restar, A. J. (2020). Methodological critique of Littman's (2018) parental-respondents accounts of "rapid-onset gender dysphoria". *Archives of Sexual Behavior*, 1–6.

Reynolds, Linda K., O'Koon, Jeffrey H., Papademetriou, Eros, Szczygiel, Sylvia, & Grant, Kathryn E. (2001). Stress and somatic complaints in low-income urban adolescents. *Journal of Youth and Adolescence*, 30(4), 499–514.

Rhee, S. H., & Waldman, I. D. (2002). Genetic and environmental influences on antisocial behavior: a meta-analysis of twin and adoption studies. *Psychological Bulletin*, 128(3), 490.

Rice, F. (2010). Genetics of childhood and adolescent depression: insights into etiological heterogeneity and challenges for future genomic research. *Genome Medicine*, 2(9), 68. https://doi.org/10.1186/gm189.

Rice, F., Harold, G., & Thapar, A. (2002). The genetic aetiology of childhood depression: a review. *Journal of Child Psychology and Psychiatry, and Allied Disciplines*, 43(1), 65–79. https://doi.org/10.1111/1469-7610.00004.

Rice, F., Riglin, L., Thapar, A. K., Heron, J., Anney, R., O'Donovan, M. C., & Thapar, A. (2019). Characterizing developmental trajectories and the role of neuropsychiatric genetic risk variants in early-onset depression. *JAMA Psychiatry*, 76(3), 306. https://doi.org/10.1001/jamapsychiatry.2018.3338.

Ridwan (1982). From Butler, N. R., & Golding, J. (1986). *From Birth to Five: A Study of the Health and Behaviour of Britain's 5 Year Olds*. Oxford, UK: Pergamon.

Riglin, L., Collishaw, S., Richards, A., Thapar, A. K., Maughan, B., O'Donovan, M. C., & Thapar, A. (2017). Schizophrenia risk alleles and neurodevelopmental outcomes in childhood: a population-based cohort study. *The Lancet Psychiatry*, 4(1), 57–62. https://doi.org/10.1016/S2215-0366(16)30406-0.

Riglin, L., Collishaw, S., Richards, A., et al. (2018). The impact of schizophrenia and mood disorder risk alleles on emotional problems: investigating change from childhood to middle age. *Psychological Medicine*, 48(13), 2153–2158. https://doi.org/10.1017/S0033291717003634.

Riglin, L., Collishaw, S., Thapar, A. K., et al. (2016). Association of genetic risk variants With attention-deficit/hyperactivity disorder trajectories in the general population. *JAMA Psychiatry*, 73(12), 1285. https://doi.org/10.1001/jamapsychiatry.2016.2817.

Riley, E. A., Sitharthan, G., Clemson, L., & Diamond, M. (2013). Recognising the needs of gender-variant children and their parents. *Sex Education*, 13(6), 644–659.

Ritschel, Lorie A., Lim, Noriel E., & Stewart, Lindsay M. (2018). Transdiagnositic applications of DBT for adolescents and adults. *American Journal of Psychotherapy*, 69(2).

Rivett, M., & Street, E. (2009). *Family Therapy 100 Key Points and Techniques.* London: Routledge.

Robertson, M. M. (2008). The prevalence and epidemiology of Gilles de la Tourette syndrome. Part 1: the epidemiological and prevalence studies. *Journal of Psychosomatic Research*, 65(5), 461–472. doi: 10.1016/j.jpsychores.2008.03.006

Rogers, C. (1976). *Client Centred Therapy.* London: Constable and Robinson.

Rosenthal, R., Archer, D., Hall, J. A., DiMatteo, M. R., & Rogers, P. L. (1979). Measuring sensitivity to nonverbal communication: the PONS test. In *Nonverbal Behavior*, pp. 67–98. Academic Press.

Routh, C. P., Hill, J. W., Steele, H., Elliot, C. E., & Dewey, M. E. (1995). Maternal attachment status, psychosocial stressors and problem behaviour: follow up Shaffer D., Gould, M. S., Brasic, J., Ambrosini, P., Fisher, P., Bird, H.,

Rust, J., & Smith, A. (2006). How should the effectiveness of Social Stories to modify the behaviour of children on the autistic spectrum be tested?: lessons from the literature. Published March 1, 2006. Research Article. https://doi.org/10.1177/1362361306062019

Rutter, M., Kreppner, J., & Sonuga-Barke, E. (2009). Emanuel miller lecture: attachment insecurity, disinhibited attachment, and attachment disorders: where do research findings leave the concepts? *Journal of Child Psychology and Psychiatry*, 50(5), 529–543.

Ryan, C., Epstein, N., Keitner, G., et al. (2005). *Evaluating and Treating Families* Hove: Routledge.

Ryan, V. (2004). Adapting non-directive play therapy for children with attachment disorders. *Clinical Child Psychology and Psychiatry*, 9(1), 75–87. https://doi.org/10.1177/1359104504039174

Ryan, V., & Wilson, K. (2005). *Play Therapy: A Non-directive Approach for Children and Adolescents.* Baillière Tindall Elsevier.

Rodriguez, A., & Bohlin, G. (2005). Are maternal smoking and stress during pregnancy related to ADHD symptoms in children? *Journal of Child Psychology and Psychiatry, and Allied Disciplines*, 46(3), 246–254.

Rosenthal, Robert (1979). *Sensitivity to Nonverbal Communication: The PONS test.* Baltimore: Johns Hopkins University Press.

Rothbaum, F., Weisz, J., Pott, M., Miyake, K., & Morelli, G. (2000). Attachment and culture: security in the United States and Japan. *American Psychologist*, 55(10), 1093–1104.

Rothman, A. D., & Nowicki, S. Jr. (2004). A measure of the ability to identify emotion in children's tone of voice. *Journal of Non Verbal Behavior*, 28(2), 67–92.

Royal College of Psychiatrists. Sleep problems in childhood and adolescence: for parents, carers and anyone who works with young people (www.rcpsych.ac.uk/healthadvice/parentsandyouthinfo/parentscarers/sleepproblems.aspx).

Rubia, K., Noorloos, J., Smith, A., Gunning, B., & Sergeant, J. (2003). Motor timing deficits in community and clinical boys with hyperactive behavior: the effect of methylphenidate on motor timing. *Journal of Abnormal Child Psychology*, 31(3), 301–313.

Rutter, M. (1993). Resilience: some conceptual considerations. *Journal of Adolescent Health.*

Rutter, M. (1998). Developmental catch-up, and deficit, following adoption after severe global early privation. English and Romanian Adoptees (ERA) Study Team. *Journal of Child Psychology and Psychiatry, and Allied Disciplines*, 39(4), 465–476. https://doi.org/10.1111/1469-7610.00343.

Rutter, M., Tizard, J., Yule, W., Graham, P., & Whitmore, K. (1976). Research report: isle of Wight studies, 1964–1974. *Psychological Medicine*, 6(2), 313–332.

Ryan, C., Russell, S. T., Huebner, R., Diaz, R., & Sanchez, J. (2010). Family acceptance in adolescence and the health of LGBT young adults. *Journal of Child and Adolescent Psychiatric Nursing*, 23(4), 205–213.

Saarni, C. (1999). *The Development of Emotional Competence*. New York: The Guilford Press.

Sadler,K., Vizard,T., Ford,T., et al. (2017). The Mental Health of Children and Young People (MHCYP) Survey NHS Digital (accessed January 8th 2020 at https://digital.nhs.uk).

Salinger, J. M., O'Brien, M. P., Miklowitz, D. J., Marvin, S. E., & Cannon, T. D. (2018). Family communication with teens at clinical high-risk for psychosis or bipolar disorder. *Journal of Family Psychology*, 32(4), 507–516. doi: 10.1037/fam0000393

Sanders, S. J., Neale, B. M., Huang, H., et al. (2017). Whole genome sequencing in psychiatric disorders: the WGSPD consortium. *Nature Neuroscience*, 20(12), 1661–1668. https://doi.org/10.1038/s41593-017-0017-9.

Satterstrom, F. K., Walters, R. K., Singh, T., Wigdor, E. M., Lescai, F., Demontis, D., ... Daly, M. J. (2018). ASD and ADHD have a similar burden of rare protein-truncating variants. *bioRxiv*. https://doi.org/10.1101/277707. http://www.ncbi.nlm.nih.gov/pubmed/277707.

Saunders, K., & Goodwin, G. (2010). *The Course of Bipolar Disorder*. Advances in Psychiatric.

Sayal, K., Prasad, V., Daley, D., Ford, T., & Coghill, D. (2018). ADHD in children and young people: prevalence, care pathways, and service provision. *The Lancet Psychiatry*, 5(2), 175–186.

Schab, D. W., & Trinh, N. H. T. (2004). Do artificial food colors promote hyperactivity in children with hyperactive syndromes? A meta-analysis of double-blind placebo-controlled trials. *Journal of Developmental and Behavioral Pediatrics*, 25(6), 423–434.

Schachar, R., & Tannock, R. (1993). Childhood hyperactivity and psychostimulants: a review of extended treatment studies. *Journal of Child and Adolescent Psychopharmacology*, 3(2), 81–97.

Scharf, J. M., Miller, L. L., Gauvin, C. A., Alabiso, J., Mathews, C. A., & Ben-Shlomo, Y. (2015). Population prevalence of Tourette syndrome: a systematic review and meta-analysis. *Movement Disorders*, 30(2), 221–228. https://doi.org/10.1002/mds.26089.

Schizophrenia Working Group of the Psychiatric Genomics Consortium (2014). Biological insights from 108 schizophrenia-associated genetic loci. *Nature*, 511(7510), 421–427.

Schlander, M., Schwarz, O., Rothenberger, A., & Roessner, V. (2011). Tic disorders: administrative prevalence and co-occurrence with attention-deficit/hyperactivity disorder in a German community sample. *European Psychiatry* , 26(6), 370–374. https://doi.org/. S0924-9338(09)00181-3 [pii].

Schneider & Jones. (2004). Chapter 3. In Geoff Goodman (Ed.), *Transforming the Internal World and Attachment* (Vol. 1, p. 62).

Schnoll, R., Burshteyn, D., & Cea-Aravena, J. (2003). Nutrition in the treatment of attention-deficit hyperactivity disorder: a neglected but important aspect. *Applied Psychophysiology and Biofeedback*, 28(1), 63–75.

Schofield, G., & Simmonds, J. (2011). "Contact for infants subject to care. *Proceedings' Family Law*, 41, 617–622.

Schore, A. N. (2003). *Affect Regulation and Disorders of the Self*. NY: W.F. Norton & Co.

Schultz, D., Izard, C. E., & Bear, G. (2004). Children's emotion processing: relations to emotionality and aggression. *Development and Psychopathology*, 16(02), 371–387.

Scott, S., Knapp, M., Henderson, J., & Maughan, B. (2001). Financial cost of social exclusion: follow up study of antisocial children into adulthood. *BMJ: British Medical Journal*, 323(7306), 191.

Scott, S., Webster-Stratton, C., Spender, Q., Doolan, M., Jacobs, B., & Aspland, H. (2001). Multicentre controlled trial of parenting groups for childhood antisocial behaviour in clinical practice; commentary: nipping conduct problems in the bud. *BMJ*, 323(7306), 194.

Scott, S. J., Stevenson, J., Taylor, E., et al. (2008). 521–542. Blackwell.

Scott, T. A., Burlingame, G., Starling, M., Porter, C., & Lilly, J. P. (2003). Effects of individual client-centered play therapy on sexually abused children's mood, self-concept, and social competence. *International Journal of Play Therapy*, 12(1), 7–30. https://doi.org/10.1037/h0088869

Sellgren, C. M., Gracias, J., Watmuff, B., et al. (2019). Increased synapse elimination by microglia in schizophrenia patient-derived models of synaptic pruning. *Nature Neuroscience*, 22(3), 374–385.269. Sensory Integration (Accessed April 2 2011) www.autism.com/fam_page.asp?PID=372.

Serrano, V. J., Owens, J. S., & Hallowell, B. (2018). Where children with ADHD direct visual attention during emotion knowledge tasks: relationships to accuracy, response time, and ADHD symptoms. *Journal of Attention Disorders*, 22(8), 752–763.

Sharpley, C. F., Bitsika, V., & Efremidis, B. (1997). Influence of gender, parental health, and perceived expertise of assistance upon stress, anxiety, and depression among parents of children with autism. *Journal of Intellectual and Developmental Disability*, 22(1), 19–28.

Shah, P. E., Fonagy, P., & Strathearn, L. (2010). Is attachment transmitted across generations? The plot thickens. *Clinical Child Psychology and Psychiatry*, 15(3), 329–345.

Sharma, A. N., Arango, C., Coghill, D., Gringras, P., Nutt, D. J., Pratt, P., Young, A. H., & Hollis, C. (2016). BAP position statement: off-label prescribing of psychotropic medication to children and adolescents. *Journal of Psychopharmacology*, 30(5), 416–421.

Shechner, T., Hong, M., Britton, J. C., Pine, D. S., & Fox, N. A. (2014). Fear conditioning and extinction across development: evidence from human studies and animal models. *Biological Psychology*, 100, 1–12. https://doi.org/10.1016/j.biopsycho.2014.04.001.

Sheridan, M. A., Fox, N. A., Zeanah, C. H., McLaughlin, K. A., & Nelson, C. A. (2012). Variation in neural development as a result of exposure to institutionalization early in childhood. *Proceedings of the National Academy of Sciences of the United States of America*, 109(32), 12927–12932. https://doi.org/10.1073/pnas.1200041109.

Sherr, L., Roberts, K. J., & Gandhi, N. (2017). Child violence experiences in institutionalised/orphanage care. *Psychology, Health and Medicine*, 22 (Supl), 31–57. https://doi.org/10.1080/13548506.2016.1271951.

Shields, J. P., Cohen, R., Glassman, J. R., Whitaker, K., Franks, H., & Bertolini, I. (2013). Estimating population size and demographic characteristics of lesbian, gay, bisexual, and transgender youth in middle school. *Journal of Adolescent Health* , 52(2), 248–250.

Shotton, G., & Burton, S. (2018). *Emotional Wellbeing: An Introductory Handbook for Schools* (2nd edition). London and New York: Routledge.

Silove, D., Alonso, J., Bromet, E., Gruber, M., Sampson, N., Scott, K., & Kessler, R. C. (2015). Paediatric-onset and adult-onset separation anxiety disorder across countries in the world mental health survey. *American Journal of Psychiatry*, 172, 647–656. https://doi.org/10.1176/appi.ajp.

Silva, R. R., Munoz, D. M., Barickman, J., & Friedhoff, A. J. (1995). Environmental factors and related fluctuation of symptoms in children and adolescents with Tourette's disorder. *Journal of Child Psychology and Psychiatry, and Allied Disciplines*, 36(2), 305–312.

Silvers, J. A., Goff, B., Gabard-Durnam, L. J., Gee, D. G., Fareri, D. S., Caldera, C., & Tottenham, N. (2017). Vigilance, the amygdala, and anxiety in youths with a history of institutional care. *Biological Psychiatry. Cognitive Neuroscience and Neuroimaging*, 2(6), 493–501. https://doi.org/10.1016/j.bpsc.2017.03.016.

Simola, P., Laitalainen, E., Liukkonen, K., Virkkula, P., Kirjavainen, T., Pitkäranta, A., & Aronen, E. T. (2012). Sleep disturbances in a community sample from preschool to school age. *Child: Care, Health and Development*, 38(4), 572–580.

Simonoff, E. , Pickles, A. , Charman, T. , Chandler, S. , Loucas, T. , & Baird, G. (2008). Psychiatric disorders in children with autism spectrum disorders: prevalence, comorbidity, and associated factors in a population-derived sample. *Journal of the American Academy of Child and Adolescent Psychiatry*, 47(8), 921–929.

Smink, F. R., Van Hoeken, D., & Hoek, H. W. (2012). Epidemiology of eating disorders: incidence, prevalence and mortality rates. *Current Psychiatry Reports*, 14(4), 406–414.

Smith, A., Taylor, E., Warner Rogers, J., Newman, S., & Rubia, K. (2002). Evidence for a pure time perception deficit in children with ADHD. *Journal of Child Psychology and Psychiatry, and Allied Disciplines*, 43(4), 529–542.

Smith, E., Meyer, B. J., Koerting, J., et al. (2017). Preschool hyperactivity specifically elevates long-term mental health risks more strongly in males than females: a prospective longitudinal study through to young adulthood. *European Child and Adolescent Psychiatry*, 26(1), 123–136.

Smythe, J., Colebourn, C., Prisco, L., Petrinic, T., & Leeson, P. (2020). Cardiac abnormalities identified with echocardiography in anorexia nervosa: systematic review and meta-analysis. *The British Journal of Psychiatry*, 1–10.

Sin, J., Spain, D., Furuta, M., Murrells, T., & Norman, I. (2017). Psychological interventions for post-traumatic stress disorder (PTSD) in people with severe mental illness. *Cochrane Database of Systematic Reviews*, 1, CD011464. Https://doi.org/10.1002/14651858.CD011464.pub2.

Singh, S. P., Paul, M., & Ford, T., et al. (2010). Process, outcome and experience of transition from child to adult mental healthcare: multiperspective study. *British Journal of Psychiatry*, 197, 305–312.

Singh, S. P., & Tuomainen, H. (2015). Transition from child to adult mental health services: needs, barriers, experiences and new models of care. *World Psychiatry*, 14(3), 358–361. doi: 10.1002/

Sobanski, E., Banaschewski, T., Asherson, P., et al. (2010). Emotional lability in children and adolescents with attention deficit/hyperactivity disorder (ADHD): clinical correlates and familial prevalence. *Journal of Child Psychology and Psychiatry, and Allied Disciplines*, 51(8), 915–923.

Social Care Institute for Excellence (2009). Think child, think parent, think family: a guide to parental mental health and child welfare. London: SCIE; Society for the Study of Behavioural Phenotypes www.ssbp.org.uk.

Sonuga-Barke, E. J. (2002). Psychological heterogeneity in AD/HD—A dual pathway model of behaviour and cognition. *Behavioural Brain Research*, 130(1–2), 29–36.

Sonuga-Barke, E., Bitsakou, P., & Thompson, M. (2010). Beyond the dual pathway model: evidence for the dissociation of timing, inhibitory, and delay-related impairments in attention-deficit/hyperactivity disorder. *Journal of the American Academy of Child and Adolescent Psychiatry*, 49(4), 345–355.

Sonuga-Barke, E. J., Brandeis, D., Cortese, S., et al. (2013). Nonpharmacological interventions for ADHD: systematic review and meta-analyses of randomized controlled trials of dietary and psychological treatments. *American Journal of Psychiatry*, 170(3), 275–289.

Sonuga-Barke, E. J., Daley, D., & Thompson, M. (2002). Does maternal ADHD reduce the effectiveness of parent training for preschool children's ADHD? *Journal of the American Academy of Child and Adolescent Psychiatry*, 41(6), 696–702.

Sonuga-Barke, E. J., Kennedy, M., Kumsta, R., et al. (2017). Child-to-adult neurodevelopmental and mental health trajectories after early life deprivation: the young adult follow-up of the longitudinal English and Romanian Adoptees study. *The Lancet*, 389(10078), 1539–1548.

Sonuga-Barke, E. J., Lamparelli, M., Stevenson, J., Thompson, M., & Henry, A. (1994). Behaviour problems and pre-school intellectual attainment: the associations of hyperactivity and conduct problems. *Journal of Child Psychology and Psychiatry, and Allied Disciplines*, 35(5), 949–960.

Sonuga-Barke, E. J., Thompson, M., Stevenson, J., & Viney, D. (1997). Patterns of behaviour problems among pre-school children. *Psychological Medicine*, 27(4), 909–918.

Sonuga-Barke, E. J. S., Daley, D., Thompson, M., Laver-Bradbury, C., & Weeks, A. (2001). Parent based therapies for pre-school Attention/Hyperactivity Disorder: a randomized controlled trial with a community sample. *American Academy of Child and Adolescent Psychiatry*, 40, 402–408.

Sood, B., Delaney-Black, V., Covington, C., et al. (2001). Prenatal alcohol exposure and childhood behavior at age 6 to 7 years: I. Dose-response effect. *Pediatrics*, 108(2), e34.

Specht, M. W., Woods, D. W., Nicotra, C. M., et al. (2013). Effects of tic suppression: ability to suppress, rebound, negative reinforcement, and habituation to the premonitory urge. *Behaviour Research and Therapy*, 51(1), 24–30. https://doi.org/10.1016/j.brat.2012.09.009.

Special Educational Needs and Disability Code of Practice: 0 to 25 years (Department of Health, Department for Education, 2014)

Spence, S. H. (2018). Assessing anxiety disorders in children and adolescents. *Child and Adolescent Mental Health*, 23(3), 266–282. doi: 10.111/camh.12251

Spence, S. H., & Rapee, R. M. (2016). The etiology of social anxiety disorder: an evidence-based model. *Behaviour Research and Therapy*, 86, 50–67. https://doi.org/10.1016/j.brat.2016.06.007.

Spencer, T. J., Biederman, J., & Mick, E. (2007). Attention-deficit/hyperactivity disorder: diagnosis, lifespan, comorbidities, and neurobiology. *Journal of Pediatric Psychology*, 32(6), 631–642.

St Pourcain, B., Robinson, E. B., Anttila, V., et al. (2018). ASD and schizophrenia show distinct developmental profiles in common genetic overlap with population-based social communication difficulties. *Molecular Psychiatry*, 23(2), 263–270. https://doi.org/10.1038/mp.2016.198.

Stahl, E. A., Breen, G., Forstner, A. J., et al. (2019). Genome-wide association study identifies 30 loci associated with bipolar disorder. *Nature Genetics*, 51(5), 793–803. https://doi.org/10.1038/s41588-019-0397-8.

Stallard, P. (1995). Parental satisfaction with intervention: differences between respondents and non-respondents to a postal questionnaire. *Journal of Child Psychology and Psychiatry*, 34(3), 397–405.

Statistical Manual of Mental Disorders 5th edition (DSMV) and the International Classification of Diseases 11th Revision ICD11.

van Steensel, F. J., Bögels, S. M., & Perrin, S. (2011). Anxiety disorders in children and adolescents with autistic spectrum disorders: a meta-analysis. *Clinical Child and Family Psychology Review*, 14(3), 302–317. doi: 10.1007/s10567-011-0097-0. PMID: 21735077; PMCID: PMC3162631.

Steensma, T. D., & Cohen-Kettenis, P. T. (2011). Gender transitioning before puberty? *Archives of Sexual Behavior*, 40(4), 649–650.

Steensma, T. D., Biemond, R., de Boer, F., & Cohen-Kettenis, P. T. (2011). Desisting and persisting gender dysphoria after childhood: a qualitative follow-up study. *Clinical Child Psychology and Psychiatry*, 16(4), 499–516.

Steensma, T. D., McGuire, J. K., Kreukels, B. P. C., Beekman, A. J., & Cohen-Kettenis, P. T. (2013). Factors associated with desistence and persistence of childhood gender dysphoria: a quantitative follow-up study. *Journal of the American Academy of Child and Adolescent Psychiatry*, 52(6), 582–590.

Steensma, T. D., van der Ende, J., Verhulst, F. C., & Cohen-Kettenis, P. T. (2013). Gender variance in childhood and sexual orientation in adulthood: a prospective study. *Journal of Sexual Medicine*, 10(11), 2723–2733.

Steimer, T. (2002). The biology of fear- and anxiety-related behaviours. *Dialogues in Clinical Neuroscience*, 4(3), 231–249. http://www.ncbi.nlm.nih.gov/pubmed/22033741.

Steinhausen, H. C., Gavez, S., & Winkler Metzke, C. (2005). Psychosocial correlates, outcome, and stability of abnormal adolescent eating behavior in community samples of young people. *International Journal of Eating Disorders*, 37(2), 119–126.

Stergiakouli, E., & Thapar, A. (2010). Fitting the pieces together: current research on the genetic basis of attention-deficit/hyperactivity disorder (ADHD). *Neuropsychiatric Disease and Treatment*, 6, 551.

Sterzer, P., Stadler, C., Poustka, F., & Kleinschmidt, A. (2007). A structural neural deficit in adolescents with conduct disorder and its association with lack of empathy. *Neuroimage*, 37(1), 335–342.

Stevenson, J. e. d. (1990). Health visitor based services for pre-school children with behaviour problems. Occasional Papers No 2, London: Association of Child Psychologists and Psychiatrists.

Stevenson, J., Buitelaar, J., Cortese, S., et al. (2014). Research review: the role of diet in the treatment of attention-deficit/hyperactivity disorder–an appraisal of the evidence on efficacy and recommendations on the design of future studies. *Journal of Child Psychology and Psychiatry, and Allied Disciplines*, 55(5), 416–427.

Stevenson, J., Sonuga-Barke, E., McCann, D., et al. (2010). The role of histamine degradation gene polymorphisms in moderating the effects of food additives on children's ADHD symptoms. *American Journal of Psychiatry*, 167(9), 1108–1115.

Stoltenborgh, M., van Ijzendoorn, M. H., Euser, E. M., & Bakermans-Kranenburg, M. J. (2011). A global perspective on child sexual abuse: meta-analysis of prevalence around the world. *Child Maltreatment*, 16(2), 79–101. doi: 10.1177/1077559511403920. Epub 2011 Apr 21. PMID: 21511741.

Stoltenborgh, M., Bakermans-Kranenburg, M. J., Alink, L. R. A., & IJzendoorn, M. H. van (2015). The prevalence of child maltreatment across the globe: review of a series of meta-analyses. *Child Abuse Review*, 24(1), 37–50. https://doi.org/10.1002/car.2353.

Stringer, H., Lozano, S., & Dodd, B. (2003). The Link between language Disorders and Behavioural Difficulties in Adolescents AFASIC Newsletter.

Sullivan, P. F., Agrawal, A., Bulik, C. M., et al. (2018). Psychiatric genomics: an update and an agenda. *American Journal of Psychiatry*, 175(1), 15–27. https://doi.org/10.1176/appi.ajp.2017.17030283.

Sullivan, P. F., Neale, M. C., & Kendler, K. S. (2000). Genetic epidemiology of major depression: review and meta-analysis. *American Journal of Psychiatry*, 157(10), 1552–1562. https://doi.org/10.1176/appi.ajp.157.10.1552.

Suris, J. C., RutishauseC, C., & Akre, C. (2015). Does talking about it make a difference? Opinions of chronically ill young adults after being transferred to adult care. *Archives De Pédiatrie*, 22, 267–271.

Swanson, J. M., Schuck, S., Porter, M. M., et al. (2012). Categorical and dimensional definitions and evaluations of symptoms of ADHD: history of the SNAP and the SWAN rating scales. *The International Journal of Educational and Psychological Assessmet*, 10(1), 51.

Swift, K. D., Sayal, K., & Hollis, C. (2014). ADHD and transitions to adult mental health services: a scoping review. *Child: Care, Health and Development*, 40, 775–786.

Sydsjö, G., Agnafors, S., Bladh, M., & Josefsson, A. (2018). Anxiety in women—a Swedish national three-generational cohort study. *BMC Psychiatry*, 18(1), 168. https://doi.org/10.1186/s12888-018-1712-0.

Sylva, K., & Lunt, I. (1982). *Child Development: A First Course Publisher*. Oxford: Wiley-Blackwell.

Szatmari, P., Saigal, S., Rosenbaum, P., & Campbell, D. (1993). Psychopathology and adaptive functioning among extremely low birthweight children at eight years of age. *Development and Psychopathology*, 5(3), 345–357.

Tarver, J., Daley, D., Lockwood, J., & Sayal, K. (2014). Are self-directed parenting interventions sufficient for externalising behaviour problems in childhood? A systematic review and meta-analysis. *European Child and Adolescent Psychiatry*, 23(12), 1123–1137.

Tarver, J., Daley, D., & Sayal, K. (2014). Attention-deficit hyperactivity disorder (ADHD): an updated review of the essential facts. *Child: Care, Health and Development*, 40(6), 762–774.

Taylor, E., & Sonuga-Barke, E. J. Disorders of attention and activity. In: M. Rutter, D. V. Bishop and D. Pine (Eds.), *Rutter's Textbook of Child Psychiatry* (5th edition). Wiley.

Taylor, M. J., Martin, J., Lu, Y., Brikell, I., Lundström, S., Larsson, H., & Lichtenstein, P. (2019). Association of genetic risk factors for psychiatric disorders and traits of these disorders in a Swedish population twin sample. *JAMA Psychiatry*, 76(3), 280. https://doi.org/10.1001/jamapsychiatry.2018.3652.

Taylor, M. J., Freeman, D., & Ronald, A. (2016). Dimensional psychotic experiences in adolescence: evidence from a taxometric study of a community-based sample. *Psychiatry Research*, 241, 35–42.

Taylor,E., Dopfner,M., Sergeant,J., et al. (2004). European Guidelines for hyperkinetic disorder-first upgrade. *European Child and Adolescent Psychiatry*, 13(Supplement 1), 7–30.

Tchanturia, K. (Ed.) (2014). *Cognitive Remediation Therapy (CRT) for Eating and Weight Disorders*. Routledge.

Tchanturia, K., Lloyd, S., & Lang, K. (2013). Cognitive remediation therapy for anorexia nervosa: current evidence and future research directions. *International Journal of Eating Disorders*, 46(5), 492–495.

Teague, S. J., Newman, L. K., Tonge, B. J., Gray, K. M., & MHYPeDD team (2018). Caregiver mental health, parenting practices, and perceptions of child attachment in children with autism spectrum disorder. *Journal of Autism and Developmental Disorders*, 48(8), 2642–2652.

Teicher, M. H. (2018). Childhood trauma and the enduring consequences of forcibly separating children from parents at the United States border. *BMC Medicine*, 16(1), 146.

Teicher, M. H., Samson, J. A., Anderson, C. M., & Ohashi, K. (2016). The effects of childhood maltreatment on brain structure, function and connectivity. *Nature Reviews. Neuroscience*, 17(10), 652–666. https://doi.org/10.1038/nrn.2016.111.

Temple Newhook, J., Pyne, J., Winters, K., et al. (2018). A critical commentary on follow-up studies and "desistance" theories about transgender and gender-nonconforming children. *International Journal of Transgenderism*, 19(2), 212–224.

Thapar, A., Zaharieva, I., Martin, A., et al. (2010). Rare chromosomal deletions and duplications in attention-deficit hyperactivity disorder: a genome-wide analysis. *The Lancet*, 376(9750), 1401–1408.

Thapar, A. (2018). Discoveries on the genetics of ADHD in the 21st century: new findings and their implications. *American Journal of Psychiatry*, 175(10), 943–950. https://doi.org/10.1176/appi.ajp.2018.18040383.

Thapar, A., Collishaw, S., Pine, D. S., & Thapar, A. K. (2012). Depression in adolescence. *Lancet (London, England)*, 379(9820), 1056–1067. https://doi.org/10.1016/S0140-6736(11)60871-4.

Thapar, A., Cooper, M., Eyre, O., & Langley, K. (2013). Practitioner review: what have we learnt about the causes of ADHD? *Journal of Child Psychology and Psychiatry, and Allied Disciplines*, 54(1), 3–16.

Thapar, A., Fowler, T., Rice, F., et al. (2003). Maternal smoking during pregnancy and attention deficit hyperactivity disorder symptoms in offspring. *American Journal of Psychiatry*, 160(11), 1985–1989.

Thapar, A., Harrington, R., & McGuffin, P. (2001). Examining the comorbidity of ADHD-related behaviours and conduct problems using a twin study design. *The British Journal of Psychiatry*, 179(3), 224–229.

Thapar, A., & Rice, F. (2006). Twin studies in pediatric depression. *Child and Adolescent Psychiatric Clinics of North America*, 15(4), 869–881. https://doi.org/10.1016/J.CHC.2006.05.007.

Thapar, A., & Rutter, M. (2019). Do natural experiments have an important future in the study of mental disorders? *Psychological Medicine*, 49(7), 1079–1088. https://doi.org/10.1017/S0033291718003896.

The Child Outcomes Research Consortium (CORC) www.corc.uk.net.

The Five Year Forward View for Mental Health (2016). NHS England.

The Independent Mental Health TaskForce to the NHS in England.

The National Committee for Primary Mental Health Workers in CAMHS and National CAMHS Support Service. (2004). The role of the child primary mental health worker, Department of Health, www.camhs.org..

Theule, J. (2016). Conduct disorder/oppositional defiant disorder and attachment: a meta-analysis. *Journal of Development and Life Course Criminology*, 2, 232–255.

Theule, J., Germain, S. M., Cheung, K., Hurl, K. E., & Markel, C. (2016). Conduct disorder/oppositional defiant disorder and attachment: a meta-analysis. *Journal of Development and Life Course Criminology*, 232–255.

Thompson, M. (2003). Working with Primary care. In Elena Garralda and Caroline Hyde (Eds.), *Assessment and Treatment in Child and Adolescent Psychiatry*. BMJ.

Thompson, M. J. J. (2001). The development of community service for young children in the new forest: joint work by a child guidance clinic with health visitors. Unpublished MD thesis University of Glasgow.

Thompson, M. J. J., Coll, X., Wilkinson, S., Uitenbroek, D., & Tobias, A. (2003) Evaluation of a mental health service for young children: development, outcome and satisfaction. *Child and Adolescent Mental Health*, 8(2), 68–77.

Thompson, M. J. J., Laver-Bradbury, C., Ayres, M., et al. (2009). A small-scale randomised controlled trial of the revised New Forest Programme for Prescholers with Attention Deficit Hyperactivity Disorder. *European Child and Adolescent Psychiatry*, 10, 605–616.

Thompson, M. J. J., Laver-Bradbury, C., Ayres, M., Poidevin, E., Mead, S., Dodds, C., ... Sonuga-Barke, E. J. S. (2009). A small-scale randomized controlled trial of the revised new forest parenting programme for pre-schoolers with an attention deficit hyperactivity disorder. *European Child and Adolescent Psychiatry*, 18(10), 605–616.

Thompson, M. J., Stevenson, J., Sonuga-Barke, E., Nott, P., Bhatti, Z., Price, A., & Hudswell, M. (1996). Mental health of preschool children and their mothers in a mixed. Urban/rural population. I. Prevalence and ecological factors. *The British Journal of Psychiatry*, 168(1), 16–20.

Thompson, M., Laver-Bradbury, C., Weeks, A., Chen, W., & Sonuga-Barke, Living with ADHD a DVD for Parents and Professionals. University of Southampton Media Services.

Thompson, M. J., Raynor, A., Cornah, D., Stevenson, J., & Sonuga-Barke, E. J. (2002). Parenting behaviour described by mothers in a general population sample. *Child: Care, Health and Development*, 28(2), 149–155.

Thomsen, P. H. (1996). Schizophrenia with childhood and adolescent onset- a nationwide register-based study. *Acta Psychiatrica Scandinavica*, 94(3), 187–193. https://doi.org/10.1111/j.1600-0447.1996.tb09847.x.

Thrive www.thriveapproach.com.

Tick, B., Bolton, P., Happé, F., Rutter, M., & Rijsdijk, F. (2016). Heritability of autism spectrum disorders: a meta-analysis of twin studies. *Journal of Child Psychology and Psychiatry, and Allied Disciplines*, 57(5), 585–595. https://doi.org/10.1111/jcpp.12499.

Tobias, A. (2019). A grounded theory study of family coach intervention with persistent school non-attenders. *Educational Psychology in Practice*, 35(1), 17–33.

Todd, R. D., Huang, H., Smalley, S. L., et al. (2005). Collaborative analysis of DRD4 and DAT genotypes in population-defined ADHD subtypes. *Journal of Child Psychology and Psychiatry, and Allied Disciplines*, 46(10), 1067–1073.

Together We Stand: The Commissioning, Role and Management of Child and Adolescent NHS Health Advisory Service thematic review National Health Service. Health Advisory Service. Thematic review Thematic review: Author: NHS Health Advisory Service: Editors: Richard Williams, Gregory Richardson: Edition: 2, illustrated: Publisher: H.M. Stationery.

Tolin, D. F., Brady, R. E., & Hannan, S. (2008). Obsessional beliefs and symptoms of obsessive–compulsive disorder in a clinical sample. *Journal of Psychopathology and Behavioral Assessment*, 30(1), 31–42.

Touchette, E., Petit, D., Paquet, J., Boivin, M., Japel, C., Tremblay, R. E., & Montplaisir, J. Y. (2005). Factors associated with fragmented sleep at night across early childhood. *Archives of Pediatrics and Adolescent Medicine*, 159(3), 242–249.

Trentacosta, C. J., & Fine, S. E. (2010). Emotion knowledge, social competence, and behavior problems in childhood and adolescence: a meta-analytic review. *Social Development*, 19(1), 1–29.

Tully, E. C., Iacono, W. G., & McGue, M. (2008). An adoption study of parental depression as an environmental liability for adolescent depression and childhood disruptive disorders. *The American Journal of Psychiatry*, 165(9), 1148–1154. https://doi.org/10.1176/appi.ajp.2008.07091438.

Van Der Kolk, B., McFarlane, A., & Weisaeth, L. (1999). *Traumatic Stress*. New York: Guildford Press.

Veale, D. (2001). Cognitive–behavioural therapy for body dysmorphic disorder. *Advances in Psychiatric Treatment*, 7(2), 125–132.

Veale, D. (2004). Advances in a cognitive behavioural model of body dysmorphic disorder. *Body Image*, 1(1), 113–125.

Verdellen, C., van de Griendt, J., Hartmann, A., Murphy, T., & Group, E. G. (2011). European clinical guidelines for Tourette syndrome and other tic disorders. Part III: behavioural and psychosocial interventions. *European Child and Adolescent Psychiatry*, 20(4), 197–207. doi: 10.1007/s00787-011-0167-3

Verdellen, C. W., Hoogduin, C. A., Kato, B. S., Keijsers, G. P., Cath, D. C., & Hoijtink, H. B. (2008). Habituation of premonitory sensations during exposure and response prevention treatment in Tourette's syndrome. *Behavior Modification*, 32(2), 215–227. doi: 10.1177/0145445507309020

Verdellen, C. W., Keijsers, G. P., Cath, D. C., & Hoogduin, C. A. (2004). Exposure with response prevention versus habit reversal in Tourettes's syndrome: a controlled study. *Behaviour Research and Therapy*, 42(5), 501–511. doi: 10.1016/S0005-7967(03)00154-2

Viding, E., Blair, R. J. R., Moffitt, T. E., & Plomin, R. (2005). Evidence for substantial genetic risk for psychopathy in 7-year-olds. *Journal of Child Psychology and Psychiatry*, 46(6), 592–597.

Vinkers, C. H., Van Gastel, W. A., Schubart, C. D., Van Eijk, K. R., Luykx, J. J., Van Winkel, R., ... Cahn, W. (2013). The effect of childhood maltreatment and cannabis use on adult psychotic symptoms is modified by the COMT Val158Met polymorphism. *Schizophrenia Research*, 150(1), 303–311.

Vlot, M. C., Klink, D. T., den Heijer, M., ... Blankenstein, M. A., Rotteveel, J., & Heijboer, A. C. (2017). Effect of pubertal suppression and cross-sex hormone therapy on bone turnover markers and bone mineral apparent density (BMAD) in transgender adolescents. *Bone*, 95, 11–19.

Wahlig, J. L. (2015). Losing the child they thought they had: therapeutic suggestions for an ambiguous loss perspective with parents of a transgender child. *Journal of GLBT Family Studies*, 11(4), 305–326.

Wallien, M. S. C., & Cohen-Kettenis, P. T. (2008). Psychosexual outcome of gender-dysphoric children. *Journal of the American Academy of Child and Adolescent Psychiatry*, 47(12), 1413–1423.

Walsh, T., McClellan, J. M., McCarthy, S. E., Addington, A. M., Pierce, S. B., Cooper, G. M., Nord, A. S., Kusenda, M., Malhotra, D., Bhandari, A., Stray, S. M., Rippey, C. F., Roccanova, P., Makarov, V., Lakshmi, B., Findling, R. L., Sikich, L., Stromberg, T., Merriman, B., Gogtay, N., Butler, P., Eckstrand, K., Noory, L., Gochman, P., Long, R., Chen, Z., Davis, S., Baker, C., Eichler, E. E., Meltzer, P. S., Nelson, S. F., Singleton, A. B., Lee, M. K., Rapoport, J. L., King, M. C., & Sebat, J. (2008). Rare structural variants disrupt multiple genes in neurodevelopmental pathways in schizophrenia. *Science*, 320(5875), 539–543. doi: 10.1126/science.1155174. Epub 2008 Mar 27. PMID: 18369103.

Ware, A. L., et al. (2013). The effects of prenatal alcohol exposure and attention-deficit/hyperactivity disorder on psychopathology and behavior. *Alcoholism: Clinical and Experimental Research*, 37(3), 507–516.

Wayman, S., Raws, P., & Leadbitter, H. (2016). *There's Nobody Is There—No One Who Can Actually Help? The Challenges of Estimating the Number of Young Carers and Knowing How to Meet Their Needs.* London: The Children's Society.

Webster-Stratton, C. (1991). Annotation: strategies for helping families with conduct disordered children. *Journal of Child Psychology and Psychiatry Newsletter*, 32(7), 1047–1062.

West, J. (1996). *Child Centred Play Therapy* 2nd Edition. London: Edward Arnold.

White, L. K., Degnan, K. A., Henderson, H. A., Pérez-Edgar, K., Walker, O. L., Shechner, T., Leibenluft, E., Bar-Haim, Y., Pine, D. S., & Fox, N. A. (2017). Developmental relations among behavioral inhibition, anxiety, and attention biases to threat and positive information. *Child Development*, 88(1), 141–155. doi: 10.1111/cdev.12696. PMID: 28042902; PMCID: PMC5215785.

White, M. (1995). *Re-Authoring Lives: Interviews & Essays.* Adelaide, Australia: Dulwich Centre Publications.

White, M., Epston, D., 1990. *Narrative Means to Therapeutic Ends.* New York: Norton.

WHO (2018). *International Classification of Diseases for Mortality and Morbidity Statistics* (11th edition). Retrieved from https://icd.who.int/browse11/l-m/en#/http%3a%2f%2fid.who.int%2ficd%2fentity%2f577470983.

Wiggs, L. (2009). Behavioural aspects of children's sleep. *Archives of Disease in Childhood*, 94(1), 59–62.

Wildeman, C., Emanuel, N., Leventhal, J. M., Putnam-Hornstein, E., Waldfogel, J., & Lee, H. (2014). The prevalence of confirmed maltreatment among US children, 2004 to 2011. *JAMA Pediatrics*, 168(8), 706–713. doi: 10.1001/jamapediatrics.2014.410. PMID: 24887073; PMCID: PMC5087599.

Wilens, T. E., Faraone, S. V., Biederman, J., & Gunawardene, S. (2003). Does stimulant therapy of attention-deficit/hyperactivity disorder beget later substance abuse? A meta-analytic review of the literature. *Pediatrics*, 111(1), 179–185. www.aimproject.org.uk.

Wilens, T. E., Kwon, A., Tanguay, S., Chase, R., Moore, H., Faraone, S. V., & Biederman, J. (2005). Characteristics of adults with attention deficit hyperactivity disorder plus substance use disorder: the role of psychiatric comorbidity. *American Journal on Addictions*, 14(4), 319–327.

Williams, N. M., Zaharieva, I., Martin, A., Langley, K., Mantripragada, K., Fossdal, R., ... Thapar, A. (2010). Rare chromosomal deletions and duplications in attention-deficit hyperactivity disorder: a genome-wide analysis. *The Lancet*, 376(9750), 1401–1408.

Willsey, A. J., Fernandez, T. V., Yu, D., King, R. A., Dietrich, A., Xing, J., Sanders, S. J., Mandell, J. D., Huang, A. Y., Richer, P., Smith, L., Dong, S., Samocha, K. E.; & Tourette International Collaborative Genetics (TIC Genetics); Tourette Syndrome Association International Consortium for Genetics (TSAICG), Neale, B. M., Coppola, G., Mathews, C. A., Tischfield, J. A., Scharf, J. M., State, M. W., & Heiman, G. A. (2017). De novo coding variants are strongly associated with tourette disorder. *Neuron*, 94(3), 486–499.e9. doi: 10.1016/j.neuron.2017.04.024. PMID: 28472652; PMCID: PMC5769876.

Wilson, K., Ruch, G., Lymbery, M., & Cooper, A. (2011). *Social Work, an Introduction to Contemporary Practice*. London: Pearsons Education Limited.

Wolfe, D. A., Crooks, C. V., Lee, V., et al. (2003). The effects of children's exposure to domestic violence: a meta-analysis and critique. *Clinical Child and Family Psychology Review*, 6, 171–187. https://doi.org/10.1023/A:1024910416164

Wolpert, M., Harris, R., Hodges, S., Fuggle, P., James, R., Wiener, A., ... Fonagy, P. (2015). THRIVE Elaborated. London: CAMHS Press.

Wonderlich, S., Klein, M. H., & Council, J. R. (1996). Relationship of social perceptions and self-concept in bulimia nervosa. *Journal of Consulting and Clinical Psychology*, 64(6), 1231.

Wong, M. M., Brower, K. J., & Zucker, R. A. (2011). Sleep problems, suicidal ideation, and self-harm behaviors in adolescence. *Journal of Psychiatric Research*, 45(4), 505–511.

Wood, H., Sasaki, S., Bradley, S. J., et al. (2013). Patterns of referral to a gender identity service for children and adolescents (1976–2011): age, sex ratio, and sexual orientation. *Journal of Sex and Marital Therapy*, 39(1), 1–6.

Woodhead, D. (2000). *The Health and Well-being of Asylum Seekers and Refugees*. London: King's Fund.

Woodruff, B. A., & Duffield, A. (2000). *Assessment of Nutritional Status in Emergency-affected Populations*. Geneva: United Nations/Sub-Committee on Nutrition.

Woolgar, M. (2013). The practical implications of the emerging findings in the neurobiology of maltreatment for looked after and adopted children: recognising the diversity of outcomes. *Adoption & Fostering*, 37(3), 237–252. doi: 10.1177/0308575913500021 Google Scholar | SAGE Journals. https://journals.sagepub.com/doi/full/10.1177/0308575920945187

Worbe, Y., Malherbe, C., Hartmann, A., Pelegrini-Issac, M., Messe, A., Vidailhet, M., ... Benali, H. (2012). Functional immaturity of cortico-basal ganglia networks in Gilles de la Tourette syndrome. *Brain*, 135(Pt 6), 1937–1946. doi: aws056 [pii] 10.1093/brain/aws056

World Health Organisation (WHO). (1992). *The ICD-10 Classification of Mental and Behavioural Disorders: Clinical Descriptions and Diagnostic Guidelines*. Geneva: World Health Organisation.

World Health Organization (1993). *The ICD-10 Classification of Mental and Behavioural Disorders: Diagnostic Criteria for Research* (Vol. 2). World Health Organization.

World Health Organization (2004). Sexual health—a new focus for WHO. *Progress in Reproductive Health Research*, 67, 1–8.

Wren, B. (2019). Notes on a crisis of meaning in the care of gender diverse children. In: L. Hertzman (Ed.), *Sexuality and Gender Now: Moving beyond Heteronormativity*, 189–212. Routledge.

Wu, P. Y., Huang, M. L., Lee, W. P., Wang, C., & Shih, W. M. (2017). Effects of music listening on anxiety and physiological responses in patients undergoing awake craniotomy. *Complementary Therapies in Medicine*, 32, 56–60. doi: 10.1016/j.ctim.2017.03.007. Epub 2017 Mar 31. PMID: 28619305.

Yang, C., Hao, Z., Zhang, L. L., Zhu, C. R., Zhu, P., & Guo, Q. (2019). Comparative efficacy and safety of antipsychotic drugs for tic disorders: a systematic review and bayesian network meta-analysis. *Pharmacopsychiatry*, 52(1), 7–15. doi: 10.1055/s-0043-124872

Yang, H., Liu, J., Sui, J., Pearlson, G., & Calhoun, V. D. (2010). A hybrid machine learning method for fusing fMRI and genetic data: combining both improves classification of schizophrenia. *Frontiers in Human Neuroscience*, 4, 192.

Yang, J., Hirsch, L., Martino, D., Jette, N., Roberts, J., & Pringsheim, T. (2016). The prevalence of diagnosed tourette syndrome in Canada: a national population-based study. *Mov Disord*, 31(11), 1658–1663. doi: 10.1002/mds.26766

Ybarra, M. L., Mitchell, K. J., Palmer, N. A., & Reisner, S. L. (2015). Online social support as a buffer against online and offline peer and sexual victimization among US LGBT and non-LGBT youth. *Child Abuse and Neglect*, 39, 123–136.

Yeung, C. K., Diao, M., & Sreedhar, B. (2008). Cortical arousal in children with severe enuresis. *New England Journal of Medicine*, 358(22), 2414–2415. doi: 10.1056/NEJMc0706528. PMID: 18509134.

Yildirim, B., Perdahli Fis, N., Yazkan Akgul, G., & Ayaz, A. B. (2017). Gender dysphoria and attention problems: possible clue for biological underpinnings. *Psychiatry and Clinical Psychopharmacology*, 27(3), 283–290.

Youngstrom, E. A., Birmaher, B., & Findling, R. L. (2008). Pediatric bipolar disorder: validity, phenomenology, and recommendations for diagnosis. *Bipolar Disorders*, 10(1 Pt 2), 194–214. doi: 10.1111/j.1399-5618.2007.00563.x

Yu, D. M., Sul, J. H., Tsetsos, F., Nawaz, M. S., Huang, A. Y., Zelaya, I., ... Toure, P. G. C. (2019). Interrogating the genetic determinants of Tourette's syndrome and other tic disorders through genome-wide association studies. *American Journal of Psychiatry*, 176(3), 217–227. doi: 10.1176/appi.ajp.2018.18070857

Zahn-Waxler, C., Cole, P. M., Welsh, J. D., & Fox, N. A. (1995). Psychophysiological correlates of empathy and prosocial behaviors in preschool children with behavior problems. *Development and Psychopathology*, 7, 27–48.

Zeanah, C., & Gleason, M. (2014). Annual research review: attachment disorders in early childhood - clinical presentation, causes, correlates, and treatment. *Journal of Child Psychology and Psychiatry*, 56(3), 207–222.

Zenner, C., Herrnleben-Kurz, S., & Walach, H. (2014). Mindfulness-based interventions in schools-a systematic review and meta-analysis. *Frontiers in Psychology*, 5, 603. doi: 10.3389/fpsyg.2014.00603. PMID: 25071620; PMCID: PMC4075476. https://www.nice.org.uk/guidance/qs53

Zucker, K. (2020). Debate: different strokes for different folks. *Child and Adolescent Mental Health*, 25(1), 36–37.

Zucker, K. J. (2017). Epidemiology of gender dysphoria and transgender identity. *Sexual Health*, 14(5), 404–411.

Zucker, K. J. (2018). The myth of persistence: response to "A critical commentary on follow-up studies and 'desistance' theories about transgender and gender non-conforming children" by Temple Newhook et al. (2018), *International Journal of Transgenderism*, 19(2), 231–245.

Multiple-Choice Answers

Chapter 3:

1) (a)
2) (c)

Chapter 5:

1) (a)
2) (e)
3) (c)
4) (b)

Chapter 7:

1) (b)
2) (a)

Chapter 9:

1) (c)
2) (a)

Chapter 10:

1) (c)
2) (b)
3) (d)
4) (c)

Chapter 12:

1) (c)
2) (e)
3) (b)
4) (a)
5) (d)

Chapter 13:

1) (a)
2) (d)
3) (b)
4) (a)

Chapter 14:

1) (c)
2) (a)
3) (c)
4) (c)

Chapter 15:

1) (b)
2) (d)
3) (a)
4) (f)
5) (d)

Chapter 16:

1) (b)
2) (d)
3) (d)

Chapter 17:

1) False
2) True
3) True
4) True
5) False

Chapter 18:

1) True
2) False
3) True
4) False
5) True

Chapter 19:

1) (d)
2) (d)
3) (e)

4) (e)
5) (b)

Chapter 20:

1) (f)

Chapter 21:

1) (d)
2) (d)
3) (d)
4) (c)
5) (e)

Chapter 22:

1) (d)
2) (c)
3) (a)

Chapter 23:

1) (d)
2) (b)
3) (d)
4) (b)
5) (b)
6) (d)
7) (c)

Chapter 24:

1) (b)
2) (c)
3) (d)

Chapter 25:

1) (b)
2) (b)
3) (a)
4) (c)
5) (b)

Chapter 26:

1) (a)

2) (b)
3) (b)

Chapter 27:

1) (c)
2) (c)
3) (a) and (b)
4) (c)

Chapter 28:

1) (c)
2) (b)
3) (a)

Chapter 29:

1) (d)
2) (b)
3) (a)
4) (c)

Chapter 30:

1) (a), (b) and (d)
2) (b)
3) (b) and (e)

Chapter 31:

1) (d)
2) (c)
3) (a)
4) (a), (c) and (e)
5) (a) and (c)

Chapter 35:

1) (d)
2) (c)
3) (a)
4) (d)

Chapter 39:

1) (a), (c) and (d)
2) (c) and (e)

3) (a) and (e)
4) (a), (c) and (d)
5) (a), (d) and (e)

Chapter 40:

1) (a)
2) (c)
3) (e)
4) (b)

Chapter 41:

1) (c)
2) (b)
3) (b)
4) (e)
5) (c)

Chapter 42:

1) (a)
2) (c)
3) (b)
4) (b)
5) (c)

Chapter 43:

1) (c)
2) (b)
3) (a)

Chapter 44:

1) (b)
2) (a)
3) (a), (b) and (d)
4) (a) and (d)
5) All

Chapter 45:

1) (d)
2) (d)
3) (c)
4) (b)
5) (a)

Chapter 46:

1) (a)
2) (c) and (d)
3) (c)
4) (a) and (d)
5) (a), (c) and (d)

Chapter 48:

1) (e)
2) (e)
3) (b)
4) (b)
5) (a)

Chapter 49:

1) (e)
2) (c)
3) (e)

Chapter 50:

1) True
2) True
3) True

Chapter 51:

1) (c)
2) (e)
3) (e)
4) (a)
5) (b)

Chapter 52:

1) (e)
2) (b)
3) False

Chapter 53:

1) (b)
2) (a)

Chapter 54:

1) (b)
2) (b)

3) (e)
4) (c)

Chapter 55:

1) (a)
2) (c)
3) (b)

Chapter 56:

1) (b)
2) (d)
3) (c)
4) (b)
5) (a)

Chapter 57:

1) (b)
2) (b)
3) (c)
4) (c)

Chapter 58:

1) (c)
2) (b)
3) (d)
4) (b)
5) (c)

Chapter 59:

1) (a)
2) (d)
3) (c)
4) (c)
5) (b)

Chapter 60:

1) (a)
2) (d)
3) (c)

Chapter 61:

1) (b)
2) (b)

3) (a)
4) (b)

Chapter 62:

1) (c)
2) (e)

Chapter 63:

1) (c)
2) (d)

Chapter 64:

1) (c)
2) (c)

Chapter 65:

1) (b)

Chapter 66:

1) (a)

Chapter 67:

1) (b)

Chapter 68:

1) (c)
2) (d)
3) (b)

Chapter 70:

1) (a)
2) (c)
3) (a)

Chapter 74:

1) (d)
2) (c)
3) (a)
4) (a)
5) (b)

Chapter 75:

1) (c)
2) (d)

Chapter 83:

1) (b)
2) (c)
3) (d)
4) (a)

Chapter 84:

1) (c)
2) (b)
3) (d)
4) (c)
5) (a)

Chapter 85:

1) (f)
2) (c)

Chapter 87:

1) (e)
2) (d)
3) (b)

Chapter 88:

1) (b)
2) (c)
3) (a)
4) (b)
5) (c)

Index

Note: page references in italics indicate figures; bold indicates tables.

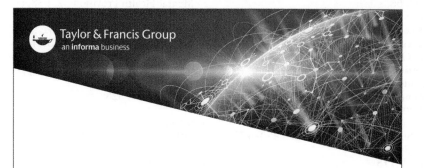